Principles and Practice of FETAL MEDICINE

DISCLAIMER

Principles and Practice of FETAL MEDICINE

Editors

Raju R Sahetya
MD DGO DFP FCPS FICOG
Obstetrician and Gynecologist
Specialist—Fertility and IVF and Fetal Medicine
President
Indian Society for Prenatal Diagnosis and Therapy (ISPAT)
Honorary Scientific Secretary
Association of Fellow Gynecologist
Pushpaa Hospital, Hinduja Hospital
Mumbai, Maharashtra, India

Jaideep Malhotra
MD (Obs & Gyn) FICMCH FIAJAGO FICOG MASRM FICMU
Director
Rainbow IVF
Infertility Consultant and Specialist
Agra, Uttar Pradesh, India

Hema Purandarey
MBBS MS FICMH PhD
Medical and Reproductive Geneticist
Founder and Director
Center of Genetic Healthcare
Director
SRL Diagnostic Services Private Limited (Genetics)
Mumbai, Maharashtra, India

Foreword

Padmashree Dr Rustom P Soonawala

JAYPEE *The Health Sciences Publisher*
New Delhi | London | Philadelphia | Panama

JAYPEE Jaypee Brothers Medical Publishers (P) Ltd

Headquarters

Jaypee Brothers Medical Publishers (P) Ltd
4838/24, Ansari Road, Daryaganj
New Delhi 110 002, India
Phone: +91-11-43574357
Fax: +91-11-43574314
Email: jaypee@jaypeebrothers.com

Overseas Offices

J.P. Medical Ltd
83, Victoria Street, London
SW1H 0HW (UK)
Phone: +44-2031708910
Fax: +44-(0)-2030086180
Email: info@jpmedpub.com

Jaypee-Highlights Medical Publishers Inc.
City of Knowledge, Building 235, 2nd Floor
Clayton, Panama City, Panama
Phone: +1 507-301-0496
Fax: +1 507-301-0499
Email: cservice@jphmedical.com

Jaypee Medical Inc.
325, Chestnut Street
Suite 412, Philadelphia, PA 19106, USA
Phone: +1 267-519-9789
E-mail: support@jpmedus.com

Jaypee Brothers Medical Publishers (P) Ltd
17/1-B, Babar Road, Block-B, Shaymali
Mohammadpur, Dhaka-1207
Bangladesh
Mobile: +08801912003485
Email: jaypeedhaka@gmail.com

Jaypee Brothers Medical Publishers (P) Ltd
Bhotahity, Kathmandu, Nepal
Phone: +977-9741283608
Email: kathmandu@jaypeebrothers.com

Website: www.jaypeebrothers.com
Website: www.jaypeedigital.com

Inquiries for bulk sales may be solicited at: jaypee@jaypeebrothers.com

Principles and Practice of Fetal Medicine

First Edition: **2017**

ISBN: 978-93-85999-69-7

Printed at: Ajanta Offset & Packagings Ltd., Faridabad, Haryana

Dedicated to

The fetus as a patient

and

All the families who have and will be benefited

by science and technology of

Prenatal Genetic Diagnosis

Contributors

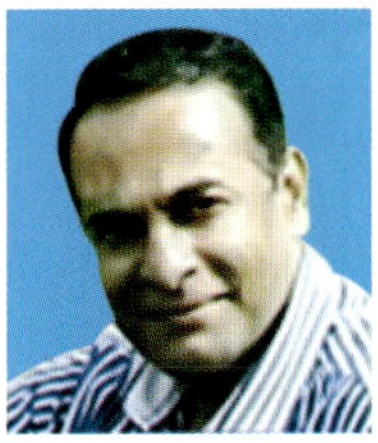

Ajit N Patil MD
Professor
Department of Obstetrics and Gynecology
DY Patil Education Society
Kolhapur, Maharashtra, India

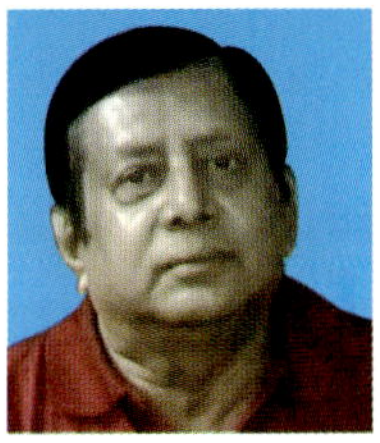

Amit Chakravarty PhD
Director/Principal
Institute of Genetic Engineering
Institute of Genetic Medicine and
Genomic Science
Kolkata, West Bengal, India

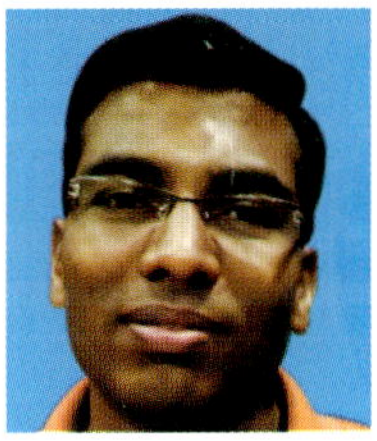

Anant Bangar DNB-Pediatric Surgery
Junior Consultant
Department of Pediatric Surgery
Lilavati Hospital and Research Center
Mumbai, Maharashtra, India

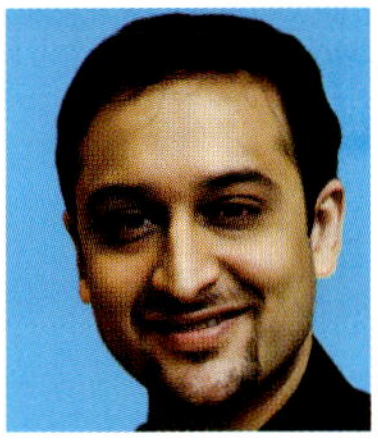

Ankesh R Sahetya DNB DGO MBBS MNAMS
Obstetrician and Gynecologist
Laparoscopic Surgeon
Consultant
Pushpaa Hospital
Thunga Hospital (Malad)
Lion Kartar Singh Hospital (Andheri West)
Assistant Honorary
Oshiwara Maternity Home
Mumbai, Maharashtra, India

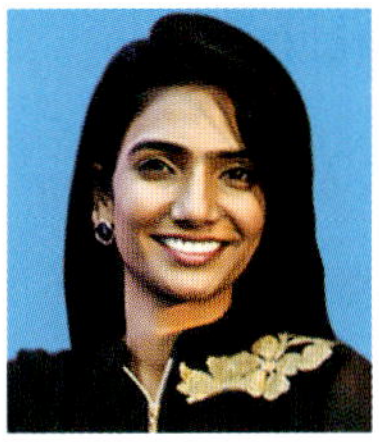

Apoorva Pallam Reddy MD DNB
Fellowship in Reproductive Medicine, Diploma in Gynec Endoscopy (Germany), Diploma in Advanced Ultrasonography
Consultant
Mathrutva Fertility Center
Bengaluru, Karnataka, India

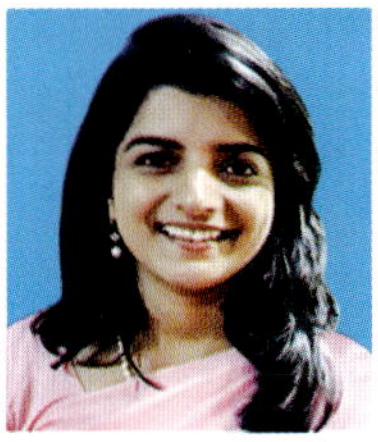

Arati Joshi DMRD
Consultant Radiologist and Sonologist
Advanced Radiology Center
Mumbai, Maharashtra, India

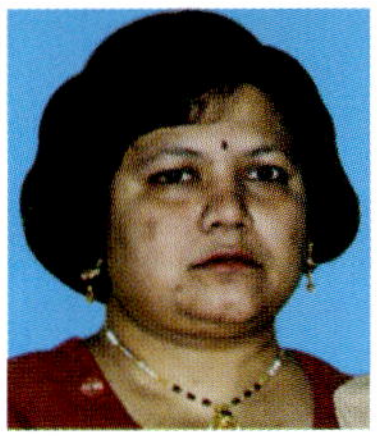

Arundhati S Athalye MSc PhD
Senior Scientific Officer/Research Officer
Department of Assisted
Reproduction and Genetics
Jaslok Hospital and Research Center
Mumbai, Maharashtra, India

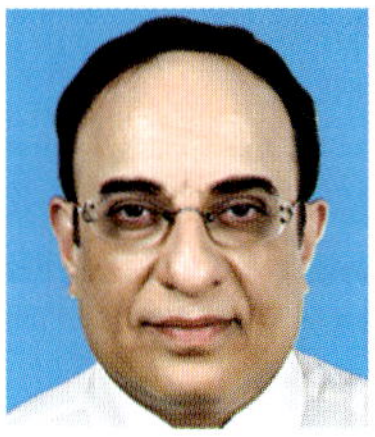

Chander Lulla MD
Consultant
Fetal Medicine Specialist and Sonologist
Ria Clinic
Head
Department of Ultrasonography
Jaslok Hospital and Research Center
Mumbai, Maharashtra, India
ISUOG Ambassador for India

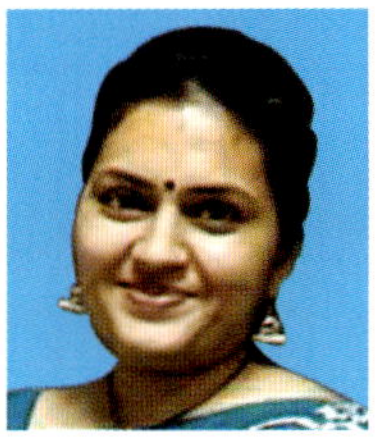

Dhanlaxmi Shetty PhD PGDHHM PGDMLS
Scientific Officer 'E'
Cytogenetics Department
Tata Memorial Center
Mumbai, Maharashtra, India

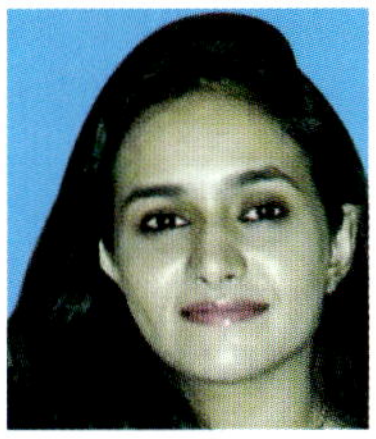

Divya A Sahetya MS
Fellowship in Reproductive Medicine (ICOG)
Obstetrician and Gynecologist
Infertility Specialist
Consultant
Pushpaa Hospital
Thunga Hospital (Malad)
Lion Kartar Singh Hospital (Andheri West)
Mumbai, Maharashtra, India

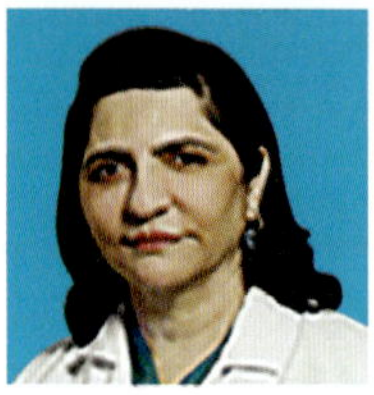

Firuza R Parikh MD DGO DFP FPCS Dip NBE
Director
Department of Assisted
Reproduction and Genetics
Jaslok Hospital and Research Center
Mumbai, Maharashtra, India

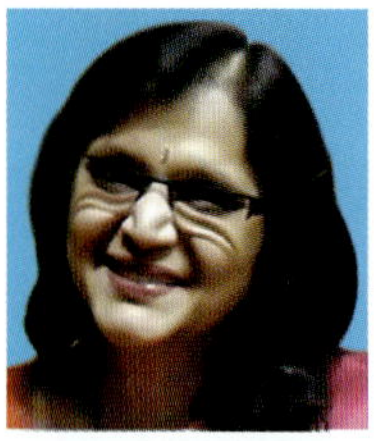

Geeta Shah MD DMRD
Medical Director
Chief Consultant Radiologist and Sonologist
Advanced Radiology Center
Mumbai, Maharashtra, India

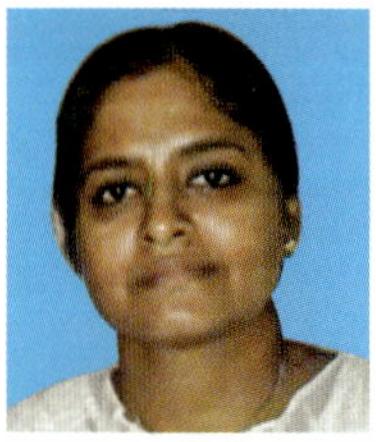

Geetha Balsarkar MD DGO DNB FCPS
Professor
Department of Obstetrics and Gynecology
Seth GS Medical College
Consultant
Nowrosjee Wadia Maternity Hospital
Mumbai, Maharashtra, India

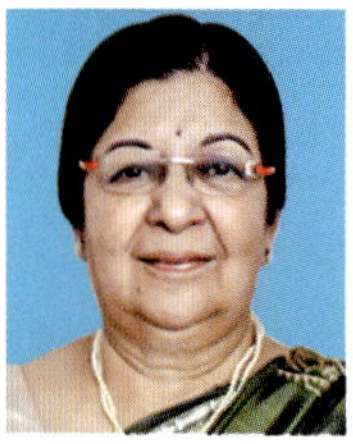

Hema Purandarey MBBS MS FICMH PhD
Medical and Reproductive Geneticist
Founder and Director
Center of Genetic Healthcare
Director
SRL Diagnostic Services Private Limited
(Genetics)
Mumbai, Maharashtra, India

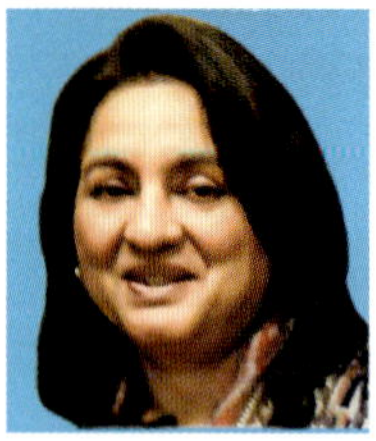

Jaideep Malhotra MD (Obs & Gyn) FICMCH
FIAJAGO FICOG MASRM FICMU
Director
Rainbow IVF
Infertility Consultant and Specialist
Agra, Uttar Pradesh, India

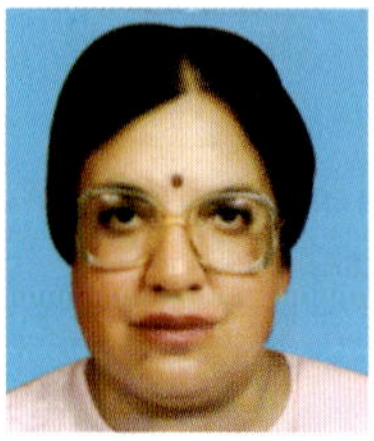

Maya Lulla MD FCPS MIAC
Consultant
Nanavati Superspecialty Hospital
Mumbai, Maharashtra, India

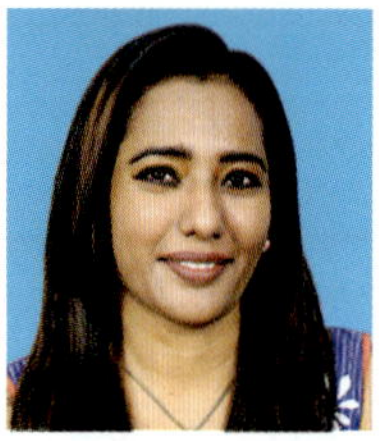

Nandini Vaz Fernandes MSc PhD
Assistant Professor
Department of Zoology
Co-Director, Human Genetic
Research Laboratory
Parvatibai Chowgule College
Margao, Goa

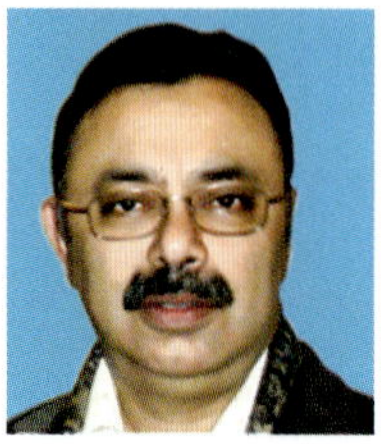

Narendra Malhotra MD FRCOG FRSH FICMCH
FICOG FICS
Director
Rainbow Hospitals
Obstetrician and Gynecologist
Agra, Uttar Pradesh, India

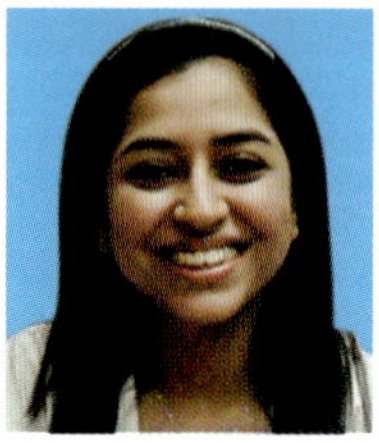

Neharika Malhotra MD (Gold Medalist) FICMCH
ICOG Fellowship in USG and Infertility
Infertility Consultant
Rainbow IVF
Agra, Uttar Pradesh, India

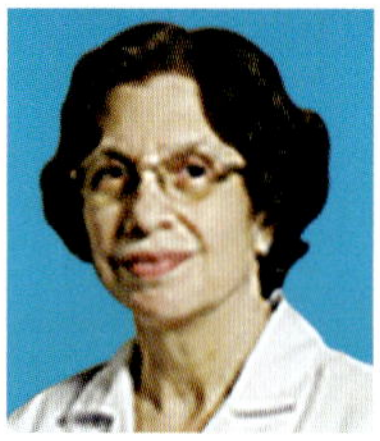

Prochi F Madon MSc PhD
Honorary Consultant Geneticist
Department of Assisted
Reproduction and Genetics
Jaslok Hospital and Research Center
Mumbai, Maharashtra, India

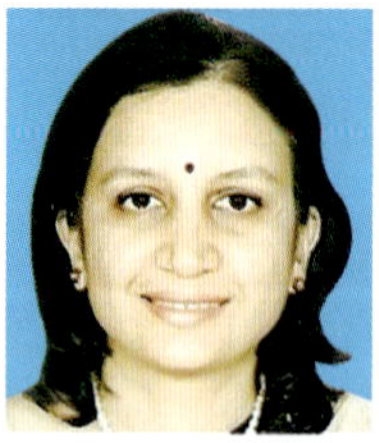

Purnima Satoskar MD DNB MRCOG (London)
Professor
Department of Obstetrics and Gynecology
Seth GS Medical College and Nowrosjee
Wadia Maternity Hospital
Consultant
Jaslok Hospital and Research Center
Mumbai, Maharashtra, India

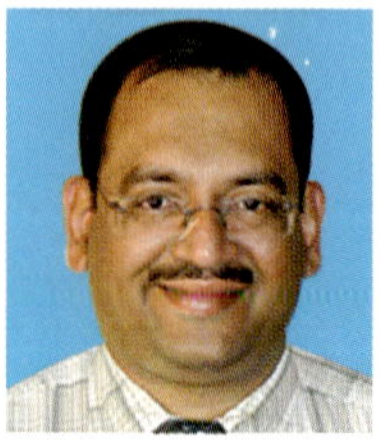

Rajeev Redkar MCH FRCS (Edin) FRCS (Glas) DNB MS
(Gen Surgery) FCPS IAS
Consultant Pediatric Surgeon
Lilavati, Shushrusha and
Wadia Children's Hospital
Mumbai, Maharashtra, India

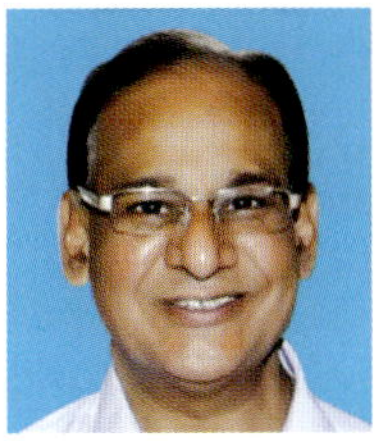

Rajendra M Jain MS (OB-GYN)
Consulting Gynecologist and Reproductive Medicine Specialist
Medical Director
Asha Fertility Center
Faculty at Aryan ART Bank
Founder Editor of AFG-Times
Treasurer of Association of Fellow Gynecologists
Mumbai, Maharashtra, India

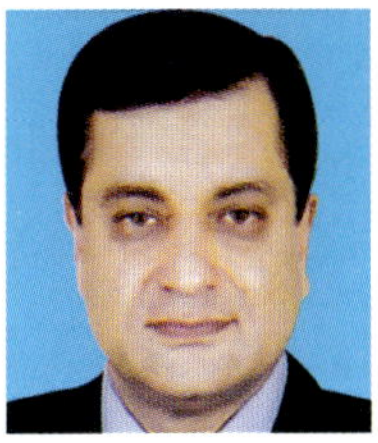

Raju R Sahetya MD DGO DFP FCPS FICOG
Obstetrician and Gynecologist
Specialist—Fertility and IVF and Fetal Medicine
President
Indian Society for Prenatal Diagnosis and Therapy (ISPAT)
Honorary Scientific Secretary
Association of Fellow Gynecologist
Pushpaa Hospital, Hinduja Hospital
Mumbai, Maharashtra, India

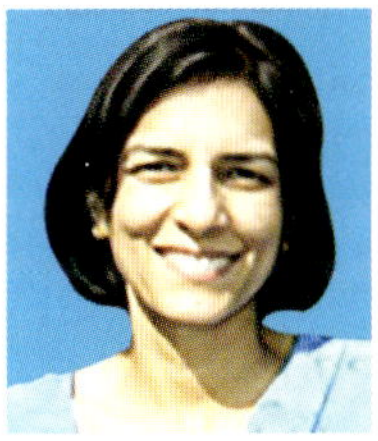

Ratna D Puri MD DM
Professor
Department of Genetics
Ganga Ram Institute of Postgraduate Medical Education and Research (GRIPMER)
Senior Consultant and Vice Chairperson
Center of Medical Genetics
Sir Ganga Ram Hospital
New Delhi, India

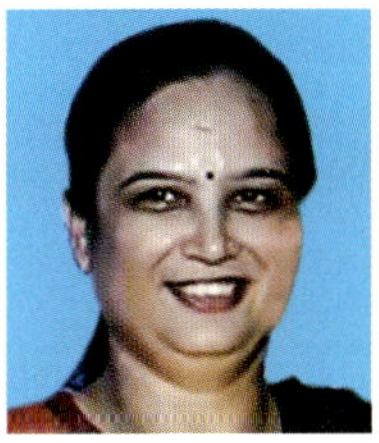

Renu Makwana MBBS MS (Obs & Gyn) FICOG
Consultant
Vasundhara Hospital and Fertility Research Center
Jodhpur, Rajasthan, India

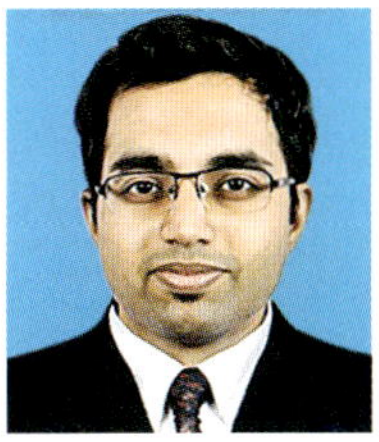

Rinoy Sreedharan MD (Obs & Gyne) MICOG
Consultant Gynecologist and Obstetrician
Krishna Multispecialty Hospital
Korba, Chhattisgarh, India

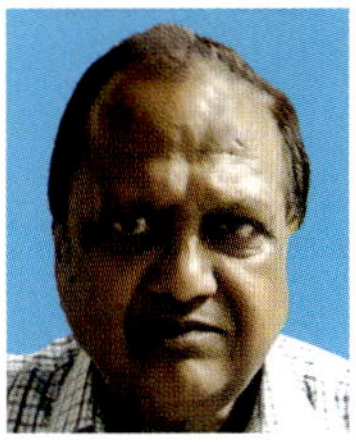

RN Goel MD DCH DGO
Member Executive Committee
Indian Society for Prenatal Diagnosis and Therapy (ISPAT)
Member
National Inspection and Monitoring Committee (NIMC) under Pre-Conception and Pre-Natal Diagnostic Techniques by Ministry of Health and Family Welfare
New Delhi
President
National Indian Federation of Ultrasound in Medicines and Biology (IFUMB)
Gynecologist and Sonologist
Agra, Uttar Pradesh, India

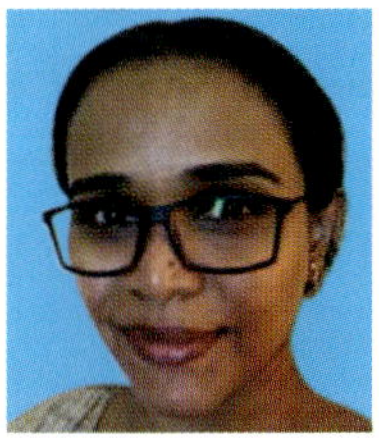

Roopa R Shinde MD (Obs & Gyn)
Fellowship (Fetal Medicine)
Consultant
Department of Fetal Medicine
Mediscan Systems
Chennai, Tamil Nadu, India

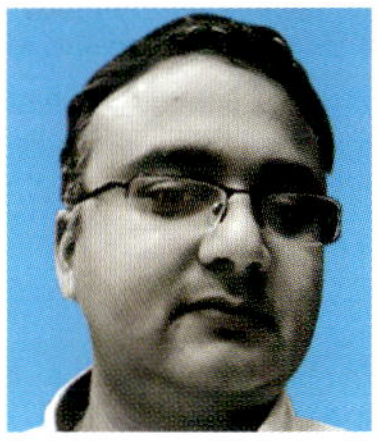

Saurabh Dani FCPS DGO
Consultant Obstetrician and Gynecologist
Ankur Hospital, Namaha Healthcare
Cloudnine Group of Hospitals
Thane, Maharashtra, India

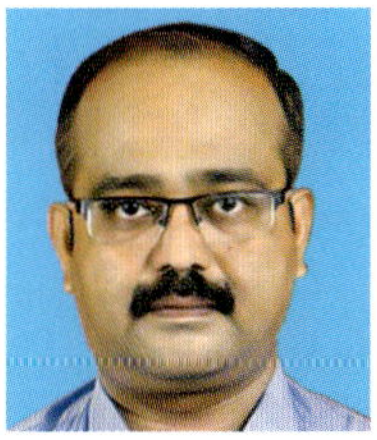

Shailesh Pande MBBS MS FDBT (Fellow DBT)
Senior Medical Geneticist and Genetic Counselor
Consultant and Head
Department of Genetics
Metropolis Healthcare Ltd
Mumbai, Maharashtra, India

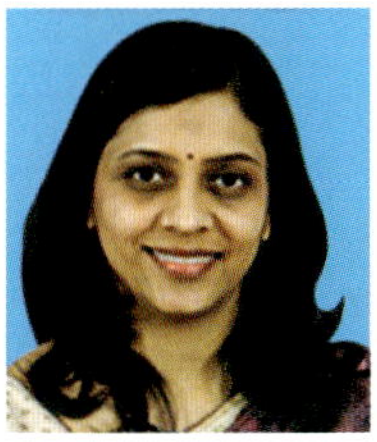

Shantala Vadeyar MD FRCOG DM RCOG
Certification in Fetal & Maternal Medicine RCOG/RCR
Certification in Advanced Obstetric Ultrasound
Consultant
Gynecology and Obstetrics
Kokilaben Dhirubhai Ambani Hospital
Medical Director
Fetal and Maternal Medicine
Cloudnine Group of Hospitals
Mumbai, Maharashtra, India

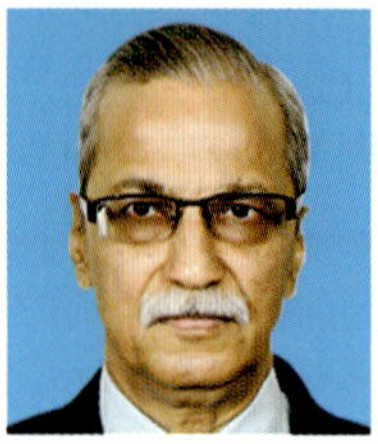

Sharad Gogate MD FCPS FICS DGO DFP
Consultant
Fetal Medicine
Obstetrics and Gynecology
Director
Fetal Medicine Consultancy Services and
Surlata Hospital
Senior Consultant
Center for Genetic Health Services
Advanced Radiology Clinic
Mumbai, Maharashtra, India

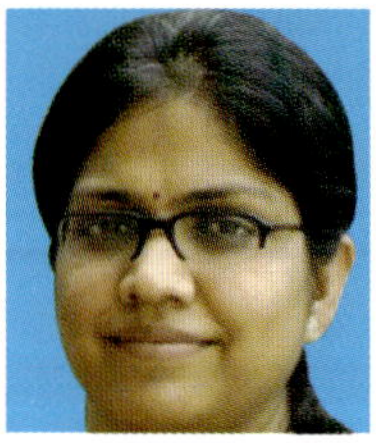

Shilpa Agrawal DGO FCPS DNB FNB
(Fellowship in High Risk Pregnancy and Fetal Medicine)
Consultant
Department of Obstetrics and Gynecology
Jaslok Hospital and Research Center
Mumbai, Maharashtra, India

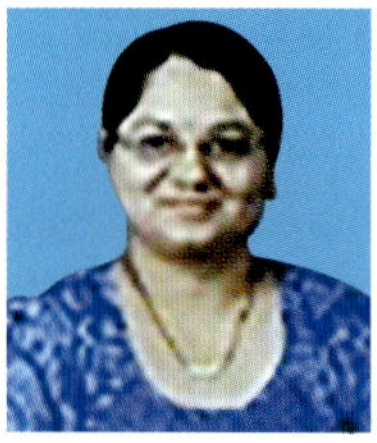

Shirin Joshi
MS (General Surgery) MCh (Pediatric Surgery)
Clinical Associate
Department of Pediatric Surgery
Lilavati Hospital and Research Center
Mumbai, Maharashtra, India

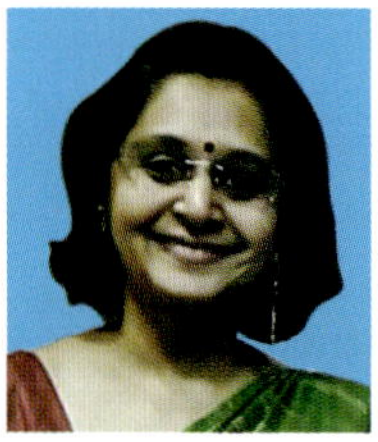

Sonali Gandhi DMRD
Consultant Radiologist and Sonologist
Advanced Radiology Center
Mumbai, Maharashtra, India

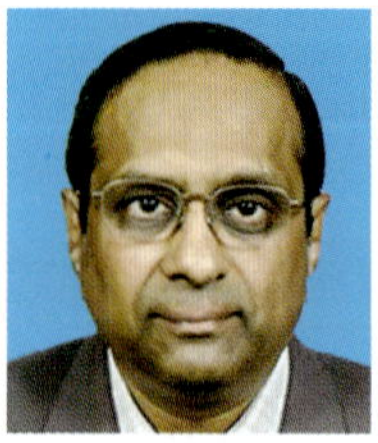

S Suresh FRCOG (Hon)
Director and Fetal Medicine Specialist
Mediscan Systems
Chennai, Tamil Nadu, India

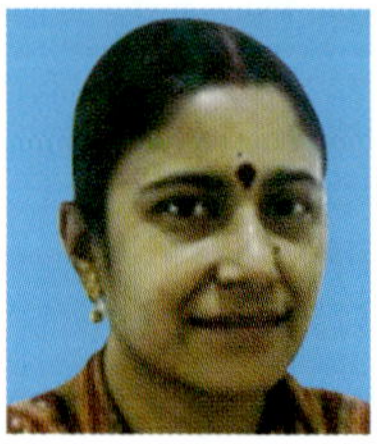

Sudipa Chakravarty PhD
Dy-Director/Vice Principal
Institute of Genetic Engineering
Institute of Genetic Medicine and
Genomic Science
Kolkata, West Bengal, India

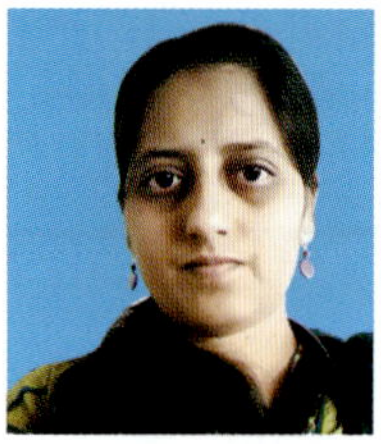

Swathi Krishna MBBS
Resident
Department of Pediatric Surgery
Lilavati Hospital and Research Center
Mumbai, Maharashtra, India

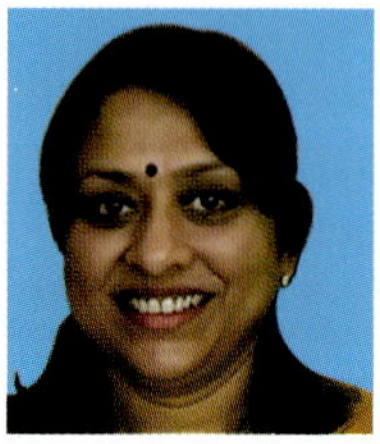

Uma Ram DGO DNB FRCOG
Director
Seethapathy Clinic and Hospital
Chennai, Tamil Nadu, India

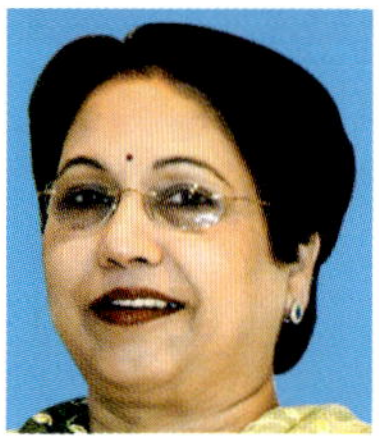

Usha P Dave PhD DHA
Medical Geneticist and Neuroscientist
Director—MILS International India
National Professor and Visiting Scientist
Haffkine Institute
Honorary Medical Geneticist
BJ Wadia Maternity Hospital
PG Research Guide of Mumbai University
Mumbai, Maharashtra, India

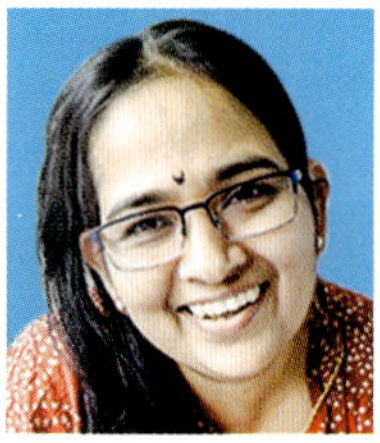

Vandana Bansal MD DGO DNB MRCOG FNB
(High Risk Pregnancy and Perinatology)
Associate Professor
Nowrosjee Wadia Maternity Hospital and
Seth GS Medical College
Consultant
Department of Fetal Medicine
Mediscan Center
Mumbai, Maharashtra, India

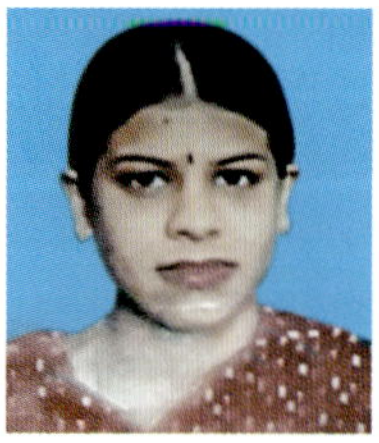

Vishalakshi Kamat MSc (Microbiology)
Quality Manager
SRL Diagnostic Services Private Limited
Center for Genetic Healthcare
Mumbai, Maharashtra, India

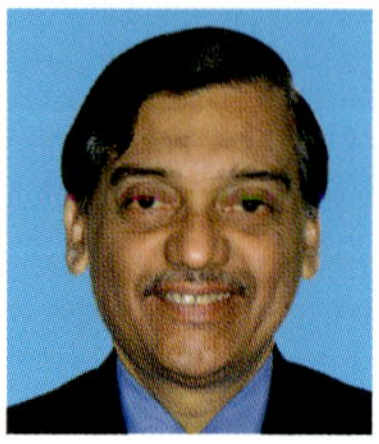

Vivek Rege MS MCh DNB (Ped. Surg) FICS
Pediatric and Neonatal Surgeon
BJ Wadia Hospital for Children
Bhatia Hospital, Saifee Hospital
Fortis Hospital, and Apollo Spectra Hospital
Mumbai, Maharashtra, India

Foreword

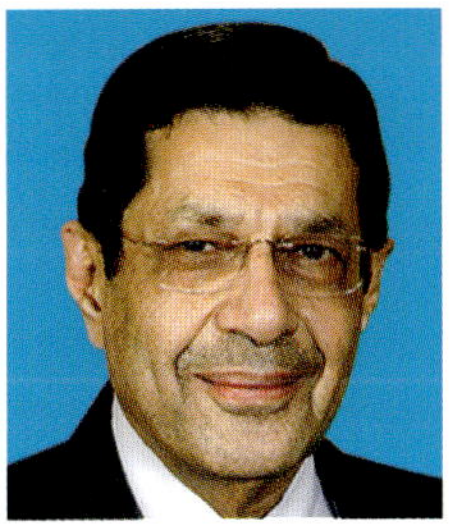

ISPAT's *Principles and Practice of Fetal Medicine* is really a big book today. Its size and scope is all the more impressive, considering the fact that just 45 years ago, it would have been a very small book, perhaps even non-existent.

Human Cytogenetics was just developing, amniocentesis for prenatal diagnosis did not appear till 1967, the use of ultrasound was limited to little more than detecting a midline shift, and talk of "The Fetus as a Patient" was yet to hear of. Yet, just 45 years later, a comprehensive book on prenatal diagnosis and associated issues requires 45 chapters to cover the relevant topics.

We are fortunate that the ISPAT's President 2014–16, Dr Raju R Sahetya and his team, joined hands with Dr Jaideep Malhotra and Dr Hema Purandarey (Co-editors) to take on this daunting task of compiling this textbook on fetal medicine.

The result provides a great service to the field by documenting how far the science of prenatal genetic diagnosis has allowed us to progress in providing prenatal care. It is a remarkable compilation authored by authorities in each topic from all over India. Thus, providing the reader a status report on the entire field of prenatal diagnosis.

The reader would do well to approach reading the book, exerting every effort to learn and understand the science of prenatal diagnosis and therapy. They can then use that understanding to work through with the patients in an ethical decision-making process in striving to provide the best care for the fetus, the child, and the mother to be.

Padmashree Dr Rustom P Soonawala
MD FRCS FRCOG FICOG
Founder President ISPAT
Head
Department of Obstetrics and Gynecology
Breach Candy Hospital
Mumbai, Maharashtra
Head
Max Healthcare
New Delhi, India
Professor Emeritus
Wadia Maternity Hospital
Mumbai, Maharashtra, India

Preface

It is with great pleasure that we introduce this first edition of ISPAT's *Principles and Practice of Fetal Medicine*. As we decided to embark on this project, we strived to ensure that this book provides the most up-to-date and comprehensive reference on this subject written in an easy-to-read style.

Prenatal genetic diagnosis will continue to focus on the wishes of all couples to have a healthy child. The past 45 years have seen the scope of the prenatal diagnosis increase from the routine to predictive diagnosis and disorders that will manifest decades after birth.

Since mid-1960s, steady progress in prenatal diagnosis has depended on basic scientific research in many related disciplines. Early attention first focused on the safety of amniocentesis and the ability to reliably cultivate amniotic fluid cells and process them for chromosomal and biochemical analyses.

The recognition of alpha-fetoprotein in 1972, as a marker for the prenatal detection of neural tube defects, opened an era of maternal serum screening.

By 1976, when the second trimester amniocentesis had shown to have an indisputably low risk, soon chorionic villus sampling (CVS) emerged as a first trimester technique, also with relative safety.

Improvement in the visualization of fetal anatomy by ultrasound imaging vastly improved accurate diagnosis. This resulted in procedural safety, optimal sampling and diagnosis of fetal malformations.

Higher resolution chromosomal analysis, newer staining techniques, and the fluorescent *in situ* hybridization significantly increased the sophistication of cytogenetic study.

In the 1990s, the use of quantitative fluorescence polymerase chain reaction (QF-PCR) to target specific whole chromosomal anomalies was introduced.

Chromosomal microarray analysis (CMA) is a relatively new test in the prenatal arena, although it has become firmly established as the frontline genetic diagnostic test.

Introduction of Noninvasive Prenatal Testing (NIPT), which analyzes cell-free fetal DNA circulating in maternal blood, is a new option in the prenatal screening and testing paradigm.

Recent developments in sequencing the fetal genome combined with progress in understanding fetal physiology using gene expression arrays indicate that we could have the technical capabilities to apply an individualized medical approach to the fetus.

The ultimate goal of the textbook is to promote improved prenatal and perinatal management of pregnancies affected by an anomalous fetus. More immediate goals include improved detection, diagnosis and understanding "Fetal Medicine and the Fetus as a Patient".

The book would not have been a reality without the support of several people, first and foremost, our families and friends who unselfishly allowed us to spend long hours away from them in completing this pleasant task.

Last but not least, we owe a great debt of gratitude to all those who have contributed by writing chapters, on subjects they specialize and practice.

Raju R Sahetya
Jaideep Malhotra
Hema Purandarey

Acknowledgments

It is my proud privilege to acknowledge the efforts put in by Drs Jaideep Malhotra and Hema Purandarey (Co-editors) and the ISPAT team 2014–16 for believing in me of making this book possible and contributing to it.

Founder President, Padmashree Dr Rustom P Soonawala, President Elect Dr Narendra Malhotra and Past President Dr Hema Purandarey for advising me from time to time, and making my task enjoyable all the way.

My son, Dr Ankesh R Sahetya, who planted the seed of an idea in my mind to bring out the book.

Contents

SECTION 4: DIAGNOSTIC TECHNIQUES: INVASIVE

SECTION 5: LABORATORY TECHNIQUES

SECTION 6: ANTENATAL USE OF FETAL THERAPY

SECTION

1

General Aspects of Prenatal Diagnosis

CHAPTER

1 Revolution in Prenatal Diagnosis

Raju R Sahetya

INTRODUCTION

Prenatal diagnosis has revolutionized prenatal care from the perspective of both the patient and the physician. For the patient, prenatal diagnosis provides genetic, anatomic, and physiologic information about the fetus or fetuses that can be used to make informed and individualized decisions regarding the pregnancy. For the physician, prenatal diagnosis provides vital information that can be utilized for better antepartum management. Information regarding specific anatomic anomalies, affords the physician the opportunity to offer the patient sophisticated prenatal procedures, such as fetal surgery or selective fetal reduction in multiple gestations. Likewise, prenatal knowledge about genetic, physiologic, and/or anatomic abnormalities enables the physician to tailor or manage the timing and mode of delivery for optimal maternal and fetal outcomes. Prenatal diagnosis also allows the neonatal and pediatric specialists to be adequately prepared for a potentially ill neonate at delivery.

HISTORICAL PERSPECTIVE IN PRENATAL DIAGNOSIS

- Modern era in 1952 by Bevus—technique of amniocentesis
- Liley in 1961—severity of erythroblastosis bilirubin level
- In 1966—fetal cells from amniotic fluid cultured and karyotyped
- In 1966—Hahnemann fetal chorionic villi [terminal villi (TV)] by hysteroscope
- In 1970, Chinese workers blind aspiration of chorionic villi for fetal sex
- In 1982, Kazy et al.—role of ultrasonography in successful chorionic villus sampling (CVS)
- In 1985, Brambati et al., rapid uncultured villi—Trisomy 21 at 11 week
- Milan group able to minimize maternal cell contamination.

Recent progresses in the fields of maternal fetal medicine, ultrasonography and human genetics have resulted in great revolution in prenatal diagnosis.

The recent major advances in the field of prenatal diagnosis are as follows:

- In recent years, there have been significant advances in antenatal screening for fetal aneuploidy. Fetal aneuploidy is defined as an abnormal number of chromosomes instead of the usual diploid complement of 46 chromosomes. One single additional chromosome is termed *trisomy* and is an important cause of congenital malformations as well as of congenital mental retardation. Down syndrome (trisomy 21), Edwards syndrome (trisomy 18), and Patau syndrome (trisomy 13) are the most common trisomies. Trisomies 18 and 13 are lethal and affect approximately 1 in 3000 and 1 in 5000 livebirths, respectively. The majority of infants with trisomy 18 die by 1 year of age, while the majority of infants with trisomy 13 die by 3 months of age. Trisomy 21 is compatible with life and affects approximately 1 in 800 to 1 in 900 livebirths. It is associated with congenital heart defects, most commonly the atrioventricular septal defect.
- Initially, prenatal diagnosis for Down syndrome constituted offering first trimester chorionic villous sampling or second trimester amniocentesis to women of advanced maternal age (age ≥35 at estimated date of delivery) and to women with a previously affected pregnancy.

BIOCHEMICAL SERUM MARKERS

In the mid-1980s, it was noted that women in the second trimester with decreased levels of maternal serum alpha fetoprotein (AFP) and increased level of human chorionic gonadotropin (hCG) were at increased risk for their pregnancy to be complicated by Down syndrome. As a result, noninvasive, first and second-trimester Down syndrome screening for the general obstetric population became feasible, and a multiple-marker serum panel, dual and triple marker, were established for this purpose.[1] Since >90% of all structural and chromosomal abnormalities derive from pregnancies without risk factors, it is reasonable that universal screening be provided.[2]

Second-trimester maternal serum screening currently includes a combination of 4 markers and is known as the "quad test". These markers include AFP, human chorionic gonadotropin (hCG), unconjugated estriol (uE3), and inhibin A.[1] For screening purposes, sonographic dating, the crown rump length (CRL) should be used instead of menstrual dating, as it optimizes the performance of the test. While screening references are available between 15 and 21 weeks' gestation, the optimal time to perform this test is between 15 and 16 weeks' gestation. In addition, laboratories adjust for factors that may affect values, such as maternal weight, multiple gestation, and history of diabetes. It is important to note that with regard to twins, the sensitivity for Down syndrome using the quad test is only 47%, with a 5% false-positive rate.[3] Maternal serum screening in multiples has been limited because of the potential for discordance between fetuses and because of the impact of the various placentas on analytes.[3,4]

In patients with a pregnancy affected by Down syndrome, the AFP and uE3 levels are lower, while the hCG and inhibin A levels are higher, than in unaffected pregnancies. In pregnancies affected by trisomy 18, the AFP, uE3, and hCG levels are all low (Fig. 1.1). The quad test can detect approximately 75% cases of Down syndrome, with a 5% screen-positive rate.[5] Meanwhile, the quad test detects 85–95% of cases in women ≥35 years of age at estimated date of delivery, with a 25% screen-positive rate.[6,7] The disadvantages of this screening method include its relatively late performance in the second trimester, resulting in definitive diagnosis by amniocentesis being provided even later in gestation. In addition, many cases of Down syndrome will not be detected with this test, and the 5% screen-positive rate indicates that many amniocenteses will be performed for every 1 case of Down syndrome identified.[8]

Abnormality	AFP	hCG	uE3
Neural tube defects	↑	—	—
Trisomy 21	↓	↑	↓
Trisomy 18	↓	↓	↓

Fig. 1.1 Serum markers at risk
Abbreviations: AFP, alpha fetoprotein; hCG, human chorionic gonadotropin

Due to the limitations of the quad test, great efforts have been put forth to devise more efficient screening protocols. Because of its ability to provide results early in pregnancy, first-trimester screening is becoming increasingly more important. First-trimester screening provides the opportunity for early risk assessment and early diagnosis of fetal aneuploidy via chorionic villus sampling (CVS). Early diagnosis allows patients privacy and for pregnancy termination earlier in gestation, if the patient so desires. In addition, earlier pregnancy termination is associated with decreased maternal morbidity and mortality.[7]

ULTRASOUND

First-trimester ultrasound is one of the greatest contributors to the recent advances in prenatal diagnosis and is rapidly becoming important for screening for fetal aneuploidy. Techniques used to evaluate risk for Down syndrome during the first trimester include nuchal translucency (NT) sonography, assay of first-trimester maternal serum markers, nasal bone sonography, and Doppler sonography of the ductus venosus.

The normal space between the spine and the overlying skin at the back of the fetal neck during the first trimester is referred to as the NT (Figs 1.2A and B). A large NT has been associated with an increased risk for aneuploidy, genetic disorders, anatomic abnormalities, and poor pregnancy outcomes.[7-9] When obtained between 10 weeks 3 days and 13 weeks 6 days' gestation, measurement of the NT has been shown to be a powerful sonographic marker for trisomy 21.[4] It is unlikely that one pathophysiologic mechanism leads to an enlarged NT. Possible etiologies include heart failure secondary to structural malformations, abnormalities in the extracellular matrix, and abnormal lymphatic development.[10-12]

Nuchal translucency sonography is technically challenging and can be obtained both transabdominally and transvaginally. The fetus should be in a perfect midsagittal view. Careful attention should be paid to distinguish the nuchal skin from the amnion. The fetus should have a neutral neck, and the image should be magnified significantly. Calipers need to be placed at the inner borders of the NT space.

In multiple pregnancy, NT appears to be a promising modality for screening for aneuploidy.

First-trimester maternal serum screening utilizes maternal serum levels of pregnancy-associated plasma protein A (PAPP-A) and free beta-hCG between 10 and 14

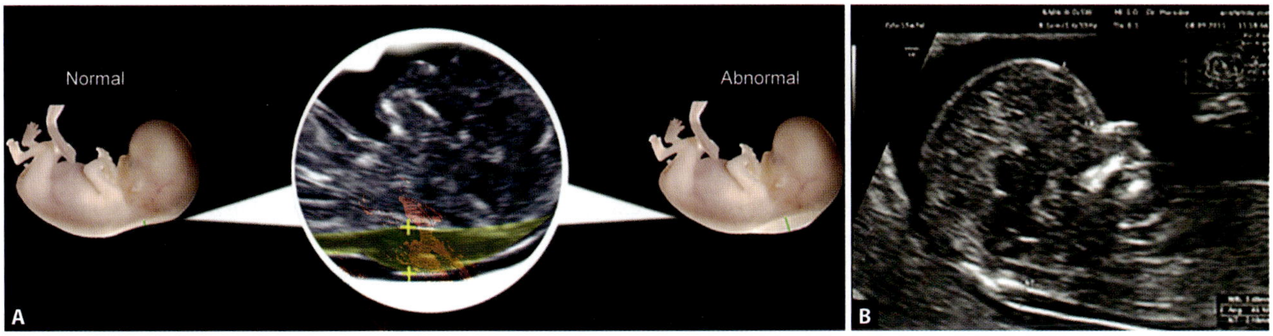

Figs 1.2A and B Nuchal translucency measurement

weeks' gestation. In pregnancies affected by Down syndrome, PAPP-A is lower compared with unaffected pregnancies at 10–14 weeks' gestation. Maternal serum levels of free beta-hCG are higher in pregnancies affected by trisomy 21 than in unaffected pregnancies. These 2 markers, combined with maternal age, can detect up to 60% of cases of Down syndrome, with a 5% false-positive rate.[13-15]

The most efficient method of first-trimester screening for aneuploidy involves combining maternal age, NT, and the serum markers PAPP-A and free beta-hCG. Between 10 and 14 weeks' gestation, this screening method may detect up to 82% of cases of trisomy 21, with a 5% false-positive rate.[4] Timing is important, as studies have shown that the accuracy of this screening protocol deteriorates over time. With this method, trisomy 21 detection rates are 87% at 11 weeks and 82% at 13 weeks, both at a 5% false-positive rate.[16]

Nasal bone sonography is another first-trimester ultrasound technique that has been proposed for screening for aneuploidy.[16,17] Similar to NT, this technique may be difficult to master and elusive to obtain. Nasal bone sonography is performed between 10 and 14 weeks' gestation. A perfect midsagittal image is required, and the fetal spine should be down with slight neck flexion. When the fetal profile is facing upwards, it may be possible to distinguish 2 echogenic lines at the fetal nose profile. The superficial echogenic line is the skin, and the deeper line is the nose bone. Failure to visualize the fetal nasal bone may be an independent risk factor for fetal aneuploidy. The studies suggesting that the absence of the fetal nasal bone may be used as a marker for trisomy 21 are limited by the fact that they are derived from high-risk populations. More recent research has suggested that nasal bone evaluation may not be useful for general population screening.[18]

Color Doppler

Doppler of the ductus venosus is another technique that has been proposed for the first-trimester screening of fetal aneuploidy (Fig. 1.3). The ductus venosus usually

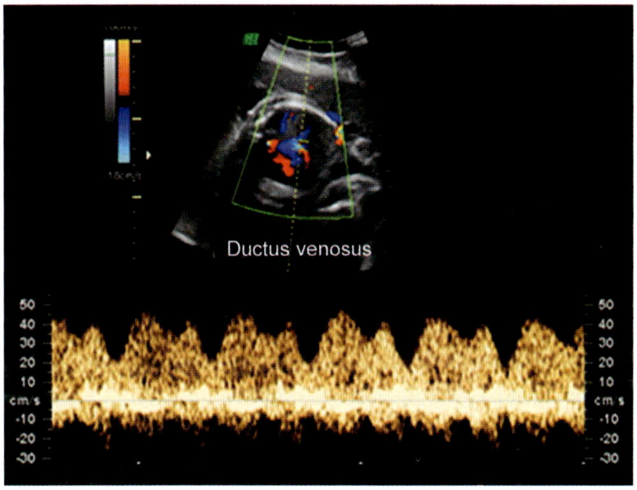

Fig. 1.3 Color Doppler ductus venosus

demonstrates a triphasic flow pattern, with forward flow reaching peaks during ventricular systole and early ventricular diastole. Absent or reversed flow at the time of atrial contraction is considered abnormal and has been suggested as a marker for aneuploidy.[19-24]

At the time of second-trimester anatomic ultrasound, any major fetal structural anomaly (such as a cardiac defect, omphalocele, diaphragmatic hernia, duodenal or esophageal atresia, renal abnormalities, clubbed or rocker-bottom feet, holoprosencephaly, meningomyelocele, and/or proboscis) should prompt immediate consultation and counseling with the genetic specialist, as these findings have been associated with trisomy. Invasive prenatal diagnosis should be offered for any major congenital anomaly. The optimal time to perform an anatomic survey is at approximately 18 weeks' gestation, as evaluation of the fetal anatomy is maximized at this time. Likewise, amniocentesis results can be obtained in a timely manner, and termination of pregnancy is still an option if the patient desires.

Second-trimester ultrasound can detect minor markers for aneuploidy.[25-27] These findings are not fetal malformations, they are specific ultrasound findings that have been associated with an increased risk for fetal aneuploidy in certain high-risk populations, such as those of advanced maternal age or those with abnormal serum screening results. The role of these markers in the low-risk population remains uncertain. These markers include nuchal thickening, mild ventriculomegaly, a short humerus or femur, echogenic bowel, enlarged cisterna magna, renal pyelectasis, echogenic intracardiac focus, hypoplastic nasal bones, a single umbilical artery, choroid plexus cysts, and overlapping fingers.

Another option for screening for aneuploidy that is gaining popularity is combining first- and second-trimester screening. Combined first-trimester NT and serum screening has shown similar results as second-trimester serum screening with the quad test with regard to screening for aneuploidy.[7] Combining first- and second-trimester screening maximizes the performance of both of these screening modalities.[28] At this point in time, patients receiving care at centers offering first-trimester screening and CVS may choose between 2 types of first- and second-trimester combined screening: Integrated screening and stepwise screening.

Integrated screening is a 2-step approach in which results are withheld until both the first- and second-trimester screening tests have been obtained, at which time a single risk assessment is provided. Patients who opt for integrated screening have NT performed between 10 and 14 weeks' gestation. A measurement of PAPP-A is also obtained during this time period. Between 15 and 16 weeks' gestation, the quad test is performed, and all results are integrated together. The trisomy 21 detection rate with this method of screening is 94%, with a 5% false-positive rate.[29]

In stepwise screening, patients undergo first-trimester testing and are given the results at that time. The second-trimester screening then utilizes the first-trimester results as the new a priori risk. The advantage of this screening method is that patients may opt for CVS in the first trimester if their screening results indicate that their pregnancy is at increased risk for aneuploidy. Otherwise, they can wait until the second-trimester screening is completed and receive results may opt for amniocentesis and afford a better Down syndrome detection rate.[30,31]

MAGNETIC RESONANCE IMAGING

Use of magnetic resonance imaging (MRI) was first described in pregnancy in 1983.[32] Its initial application was for maternal and placental abnormalities. Fetal MRI was initially limited because of fetal motion artifact. In the 1990s, fetal MRI became practical because of the development of single-shot rapid acquisition sequence with refocused echoes. This high-quality T2-weighted sequence has a slice acquisition time of <1 second and essentially "freezes" fetal motion.[33] As a result, excellent fetal imaging can now be obtained without maternal or fetal sedation (Figs 1.4A to F).

The main indication for fetal MRI is further evaluation of inconclusive ultrasound findings. It is also useful for evaluation prior to fetal surgery. Fetal MRI has proven to be extremely helpful for the examination of many suspected fetal anomalies.

Fetal MRI has been particularly helpful with the diagnosis and management of suspected fetal central nervous system (CNS) abnormalities and is suggested, if a CNS abnormality is suspected on prenatal ultrasound. Fetal MRI can aid in the diagnosis of ventriculomegaly, agenesis of the corpus callosum, posterior fossa abnormalities, cortical gyral malformations, hemorrhage, holoprosencephaly, arachnoid cysts, neural tube defects, and vascular malformations.[34] In fact, MRI has changed the diagnosis and aided in the management of many cases of suspected CNS abnormalities on ultrasound.

Similar to MRI, three-dimensional (3D) ultrasound allows for multiplanar imaging and allows the examiner to move back and forth between different planes because of the capability of viewing the fetus in 3 rather than 2 spatial planes (Figs 1.5A to F). Images can be reconstructed, and the examiner can move the fetus into desired positions that are often not possible with conventional ultrasound. In addition, 3D scanning enhances imaging capabilities by permitting surface rendering of a structure.

Preimplantation Genetic Diagnosis

In the field of reproduction endocrinology, preimplantation genetic diagnosis (PGD) (Figs 1.6A to G) is one of the most exciting new advances.[35] This technique allows for genetic testing prior to embryo transfer in patients undergoing assisted reproductive technology (ART). One or two cells are biopsied from embryos at the 6- to 8-cell stage and are analyzed for chromosomal abnormalities or for single-gene disorders. Alternatively, polar bodies can be biopsied from oocytes for genetic testing as well. Preimplantation genetic diagnosis has been used for couples at risk for having pregnancies affected by single-gene or X-linked disorders. It has also been used for couples with an age-related risk for aneuploidy and for couples who carry balanced chromosomal rearrangements.[36] In addition, it is thought that patients who have experienced many failed *in vitro* fertilization (IVF) cycles or who have experienced recurrent early pregnancy loss may benefit from PGD. Only embryos free of the genetic abnormalities under evaluation are replaced at the time of embryo transfer. The main drawback to this procedure is that patients must undergo IVF in order to have PGD even if they do not have any fertility issues.

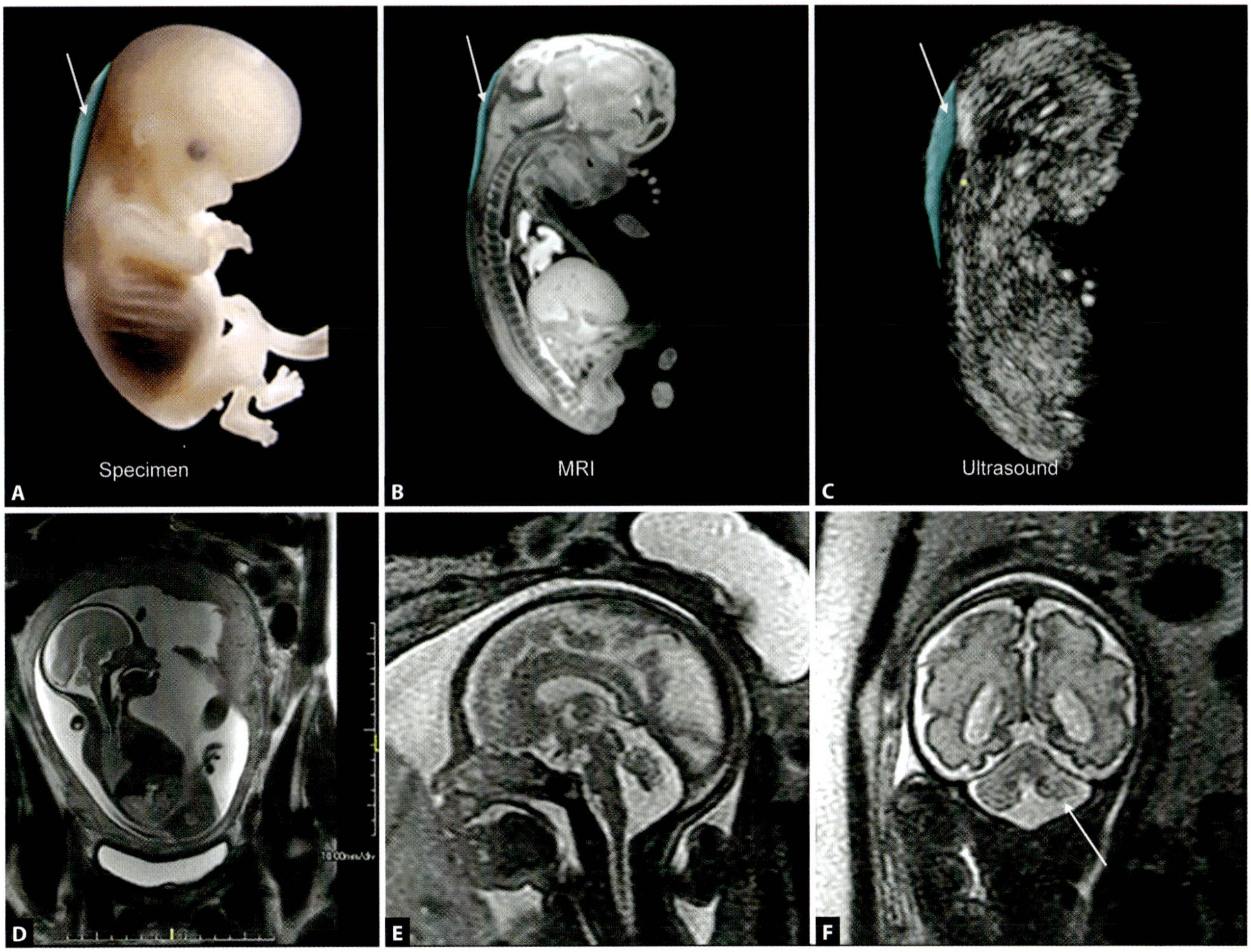

Figs 1.4A to F Fetal magnetic resonance imaging

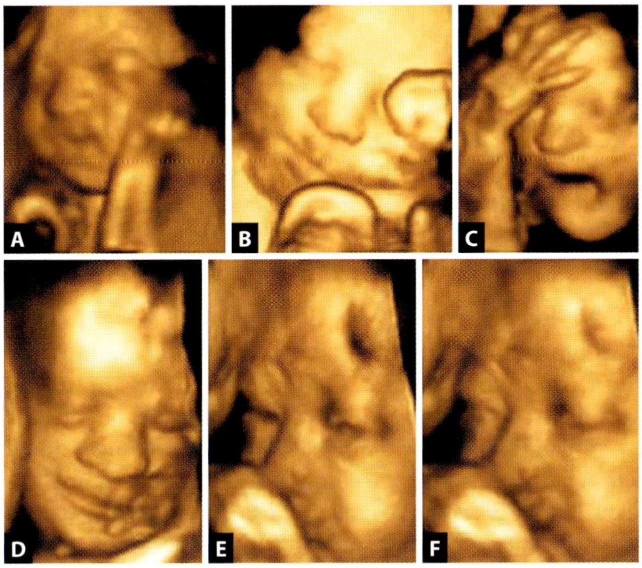

Figs 1.5A to F 3D/4D imaging and surface rendering of structure

Fetal Cells and DNA in Maternal Circulation

Noninvasive prenatal genetic diagnosis is an important area of research, as it would be preferable to invasive methods such as amniocentesis and CVS, which carry a small but definitive risk for fetal loss. Isolating fetal cells or free fetal DNA from maternal plasma is currently an exciting and promising area of research (Fig. 1.7). However, these techniques are extremely challenging. Many different protocols have been developed using one or more techniques, such as fluorescence-activated and magnetic-activated cell sorting, to recover fetal cells after separation from whole blood.[37] Practical applications for the clinician have not yet been developed. One of the main limiting factors seems to be the rarity of such cells in the maternal circulation. Enrichment techniques are needed help increase the yield. Estimates of the number of fetal cells in the maternal circulation vary depending on the gestational age and the technique used to obtain the cells.[2]

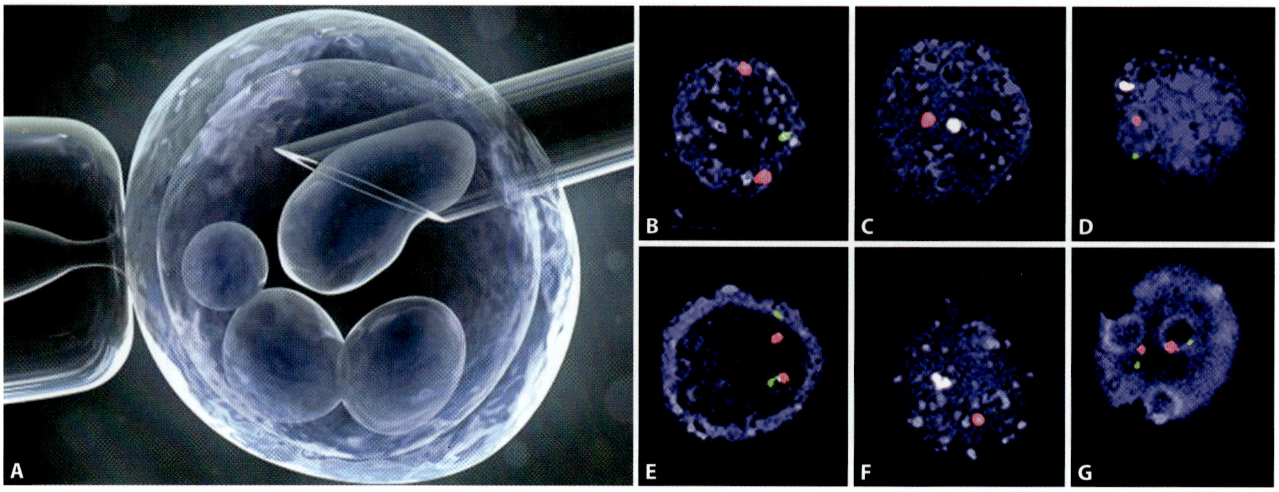

Figs 1.6A to G Biopsy for preimplantation genetic diagnosis and fluorescent *in situ* hybridization (FISH)

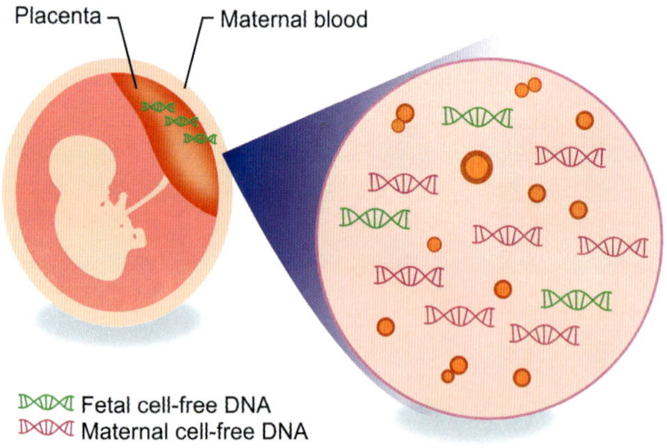

Fig. 1.7 DNA from maternal plasma

Current potential applications for analysis of fetal cells and of cell-free fetal DNA in maternal circulation include noninvasive detection of certain paternally inherited genetic traits and noninvasive detection of fetal Rhesus (Rh)D genotype in Rh(D)-sensitized patients. Noninvasive fetal genotyping would be useful for the management of Rh(D)-sensitized patients whose partners are heterozygous for the Rh(D) gene because no further diagnostic or therapeutic procedures would be necessary, if the fetus was confirmed Rh(D)-negative. In X-linked genetic disorders, in which half of the fetuses will be female and unaffected, fetal DNA determination of the fetal sex could reduce the number of invasive procedures required for the diagnosis of X-linked genetic disorders by 50%.[38] Additional clinical applications of fetal cells and fetal DNA in maternal circulation may include screening for aneuploidy, pre-eclampsia, or preterm labor.[39,40] These applications currently rely on the detection of Y-chromosomal sequences and are limited to male fetuses.[41] The above noninvasive diagnostic methods are not yet in clinical use but offer extremely exciting options for the future.[2,42]

Noninvasive Diagnosis of Fetal Anemia by Doppler Ultrasound

Previously, the diagnosis of fetal anemia required percutaneous umbilical blood sampling (PUBS), an invasive procedure with an inherent risk for fetal loss. Doppler measurements of the middle cerebral artery peak systolic velocity can now be used to noninvasively diagnose anemia in fetuses without hydrops who are at risk for anemia secondary to conditions such as Rh(D) sensitization and parvovirus B19 infection (Fig. 1.8).[43,44] This noninvasive method of detecting fetal anemia decreases the number of invasive PUBS procedures needed in these high-risk patients.

Normal Doppler of the middle cerebral artery peak systolic velocity at 18 weeks 3 days' gestation in a pregnancy.

The Use of Chromosomal Microarray Analysis in Prenatal Diagnosis

Chromosomal microarray analysis is a technique that identifies chromosomal abnormalities, including submicroscopic abnormalities that are too small to be detected by conventional karyotyping (Fig. 1.9). Like conventional fetal karyotyping, prenatal chromosomal microarray analysis requires direct testing of fetal tissue and thus can be offered only with chorionic villus sampling or amniocentesis.

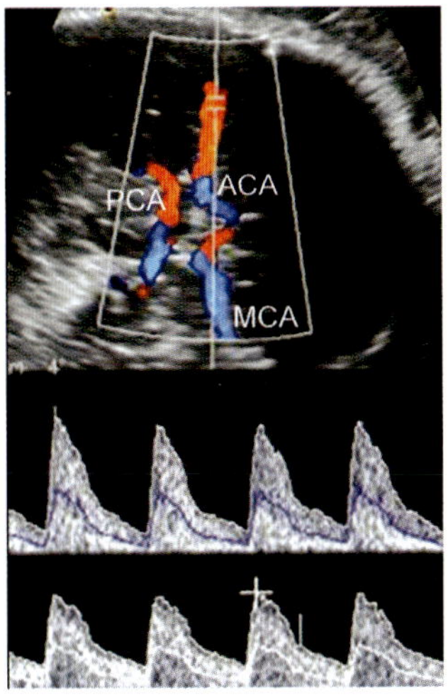

Fig. 1.8 MCA in Rh(D) sensitization
Abbreviations: PCA: posterior cerebral artery; ACA: anterior cerebral artery; MCA: middle cerebral artery

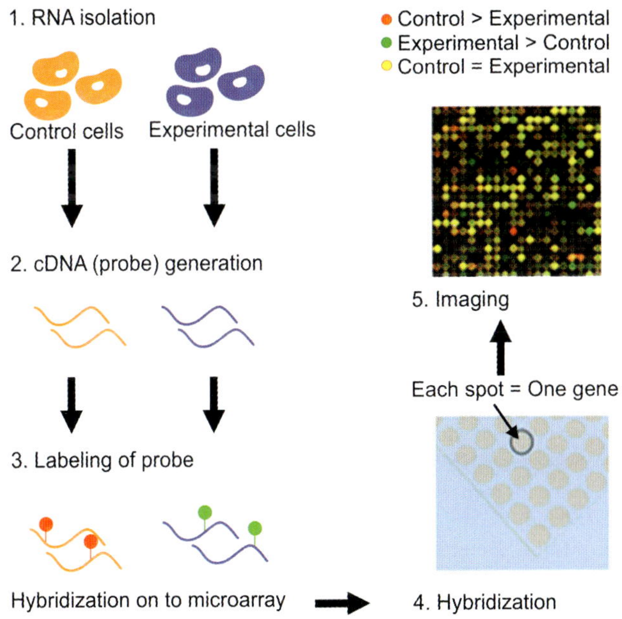

Fig. 1.9 Microarray for prenatal diagnosis

Prenatal chromosomal microarray analysis is most beneficial when ultrasonographic examination identifies fetal structural anomalies. The potential for complex results and detection of clinically uncertain findings identified by prenatal chromosomal microarray testing can result in substantial patient anxiety.

This underscores the critical need for comprehensive patient pretest and post-test genetic counseling from qualified personnel about the benefits, limitations, and results of testing so that patients can make informed decisions.

CONCLUSION

While there have been exciting advances in the field of prenatal diagnosis within the past few years, the future holds the promise of great breakthroughs. Advances in the areas of genomics, proteomics, and stem-cell research are anticipated.

It is expected that imaging modalities will continue to improve, and it is hoped that techniques used in the fields of noninvasive prenatal diagnosis and in preimplantation genetic diagnosis will continue to advance.

Accurate prenatal diagnosis of fetal abnormalities improves patient care by optimizing patient counseling and allowing for informed patient and physician decision making.

REFERENCES

1. Wald NJ, Densem JW, George L, et al. Prenatal screening for Down's syndrome using inhibin-A as a serum marker. Prenat Diagn. 1996;16:143-53.
2. Kumar S, O'Brien A. Recent developments in fetal medicine. BMJ. 2004;328:1002-6.
3. Cuckle H. Down's syndrome screening in twins. J Med Screen. 1998;5:3-4.
4. Malone FD, D'Alton ME, for the Society for Maternal Fetal Medicine. First trimester screening for Down syndrome. Obstet Gynecol. 2003;102:1066-79.
5. Wald NJ, Huttly WJ, Hackshaw AK. Antenatal screening for Down's syndrome with the quadruple test. Lancet. 2003;361:835-6.
6. Haddow JE, Palomaki GE, Knight GJ, et al. Prenatal screening for Down's syndrome with use of maternal serum markers. N Engl J Med. 1992;327:588-93.
7. ACOG Committee Opinion #296: First-trimester screening for fetal aneuploidy. Obstet Gynecol. 2004;104:215-7.
8. Malone FD, Berkowitz RL, Canick JA, D'Alton ME. First-trimester screening for aneuploidy: Research or standard of care? Am J Obstet Gynecol. 2000;182:490-6.
9. Nicolaides KH, Heath V, Cicero S. Increased fetal nuchal translucency at 11-14 weeks. Prenat Diagn. 2002;22:308-15.
10. Nicolaides KH. Nuchal translucency and other first trimester sonographic markers of chromosomal abnormalities. Am J Obstet Gynecol. 2004;191:45-67.
11. Snijders RJ, Thom EA, Zachary JM, et al. First trimester trisomy screening: Nuchal translucency measurement training and quality assurance to correct and unify technique. Ultrasound Obstet Gynecol. 2002;19:353-9.
12. Haddow JE, Palomaki GE, Knight GJ, et al. Screening of maternal serum for fetal Down's syndrome in the first trimester. N Engl J Med. 1998;338:955-61.
13. Welch KK, Malone FD. Nuchal translucency-based screening. ClinObstet Gynecol. 2003;46:909-22.
14. Malone FD, Ball RH, Nyberg DA, et al. First trimester cystic hygroma—Apopulation based screening study (the FASTER Trial). Am J Obstet Gynecol. 2001;185:S99.

15. Canick JA, Kellner LH. First trimester serum screening for aneuploidy: Serum biochemical markers. Semin Perinatol. 1999;23:359-68.
16. Malone FD, Wald NJ, Canick JA, et al. First- and second-trimester evaluation of risk (FASTER) trial: Principal results of the NICHD multicenter Down syndrome screening study. Am J Obstet Gynecol. 2003;189(6 suppl):S56.
17. Cicero S, Curcio P, Papageorghiou A, et al. Absence of nasal bone in fetuses with trisomy 21 at 11-14 weeks of gestation: An observational study. Lancet. 2001;358:1665-7.
18. Malone FD, Ball RH, Nyberg DA, et al. First-trimester nasal bone evaluation for aneuploidy in the general population. Obstet Gynecol. 2004;104:1222-8.
19. Bilardo CM, Muller MA, Zikulnig L, et al. Ductusvenosus studies in fetuses at high risk for chromosomal or heart abnormalities: Relationship with nuchal translucency measurement and fetal outcome. Ultrasound Obstet Gynecol. 2001;17:288-94.
20. Antolin E, Comas C, Torrents M, et al. The role of ductus venosus blood flow assessment in screening for chromosomal abnormalities at 10-16 weeks of gestation. Ultrasound Obstet Gynecol. 2001;17:295-300.
21. Matias A, Gomes C, Flack N, et al. Screening for chromosomal abnormalities at 10-14 weeks: The role of ductusvenosus blood flow. Ultrasound Obstet Gynecol. 1998;12:380-4.
22. Mavrides E, Sairam S, Hollis B, et al. Screening for aneuploidy in the first trimester by assessment of blood flow in the ductusvenosus. Br J Obstet Gynaecol. 2002;109:1015-9.
23. Murta CG, Moron AF, Avila MA, Weiner CP. Application of ductusvenosus Doppler velocimetry for the detection of fetal aneuploidy in the first trimester of pregnancy. Fetal Diagn Ther. 2002;17:308-14.
24. Zoppi MA, Putzolu M, Ibba RM, et al. First-trimester ductus venosus velocimetry in relation to nuchal translucency thickness and fetal karyotype. Fetal Diagn Ther. 2002;17:52-57.
25. Nyberg DA, Souter VL, El-Bastawissi A, et al. Isolated sonographic markers for detection of fetal Down syndrome in the second trimester of pregnancy. J Ultrasound Med. 2001;20:1053-63.
26. Filly RA, Benacerraf BR, Nyberg DA, Hobbins JC. Choroid plexus cyst and echogenic intracardiac focus in women at low risk for chromosomal anomalies. J Ultrasound Med. 2004;23:447-9.
27. Bromley B, Lieberman E, Shipp TD, Benacerraf BR. The genetic sonogram: A method of risk assessment for Down syndrome in the second trimester. J Ultrasound Med. 2002;21:1087-96.
28. Wald NJ, Rodeck C, Hackshaw AK, et al. First and second trimester antenatal screening for Down's syndrome: The results of the Serum, Urine, and Ultrasound Screening Study (SURUSS). Health Technol Assess. 2003;7(11):1-77.
29. Wald NJ, Watt HC, Hackshaw AK. Integrated screening for Down's syndrome on the basis of tests performed during the first and second trimesters. N Engl J Med. 1999;341:461-7.
30. Coakley FV, Glenn OA, Qayyum A, et al. Fetal MRI. A developing technique for the developing patient. AJR Am J Roentgenol. 2004;182:243-52.
31. Garel C, Brisse H, Sebag G, et al. Magnetic resonance imaging of the fetus. Pediatr Radiol. 1998;28:201-11.
32. Smith FW, Adam AH, Phillips WD. NMR imaging in pregnancy. Lancet. 1983;1:61-62.
33. Kiefer B, Grassner J, Hausman R. Image acquisition in a second with half Fourier acquisition single-shot turbo spin-echo. J MagnReson Imaging. 1994;4(P):86-87.
34. Levine D. Magnetic resonance imaging in prenatal diagnosis. CurrOpin Pediatr. 2001;13:572-8.
35. Sermon K, Van Steirteghem A, Liebaers I. Preimplantation genetic diagnosis. Lancet. 2004;363:1633-41.
36. Sampson JE, Ouhibi N, Lawce H, et al. The role for pre-implantation genetic diagnosis in balanced translocation carriers. Am J Obstet Gynecol. 2004;190:1707-11.
37. Bischoff FZ, Hahn S, Johnson KL. Intact fetal cells in maternal plasma: Are they really there? Lancet. 2003;361:139-40.
38. Jackson L. Fetal cells and DNA in maternal blood. Prenat Diagn. 2003; 23:837-46.
39. Farina A, LeShane ES, Lambert-Messerlian GM, et al. Evaluation of cell-free fetal DNA as a second- trimester maternal serum marker of Down syndrome pregnancy. Clin Chem. 2003;49:239-42.
40. Wataganara T, LeShane ES, Farina A, et al. Maternal serum cell-free fetal DNA levels are increased in cases of trisomy 13 but not trisomy 18. Hum Genet. 2003;112:204-8.
41. Pertl B, Bianchi DW. Fetal DNA in maternal plasma: Emerging clinical applications. Obstet Gynecol. 2001;98:483-90.
42. Bianchi DW, Simpson JL, Jackson LG, et al. Fetal gender and aneuploidy detection using fetal cells in maternal blood: Analysis of NIFTY I data. National Institute of Child Health and Development Fetal Cell Isolation Study. Prenat Diagn. 2002;22: 609-15.
43. Mari G, Deter RL, Carpenter RL, et al. Noninvasive diagnosis by Doppler ultrasonography of fetal anemia due to maternal red-cell alloimmunization. Collaborative Group for Doppler Assessment of the Blood Velocity in Anemic Fetuses. N Engl J Med. 2000;342:9-14.
44. Cosmi E, Mari G, DelleChiaie L, et al. Noninvasive diagnosis by Doppler ultrasonography of fetal anemia resulting from parvovirus infection. Am J Obstet Gynecol.2002;187:1290-3.

CHAPTER

2 Multidisciplinary Approach for Prenatal Screening and Diagnosis

Apoorva Pallam Reddy, Narendra Malhotra, Jaideep Malhotra

INTRODUCTION

The exhilaration at the thought of being a mother is more often than not plagued by the worries of the well being and normalcy of the fetus. "Is my baby doing alright?" is the most common question fired at any obstetrician. In spite of the extensive line up of investigations available, there are always asterisk (*) signs saying that 'all risks cannot be ruled out'.

Apart from the most frequently occurring fetal aneuploidies like trisomies 21, 18, and 13 there are many more structural defects that can be detected by prenatal screening. Various congenital cardiac anomalies, abnormalities of the chest and gastrointestinal tract, urinary tract abnormalities, anomalies of the central nervous system, externally visible body defects and skeletal abnormalities can be detected by antenatal ultrasonography.

The diagnosis of these anomalies is essential not only to detect the fetuses that are not viable but more importantly identify the ones that need extra support for viability. Under such circumstances having a multidisciplinary approach that involves adequate counseling and active involvement of the parents in their baby's care is the only way forward.

In this chapter, we discuss about all the members that need to come together to form an ideal prenatal management team and regarding their role in improving the fetal outcome. (Flow chart 2.1).

PRENATAL SCREENING COUNSELOR

Prenatal screening should not be considered as yet another routine antenatal investigation, added to the pre-existing long list of tests, as the results can potentially change the course of pregnancy. It is important for health care professionals to both ***offer*** the screening tests available and ***discuss*** their implicatiosn with all pregnant women. Information pamphlets, in their native language, can also be helpful in explaining the purpose and limitations of the tests. The decision for screening is entirely voluntary and should be documented.

Tips for Prescreening Counseling[1]

- Counsel your patient that all pregnant women have some risk of having a fetus affected by trisomy 21, 18, or 13 or other structural defects.
- Explain that prenatal screening will use specific maternal and pregnancy factors (e.g. age, ethnicity) to assess her individual risk of having an affected fetus with maternal age being an important effector for risk.
- Emphasize that a positive screen will mean that her risk is above a predetermined cutoff (set by regional programs), not that her fetus is necessarily affected. Distinguish clearly between a screening test and a diagnostic test.

Flow chart 2.1 Essential members of the multidisciplinary team for prenatal screening and management

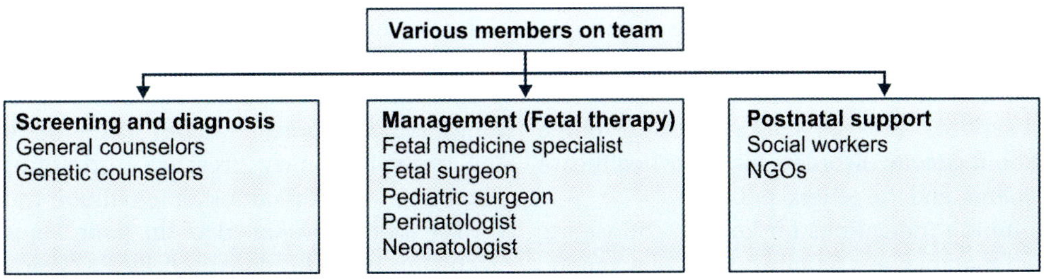

- Give simple examples while explaining the specific and personalized risk. For example, a risk of 1:100 means that for one woman carrying an affected fetus, there are 99 women carrying a fetus that is not affected.
- Discuss options and the invasive prenatal testing that may need to be considered after screening.
- *Screen negative:* Explain that if screening is negative, no further testing is indicated other than routine second trimester ultrasound screening but does not guarantee the birth of a healthy baby.
- *Screen positive:* Inform your patient that if the screening test is positive she is eligible for diagnostic testing.
- *Diagnostic testing:* Ensure your patient is aware that diagnostic testing is entirely voluntary. This testing would be done by amniocentesis in 2nd trimester or late 1st trimester, which carries a procedural risk of 1/100 to 1/175 for loss of the pregnancy or by chorionic villus sampling, in early 1st trimester which carries a procedural risk of 1/100 for loss of the pregnancy.
- *Decide for or against termination:* Ensure your patient knows that she has the option of continuing or terminating the pregnancy, if the test shows that her fetus has an aneuploidy or another significant chromosomal anomaly. It is a common misconception that screening is offered only to patients who would terminate a pregnancy if an anomaly were found. It is important to tell patients who may choose to continue the pregnancy that their fetus will be given the best care possible.
- In the case of chromosomal anomalies that have an extremely poor prognosis, this may include referring the patient to a neonatologist to discuss palliative.

GENETIC COUNSELORS[2]

Genetic counselors work as part of a healthcare team, providing information and support to families affected by or at risk of a genetic disorder. They help to identify families at possible risk of a genetic disorder, gather and analyze family history and inheritance patterns, calculate risks of recurrence, and provide information about genetic testing and related procedures.

Genetic counselors also provide supportive counseling services, serve as patient advocates, and refer individuals and families to other health professionals and community or state support services. They serve as a central resource of information about genetic disorders for other healthcare professionals, patients, and the general public.

The most common indications for genetic counseling include advanced maternal age, family history of a genetic condition, and suspected diagnosis of a genetic condition.

The post-test session involves more than the provision of medical information and often focuses on helping families cope with the emotional, psychological, medical, social, and economic consequences of the test results. In particular, psychological issues such as denial, anxiety, anger, grief, guilt, or blame are addressed and, when necessary, referrals for in-depth counseling are offered. Information about community resources and support groups are provided to the patient/family.

If the genetic test is positive, testing should be considered in additional relatives of this individual.

At the conclusion of the genetic counseling sessions, the patient should be offered a written summary of the major topics discussed. The summary is often provided in the form of a letter which serves as a permanent record of the relevant information discussed, as well as relaying additional information that may have become available after the final counseling session.

Fetal Therapy

Fetal therapy was introduced as early as 1952 by Brevis as amniocentesis for management of rhesus isoimmunization and is currently a very well-established field.

Definition

A therapeutic intervention for the purpose of correcting or treating a fetal anomaly or condition. In almost every case, the fetus is at risk of intrauterine death from the abnormality. Advances in fetal therapy have enabled us to prevent and treat potentially life-threatening conditions and improve outcome.

FETAL MEDICINE PHYSICIAN

Fetal medicine specialists use ultrasound, blood tests, and procedures such as fetoscopy to evaluate the developing fetus.

They perform diagnostic procedures like chorionic villous sampling, amniocentesis and fetal blood sampling as well as therapeutic interventions like laser ablation of AV anastomosis in twin to twin transfusion syndrome, twin reversed arterial perfusion syndrome or selective fetal reduction of the anomalous twin.

Tracheal occlusion in fetuses with congenital diaphragmatic hernia, aims at blocking the outlet of the lung-fluid, which accumulates within the lungs increasing the transpulmonary pressure, promoting lung growth. Percutaneous fetal endoscopic balloon tracheal occlusion (FETO) is being evaluated for the same. Fetuses with tracheal occlusion must be delivered by EXIT procedure (partial delivery of the fetus, removal of the tracheal occlusion, administration of surfactant and institution of assisted ventilation while the infant is still on placental support).

In very severe cases of erythroblastosis fetalis fetal intrauterine transfusion can be performed to treat the hemolytic anemia. A pediatric hematologist can be involved in decision making.

FETAL SURGEON[3]

Rare fetal tumors like congenital cystic adenomatoid malformation of the lung (CCAM) and sacrococcygeal teratoma (SCT) cause almost 100% fetal mortality when associated with hydrops fetalis. These tumors cause hydrops by either venous obstruction due to mediastinal shift (CCAM) or high output heart failure (SCT). Operative removal of these tumors has resulted in survival of ~50% of the affected fetuses.

Intrauterine repair of myelomeningocele decreases the incidence of hindbrain herniation and shunt-dependent hydrocephalus in infants with spina bifida, but increases the incidence of premature delivery [Management of Myelomeningocele Study (MOMS)].

Aspiration of fetal ovarian cysts larger than 30 mm to prevent torsion and avoid neonatal surgery is being evaluated in France.

PEDIATRIC SURGEON

- *Diaphragmatic hernia:* The outlook for babies born with CDH is increasingly positive with new surgical techniques and ways to support babies as they heal. Surgery is performed after delivery as soon as the lungs can maintain good blood flow through the vessels prior to the operation.
- *Duodenal atresia:* Duodenal atresia is often characterized by a "double bubble" on prenatal ultrasound. One bubble represents air in the stomach and the other bubble represents the first part of the duodenum, with no air past that. Surgery is required to treat duodenal atresia, usually within the first few days of life.
- *Esophageal atresia:* VACTERL association because of the possible involvement of vertebral column, anorectal, cardiac, tracheal, esophageal, renal (kidney), and limbs require early management of neonate for better prognosis.
- Management of nonfatal cosmetic conditions like cleft lip, cleft palate, congenital tallipes should be discussed clearly as soon as the diagnosis is made.

PERINATOLOGIST AND NEONATOLOGIST

In cases where antenatal screening has not been done or has not picked an anomaly, pediatricians often face the responsibility of revealing the diagnosis to the parents and dealing with the emotional overture. They also have to deal with complications in the neonatal period (IUGR, congenital anomalies) and various comorbidities (hypothyroidism, recurrent otitis media, atlantoaxial instability, transient myeloproliferative disorders). The perinatologist should be involved in the decision making of mode of delivery for anomalous fetuses along with the couple.

SOCIAL WORKERS AND SUPPORT GROUPS[4]

Despite the best efforts and elaborate investigations 1 in 1000 live births result in a Downs baby. For a couple waiting to hold their newborn close, the idea of an 'abnormal' fetus is always shattering. Lack of knowledge on the routine management and anticipated medical problems only compounds the emotional turmoil. Thankfully there are a lot of Down's syndrome support groups both nationally and internationally helping many Downs babies lead a life as close to normalcy as possible. A case report of a 25-years-old married Downs lady delivering a healthy term baby only emphasizes the importance of familial and social support.

NONVIABLE TO VIABLE: YES WE CAN!!

Since 2012, donation possibilities for babies, specifically babies with anencephaly, have expanded and currently there are more potential for donation than ever before. Although each particular case is unique, and each potential donation has various criteria that must be met, donation is a very viable option for a baby with anencephaly, if families wish to pursue this option. Donation can be used either for transplant or research.

The recent story of Teddy, the anencephalic twin, donating kidney and heart valves to an adult suffering from renal failure is no less than a heroic act.

Currently, India does not have any legislation over organ donation in anencephalus fetuses. With an extremely poor national organ donation rate of 0.26 per million population, it is indeed essential to tap into the possibility of organ donation from anomalous fetuses.

Where Do You, As An Obstetrician, Stand in All This?

Just like the conductor of a symphony orchestra unifies the performers and executes clear preparations to shape the sound of the ensemble, the obstetrician plays the key role of coordinating all the events in prenatal screening, diagnosis and management and bringing out the entire team as one unit.

CONCLUSION

A multidisciplinary yet integrated approach for prenatal screening and diagnosis with expert counseling and close follow-up after delivery for appropriate medical support not only improves the chance of healthy viable fetus but also decreases the anxiety levels for the parents.

REFERENCES

1. Lola Cartier, et al. SOGC Committee Opinion Counseling Considerations for Prenatal Genetic Screening, 2012(277).
2. Understanding Genetics: A District of Columbia Guide for Patients and Health Professionals.
3. Joseph P Bruner, et al. Fetal surgery for myelomeningocele and the incidence of shunt-dependent hydrocephalus. The Journal of American Medical Association, 1999.
4. Kaushal M, Baxi A, Kadi P, et al. Woman with Down syndrome delivered a normal child. IJIFM. 2010;1(1):45-7.

CHAPTER

3 Goals and Issues in the Delivery of Genetic Services in India

Hema Purandarey

The Indian subcontinent comprises of four countries—India, Pakistan, Sri Lanka, and Bangladesh.[1] Of which, inhabited by over 1 billion people, *India* is a vast landmass with rich and varied heritage. It is a land of diverse social, religious and cultural practice. With considerable improvement in infection control and malnutrition, genetic disorders have now become more apparent.

Any deviation from normal physical and/or mental development is broadly classified into various categories.

The following terminology is used in medical genetics to understand the internal differences:

Birth defects: Any type of functional or structural abnormality determined largely by factors operating before birth, *in utero* or in the immediate postnatal period.[2]

Congenital malformations: These are structural abnormalities present at birth and may or may not have a genetic component.[2]

Genetic disorders: These are conditions in which a defect lies in the DNA and plays a major role in causation of pathological conditions. They can be inherited or sporadic.[2] Some conditions are of late onset, but once detected in the index case, it can be diagnosed *in utero* as early as 10 weeks.

Genetic disorders are classified as:

- *Chromosomal abnormalities:* A human cell contains 23 pairs of chromosomes. 22 pairs of autosomes and 1 pair of sex chromosomes - XX in females and XY in males. Any alteration in the number or structure of chromosomes can lead to chromosomal abnormalities.[2] They are mainly caused by random errors of cell division in gamete formation or are sporadic and can be transferred to the next generation.
- *Single gene disorders:* They are caused by mutations in a single major gene. The clinical manifestations are variable depending on the function of the normal gene. These are inherited as dominant, recessive, autosomal or X-linked inheritance.[2]
- *Multifactorial conditions:* These are caused due to interaction of several genes and/or environmental factors.[2]
- *Environmentally influenced conditions:* These are birth defects caused due to interference of the environmental factors with normal embryogenic or fetal development. These include physical agents, chemicals and infections.[2]

PREVALENCE OF GENETIC DISORDERS, BIRTH DEFECTS AND CONGENITAL MALFORMATIONS

The prevalence of birth defects, congenital malformations and genetic defects in India[3] majorly appears to be due to the practice of consanguineous marriages in certain communities, large population, and occurrence of different genetic disorders in different communities due to the multicultural population (Table 3.1).

Frequency of birth and genetic defects in a developing country like ours is often underestimated due to lack of availability of diagnostic capacities, unreliable health records, statistics and management. The rate of morbidity and mortality perinatally due genetic and birth defects is steadily on a rise.

Table 3.1 Prevalence of genetic disease at birth in India[4]

Disorder	Incidence	Estimated cases/year
Congenital malformations	1 in 50	495,096
G6PD deficiency	1:35 to 1:10 (M)	390,000
Down syndrome	1:1139	21,412
β-thalassemia	1:2700	9,000
Sickle cell disease	1:1200	5,200
Amino acid disorders	1: 2347	9,760
Other metabolic disease	1:2500	9,000
Duchenne muscular dystrophy	1: 5000 (M)	2,510
Spinal muscular atrophy	1:10,000	2,510

Table 3.2 Prevalence of common malformations in India (Verma et al. 1998)[5]

Malformations	Cases per 10,000	Estimated births
Neural tube defects	36.3	88,532
Talipes	14.5	35,364
Polydactyly	11.6	28,364
Hydrocephalus	9.5	23,169
Cleft lip end/or palate	9.3	22,681
Congenital heart disease	7.1	17,316
Hypospadias	5.0	12,194
Tracheoesophageal fistula	3.7	9,023
Diaphragmatic hernia	2.6	6,341
Anorectal atresia/stenosis	2.4	5,853
Microcephaly	2.2	5,365
Cleft palate alone	1.7	4,146
Intersex and cryptorchidism	1.6	3,902
Intestinal atresia/stenosis	1.2	2,926
Anophthalmia/ microphthalmia	1.0	2,438

Global prevalence of birth defects, genetic disorders and congenital malformations in India are similar to that of the developed countries with a few regional differences (Table 3.2).

Globally, about 7.9 million children are born annually with a serious genetic disorders, birth defects and congenital malformations which accounts for 6% of the total births.

At least 3.3 million children under 5 years die from birth defects every year and 3.2 million of those who survive may be disabled for life.

7.9 per 1000 infants have *cardiovascular defects*, 4.7 have *neural tube defects* and 1.2 have some form of *hemoglobinopathy*, 1.6 have *Down's syndrome* and 2.4 have *G6PD deficiency*.

India accounts as one of the highest shares of birth defects in the world. There are about 1.7 million babies born with birth defects annually.

In the study conducted by National Neonatology Forum, congenital malformations were the second most common cause (9.9%) of mortality among stillbirths and the fourth most common cause (9.6%) of neonatal mortality and that accounted for 4% of under five mortality.[2]

Congenital hypothyroidism: 1 in 1000 livebirths.

1 in 1000 was reported for *Down's syndrome* in India.

Failure of specific and timely intervention can cause irreversible life-long mental, physical, auditory or visual disability.

SOME GOALS AND STRATEGIES NEED TO BE FORMULATED IN ORDER TO REDUCE THE PREVALENCE

In genetics, healthcare is offered at three levels:

Primary Healthcare Level

It is the backbone of all genetic services. Programs employing low technology and reach a large population must be incorporated. Some actions at the primary healthcare level are:[2]

- Public education and awareness in genetics
- Carrier and genetic risk detection in the community for its prevalence by appropriate genetic techniques.
- Prenatal screening for maternal biochemical markers for prevalent genetic risks
- Genetic counseling
- Rubella immunization
- Prevention of fetal alcohol effects
- Encouragement of reproduction at optimal maternal ages
- Prenatal screening for maternal biochemical markers for Down syndrome risk.

The sites for provision of primary healthcare services in medical genetics are community health centers, clinics and hospitals, medical professionals and schools. The primary healthcare service providers are medical practitioners with task-oriented basic training in applied genetics.[2]

Secondary Healthcare Level

It is based in medium sized hospitals with medical specialists and better technology like a general clinical laboratory, radiology and ultrasound facilities.

It deals with genetic problems of intermediate complexity that cannot be solved at primary healthcare level. They mainly deal with confirmation of suspected diagnosis, follow-up of initial screening tests, management of specific conditions and genetic counseling, done by professionals trained in applied genetics and genetic counseling. Fetal ultrasound and prenatal diagnostic procedures are performed in this level.[2]

Tertiary Healthcare Level

It is the best available care for genetic disorders and birth defects. It rendered in a medical genetics center located in a university hospital and tertiary health center in a major city. It is mostly concentrated on diagnostic services, provision of complex counseling and care to patients suffering from severe genetic disorders and their families. They are also involved in development of research and training programs in the field.[2]

The delivery of genetic services must be organized at all levels of care for the complete advantage of the existing resources to maximize their efficiency.

Genetic services deal with genetic disorders, birth defects and congenital malformations. The major goals of genetic services are prevention, management and treatment of birth defects caused due to genetic factors.

Prenatal genetic diagnosis is an important service to be offered. The goal is to provide information about the fetus' status to parents at risk for a specific genetic condition in the fetus and also alternate reproductive options available. Maternal genetic diseases are also taken into account while testing.

When targeted to families, the goal of the genetic services is to help people with a genetic disadvantage to live and reproduce as healthily as possible.

Another goal of genetic testing in targeted population, is that they acquire a public health goal to reduce the burden of genetic defects on the population.

A healthy progeny needs a healthy conception safeguarding the fetal health.

These services are provided by trained clinical geneticists with a certified genetic counselor. Access to pathology, radiology, ultrasound, oncology, neurology, ophthalmology must be provided. The medical geneticist should be trained to treat selected conditions.

HEALTHCARE SYSTEMS IN INDIA WITH RESPECT TO GENETIC SERVICES

Different healthcare systems are adopted by individual states. Public health sectors and hospitals are funded by the state government. The central government formulates comprehensive health policies and plans under Ministry of Health and Family Welfare. The central government funds many healthcare projects like National Rural Health Mission, control programs for cancer, iodine deficiency disorders, etc.[5] Medical education and medical profession have a shared responsibility of the central and state government.

There is a two-tier healthcare system present in India – difficult cases are transferred to urban hospitals and routine medical healthcare is provided in rural areas. There has been established a network of village healthcare centers, subcenters, primary centers, community health centers, district hospitals and medical colleges;[5] but genetic healthcare is often put on an backburner in these centers, which leads to missing out on diagnosis of manageable genetic disorders. Moreover, inadequacy of trained staff and facilities leads to further lag in the implantation of the schemes.

Challenge for India is providing healthcare to a vast rural, urban and urban poor population.[5] The rural population has limited access to medical facilities. In urban areas, healthcare services are obtained from the best institutions only to the part of population which can pay for it.[5] The urban poor cannot avail such health facilities for prevention and care of children with birth defects. Even in health insurance, genetic disorders are not usually covered.

Diagnosis and management of genetic disorders, congenital malformations and birth defects is possible in urban settings, but since majority of the Indian population lives in rural and remote areas with poor access to healthcare infrastructure, efforts need to be made to help the diagnostic and management facilities to reach them.

The National Rural Health Mission (NRHM) helps in improvement of availability and access to quality healthcare to people from rural areas and also from low income backgrounds.[5]

In 2013, the Maharashtra government under the guidance of NRMH established the Rashtriya Bal Swasthya Karyakram for provision of adequate and quality genetic healthcare services to the rural population. Under this scheme 30 different and highly prevalent genetic disorders, congenital malformations and birth defects are covered for identification by screening, free treatment and management.

Center for Genetic Healthcare (CGHC) has taken a step for provision of genetics services for awareness, diagnosis and management, in the interiors of Maharashtra like Sindhudurg by identifying prevalent disorders and organizing various camps for spreading awareness in association with District civil hospitals, collectors with the help of medical fraternity of Sindhudurg.

A lot of support groups have been set up in India which are working zealously nationwide, operating with doctors, drug companies, laboratories and other NGOs to create awareness of genetic disorders, organize counseling services and centers for diagnosis and treatment. They also support people from low income groups to gain access to the best available healthcare facilities.

COMPONENTS OF GENETIC SERVICE

Genetic services have following integral components: Carrier screening, facilities for genetic counseling and facilities for sound diagnosis and establishment of laboratories for confirmation of the diagnosis. These need to be developed as a composite unit for effective genetic services. Specialized laboratories are needed for genetic diagnosis, which should be centralized to ensure minimum workload, quality monitoring and cost effectiveness. The biggest challenge is the establishment of laboratories for molecular genetics, cytogenetics, biochemical genetics and immunogenetics for analysis of parent as well as fetal samples.

With very few centers undertaking such kind of testing, it is grossly inadequate for a population of 1.15 billion and therefore better means to give access to majority of the people is of utmost importance.[5]

This challenge can however be overcome by an urban-rural partnership set up. Genetic samples are resistant to environmental and transportation damage, hence a system to collect the samples can be developed in the rural areas and then those samples can be transported to the cities with genetic testing infrastructures for confirmation of diagnosis and testing.

Making genetic counseling a part of preventive services is an urgent need as it helps educate patients about their risks, which in turn helps them to plan an appropriate test regarding tissue and timing. On the basis of the results obtained, post-test counseling will help them make informed choices. Unfortunately in India, there are very few diagnostic centers and fewer counselors and thus education of healthcare professionals, health authorities and public on genetic risks is one of the most essential components of genetic services.

Screening and Diagnostic Programs

There are different screening and diagnostic tests available for various genetic disorders worldwide and in India (Table 3.3).

The major types are:

Newborn Screening

Out of 25 million babies born annually in India, every 1 in 2000 newborns suffers from a metabolic disorder. It differs from community to ethnicity to location. But, currently there is no universal newborn screening program in India. It is done in some private hospitals with their own screening policies. The issue with such unstructured screening program is that many newborns with treatable or manageable disorders are missed. There is a dearth of standardized laboratory services, absence of quality control and improper surveillance. But now steps are being taken to hold nationwide mass screening programs, with a hope for creating better infrastructure for the screening.

Carrier Screening

It is part of population screening. It is done to test the prevalence of a specific disorder in a particular region or community.

In India, thalassemia is one of the most prevalent genetic disorders with several different mutations. Now techniques have developed to see the common mutations for thalassemia for its control and prevention, with a long time vision of a thalassemia-free India.

Table 3.3 Identified health conditions for child health screening and early intervention services[3]

Defects at birth	Deficiencies
• Neural tube defect • Down's syndrome • Cleft lip and palate/cleft palate alone • Talipes (club foot) • Developmental dysplasia of die hip • Congenital cataract • Congenital deafness • Congenital heart diseases • Retinopathy of prematurity	• Anemia especially severe anemia • Vitamin A deficiency (Bitot spots) • Vitamin D deficiency (rickets) • Severe acute malnutrition • Goiter
Childhood diseases	**Developmental delays and disabilities**
• Skin conditions (scabies, fungal infection and eczema) • Otitis media • Rheumatic heart disease • Reactive airway disease • Dental caries • Convulsive disorders	• Vision impairment • Hearing impairment • Neuromotor impairment • Motor delay • Cognitive delay • Language delay • Behavior disorder (autism) • Learning disorder • Attention deficit hyperactivity disorder • Congenital hypothyroidism. Sickle cell anemia, beta-thalassemia (optional)

Prenatal Screening

Using ultrasound: It is the most basic form of screening available today even accessible to the remotest areas. It is the first point contact in screening for any fetal wellbeing. It can be used for screening as early as 11–13.6 weeks and 18 weeks for fetal growth, development and anomalies.

Maternal serum screening: It is now a common investigation offered to all pregnant women to pick up at risk cases for chromosomal aneuploidies.

In case of high-risk cases, confirmatory diagnostic tests like chorion villus sampling and amniocentesis can be offered.

The diagnostic tests are offered to women who are at increased risk for genetic disorders in the fetus due to positive screening tests, previously affected child, family history and personal medical history and bad obstetric history.

The tests are offered after giving them complete information about the disorder in question for diagnosis by way of pre-test counseling prognosis and management.

The obstetric procedures involved in fetal screening are:

Chorion villus sampling—11-13.6 weeks, amniocentesis - 15-17 weeks.

Laboratory tests are based on the type of disorder namely chromosomal, molecular or biochemical.

Informed written consent is necessary in all the cases. In India, prenatal diagnostic testing is governed under Pre-Conception and Pre-Natal Diagnostic Techniques Act, 1994 (PCPNDT)

Evaluating the affecting: Many genetic disorders can only be diagnosed after evaluating the affected child or the affected family member.

Accreditations

Accreditation of laboratories is not mandatory in India. There is however a voluntary accreditation program available.[5] An autonomous body - National Accreditation Board for Testing and Calibration Laboratories (NABL) is a sole government-authorized accreditation body in India. Accreditation should be made mandatory to ensure proper quality control in the services offered especially in prenatal diagnosis. It is always important to get tested at accredited laboratories as results of prenatal diagnosis are irreversible and any error can lead to wrongful birth and wrongful life.

Birth Defects Registry: The Need

In India so far, there is no uniform method for surveillance and recording of birth defects. Therefore incidence of genetic defects could be much higher than quoted. Steps have been taken to create national database of prevalence of different genetic defects and malformations in the Indian population. Not only the birth records, but also establishment of this database is recording of the number of pregnancies terminated owing to a malformed fetus, is important. Steps need to be taken to account for the causes of those malformations to get an accurate data for identifying pockets of specific disorders and launching preventive and management programs and research.

Training

Compared to developed countries, even today, the teaching of genetics in medical colleges is inadequate in India. This leads to lack of understanding and sensitivity among the medical practitioners about genetic disorders and their management. There is a pressing need for improvement in teaching the importance of genetics starting from school level extending up to medical colleges.

Since the last decade, a few medical schools in India have started taking courses in clinical genetics for medical students as well as physicians and allied health personnel. Courses and workshops have also been organized to train medical and other health professionals in medical genetics.

In India, ISPAT (Indian Society of Prenatal Diagnosis and Therapy) is one such pioneer institution dedicated to prenatal services, which is involved in spreading awareness, organizing training programs and workshops in medical genetics to sensitize the healthcare professionals, obstetricians and others involved in prenatal healthcare, towards birth defects, congenital malformations and genetic disorders.

Opportunities in genetics are not only limited to medical fields but also present in the fields of Agriculture and wildlife management, Computational biology (Bioinformatics), Law and Justice, Business and Engineering, Bioscience communication, History and anthropology, Space exploration.

More people should be made aware about the plethora of opportunities present in the field in India.

Public-Private Partnerships

Though large and widespread, the current health infrastructure present in India cannot cope with meeting newer health challenges especially in the area of genetics. Public sector hospitals have insufficient funds to be updated with technological advancements. Private sector is now growing rapidly and many genetic healthcare centers have been established, with expensive technologically updated equipment and expertise. Public-Private Partnerships is the perfect solution for lack of infrastructure, resources faced by the public sector.

The CGHC is also participating by offering genetic services at lower cost to municipal and government hospitals. It allows undiscriminated utilization of expertise and services available.

Center for Genetic Healthcare

In the view of the gravity of need of genetic services, Center for Genetic Healthcare was established in 1981 to provide genetic diagnostic facilities in the country. The center has a team of dedicated experts from fields of obstetrics, sonology, fetal medicine, pediatrics. Not only are the services provided in Mumbai, Maharashtra, but samples are also received from all over the country and especially from the rural areas of Maharashtra for genetic testing, prenatal diagnosis. Genetic counseling is also sought for the center has been accredited by NABL and CAP (College of American Pathology), to ensure optimum standards in quality.

Individuals with genetic disorders are guided for prognosis, significance of the disorder, recurrence risk for progeny, prevention, alternate reproductive options and prenatal diagnosis for improved outcome.

Prenatal diagnosis is an important component of genetic services and also forms a large part of cases seen at the center. Major indications for the test and genetic counseling were advanced maternal age, maternal serum markers, abnormal ultrasound findings, single gene disorders, repeated pregnancy wastage and family history. Chromosomal abnormalities and variants were found in approximately 6% of the cases.

Various camps were held for awareness, screening, diagnosis and management of genetic disorders like club foot, congenital heart disease across Maharashtra and also make genetic services accessible to them.[6]

CONCLUSION

Though genetic disorders are individually rare, collectively they are a burden on the population.

The observed birth prevalence of genetic disorders and birth defects is only the tip of the iceberg of the overall prevalence of these conditions.

With explosive advancement in technology and extensive research in the field and awareness due to easily available information through the internet, resolution of the problem is not far away. But, since most genetic disorders are multisystem and lifelong, genetic services alone cannot have a foothold, but must be integrated with related medical services like prenatal health, preconception planning, child development monitoring, special clinics and rehabilitation centers involving various medical professionals.

To evaluate the adequacy of a genetic program, assessment between genetics and health for single gene disorders and non-communicable diseases is essential. This needs assessment evaluates the availability of quality genetic resources in the community, appropriateness of genetic services offered, its accessibility, cost benefit and community's knowledge of using genetics for improved health. It alerts the authorities for need of better provision of services.

A major part of care and prevention of birth defects needs to be implemented through the primary healthcare programs in India.

We should start with prevalent birth defects like Down's syndrome, congenital heart defects, thalassemia, neural tube defects, cleft lip/palate and move to the uncommon but present ones. The strategies may differ from location to location and presence of specific community-related disorders. Samples for genetic testing can be transported by courier services even from the remotest areas to any genetic center.

There also need to provisions to improve on the maternal nutrition, fortification of food with folic acid and prevention of maternal infections. Training of medical and paramedical personnel is of utmost importance for sound diagnosis.

Prenatal screening between 11 and 14 weeks of gestation by, ultrasound and maternal serum screening for early detection of fetal anomalies and risk for chromosomal disorders can prove cost-effective in the long run, and thus must be readily available and accessible.

Patients need to be provided with appropriate preconception and antenatal counseling and postnatal management of children with birth defects.

Counseling about teratogens is vital for prevention of birth defects as exposure can lead to malformations. Since exposure to teratogens is very common, counseling gives an objective proof which may help in prevention of unfounded pregnancy terminations.[2]

Lastly education and sensitization of doctors especially pediatricians and obstetricians is paramount as they are the first contact with patients.

REFERENCES

1. Muin J. Khoury, Wylie Burke, Elizabeth J (Eds). Genetics and Public Health in the 21st century. Thomson. Oxford University Press, 2000.
2. Services for the prevention and management of genetic disorders and birth defects in developing countries. Report of a joint WHO/WAOPBD meeting, 1999.
3. Rashtriya Bal Swasthya Karyakram (RBSK). Child health screening and early intervention services under NRHM.
4. Genetic Disorders of the Indian Subcontinent. Dhavendra Kumar. Kluwer (Ed) Academic Publishers, 2004.
5. Genomics and Healthcare in the developing world. Dhavendra Kumar (Ed). Oxford University Press.
6. Camps by Centre for Genetic Healthcare:
   - Red Cross Paediatric ECHO Camp and Janukiya Samupadeshan Shibir, 2014.
   - Prevention of Birth defects in Sindhudurg (CTEV and CP) in Association with Oras Hospital, Sindhudurg, 2010.
   - Janukdosh and janmavikruti salla nidan pratibandh and vandhyatva shibir, with Red Swastik Society and Gynec Society, Parbani, 2004.
   - Janukdosh and janmavikruti salla nidan pratibandh and vandhyatvashibir, with Red Swastik Society and Dr. Kailas Sachdeo, Jalna, 2003.

CHAPTER

4 Prenatal Diagnosis: Challenges and Opportunities Obstetrician Perspective

Rajendra M Jain, Raju R Sahetya

INTRODUCTION

The goal of prenatal diagnosis is to help parents learn what they need to know about the health of their unborn child, to help them make informed decisions for themselves and their family within the context of their own ethical value system. Obstetrician can use a wide variety of screening and diagnostic tests to assess health of a fetus to manage the pregnancy, to determine potential outcomes, to plan for complications at birth, to decide whether to continue the pregnancy and to discover conditions that may impact future pregnancies. Use of non-judgmental, non-directive genetic counseling is important in helping families make the best choice for them. The obstetrician and geneticist have also to provide risk assessment for other family members. The decision to terminate or continue a pregnancy is based on prenatal diagnostic findings and is not an easy decision because we need to address ethical, legal, social issues. In last four decades, the availability of biochemical and ultrasonography screening and explosion of laboratory techniques has revolutionized the approach altogether.

HISTORICAL PERSPECTIVE OF PRENATAL DIAGNOSIS: FROM EARLY 1980S TO RECENT PAST (FIG. 4.1)

The history of amniocentesis and chorionic villus sampling indicates that women have played various roles in the developmental and diffusion stages of both procedures. Effective policies regarding the impact of prenatal diagnosis on women can be shaped on the basis of lessons learned from that history.

Prenatal Diagnosis Sensitivity

First trimester sensitivity, second trimester sensitivity and diagnostic testing are given in Table 4.1.

FETAL MEDICINE TEAM (FIG. 4.2)

Goal of healthy baby requires an integrated approach. Obstetricians, geneticists, genetic counselor, genetic laboratory, fetal medicine specialists and pediatrician, ensure maximum opportunities and appropriate care that will create positive impact on public health.

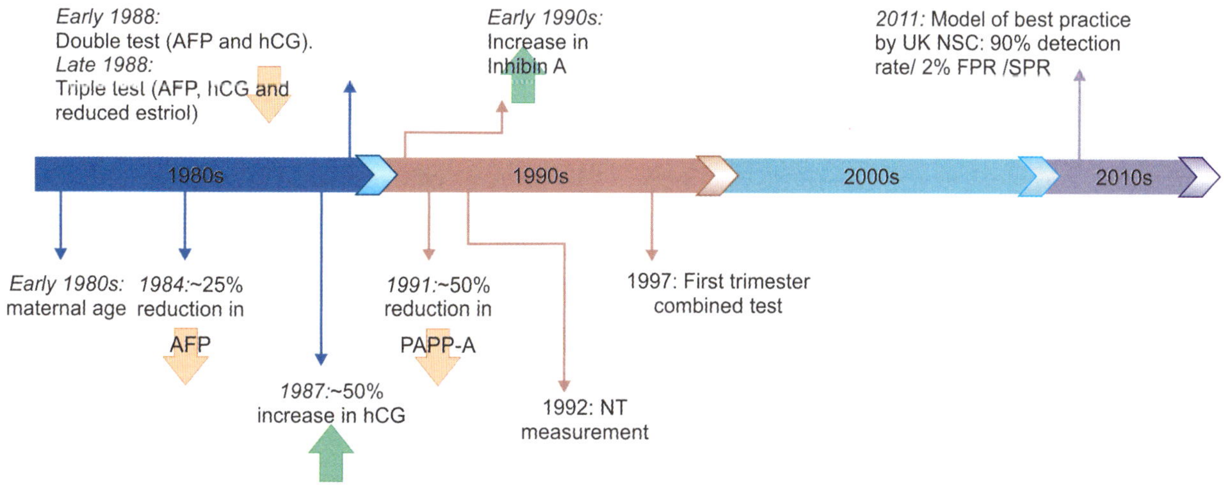

Fig. 4.1 Historical perspective in prenatal diagnosis

Table 4.1 Prenatal diagnosis sensitivity

First trimester	%
• Maternal age	30–50
• PAPP-A, hCG, MA	60–63
• NT measurement and MA	74–80
• Combined test (NT, PAPP-A, hCG, MA)	86–90
• Combined test plus nasal bone, tricuspid flow, ductus venosus and facial angle	95
Second trimester	
• Maternal age	30–50
• 2nd trimester double test (AFP, hCG, MA)	60
• Triple test (AFP, hCG, E3, MA)	68
• Quadruple test (AFP, hCG, E3, Inhibin A, MA)	79
• Ultrasound (16–23 weeks) with anomaly screening	75
Invasive diagnostic testing	
• Chorionic villus sampling	close to 100
• Amniocentesis	close to 100

Abbreviations: PAPP-A, pregnancy associated plasma protein-A; MA, maternal age; NT, nuchal translucency; hCG, human chorionic gonadotropin; AFP, alpha-fetoprotein

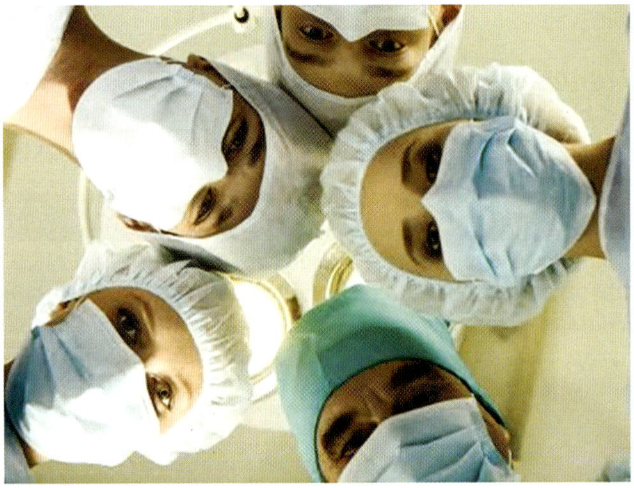

Fig. 4.2 The fetal medicine team

Reducing Burden of Abnormal Children

Complexity of genetic information has generated huge scope but frontline obstetrician or fetal medicine expert has no time to explain nuances of emerging science of prenatal diagnosis, hence need for genetic counselor is more relevant in current scenario, and it is observed that counselor some time know better than treating clinician about genetic disorders.

Ultimately, benefit from prenatal diagnosis is observed in advanced maternal age (>35 years) couple, ethnicity at increased risk for genetic disease, known family history of genetic disease or multifactorial disorders, history of multiple pregnancy losses, exposure of teratogen during early pregnancy, abnormal ultrasound findings, abnormal maternal serum screen results.

Obstetrician's duty is to explain about types of birth defects such as structural defects, genetic syndromes, chromosomal disorder to the couple. Experience has shown that the care and prevention of birth defects is feasible and cost-effective and requires comprehensive approach about maternal and child health programs and also provision of basic medical genetic services to ensure that people with birth defects or at reproductive risk of having children with birth defects can reproduce as normally as possible.

Established prenatal diagnosis techniques are maternal serum screening tests, visualization of the fetus by ultrasound (2D and 3D) and by fetoscopy, genetic and biochemical studies of fetal cells by chorionic villus sampling/amniocentesis/ fetal blood sample (percutaneous umbilical sample)/ circulating fetal cells or cell free fetal DNA in maternal blood. Therefore obstetrician must familiarize to these prenatal diagnostic procedures to discharge his obligation in proper way. Therefore goal of healthy baby requires an integrated team approach involving the patient, obstetrician, genetic professional, genetic laboratory, fetal medicine specialists and pediatricians to ensure maximum options and appropriate care and that will create positive impact on public health by reducing burden of abnormal children.

Birth Defect

Birth defects are defined as abnormalities of structure or function, including metabolism, which are present from birth.Serious birth defects are life threatening or have the potential to result in disability which may be physical, intellectual, visual or hearing impairment or epilepsy. More than 7000 different birth defects have been identified to date. Some birth defects are clinically obvious at birth and others may only be diagnosed later in life. The spina bifida is one example of a structural defect that is obvious at birth whereas hemophilia is a functional defect usually not clinically obvious until infancy or childhood (Table 4.2 and Fig. 4.3).

Challenges of Prenatal Diagnosis

All couple want a healthy baby, but 2–3% of children is born with a birth defect is a universal fact. Two basic questionnaire required to be answered.

Can we offer prenatal diagnosis to all pregnant women?

- 90% of structural and chromosomal abnormal fetus are born to "low-risk women"
- Maternal age alone is "poor screening tool" (detects ~ 30% of all Down's syndrome cases)

Table 4.2 Aneuploidies interpretation

Aneuploidies	AFP	Estriol	hCG	Inhibin A	Mnemonic
Down's syndrome	Low	Low	High	High	High
Turner's syndrome	Decreased	Decreased	Very high	Very high	High
Edward's syndrome	Unchanged	Low	Very low	Unchanged	HE is low
Patau's syndrome	Increased	Normal	Normal	Normal	AFPatau is high

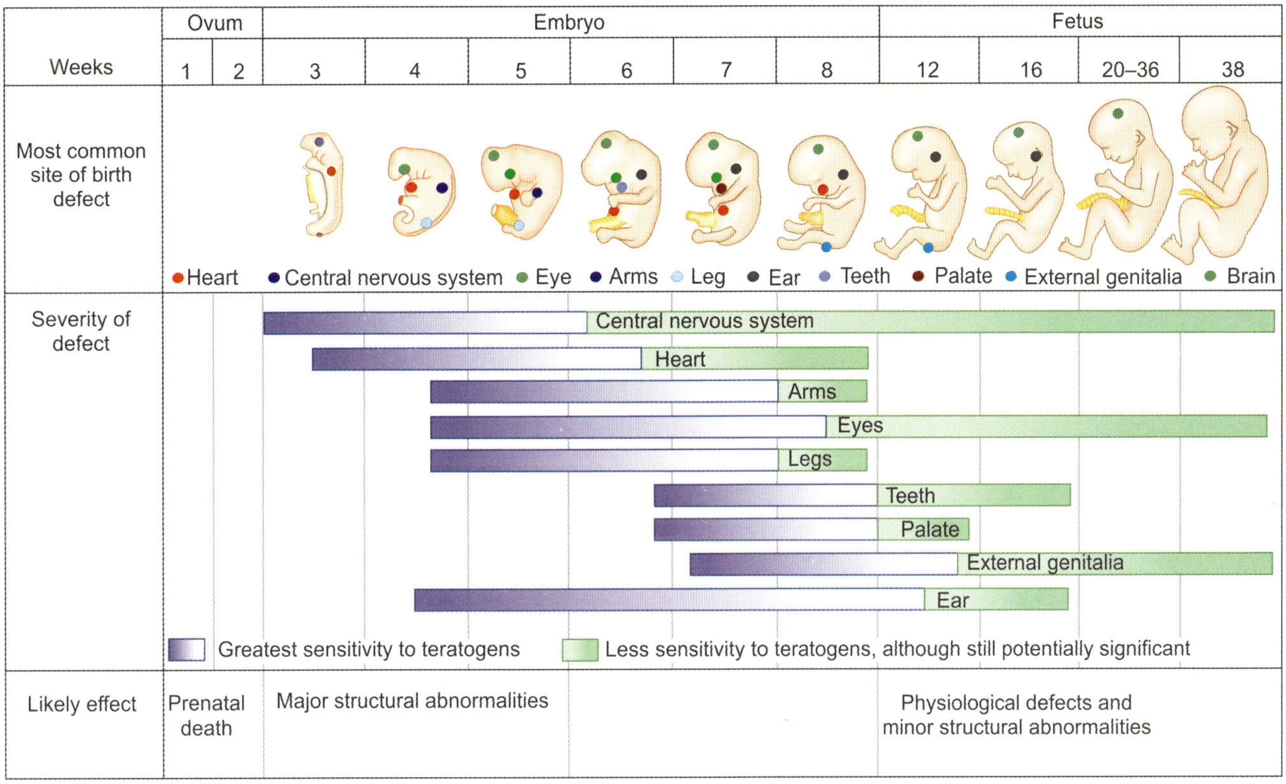

Fig. 4.3 Teratogen sensitivity timeline

- "Acceptance and tolerance of genetic risk" differ between elderly primigravida and multigravida
- Birthing trend in society (1–2 child norm)
- *1970:* ~5% birth to women over 35 years
- *1990:* ~10% birth to women over 35 years
- *2015:* ~15% birth to women over 35 years.

If abnormality is detected by screening test then what?

- Further confirmatory testing is required (CVS/amniocentesis).
- Referral to tertiary care center.
- Genetic counseling and altered obstetric management (MTP/NICU care).
- Preparation for special needs for neonatal or child management.

Window of Opportunities During Preconception Period

- Balanced diet with adequate micronutrient and folic acid 400 µg (FIGO recommendation) + B_{12} + B_6 combination (for prevention of NTD and hemocysteinemia)
- Rubella status of woman and vaccination (for prevention of structural defects)
- Torch panel (to know Toxoplasmosis and Rubella and Syphilis status)
- Diabetes control is essential ($HBA_{1C} < 6.0$) (for prevention of structural defects)
- Minimize or avoid teratogenic drugs (isotretinoin, phenytoin, thalidomide, valproic acid, streptomycin, lithium)

- Screening for abnormal hemaglobinopathies (sickle cell, thalassemia trait)
- G6PD deficiency
- Ethnicity for increased risk for genetic disease (Pan ethnic screening program)
- Review of past obstetric record (POC report in cases of RPL)
- Educate the public about birth defects (what steps to be taken by couple to maximize the chances of a healthy pregnancy).

THALASSEMIA TRAIT

Mentzer Index

- The index is calculated from the results of a complete blood count.
- If the quotient of the mean corpuscular volume divided by the red blood cell count is less than 13, thalassemia is said to be more likely. To confirm requires Hb electrophoresis. Fetal Hb > 3.5
- If the result is greater than 13, then iron-deficiency anemia is said to be more likely.

G6PD Deficiency

How do one get G6PD deficiency?

What are the chances of passing it on to the child?

- If the father is unaffected (healthy) and the mother is a carrier (no clinical symptoms):
  - One daughter out of two will be a carrier
  - One son out of two will be G6PD deficient
- If the father is G6PD deficient and the mother is unaffected:
  - All daughters will be carriers
  - All sons will be unaffected.

Pan Ethnic Program (Table 4.3)

- Are public policies catching up with technological reality?
- Is there any connection between high-risk and actual risk after screening?

Table 4.3 Problems with Pan ethnic program are required to be answered (1970: Simple screening program)

Ethnicity	Carrier testing
European/Caucasian	Cystic fibrosis
Eastern European Jewish	Ashkenazi Jewish Panel
French Canadian	Cystic fibrosis, Tay-Sachs
Mediterranean/Middle Eastern	Cystic fibrosis, hemoglobinopathies
Hispanic African, African-American	Hemoglobinopathies
Caribbean, Asian	Hemoglobinopathies

- An Ashkenazi panel 1–3 tests in '1970' has gone up to 18 tests 'currently' as routine test offerings.
- Is it cost effective to offer screening for everything to everyone?
- Nowadays patient come to clinic tells us that they tested for everything. Is it true in real sense?

Window of opportunities in the ART/IVF clinic: Maintenance of genomic integrity during gametogenesis, fertilization and embryo cleavage is essential for normal human embryogenesis.

Various ART clinics scenario where opportunity arises:

- Male partner with severe oligospermia or obstructive azoospermia, there is role of cytogenetics and Y-microdeletion study and molecular genetics.
- Female partner with unexplained low ovarian reserve may have mosiac turner XX/XO and Fragile X syndrome-FMR-1 mutation carrier status and that to be investigated.
- All elderly couple (female >35 years) is usually asked to undergo first trimester screening.
- Donor of gametes are screened for Pan ethnic panel and infectious diseases as per ICMR guidelines of India.

Preimplantation genetic screening:

- Biopsy of embryos and molecular cytogenetic genetic analysis (spectral karyotyping) offered to couple having translocation, XXY problems, cystic fibrosis, Tay-Sachs disease.

Window of opportunities during 1st month of gestation:

Dating, viability and chorionicity scan (TVS): The purpose of the dating scan is to:

- How many week pregnancy and to work out due date (EDD).
- Check whether twins or multiple pregnancy.
- Check for intrauterine or extrauterine pregnancy.
- Check for fetal development.

Give attention to multiple pregnancy especially monozygotic twin (MZT) (Figs 4.4 and 4.5):

- ~ 3% of all birth is twin and ~1% are monozygotic in USA
- Risk of abnormal child is increased approximately twice in MZT than age related risk
- Diagnosing vanishing twin (Mosiacism on CVS karyotyping report create confusion)

Window of opportunities during 2nd month of gestation:

Noninvasive prenatal screening with cell free fetal DNA (cff-DNA) (NIPT test) (Table 4.4):

- 1997, Introduction of NIPT as routine antenatal care thus need for invasive diagnostic test for aneuploidy can be avoided.

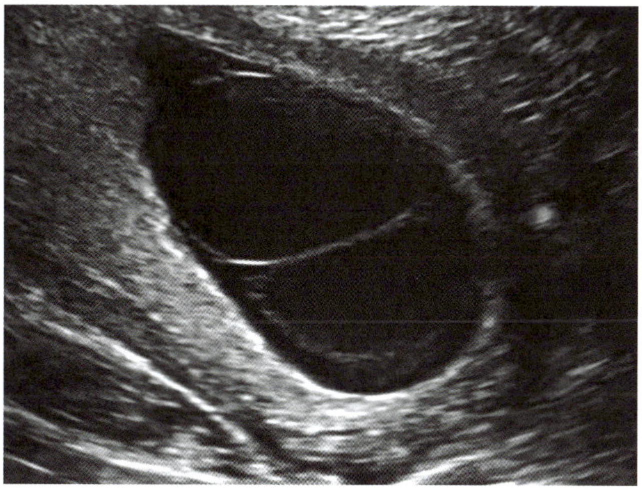

Fig. 4.4 T sign = Monochorionic diamniotic twins

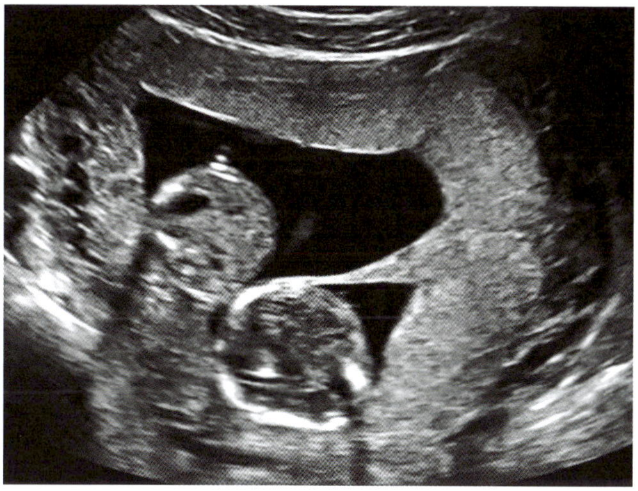

Fig. 4.5 Lambda sign = Dichorionic diamniotic twins

Table 4.4 Clinical trials validated cffDNA analysis for detection of fetal aneuploidies

Studies	Trisomy 21		Trisomy 18		Trisomy 13	
	Sensitivity % (95% CI)	Specificity (95% CI)	Sensitivity % (95% CI)	Specificity (95% CI)	Sensitivity % (95% CI)	Specificity (95% CI)
Palomaki et al., 2011	98.6 (95.9–99.7)	99.8 (99.4–99.9)	—	—	—	—
Palomaki et al., 2012	—	—	100 (93.9–100)	99.7 (99.3–99.9)	91.7 (61–99)	99.1 (98.5–99.5)
Bianchi et al., 2012	100 (95.9–100)	100 (99.1–100)	97.2 (85.5–99.9)	100 (99.2–100)	78.6 (49.2–99.9)	100 (99.2–100)
Dan et al., 2012	100	99.96	100	99.96	—	—
Norton et al., 2012	100 (99.5–100)	99.97 (99.8–99.99)	97.4 (86.5–99.9)	99.93 (99.75–99.98)	—	—
Ashoor et al., 2012	100	100	98	100	—	—
Spans et al., 2012	100	99.2	100	100	—	—
Ashoor et al., T 13; 2012	—	—	—	—	80 (49–94.3)	99.9 (99.7–100)
Nicolaides et al., 2012	99	99.9	99	99.9	—	—

Abbreviation: CI, confidence interval

- Test prices for NIPT screening test is varied from $US 350 to $US 900.
- Presently high test prices limits or restricts widespread use of NIPT
- In India, PC-PNDT Act restricted use of this technique especially in Maharashtra state.

Couple having family history of congenital anomalies (e.g. retinitis pigmentosa).

Importance of History Taking and Pedigree Chart (Fig. 4.6)

The incidence of primary retinitis pigmentosa (RP) is approximately 1 in 4000. To date, more than 70 different genetic defects have been identified.

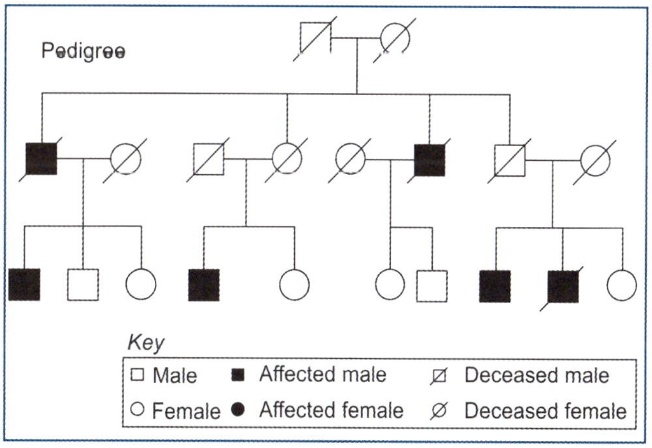

Fig. 4.6 Pedigree charting

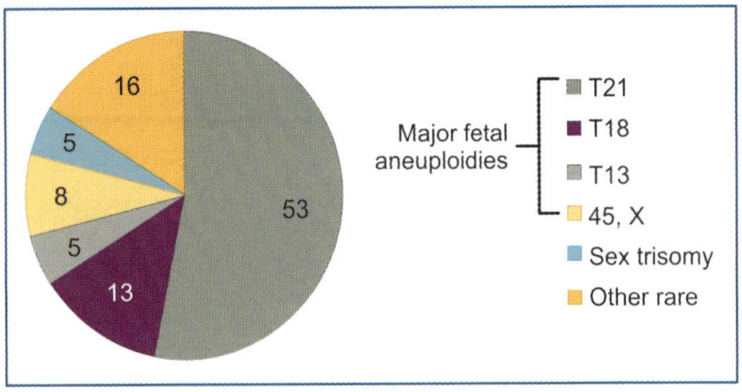

Fig. 4.7 Major fetal aneuploidies

Following are defects:

- X-linked (~9%)
- Autosomal recessive (~16%)
- Autosomal dominant (~22%)
- Remaining cases (~53%) are primary RP or RP simplex

Early referral to geneticist is of paramount importance to know inheritance pattern and advice for prenatal diagnosis (Fig. 4.7).

Window of opportunities during 3rd month of gestation:

- NT scan with nasal bone visualization between 11 and 14 weeks (Fig. 4.8)
  - 11–13 weeks and 6 days.
  - Crown-rump length between 45 and 84 mm.
  - *Magnification:* The fetal head and thorax occupy the whole screen.
  - A mid-sagittal view of the face should be obtained.
  - This is defined by the presence of the echogenic tip of the nose and rectangular shape of the palate anteriorly,
  - The translucent diencephalon in the center and the nuchal membrane posteriorly.
  - The fetus should be in a neutral position, with the head in line with the spine.
  - Care must be taken to distinguish fetal skin and amnion.
  - The widest part of translucency must be measured.
- Neurosonogram or structural defect scanning
  - Anencephaly (Frog eye appearance)
  - Holoprosencephaly (trisomy 13)
  - Cystic hygroma (abnormal outcome in ~86% of fetuses) (45XO, trisomy18)
  - Distended bladder (trisomy 18).
- Dual screening test (PAPP-A and free β-hCG level in maternal serum).

Where do all these markers come from? (Fig. 4.9)

- Opportunity to carryout CVS procedure (FISH/structural karyotyping)

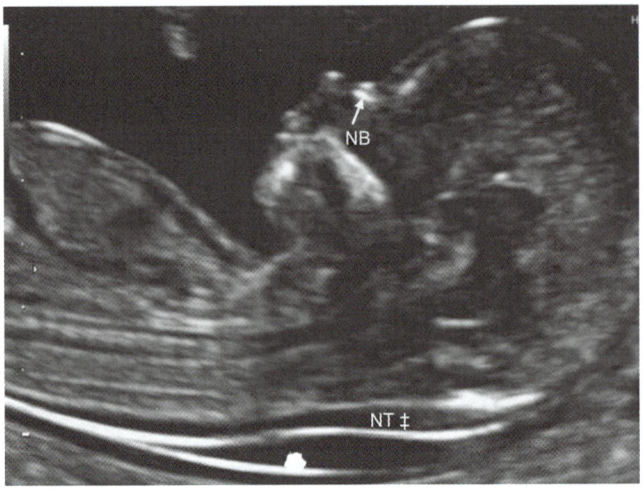

Fig. 4.8 Protocol for measurement – FMF – NT and nasal bone

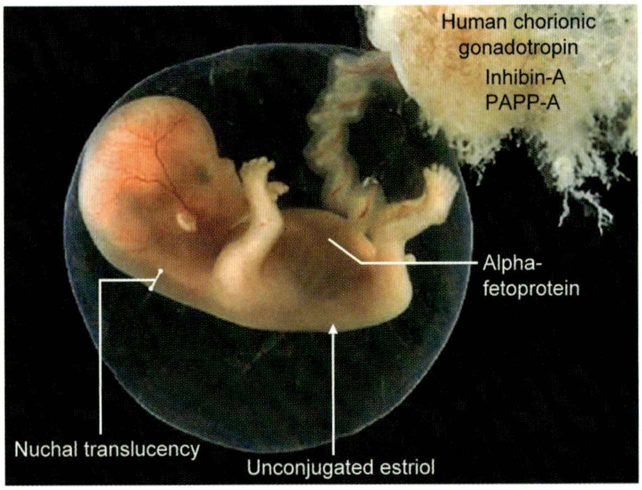

Fig. 4.9 The source of biochemical markers

- Fetal reduction offered for multiple pregnancy
- Send Product of conception if miscarriage for cytogenetic and FISH study to explain the cause for abortion to bereaved couple.

Neurosonogram (Anencephaly)

Anencephaly is the most severe form of cranial neural tube defect (NTD) and is characterized by absence of cortical tissue (brain stem and cerebellum may be variably present) as well as absence of the cranial vault. Incidence is around 1:1000 and female predilection with a F : M of ~4:1. Anencephaly may be sonographically detectable as early as 11 weeks and has an accuracy of approximating 100% at 14 weeks. Anencephaly is incompatible with life. Folic acid therapy may reduce risk

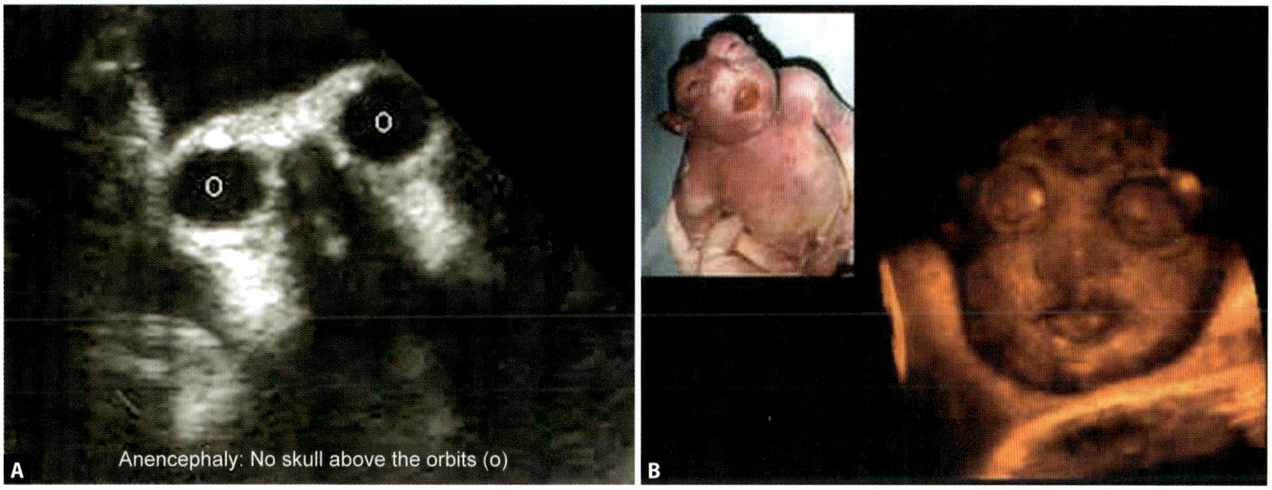

Figs 4.10A and B Anencephaly. (A) Ultrasound; (B) Post-delivery and 3D image

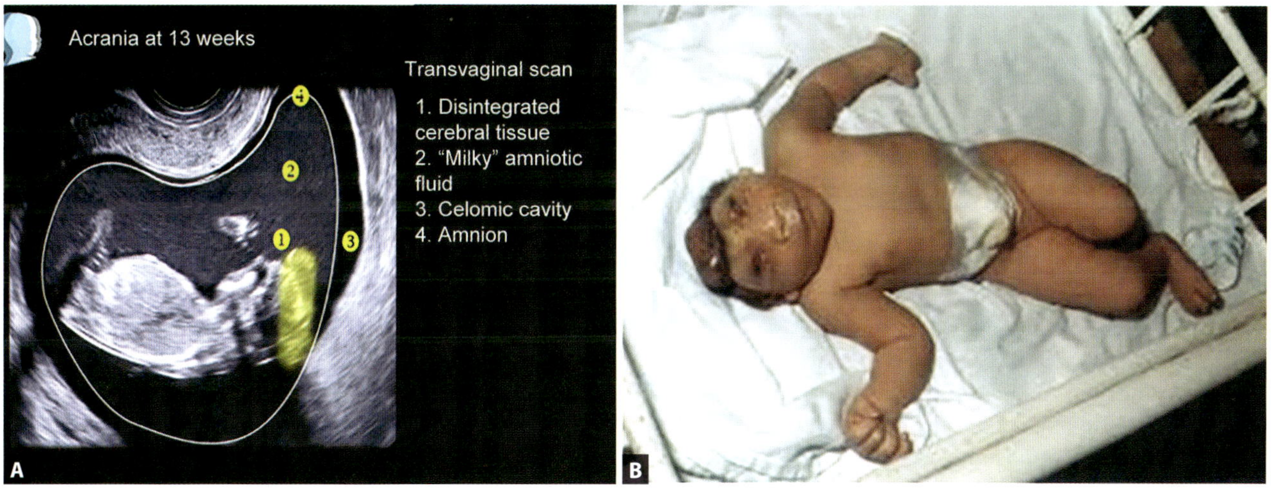

Figs 4.11A and B Acrania, an MRI image and after birth

of recurrence. There is a slight risk ~2.5% in recurrence of a neural tube defect in future pregnancies (Figs 4.10A and B).

Neurosonogram (Acrania)

Acrania is a rare congenital disorder that occurs in the human fetus in which the flat bones in the cranial vault are either completely or partially absent. The cerebral hemispheres develop completely but abnormally. The condition is frequently, though not always, associated with anencephaly. Fetal acrania can be diagnosed from 11 weeks onward. At 11–14 weeks gestation, no vault ossification is visible in the midline on a perfect mid-sagittal image.

Tricuspid regurgitation present in the first-trimester fetus increases the risk for Down's syndrome and other chromosomal abnormalities (Figs 4.11A and B).

Summary of first trimester opportunities: 95% of high-risk and 80% of low-risk women preferred first trimester screening. Early risk assessment between 11 and 14 weeks by sonography for structural defects (an abnormality of the formation of a specific organ or body part) such as:

- Hydrocephalus/anencephaly/acrania/spina bifida
- Several kidney abnormalities
- Clubbed foot/cleft lip/various types of heart defects.

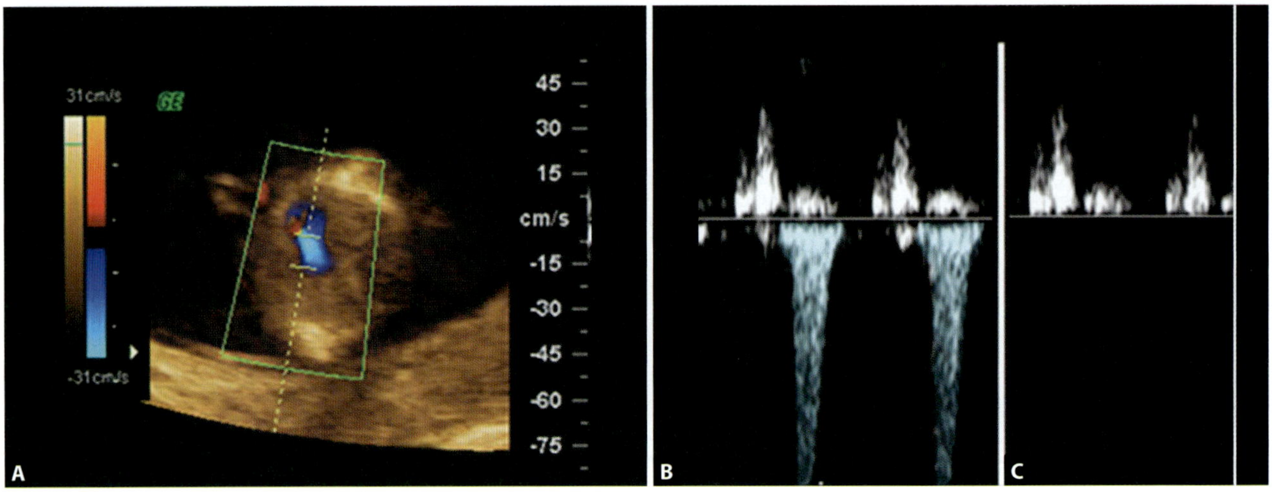

Figs 4.12A to C (A) Color Doppler; (B) Tricuspid regurgitation; (C) Normal

Offering *carrier testing* based on ethnicity and to identify genetic syndromes prenatally by family history of both parents and by drawing pedigree chart to know type of pattern of inheritance.

- Autosomal dominant disorders (vertical pattern of inheritance)
- Autosomal recessive disorders (horizontal pattern of inheritance)
- X-linked disorders (knights move pattern of inheritance)

Genetic abnormalities mostly results in miscarriage therefore POC study is useful for counseling.

Approximately half of recognized miscarriages are due to chromosome abnormalities of these 2% have unbalanced translocations. The balanced translocation carriers may be interested in fetal chromosome analysis by CVS procedure during future pregnancies (Gardner and Sutherland, 1996). Some abnormal fetuses are carried to term and can have varying degrees of problems after birth such as Trisomy 21,13,18, X, Y, hence early diagnosis by CVS or NIPT is indicated in elderly female. The karyotypes may also reveal other structural chromosome abnormalities such as translocations, inversions, insertions, deletions or rings.

Window of Opportunities during 4th Month of Gestation

Anomaly Scan

Ultrasound may suggest the presence of chromosomal aneuploidies such as Down syndrome, genetic syndromes such as dwarfism, hereditary renal disorders or isolated birth defects. The abnormal ultrasound findings may prompt "Amniocentesis" if fetal structural abnormalities or markers associated with chromosome conditions are identified (Figs 4.12A to C).

Some common conditions detected by ultrasound (anomaly scan) such as:

- Neural tube defects/ventriculomegaly
- Body wall defects/diaphragmatic hernia
- Major organ abnormalities
- Oligo or polyhydramnios

Major Limb

- Abnormalities
- Growth disturbances

Single echogenic intracardiac focus (EIF) is seen in 3–4% of normal fetuses and is common in Asian patients. An isolated, single, small EIF with no associated fetal anomalies is of no clinical significance.

Echogenic bowel is a nonspecific finding observed during 0.2–1.8% of routine second-trimester ultrasound examinations (Figs 4.13A and B).

AMNIOCENTESIS

Amniocentesis is carried out between 14–18 weeks of pregnancy. Amniotic fluid sent to a genetic diagnostic lab for high resolution karyotyping. This procedure requires no anesthesia and lab result is usually obtained in about 3–4 weeks. When the test is carried out by experienced obstetrician, the risk of a miscarriage related to the test is about 1%. Potential disadvantages of techniques include maternal cell contamination, placental mosaicism and failure to obtain an adequate specimen which may result in the need for a repeat amniocentesis (Figs 4.14A and B).

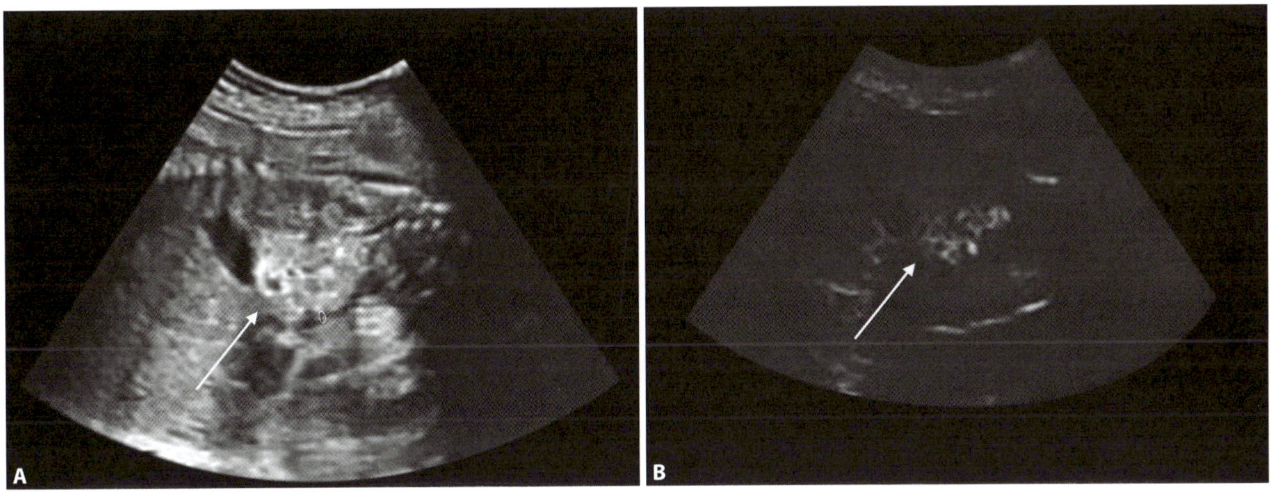

Figs 4.13A and B Ultrasound imaging of suspected echogenic bowel in the second trimester. (A) A fetus with echogenic bowel seen using normal ultrasound gain setting; (B) Same finding demonstrated as a lower gain

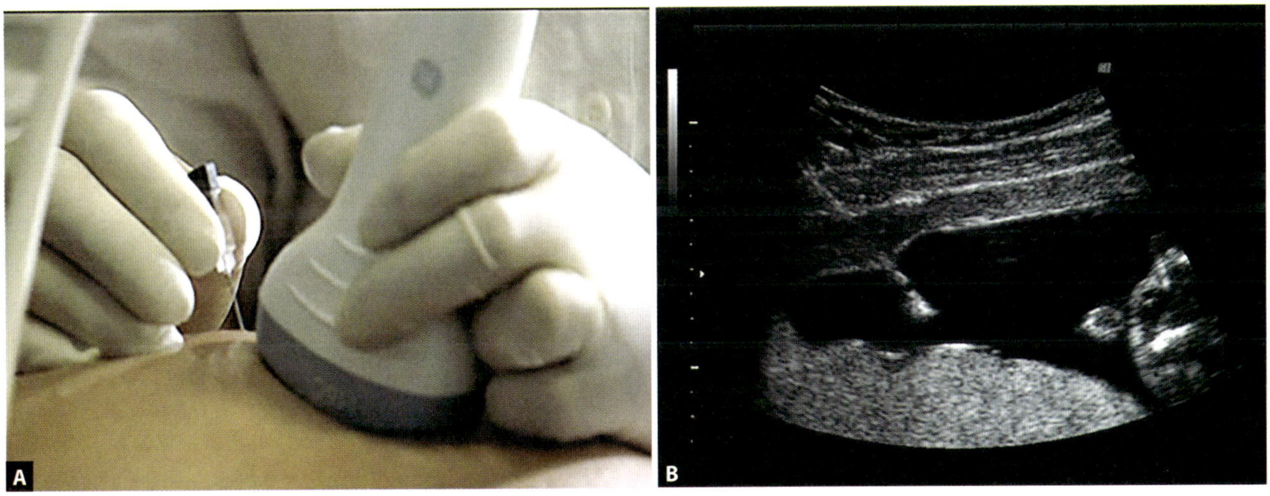

Figs 4.14A and B Ultrasound guided amniocentesis

Window of Opportunities during 5th Month of Gestation

Repeat anomalies scan for:

- *Diaphragmatic hernia:* Normal sonographic studies during the first half of pregnancy do not exclude the subsequent development of congenital diaphragmatic hernia, therefore advisable of repeat ultrasonography examinations at 22 weeks.
- *Cardiac scan:* Fetal cardiac anomalies are common, with half of them being lethal or requiring complex surgeries (Figs 4.15A and B).

Early detection of these anomalies enables early referral to tertiary care centers with adequate expertise. A routine antenatal ultrasound performed between 18-22 weeks enables detection of most of these malformations. Further comprehensive evaluation can be performed with a dedicated fetal echocardiography.

Window of Opportunities During 6th Month of Gestation

Rule out renal anomalies and urogenital sinus abnormalities by USG between 24-28 weeks. The persistent urogenital sinus and associated renal anomalies are usually diagnosed prenatally between 25-30 weeks gestation. It is important to diagnose type of intrauterine growth restriction (IUGR) and its relevance to genetic abnormalities.

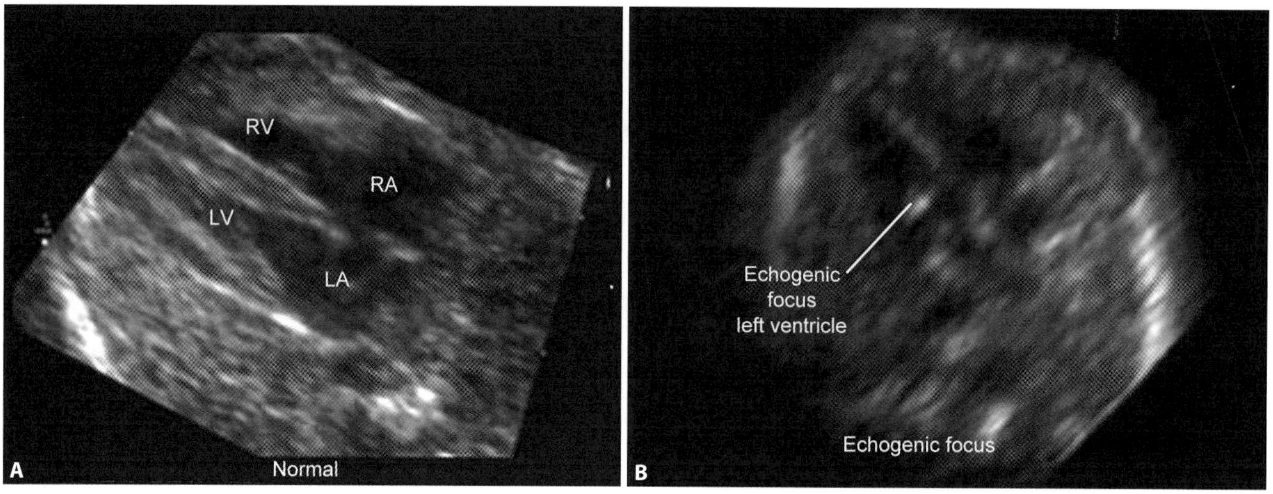

Figs 4.15A and B Echogenic intracardiac focus (EIF), seen in the left ventricle

Congenital hydrocephalus is another condition which to be looked for.

Developmental renal defects include:

- Bilateral/unilateral renal agenesis
- Renal hypodysplasia with or without cysts
- Multicystic dysplastic kidney.

Prenatal diagnostic studies of genetic syndrome involving renal abnormalities are:

- Meckel syndrome
- Robert's syndrome
- Bilateral renal agenesis.

Looking for sign of IUGR/oligohydramnios: Oligohydramnios is inadequate volume of amniotic fluid (amniotic fluid index < or = 5 cm). Oligohydramnios results in poor development of the lung tissue and can lead to fetal death and commonly observe in renal anomalies, fetal demise, trisomy 13/18/ triploidy, premature rupture of membrane.

Congenital hydrocephalus: Hydrocephalus is one of the most common congenital anomalies affecting the nervous system, and incidence of 0.3–2.5 per 1,000 livebirths. Common causes are aqueductal stenosis, Dandy-Walker syndrome, spina bifida, Chiari II malformation.

Classic X-linked recessive aqueduct stenosis hydrocephalus (Bickers-Adam syndrome) represents ~ 7 % of male hydrocephalus. Hydrocephalus may also be present in a number of major and minor chromosomal aberrations affecting chromosome 8, 9, 13, 15, 18 or 21.

Prenatal diagnosis is carried out by using sonographic measurements of the enlarged ventricles. Ratio of LVH/HW had the highest diagnostic accuracy of 97.1% between 19–21 weeks and 100% between 22 and 24 weeks. Fetal MRI is a more anatomically precise modality for prenatal neuroimaging. Amniocentesis is offered for viral cultures, chromosomal analysis and alpha-fetoprotein levels.

Window of Opportunities during Third Trimester

Skeleton Dysplasia (Figs 4.16A to D)

Ultrasound examination during third trimester can demonstrate the osteochondro-dysplasias or skeletal dysplasias, which are a genetically *heterogeneous group* of over 350 distinct disorders. It is essential to differentiating "lethal" skeletal dysplasias (by appearance of the chest) from "nonlethal" disorders and to determine post-delivery management plans. The skeletal dysplasias can be inherited as autosomal dominant, autosomal recessive, or X-linked disorders, and occasionally from imprinting errors, somatic mosaicism, and teratogen exposure.

The molecular defect has been identified in almost half of the well-recognized skeletal dysplasias. However, the application of these findings to direct patient care is not yet possible for many of these disorders. The mothers who themselves have skeletal dysplasias need consultation with obstetricians and anesthetist regarding optimal management, including mode of delivery

X-ray of the Fetus

- X-ray of the affected fetus is mandatory
- X-ray can detect 247 skeletal disorders

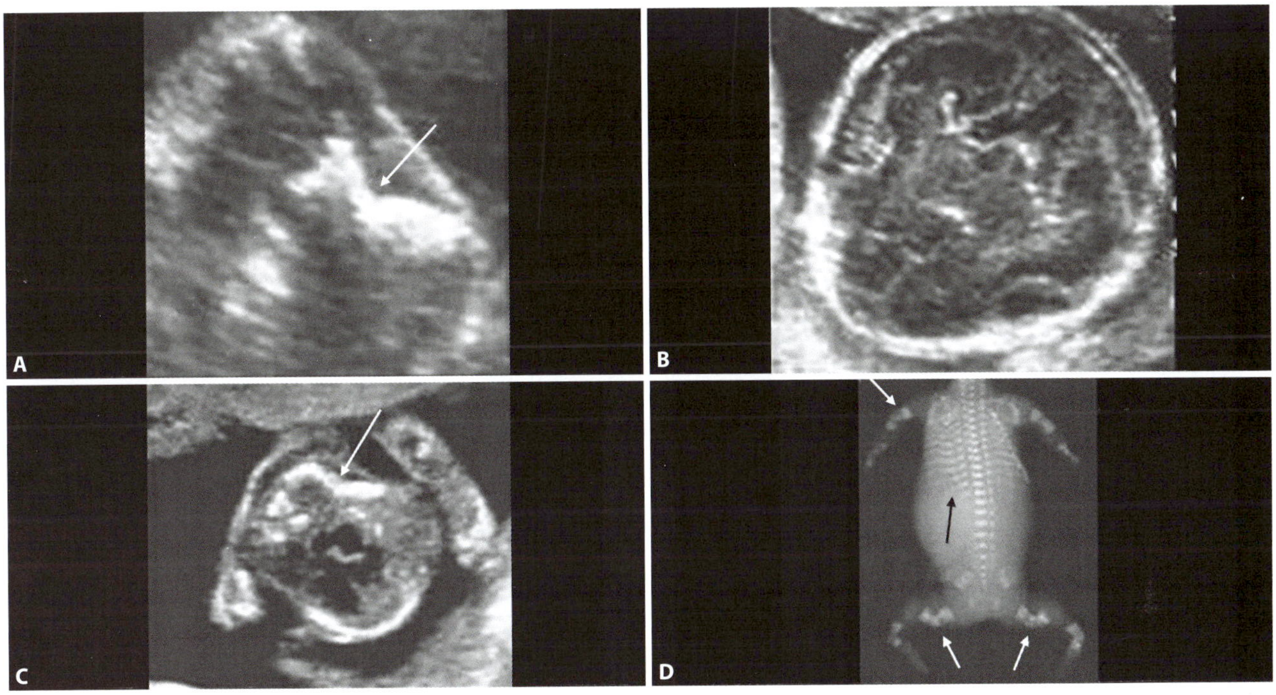

Figs 4.16A to D Skeletal dysplasia. (A) The femoral irregularity and angulation (arrow), a finding that is consistent with fractures; (B) The decreased skull ossification which allows easy visualization of the intracranial structures; (C) Irregular shape of the ribs (arrow), a finding that also suggests fractures; (D) Postmortem radiograph shows wavy ribs (black arrow) and irregular deformed long bones (white arrows) due to multiple fractures

- X-ray can identify gene mutation
- X-ray can do skeletal survey
- X-ray can evaluate bone mineralization.

Fetal middle cerebral artery Doppler assessment for (Fig. 4.17):

- Fetal cardiovascular distress
- Fetal anemia
- Fetal hypoxia
- Intrauterine growth restriction (IUGR)
- Twin-to-twin transfusion syndrome (TTTS) and twin anemia polycythemia sequence (TAPS).

There are a variety of noninvasive and invasive techniques available for prenatal diagnosis and each of them can be applied only during specific time periods during the pregnancy for maximum utility. Knowing about problems before the neonate is born may help parents make decisions about health care for their neonate and some problems can be treated before the fetus is born, while other problems may need special treatment right after delivery but in some cases intending couple may decide not to continue the pregnancy (Fig. 4.18).

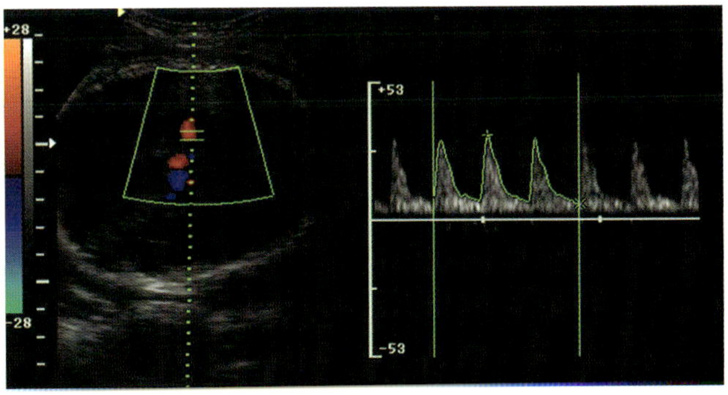

Fig. 4.17 Color Doppler—middle cerebral artery

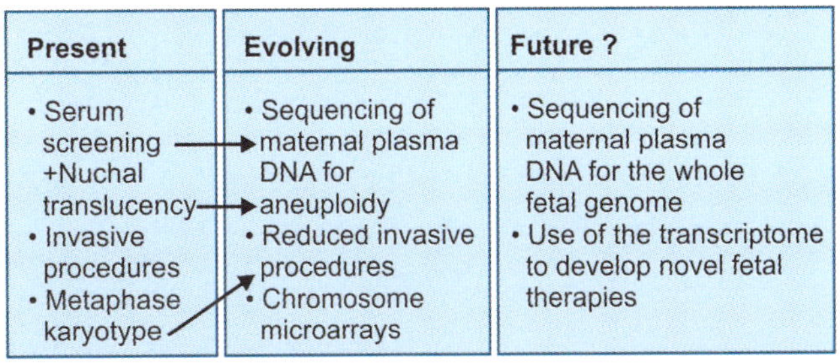

Fig. 4.18 Present evolving and future of prenatal diagnosis

BIBLIOGRAPHY

1. Abruzzo MA, Hassold TJ. The etiology of nondisjunction in humans. Environmental and Molecular Mutagenesis. 1995;25(Suppl 2):38-47.
2. Antepartum and intrapartum consensus guideline. J Obstet Gynaecol Can. 2007;29(9 Suppl 4):S3-56.
3. Benn P, Curnow KJ, Chapman S, Michalopoulos SN, Hornberger J, Rabinowitz M. An economic analysis of cell-free DNA non-invasive prenatal testing in the US general pregnancy population. PLoS ONE. 2015;10(7):e0132313.
4. Burton BK, Schulz CJ, Burd LI. Limb anomalies associated with chorionic villus sampling. Obstetrics and Gynecology. 1992;79:726-30.
5. Feichtinger M, Stopp T, Göbl C, Feichtinger E, Vaccari E, Mädel U, et al. Increasing live birth rate by preimplantation genetic screening of pooled polar bodies using array comparative genomic hybridization. 2015.
6. Ferguson-Smith M, Yates RW. Maternal age specific rates for chromosome aberrations and factors influencing them: report of a collaborative European Study on 52 965 amniocenteses. Prenatal Diagnosis. 1984;4(Spec no):5-44.
7. Firth HV, Boyd PA, Chamberlain P, et al. Severe limb abnormalities after chorionic villus sampling at 56-66 days' gestation. Lancet. 1991;337:762-3.
8. Gardner RJM, Sutherland GR. Chromosome Abnormalities and Genetic Counseling, 2nd edn. Oxford: Oxford University Press; 1996.
9. Guedj F, Bianchi DW. Noninvasive prenatal testing creates an opportunity for antenatal treatment of Down syndrome. Prenat Diagn. 2013;33(6):614-8.
10. Hook EB, Chamber GM. Estimated rates of Down syndrome in live births by one year maternal age intervals for mothers aged 20-49 in a New York State Study: implications of the risk figures for genetic counselling and cost-benefit analysis of prenatal diagnosis programs. Birth Defects Original Article Series. 1977;13(3A):123-41.
11. Hook EB. Chromosome abnormalities in older women by maternal age: evaluation of regression-derived rates in chorionic villus biopsy specimens. American Journal of Medical Genetics. 1990;35:184-7.
12. Hook EB. Rates of chromosomal abnormalities of different maternal ages. Obstetrics and Gynecology. 1981;58:282.
13. Jones KL. Smith's Recognizable Patterns of Human Malformation, 5th edn. London: WB Saunders; 1997.
14. Kitzman JO, Snyder MW, Ventura M, Lewis AP, RuolanQiu, Simmons LE. Noninvasive whole-genome sequencing of a human fetus. Sci Transl Med. 2012;4(137):137ra76.
15. Milachich T. New advances of preimplantation and prenatal genetic screening and noninvasive testing as a potential predictor of health status of babies. Biomed Res Int. 2014;2014:306505.
16. Minear MA, Lewis C, Pradhan S, Chandrasekharan S. Global perspectives on clinical adoption of NIPT. Prenat Diagn. 2015;35(10):959-67.
17. Moore KL, Persaud TVN. The Developing Human: Clinically Oriented Embryology, 6th edn. London: WB Saunders; 1998.
18. Norwitz ER, Levy B. Noninvasive prenatal testing: the future is now. Rev Obstet Gynecol. 2013;6(2):48-62.
19. Reece EA, et al. Early prenatal diagnosis of hydrocephalus. Am J Perinatol. 1997;14(2):69-73.
20. Reed S. Counselling in Medical Genetics. London: WB Saunders. 1955.
21. Sherman SL, Petersen MB, Freeman SB, et al. Nondisjunction of chromosome 21 in maternal meiosis I: evidence for a maternal-age dependent mechanism involving reduced recombination. Human Molecular Genetics. 1994;3: 1529-35.
22. Tongsong T, Wanapirak C, Kunavikatikul C, et al. Cordocentesis at 16-24 weeks of gestation: experience of 1320 cases. Prenatal Diagnosis. 2000;20:224-8.
23. XinGuo, Bayliss P, Damewood M, Varney J, Ma E, Vallecillo B, Dhallan R. A noninvasive test to determine paternity in pregnancy. N Engl J Med. 2012;366(18):1743-5.

SECTION

2

Prenatal Genetic Counseling

CHAPTER

5

Genetic Counseling

Divya A Sahetya, Ankesh R Sahetya

INTRODUCTION[1,2]

Genetic counseling is a vital part of the field of medical genetics. Genetic counselors are trained in the fields of genetics and psychosocial counseling, and act as advocates for families affected by genetic disorders, helping them to understand the concepts of heredity and assisting them in planning for treatment of affected individuals as well as providing options for future offspring.

The discovery of the structure of deoxyribonucleic acid (DNA) in 1953, the chromosomal basis of Down syndrome in the late 1950s, and the rediscovery of Mendel's work catalyzed an explosion in the understanding of genetics and heredity. In the early 1970s the technique of amniocentesis allowed prenatal diagnosis of chromosome abnormalities and certain biochemical disorders. The development of molecular genetic technology in the past two decades has increased our knowledge of DNA and single gene mutations exponentially. The Human Genome Project, a collaborative effort of the 1990s to sequence the entire human genome, currently identifies new disease genes regularly. This explosion of knowledge has led to the need for trained individuals who can interpret complex information for families and help them to understand its implications. Thus, the field of genetic counseling as a profession was born. The first class of genetic counselors graduated from Sarah Lawrence College in 1971.

DEFINITION[1]

Genetic counseling is a communication process, which aims to help individuals, couples and families understand and adapt to the medical, psychological, familial and reproductive implications of the genetic contribution to specific health conditions.

This process integrates the following:

- Interpretation of family and medical histories to assess the chance of disease occurrence or recurrence.
- Education about the natural history of the condition, inheritance pattern, testing, management, prevention, support resources and research.
- Counseling to promote informed choices in view of risk assessment, family goals, ethical and religious values.
- Support to encourage the best possible adjustment to the disorder in an affected family member and/or to the risk of recurrence of that disorder.

Modern genetic counseling is a communication process between a healthcare professional trained in genetics and an individual and family affected by or at risk for an inherited disorder. The goals of this process include promoting awareness of the medical facts of the condition, understanding the role of heredity in the expression of the condition and its risk of recurrence, discussing the options available for dealing with the disorder, and assisting families in choosing the options that are most appropriate for them.

INDICATIONS: NEED FOR GENETIC COUNSELING[2]

Genetic counseling is imperative for any individual, family or couple who has:

- Given birth to a child with a congenital anomaly or known genetic disease.
- A family history of an inherited condition.
- A family history of intellectual impairment or developmental delay.
- A child with short stature, growth delay or overgrowth syndrome.
- A child with a chromosome abnormality.
- A history of infertility or multiple pregnancy losses.
- A strong family history of cancer.
- Pregnancy at age 35 years or older.

Each group noted above can benefit from counseling services in varying ways. The first group mentioned are new parents who have just learned that their baby has a serious and possibly life-threatening condition. Initial thoughts often expressed are: 'Why did this happen and was there something I did to cause it to happen?' Trained genetic counselors help to allay some of these initial fears. They take time to ensure that families understand the known causes of the condition or the sporadic nature of a defect that is perhaps not well understood. Others referred for consultation may wish to know their risk of genetic disease given a documented family history.

Couples who suffer from infertility or recurrent pregnancy loss may wish to know what options exist to help them achieve a pregnancy. Because pregnant women who are 35 years of age and older are at increased risk for having a child with a chromosome abnormality, they need genetic counseling to understand the actual risks of chromosomal aneuploidy and the options for prenatal diagnosis. These couples frequently require information and assistance in deciding whether or not to pursue this type of testing.

ROLE OF THE GENETIC COUNSELOR[2,3]

By definition, genetic counseling is nondirective. This means that counselors provide the family with all the available options free from the biases of an individual counselor or from preconceived ideas the counselor may have about the family. The counselor must assist the family by allowing them to express all their fears and concerns in a nonthreatening atmosphere. Genetic counselors assist families in coping with the emotional burden of caring for a child with a chronic handicapping condition by assessing their coping skills. A genetic counselor helps families to address issues that may be far reaching, as the information covered in a genetic consultation may impact other family members who are not present at the time.

In most of the major hospitals which offer genetic services, counselors may be part of the pediatrics department, a maternal—fetal medicine department, oncology department or neurodevelopment center. Each of these groups may have one or more genetic counselors, based on the volume of patients. Some genetic counselors work for private corporations. Commercial laboratories hire genetic counselors to assist in the interpretation of genetic test results. A few genetic counselors work in private practice and assist any family referred to them. All counselors work as part of a team of healthcare providers, which may include physicians trained in genetics, nurses, social service case managers and others.

PRINCIPLES OF GENETIC COUNSELING[2,4]

To provide appropriate information for families, genetic counselors follow several guiding principles. These include providing an accurate diagnosis, education of family members, supportive counseling, and follow-up.

DIAGNOSIS[3,4]

The single most important aspect of genetic evaluation is that of establishing an accurate diagnosis for the affected individual. Without this cornerstone, the information provided to the family could be inaccurate and thus inappropriate, and could result in further harm. To determine a diagnosis, the genetics team must gather information. The first step in a consultation involves eliciting a detailed family history with pedigree construction for at least three generations. Counselors perform this task, paying careful attention to occurrences such as unexplained infant deaths and multiple pregnancy losses. Counselors may need to request medical records or autopsy results on relatives with a known or suspected diagnosis. A positive family history helps to support a suspected diagnosis. Often, however, the patient in question is the first person in the family to be affected, the index case. A negative family history can also help in the interpretation of inheritance patterns. Counselors pay careful attention to a mother's pregnancy when assisting in the evaluation of a newborn or young child. Questions regarding the woman's reproductive history, illnesses during her pregnancy and possible exposures to teratogens (substances known to increase risks of birth defects) at work or in the home, and any underlying medical conditions may help in determining a cause for the child's condition. As the consultation continues, questions regarding the child's attainment of developmental milestones help in pin pointing whether the condition was present prenatally or developed postnatally.

Each affected individual should have a detailed physical examination by a physician trained in dysmorphology (the identification and interpretation of patterns of structural defects). This examination may indicate the necessity of evaluating other family members for signs of an inherited condition.

After analysis of the information gained during the consultation, the genetics team may order diagnostic testing for a suspected condition. Counselors inform families of the benefits, risks and limitations of such testing before testing begins. Counselors assist families in understanding the informed consent process. They must ensure that families comprehend the ramifications of test results, whether they are positive or negative. This complete evaluation can establish a diagnosis of an inherited condition, but may also rule out heredity as a cause and greatly reduce a family's risk of recurrence.

EDUCATION[3,4]

After establishing an accurate diagnosis, counselors begin the process of educating the family. The genetics teamshares with the family the known and unknown aspects of aparticular disorder. Important topics for discussion include the incidence of the condition in the general population, its natural history, prognosis for affected individuals, and existing treatment and/or management options. Counselors assess the level of comprehension in the family. Explaining medical information requires genetic counseling technical terms and counselors must vary the method of delivering complex information to ensure patient understanding.

For inherited disorders, a discussion of the mode of transmission is essential. Simple drawings of dominant, recessive and sex-linked inheritance are often helpful. As the family assimilates the information, the realization that the condition could occur again prompts questions on actual recurrence risks. For genetic conditions the recurrence risks can vary, be as high as 50%, or 1 in 2, for a fully penetrant, autosomal dominant disorder. Recurrence risks may be no higher than the occurrence in the general population for sporadic conditions. For multifactorial birth defects (caused by genetic and environmental factors), such as isolated neural tube defects, the recurrence risks are based on empirical data and usually range between 3% and 10%. Counselors often use the technique of quoting the chance for having a child without the disorder in a future pregnancy. For example, when a couple has had a child with cystic fibrosis they would have a 25% recurrence risk in any future pregnancy. They would also have a 75% chance of having a child without cystic fibrosis. If counselees cannot comprehend percentages, counselors must utilize other methods for relaying this vital information. Sometimes it is impossible to pinpoint the exact inheritance of a disorder. In these instances it becomes more appropriate to quote a range of risk. Even in seemingly straightforward cases, additional information gleaned from the family history may modify a family's recurrence risks. For some conditions, genetic test results may not identify 100% of affected or carrier individuals. A negative test result does not mean that an individual is free from that diagnosis. Counselors often utilize complex statistical analyses for better definition of recurrence risks within a family. A complete evaluation may reveal that there is no increased risk of recurrence within the family.

Families often base their decisions for future pregnancies on the perceived burden of the disorder on the family. A family's perceptions, however, are often shaped by their cultural background, lifestyle, economic status, and previous experience with the particular disorder. Counselors attempt to assist families in examining all these issues and to guide them in choosing reproductive options that are most appropriate for them.

SUPPORTIVE COUNSELING[2,3]

Upon learning that a newborn has a genetic disease or a major birth defect, a parent's first reaction may be one of guilt or shame, followed shortly by grief and anger. The couple has lost the normal baby they had planned. These parents experience a mourning process very similar to that seen with a stillbirth or infant death. The emotional burden of coping with a chronic, handicapping condition is tremendous. Genetic counselors address these issues with families, provide supportive counseling, and help families to identify resources for dealing with thediagnosis.

Counselors help families to express the concerns and feelings they have surrounding a diagnosis. Often feelings of guilt, denial, anger, depression and concerns about potential discrimination surface. Counselors validate these emotions and assure families that they are quite normal under the circumstances. Counselors respect the individuality of each family member and recognize that each one may express different emotions at different times. Assessment of family support systems and coping skills helps to guide families in working through the grief process.

Due to the inheritance of certain conditions, families may need to share important and possibly life-altering information with extended family members. The confidentiality of genetic information prevents counselors from contacting anyone other than those being counseled unless they obtain written permission. Counselors emphasize the importance of sharing this information andassist individuals in determining how and when to contact other family members at risk.

FOLLOW-UP[3,4]

The final step in the genetic counseling process is that of follow-up. Counselors often summarize the important medical and genetic information in a letter to the family so that it can be accessed at any time. This aids in understanding as the material can be studied in a less stressful atmosphere. Inclusion of the results of tests that confirm the diagnosis is helpful for future generations. Individuals are encouraged to return for further counseling if questions arise or emotional issues become overwhelming.

Due to the psychological impact of genetic disease and its long-term effects on families, counselors make referrals to other professionals when appropriate. Referrals to local clergy, mental health professionals and social service agencies may be beneficial. In addition, national and local support groups exist for many genetic disorders and provide up-to-date information to members. Counselors often handle requests for family-to-family contacts so that experiences can be shared.

Counselors often recommend that families genetic counseling recontact them periodically to learn whether any new treatment, such as gene therapy, has become available. An individual seen 5 years ago and diagnosed with a genetic disorder may benefit from information provided by a new diagnostic test. Other family members may be relieved to know that carrier testing or prenatal diagnosis for the condition is now available. Counselors should notify families as new treatments, such as gene therapy, become available. The process of genetic counseling is a multistep one which may require multiple visits. Families need time to digest the information provided with ample opportunity to have all their questions answered and concerns addressed.

The term nondirective describes the genetic counseling process. This means that the interaction between counselor and client is free from counselor biases and from coercion by health care providers to choose a course of action. Counselors discuss all aspects of a condition as well as the known benefits, risks and limitations of testing or treatment options. Careful attention is paid to family value systems. Counselors support families in the choices they make, recognizing that there are no right or wrong answers—just difficult decisions.

EMPIRICAL RISKS[5,6]

One of the most important facts that genetic counselors share with families is that in every pregnancy there exists a chance for having a child with an identifiable birth defect or inborn error of metabolism. This risk is referred to as the general population risk for birth defects, which is approximately 3-5%. These numbers stem from empirical data of observed numbers of affected individuals from population studies. On first glance the numbers appear high, but included in the risk are minor malformations such as polydactyly (extra digits). These minor findings are quite common, whereas major malformations (e.g. congenital heart defects, cleft lip and/or palate) occur much less frequently. Attending pediatricians should seek a genetics consultation for any child born with one major malformation or three or more minor malformations.

MALFORMATION WITH INCIDENCES[6]

- Cleft lip with or without cleft palate: 1 in 1000
- Cleft palate only : 1 in 25
- Clubbed foot: 1-4 in 1000
- Congenital heart defect (isolated): 1 in 200
- Dislocation of hip: 1-5 in 1000
- Hypospadias neural tube defect: 1 in 50
- Pyloric stenosis: 1 in 330

REPRODUCTIVE OPTIONS[4-6]

A multitude of reproductive choices now exists for families who find themselves at an increased risk for having a child with a genetic disease or birth defect. Available options include screening tests, invasive diagnostic tests, and a wide range of assisted reproductive technologies. Genetic counselors educate families about all their options as well as the benefits, risks and limitations of each option. Counselors must obtain informed consent before testing can begin.

DIAGNOSTIC TESTS

Any couple at a high-risk for having a child with a chromosome abnormality or detectable single gene defect may choose prenatal diagnosis by amniocentesis at approximately 16 weeks' gestation (Fig. 5.1) or chorionic villus sampling as early as 10 weeks of pregnancy (Fig. 5.2). Normal test results have the potential to relieve tremendous anxiety and allow couples to relax for the remainder of the pregnancy. If testing reveals an abnormality, the couple must consider what to do with that information. Counselors take great care when delivering this information to families. While being nondirective, counselors discuss the impact of having an affected child. Some couples may choose to continue the pregnancy and prepare for the birth of an affected child. Others may decide that they wish

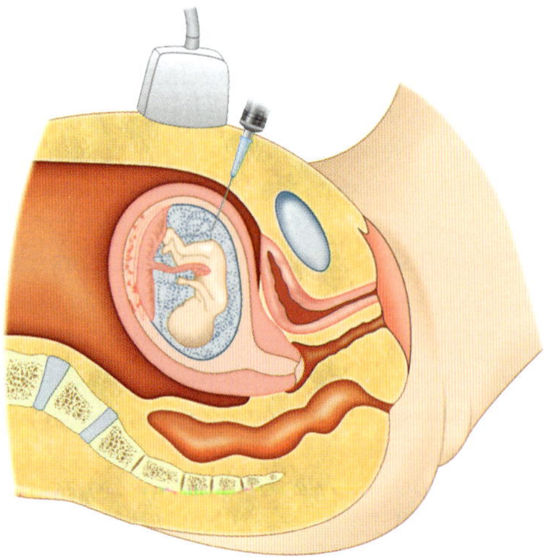

Fig. 5.1 Ultrasound-guided amniocentesis

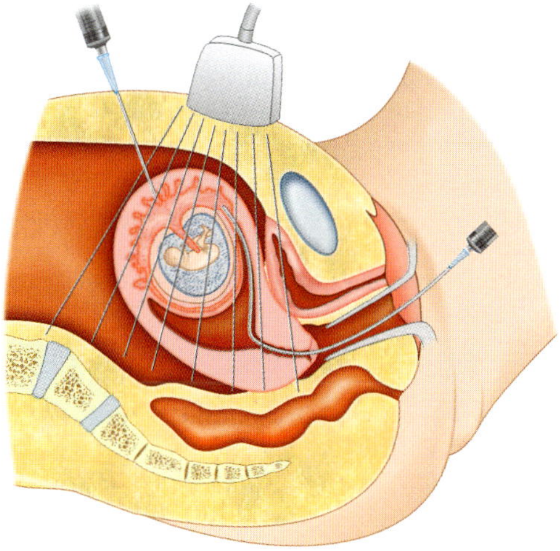

Fig. 5.2 Ultrasound-guided chorionic tissue biopsy

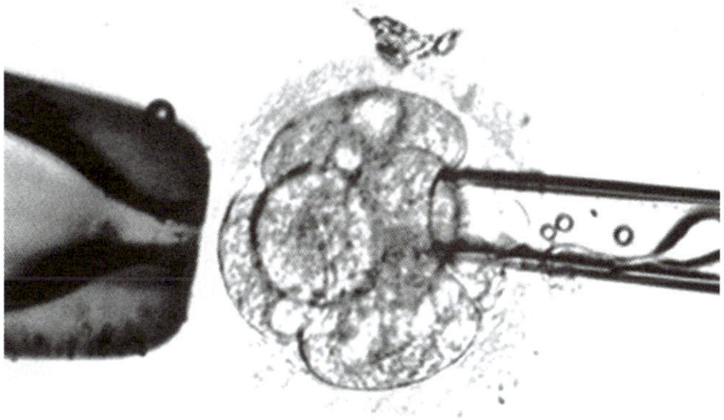

Fig. 5.3 Preimplantation genetic diagnosis

to terminate an affected pregnancy. This is one of the most difficult and emotional decisions a couple may ever face. Genetic counselors assist families in making a choice that best accommodates their beliefs and values.

Some families would never choose to end a pregnancy regardless of prenatal test results due to ethical, moral and/or religious beliefs. Often these couples will decline prenatal diagnosis and take the risk of having an affected child. However, some would choose to proceed with testing so that they might ready themselves for dealing with the situation at, or possibly before, delivery. For certain disorders prenatal treatment may exist. These situations are rare but counselors discuss these options with families. If no antenatal treatment is available, counselors assist families in creating a management plan for their newborn. Taking families for a tour of the neonatal intensive care unit and arranging consultations with neonatologists and surgeons before delivery allows parents to make treatment choices in advance.

Other families make a decision to terminate an affected pregnancy. Counselors discuss the methods of pregnancy termination and any risks posed to the mother. Depending upon the center performing the termination, parents may have some options regarding this procedure. In the United States, state laws govern the gestational age at which termination is no longer an option. This varies between states but generally the limit is 20–24 weeks' gestation. Physicians perform two types of pregnancy termination in the second trimester of pregnancy. The first option is that of an outpatient surgical procedure known as dilation and evacuation (D+E). The second procedure involves induction of labor and delivery. There are advantages and disadvantages to both procedures, and counselors address these issues with families as well. Whatever choice a couple makes, they will need supportive counseling, which genetic counselors provide.

Some families with one affected child may desire future healthy children but pregnancy termination is not an option for them. In the past these couples had only two options: to attempt a pregnancy and hope for an unaffected child, or adopt a healthy child. Often these couples would choose methods of permanent sterilization to prevent further affected offspring. There are other options available for them today. Assisted reproductive technologies give these couples more choices. If one or both parents carry a single gene mutation they may choose to use donor sperm or donor egg to conceive a pregnancy. Genetic testing can assure couples that the donor does not carry the known mutation.

The most recent technology, preimplantation genetic diagnosis (PGD) allows genetic testing as an embryo reaches the six- to eight-cell stage of development. The procedure begins with standard *in vitro* fertilization techniques. As the embryo reaches the six- to eight-cell stage, technologists remove one cell and analyse it for the presence of a mutant gene, a chromosome abnormality or fetal sex if a sex-linked disorder exists (Fig. 5.3). Several Center's in the USA and abroad currently offer PGD for chromosomal aneuploidy, inherited unbalanced translocations, and common single gene disorders such as Tay-Sachs, thalassemia and cystic fibrosis. The applications for PGD are wide ranging as molecular technologies increase our ability to identify more and more disease-causing mutations.

CONCLUSION[1,7,8]

Over the past decades, a growing number of risk factors in pregnancies and health of the (unborn) child have been identified in medical research. The effects of many pre-existing medical conditions, external exposures and medications used in pregnancy have become clearer. As reviewed in various studies, strict blood glucose levels for diabetes, for example, or medication adjustments for women with epilepsy can reduce the number of congenital disorders. The use of folic acid preconceptionally may prevent neural tube defects and family history may unveil other issues to discuss. By empowering women/couples with information about their potential risk factors as well as recommendations prior to attempting a pregnancy, they can make informed and autonomous decisions about their future reproductive planning in keeping with their value and belief systems.

REFERENCES

1. Emery AEH, Rimoin DL. Principles and Practice of Medical Genetics, 3rd edn. Edinburgh: Churchill Livingstone. 1997.
2. Fuhrmann W, Vogel F. Genetic Counseling. New York: Springer. 1983.
3. Harper PS. Practical Genetic Counseling, 3rd edn. London: Wright. 1988.
4. Leonard CO, Chase GA, Childs B. Genetic counseling: a consumer's view. New England Journal of Medicine. 1972;287(9):433-9.
5. Reed SC. A short history of genetic counseling. Social Biology. 1974;21(4):332-9.
6. Robinson A, Linden MG. Clinical Genetics Handbook, 2nd edn. Boston: Blackwell Scientific. 1993.
7. Thompson MW, McInnes RR, Willard HF. Thompson and Thompson: Genetics in Medicine, 5th edn. Philadelphia: WB Saunders. 1991.
8. Zuckerman B, Frank DA, Hingson R, Amaro H, Levenson SM, Kayne H, et al. Effects of maternal marijuana and cocaine use on featl growth. N Engl J Med. 1989;320:762-68.

CHAPTER

6 Premarital and Preconception Counseling

Ankesh R Sahetya

DEFINITION[1]

Premarital counseling is a type of therapy that helps couples prepare for marriage. Premarital counseling can help ensure that you and your partner have a strong, healthy relationship — giving you a better chance for a stable and satisfying marriage. Premarital counseling can also help you identify weaknesses that could become problems during marriage.

Premarital counseling is often provided by licensed therapists known as marriage and family therapists. These therapists have graduate or postgraduate degrees. Premarital counseling might be offered through religious institutions as well. In fact, some spiritual leaders require premarital counseling before conducting a marriage ceremony.

INDICATIONS[1,2]

Premarital counseling can help couples improve their relationships before marriage. Through premarital counseling, couples are encouraged to discuss topics related to marriage, such as:

- Finances
- Communication
- Beliefs and values
- Roles in marriage
- Affection and sex
- Children and parenting
- Family relationships
- Decision-making
- Dealing with anger
- Time spent together.

Premarital counseling helps partners improve their ability to communicate, set realistic expectations for marriage and develop conflict-resolution skills. In addition, premarital counseling can help couples establish a positive attitude about seeking help down the road.

Keep in mind that you bring your own values, opinions and history into a relationship, and they might not always match your partner's. In addition, many people go into marriage believing it will fulfill their social, financial, sexual and emotional needs—and that is not always the case. By discussing differences and expectations before marriage, you and your partner can better understand and support each other during marriage.

Early intervention is important because the risk of divorce is highest early in marriage.

PROCEDURE[3,4]

The only preparation needed for premarital counseling is to find a therapist. Loved ones and friends might have recommendations. Your health insurer, employee assistance program, clergy, or state or local mental health agencies also might offer recommendations.

Before scheduling sessions with a specific therapist, consider whether the therapist would be a good fit for you and your partner. It is very important to know the education and experience of the concerned therapist.

EXPECTATIONS[1,5]

Often in premarital counseling, each partner is asked to separately answer a written questionnaire to assess their perspectives of one another and their relationship. These questionnaires can also help identify a couple's strengths, weaknesses and potential problem areas. The aim is to foster awareness and encourage couples to address concerns proactively. Your counselor can help you interpret your results together, encourage you to discuss areas of common unhappiness or disagreement, and set goals to help you overcome challenges.

Your counselor might also have you and your partner use a tool called a couples resource map—a picture and scale of your perceived support from individual resources, relationship resources, and cultural and community resources. You and your partner will create separate maps at first. Following a discussion with your counselor about differences between the two maps, you will create one map as a couple. The purpose is to help you and your partner remember to use these resources to help manage your problems.

In addition, your counselor might ask you and your partner questions to find out your unique visions for your marriage and clarify what you can do to make positive changes in your relationship.

Remember, preparing for marriage involves more than throwing a party. Take the time to build a solid foundation for your relationship

PRECONCEPTION COUNSELING

Preconception counseling (also called **preconceptual counseling**) is a meeting with a health-care professional by a woman before attempting to become pregnant. It generally includes a **preconception risk assessment** for any potential complications of pregnancy as well as modifications of risk factors, such as increasing folic acid intake to reduce the risk of neural tube defects and counseling on smoking cessation, alcohol reduction, and medications that may compromise fetal development.

Physicians, midwives and baby experts recommend that a woman visit them as soon as the woman is contemplating having a child, and optimally around 3–6 months before actual attempts are made to conceive.[6] This time frame allows a woman to better prepare her body for successful conception and pregnancy, and allows her to reduce any health risks, which are within her control. Obstetricians have developed comprehensive checklists and assessments for the woman who is planning to become pregnant.

In one sense, preconception counseling and assessment can be compared to a well-baby visit in which a baby is screened for normal health, normal development, with the benefit of identifying emerging problems that may have gone unnoticed in an infant.

For a woman, the preconception counseling assessment and screening is intended to assess normal health of a child-bearing woman, while at the same time identifying:[7]

- Existing or emerging illness or disease which may have gone undetected before,
- Existing risks for the woman who may become pregnant, and
- Existing risks which may affect a fetus if the woman does become pregnant.

Obstacles to Preconception Counseling

A common obstacle to preconception counseling and assessment is that many pregnancies are still unplanned. Globally, 38% of pregnancies are unintended.[8] For this reason, many experts recommend that all women of childbearing age be offered preconception care counseling regardless of intent to become pregnant.[9]

Another common obstacle to pre-conception counseling and assessment is of women not knowing, realizing, or understanding the benefits of visiting their physician or midwife before trying to become pregnant. Most women still take for granted the biological aspects of becoming pregnant, and do not consider the value of prescreening before becoming pregnant. Most women who want and anticipate having a baby are naturally prone to thinking in terms of having a well baby. In the majority of cases, women do not think about having a baby who has any kind of problem. Most women do not know how their own medical history could pose risks to a developing fetus. Likewise, they may not understand that pregnancy carries a certain number of risks as well. When family history risks and pregnancy risks are considered together, it may point to potential problems for that particular woman, or to her unborn baby once she becomes pregnant.

Systematic Compilation of Preconceptional Counseling

Questionnaire

Prescreening covers many body-system areas (not just the reproductive organs), as well as aspects of the woman's lifestyle, and family history information. It begins with basic information and becomes more in-depth, especially if the woman has had previous illnesses, diseases, etc. Prescreening assessments begin with a questionnaire, which the woman fills out, generally before seeing the physician or midwife. Some offices have the woman go over parts of the questionnaire with a nurse practitioner, if available.

BLOOD WORK

Certain blood work may be ordered. This often includes a CBC (complete blood count), which can show anemia. A CBC includes WBC (white blood cell count), which can show the presence of infection. Anemia and infection, indicating problems with the woman's overall health at that moment, can both affect a woman's ability to become pregnant at that time as well as affect the stability of the pregnancy and health of the fetus. Fortunately in the majority of cases, both infection and anemia can be treated once the cause is identified. Anemia may require ongoing evaluation and iron supplement. The triple H testing, that is HIV 1 and 2, Hepatitis B and Hepatitis C are of great importance. Also checking for Diabetes, HbA1C and thyroid status, US TSH, of the would be mother is of great value. It is also very important to know about rubella immunity.

Urinalysis

Urine sample or urinalysis can reveal the presence of proteinuria (protein in the urine), a possible indicator of infection or kidney disease, or the presence of blood which can indicate a urinary tract infection. Urinalysis might also show the presence of glucose (glycosuria), but women of childbearing age are unlikely to have undiagnosed diabetes (this is separate from gestational diabetes that may occasionally develop during the course of a subsequent pregnancy).

PHYSICIANS

When women have pre-existing illnesses/conditions/diseases, these may add to prenatal risks and will need ongoing evaluation. Also any medications which are used to treat these conditions will need monitored and possibly reduced or increased.

The presence of diabetes remains a huge risk for the unborn child, and a woman will be screened specifically for this condition. Known diabetics will need monitored closely.[10]

THE WOMAN'S ROLE

A woman may need to adjust certain aspects of her health and well-being which are in her control. These usually include aspects of lifestyle, drug and alcohol use, exercise, rest and stress reduction. In addition, she may need to discontinue certain herbs or over-the-counter medications as recommended by her healthcare provider. Many physicians will also recommend prenatal vitamins before a woman actually conceives in order to boost her overall health.

Preconception counseling in the tertiary care centers in developed countries is recommended to include:[11]

- Height and weight to calculate BMI
- Blood pressure
- Medical history
- Abdominal and pelvic examination
- Rubella screening
- Varicella screening
- Domestic violence screening
- Depression screening
- Testing for *Gonorrhea* and *Chlamydia* for women at high risk for STDs.

REFERENCES

1. Abd-Al-Azeem ST, Elsayed ET, El-Sherbiny NA, Ahmed LA. Promotion of knowledge and attitude towards premarital care: An interventional study among medical student in Fayoum University. Retrieved June 10th, 2011 from *http:// www.academicjournals.org/jphe.*
2. Baron-Epel O. Consumer-oriented evaluation of health education services. Patient Education and Counseling Journal. 2003;139:497-9.
3. El-Hazmi MA. Pre-marital examination as a method of prevention from blood genetic disorders. Community views. Saudi Medical Journal. 2006;27(9):1291-5.
4. Castilla EE. How to apply epidemiological information from malformations registries to the practice of primary prevention of birth defects and the care of the affected. Paper presented at the joint WHO/WAOPBD meeting on Prevention and Care of Genetic Disorders and Birth Defects in Developing Countries. The Hague, Netherlands. 1999. pp. 5-7.
5. Jennings B. Genetic literacy and citizenship: possibilities for deliberative democratic policymaking in science and medicine. Good Social Journal. 2004;13:38-44.
6. Williams L, Zapata D'A, Morrow H. Associations between preconception counseling and maternal behaviors before and during pregnancy. Matern Child Health J. 2012;16:1854-61. doi:10.1007/s10995-011-0932-4. Cite uses deprecated parameter |coauthors= (help).
7. Get Ready for Pregnancy March of Dimes. October 2013. Retrieved. 2014-11-04.
8. Speidel JJ, Harper CC, Shields WC. The potential of long-acting reversible contraception to decrease unintended pregnancy. Contraception. 2008;78(3):197-200. doi:10.1016/j.contraception.2008.06.001. PMID 18692608.
9. Kevan C, Allison S. The challenge of preconception counseling: Using reproductive life planning in primary care. Journal of the American Association of Nurse Practitioners. 2013. pp. 108. doi:10.1002/2327-6924.12054.
10. William H, Charron-Prochownik D. Preconception counseling: An opportunity not to be missed. Clinical Diabetes. 2000;18(3):122.
11. Healthcare Guideline: Routine Prenatal care. 14th edn by the Institute for Clinical Systems Improvement. July 2010.

CHAPTER

7

Genetic Counseling in Prenatally Diagnosed Chromosomal Abnormalities

Hema Purandarey

INTRODUCTION

Prenatal diagnosis (PND) aims to consider pregnancies/couples at an increased risk for genetic disorders and offer them choices by summarizing the associated clinical problems, plan an appropriate confirmed prenatal diagnostic test, communicate and interpret the results, and assist in the decision making by way of nondirective genetic counseling. Genetic counseling is always offered at two levels, pre-test counseling and post-test counseling. The advice also includes cost-effectiveness and discusses supportive measure.

There are three components to PND namely:

1. Choosing the right confirmatory diagnostic test
2. Selecting an appropriate tissue at an appropriate gestational age
3. Interpretation of the results.

Post results, couples are generally interested in prognosis after the diagnosis.

The commonly used tissues for PND are obtained by invasive procedures such as chorionic villus sampling (CVS), amniocentesis and cord blood sampling. These invasive techniques though are safe for the mother and the fetus, even in experienced hands, carry a small risk of miscarriage (1%). The laboratory test is always planned as per the specific underlying genetic problem namely chromosomal, metabolic or molecular disorder. Amongst all the incidences, cytogenetic disorders is highest in population thus fetal karyotyping is still the most frequent request for PND.[1] Present chapter deals with the indications for prenatal cytogenetic studies, types and selection of tissues used, interpreting the results and most importantly resolving the problem karyotypes and prognostic implications.

Obstetrician and genetic counselor share this huge responsibility by comprehending the implications of observed chromosomal abnormalities in prenatal fetal tissue samples, the need for any supplementary follow-up test. The chromosomal abnormalities are the greatest contributors to fetal morbidity and mortality. As the chromosomal disorders are not correctable, decision of continuation or termination of pregnancy has to be done very carefully. The genetic counselor also provides reassurance and reduces level of anxiety in a couple with normal fetal karyotypes.

INDICATIONS FOR PRENATAL DIAGNOSIS

Indications for PND are advanced maternal age, previous child or family history of a chromosomal defect, or repeated pregnancy wastage in a couple, maternal serum screening tests, noninvasive prenatal test, abnormal ultrasound findings, parental inversions and heteromorphic variations, families at risk for fragile-X, supernumerary/marker chromosome, chromosomal instability syndrome. The following are discussed in detail.

Advanced Maternal Age

Maternal age was the most common indication considered for PND in chromosomal aneuploidy mainly in Down syndrome. The risk is related with maternal age at delivery and increases with advancing maternal age. Other chromosomal aneuploidies of chromosome 13, 18 and sex chromosomes are also associated with increasing maternal age. Throughout the world reported population risk for Down syndrome is 10 per 10,000 livebirths.[2] However, aneuploidy rate at conception is still higher as seen from the aborted specimens and CVS samples. This is because majority of aneuploid fetuses do not reach term.[3,4]

Paternal age though not a well-established factor for Trisomy 21 risk but in combination with advanced maternal age 40 and above has 50% contribution towards fetal Trisomy 21. Paternal age is also known to be associated with post-zygotic errors and other chromosomal abnormalities like deletion, inversion, translocation, supernumerary marker chromosomes, polyploidy, triploidy, 47,XYY and 45,X.

Previous Child or Family History of a Chromosomal Defect, or Repeated Pregnancy Wastage in a Couple

If there is a previous child with chromosomal disorder or any history of repeated abortions or a family member with a chromosomal disorder, the risk to the couple increases in subsequent pregnancies. The prior risk to the couple increases if either of the parent has a chromosomal rearrangement. Down syndrome is an example for this with varied recurrence risks. Evaluation of the index case and parental karyotyping therefore should always be undertaken to assess the chromosomal pattern and for recurrence risk estimation and for appropriate PND. In a carrier parent, this is an important indication of PND.

Maternal Serum Screening Tests

Maternal serum screening helps to identify pregnancies at risk for common chromosomal aneuploidies namely Trisomy 13, Trisomy 18, Trisomy 21 and NTD (open neural tube defects). The test is performed in 1st or 2nd trimester of the pregnancy. First trimester screening (dual marker) are offered in the 10–13 weeks of pregnancy by using two serum analytes PAPP-A and fb-hCG in combination of fetal nuchal translucency measurement on ultrasound. Second trimester screening (triple and quadruple marker) is offered between 15 weeks and 21 weeks. Triple marker is a statistical evaluation of combining three serum analytes namely serum alpha feto-protein (AFP), human chorionic gonadotropin (hCG) and serum estriol (uE3). An additional serum analyte Inhibin A (Inh-A) is added in the quadruple test.

The predictive values of these test ranges between 84% and 94% are shown in Table 7.1. Maternal factors like date of birth, age at delivery, weight, diabetes and smoking status, number of fetuses, Conception (Natural/IVF) and ethnicity are important factors considered in statistical calculations.

Noninvasive Prenatal Screening (NIPS)

Noninvasive maternal plasma screening analyzes fetal DNA for chromosomal aneuploidy 13, 18, 21, sex chromosomes and triploidy is now used in prenatal testing and is high predictivity test for trisomies 21 and 18 and is less for sex chromosomal aneuploidy or triploidy. The validity is between 10 and 24 weeks for singleton pregnancies. All high-risk cases needs confirmation by invasive tests. Thus, NIPT is considered as a high end screening test and not a diagnostic test.

Abnormal Ultrasound Findings

With high-resolution ultrasound many systemic markers for underlying chromosomal disorders are observed. Figures 7.1A to F show the presence of a chromosomal marker and its association with specified chromosome. Structural anomalies detected on ultrasound scan indicate much higher risk for a fetal chromosomal anomaly than the risk of maternal age or previous birth history of a trisomic child. In case of a normal fetal karyotype, pre- or post-surgical correction, mode and time of delivery is planned together in consultation with a pediatric surgeon and an obstetrician. In case of skeletal dysplasias even in a normal karyotype, molecular testing like FGFR3 mutations, is suggested. It is important that babies with treatable congenital malformations be delivered at newborn special care unit.

Table 7.1 Maternal serum screening—right test at right time

Option	First trimester	First and second trimester combined			Second trimester
	First screen	Sequential screen	Integrated screen	Serum integrated screen	Afp4
Benefits	The highest detection rate in the first trimester	Early answer and high detection rates	The highest detection rates	The highest detection rates without NT	The best second trimester screening
Down syndrom detection rate	83%	90.4%	92%	87%	81%
FPR	5%	3.7%	5%	5%	5%
OAPR	1 in 3	1 in 7/1.16	1 in 21	1 in 22	1 in 23
Trisomy 18 detection rate	80%	90%	90%	90%	90%
ONTD detection rate	—	80%	80%	80%	80%
Marker	NT, PAPP-A, hCG	NT, PAPP-A, hCG, AFP, hCG, uE3, inhibitin	NT, PAPP, AFP, hCG, uE3, inhibin	PAPP, AFP, hCG, uE3, inhibin	AFP, hCG, uE3, inhibin
Timing	10–13 weeks	10–13 weeks 15–21 weeks	10–13 weeks 15–21 weeks	10–13 weeks 15–21 weeks	15–21 weeks

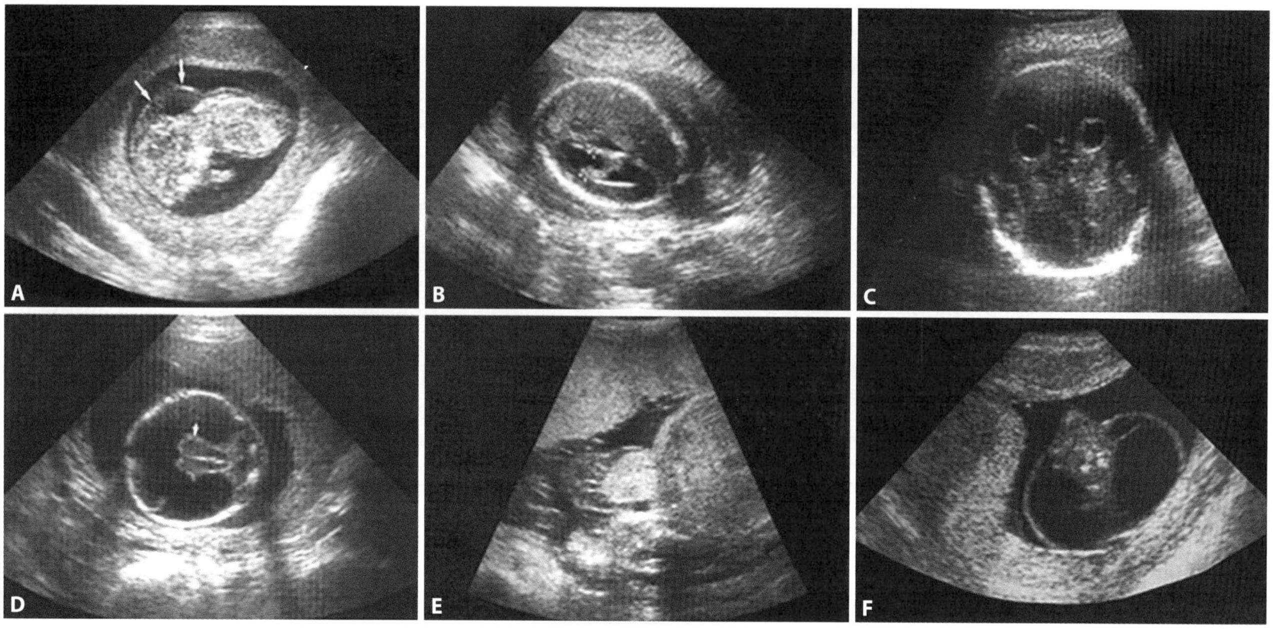

Figs 7.1A to F USG soft markers. (A) Nuchal translucency trisomy 21, 45, X; (B) Ventriculomegaly trisomy 13, 18, 21; (C) Choroid plexus cyst trisomy 18; (D) Holoprosencephaly trisomy 13, 15; (E) Exomphalos trisomy 18; (F) Cystic hygroma 45, X

Some prenatally diagnosed conditions having normal karyotypes managed in prenatal and neonatal period such as—hydrocephalus obstructive uropathy, diaphragmatic hernia, nonimmune hydrops, hemolytic anemia.

Parental Translocations, Inversions and Heteromorphic Variations[2]

Parental chromosomal translocations are often detected in cases of cytogenetic studies in a bad obstetric case or evaluation of a parent due to known family history of chromosomal disorders or infertility work-up and becomes an indicator for fetal chromosomal studies.

In maternal chromosomal rearrangement the risk of chromosomal disorder in the progeny is higher as compared to paternal rearrangement and is due to difference in the frequency of maternal and paternal nondisjunction errors at meiosis, as males and females have different underlying biological process.

Inversion

There are two types of inversions—pericentric and paracentric.

Some inversions have no risk to a carrier and consequences in the progeny are not always pathological. Chromosome 1, 9, Y fall in this category. Other will have varied risk and are associated with birth of a handicapped child due to duplication and deficiencies at crossing over within the pericentric loop formed at meiosis in a carrier parent. Others are either stable or lethal leading to early pregnancy loss.

Families at Risk for Fragile-X

Prenatal diagnosis in a female with a family history of or a previous child with fragile-X is undertaken only when her carrier status is proved by molecular method of polymerase chain reaction (PCR) for CCG repeats.

Fragile-X is a modified X-linked recessive inheritance disorder and a common cause of mental retardation next to Down syndrome. Most affected individuals are males.

However, 30% of the females too can be affected. Fragile-X chromosome may not be always detected by special folic acid deficient medium and needs molecular testing for confirmation (PCR for CCG repeats) as it is a disorder of triplet repeat.

Supernumerary or Marker Chromosome

Marker chromosomes are small supernumerary marker chromosomes (SMC) of heterogeneous origin. Marker chromosome can be harmful or in a phenotypically normal parent transmitted from generation to generation with no significant phenotypic abnormality. There is a 50% risk that the child will inherit the marker, and have harmful effects if the parents carry an SMC in all the cells. The risk is greater in maternal transmission.

Chromosomal Instability Syndrome

In a pregnancy at risk of chromosome breakage syndrome, prenatal diagnosis can be attempted with appropriate media and controls.

INTERPRETATION OF PRENATAL KARYOTYPES

Interpretation of prenatal karyotype plays a significant role in the management of a high risk pregnancy as the decision of continuation or termination of pregnancy is dependent on the same and the act is irreversible.

Few questions linger around after an abnormal karyotype is observed:

- Is the karyotype indicating any true chromosomal abnormality in the fetus?
- Is the abnormality confined to the placenta?
- What will be the severity of the phenotype caused by the abnormality?
- Should anything be offered to confirm the same?

Table 7.2 gives the karyotypes, interpretation and resolving problems.

TYPES OF ABNORMALITIES OBSERVED IN PRENATAL TISSUES

Mosaicism

Presence of mosaicism in a karyotype is reported when two or more cell lines with different chromosomal patterns are present in the same specimen. In prenatal samples, it carries more significance as prognosis and continuation or termination of pregnancy largely depends on this.[5] For interpretation of the results it is important to distinguish true mosaicism from pseudomosaicism by analyzing it in a different fetal tissue. In true chromosomal mosaicism different cell lines originate, during early postzygotic development and seen in the fetus.

Postzygotic nondysjunction is restricted to trophoblast and extraembryonic membranes. Contamination with maternal tissue can also show a mosaic cell line for fetal and maternal cells and is called as confined placental mosaicism. Major autosomal trisomies, sex chromosome anomalies, chromosomal rearrangement and polyploidies can occur in the mosaic form.[6]

Mosaicism in a CVS sample is more common and should be resolved by comparing short and long-term cultures as well as follow-up by amniotic fluid studies. In amniotic fluid mosaicism fetal blood sampling is recommended. If there is a sex chromosomal anomaly genotype-phenotype correlation by ultrasound is suggested.

Maternal Cell Contamination

Problem of maternal cell contamination is largely associated with CVS cultures, especially sex chromosomal mosaicism (46,XX/46,XY Mosaicism), however, other chromosomes, can also be involved. In severe cases 46,XX karyotype can be seen, where the true fetal karyotype is 46,XY or an abnormal karyotype. Some chromosomal abnormalities are confined to placenta having different fetal karyotypes (Figs 7.2A to D).

Tissue Specific Mosaicism

Tetrasomy of 12p a chromosomal disorder if observed in amniotic fluid culture, needs a special mention. The consequences of this are mental retardation, seizure, streaks of hypo- or hyperpigmentation and dysmorphic features and diaphragmatic hernia. The syndrome is known as Pallister-Killian syndrome.[7] This is tissue specific and is in a mosaic form in the body (Fig. 7.3). Correlation with ultrasound findings, especially for diaphragmatic hernia is important. Fetal blood karyotype in these cases will not confirm the tetrasomy of 12p as this chromosomal abnormality is only expressed in fibroblast culture. The confirmation until late was possible by skin biopsy fibroblast culture only.[8] Currently, CGH array on the fetal blood is being used for prenatal diagnosis allowing confirmation of tetrasomy of 12p.

Placental Mosaicism

IUGR: Intrauterine growth retardation, *TMT:* Triple marker test, *DMT:* Double marker test, *AF:* Amniotic fluid, *AMA:* Advanced maternal age, *CVS:* Chorionic villus sampling, *POC:* Products of conception.

CONFINED PLACENTAL MOSAICISM

Same mosaic cell lines can be found in multiple tissues. In all the cases of mosaicism, karyotype from other tissue is recommended.

Table 7.2 summarizes the abnormalities observed and resolving the problem.

Autosomal Trisomies

Autosomal trisomies for chromosomes 13, 18, 21 and sex chromosomes result in a clinically significant syndrome seen postnatally. They have a severe impact on physical and mental development. Trisomies of involvement of 2, 3, 14, 15, 16, 20 and 22 have high risk of pseudomosaicism and are of trophoblastic and extraembryonic origin. Trisomies of

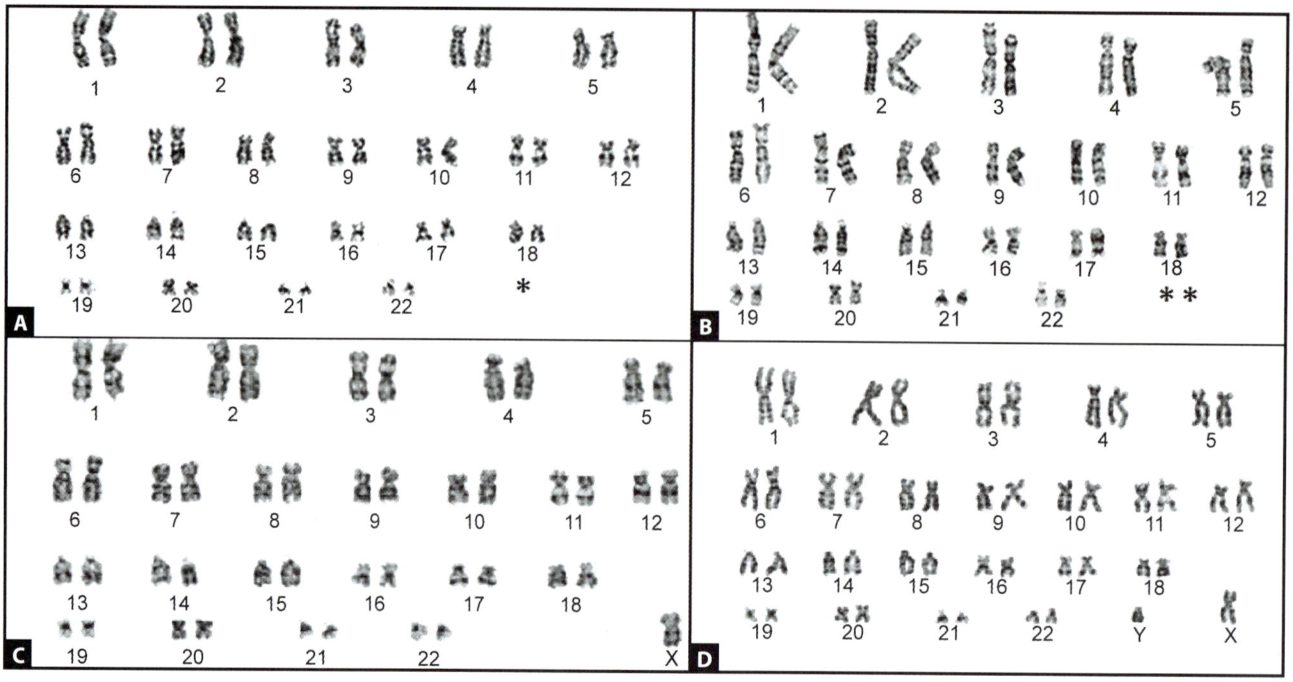

Figs 7.2A to D A case of placental mosaicism—CVS karyotype of a 32-year-old primi with increased risk for Trisomy 21. Karyotype revealed (A) Monosomy for sex chromosome 45,*; (B) Confirmation by amniotic fluid 46,**; (C) Placenta at birth (Left side) 45, X; (D) Right side 46,XY. Sex Chromosome in prenatal diagnosed cases are not revealed as per the PCPNDT Act in Figure (A) and (B)

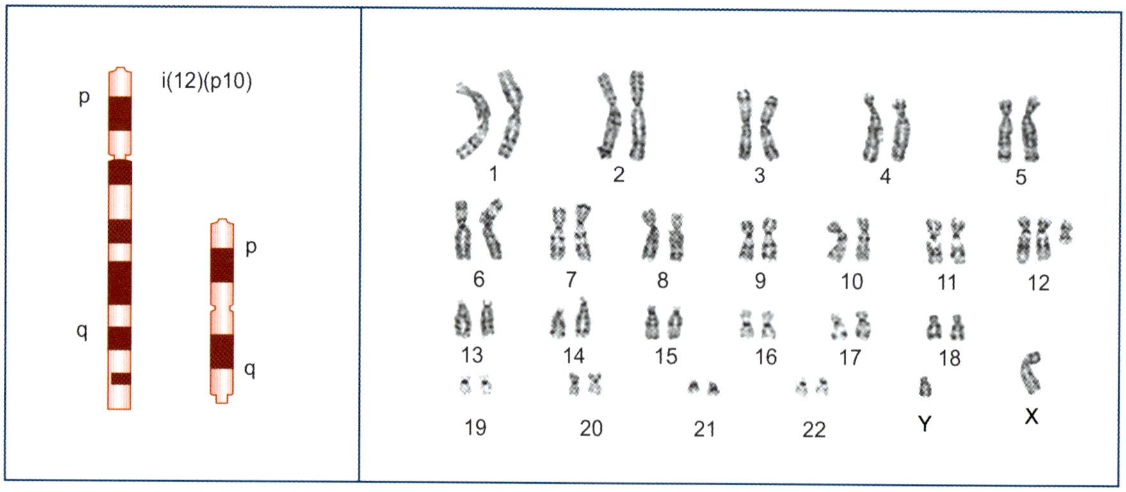

Fig. 7.3 Karyotype of Pallister-Killian syndrome case. This karyo shows isochromosome for short arm of chromosome 12 (duplication of short arm of chromosome 12) mosaic 47,XY,+i(12)(p10)[03]/46,XY[02]

chromosome number, 3, 14, 16 and 22 are of placental origin hence seen more often in CVS samples, while trisomies for chromosome number 2 and 20 occur frequently in amniotic fluid cultures. Trisomy for chromosome number 20 may be detected in specific fetal tissues such as kidney, rectum, esophagus and placenta.[6,10] It suggests that trisomy 20 is confined to specific fetal tissues (Figs 7.4 and 7.5).

Trisomy of Clinically Recognized Syndromes

Trisomies in the clinically recognized syndrome can also be present in the mosaic form and the risk to the fetus is still high. Pseudomosaicism has been demonstrated for Tri 13, 18 and for mosaic trisomies of chromosomes 7, 8, 9, 13, 18, 21. Follow-up by amniocentesis or fetal blood sampling is recommended in such cases.

Table 7.2 Interpretation and resolving problems in fetal karyotypes

Karyotype	Tissue	Consequences	Resolving problem
Recognized chromosomal abnormality (Mosaic and Nonmosaic) 13,18,21	CVS/PB Amnio	Syndrome association clear prognosis. True mosaics are known	Correlate with maternal serum marker and ultrasound. In mosaic cell line (Placental mosaicism to be excluded by amnio or fetal blood sampling Correlate with known syndrome
Nonrecognized chromosomal abnormality	CVS, Amnio	No syndrome is known Majority are false positive	Fetal blood sampling for confirmation
Polyploidy Triploidy	CVS, Amnio	Leads to IUGR , viability questionable	USG to rule out multiple pregnancy FBS to rule out cultural artefacts
Tetraploidy—92,XXXX or XXYY	CVS/PB, Amnio	Majority are endoreduplication	Confirmed by FBS to rule out cultural artefacts
Sex chromosomal abnormalities 46,XX/46,XY	CVS/PB, Amnio	Fertility issues, development of sexual organs affected, secondary sexual characters, can be ambigous or no genotype-phenotype correlation. Maternal contamination/twin or true hermaphrodite	Check maternal markers if any. USG for genitalia genotype-phenotype correlation) confirmation by fetal blood sample
45,X/46,XX/47,XXX,45,X/46,XY/47,XXY 46,XY/47,XXY 46,XX/47,XXX	CVS/PB, Amnio	Known sex chromosomal syndrome Confined to placental anomaly, true fetal mosaics	Further sampling for confirmation, FBS if required
Supernumerary marker chromosome	CVS/PB, Amnio	De novo can have phenotypic abnormalities or familial	Parental karyotype to check if its familial, if not FBS for continuation
Pallister-Killian syndrome	Amnio	Present in amniotic fluid culture in mosaic form	Not present in,fetal blood karyotyping does not show. USG for diaphragmatic hernia and fetal blood for array CGH is useful
Translocations • Robertsonian • Balanced translocations • Unbalanced translocations	CVS, Amnio, FBS CVS, Amnio	Carrier unaffected False positive False positive	Check parental karyotype de novo or familial, fetal blood sampling,balanced, FBS only if it appears de novo or unbalanced
Inversions • Pericentric nonheterochromatic • Pericentric heterochromatic • Inversions paracentric		Variants 9 and Y may be false positive	 Parental karyotype Parental karyotypes
Ring • mosaic • nonmosaic			Parental karyotypes to see if a parent has the ring in mosaic form FBS to confirm Parental karyotypes to see if a parent has the ring in mosaic form FBS to confirm
Fragile-X		May be limited to a few cells Test several hundred cells	Family history,test mother and other family members Ensure 5% cells have Fra X, FBS.
Fetuses at risk for Fra X		Risk of false -ves	FBS most accurate. check several hundred cells in stringent culture conditions

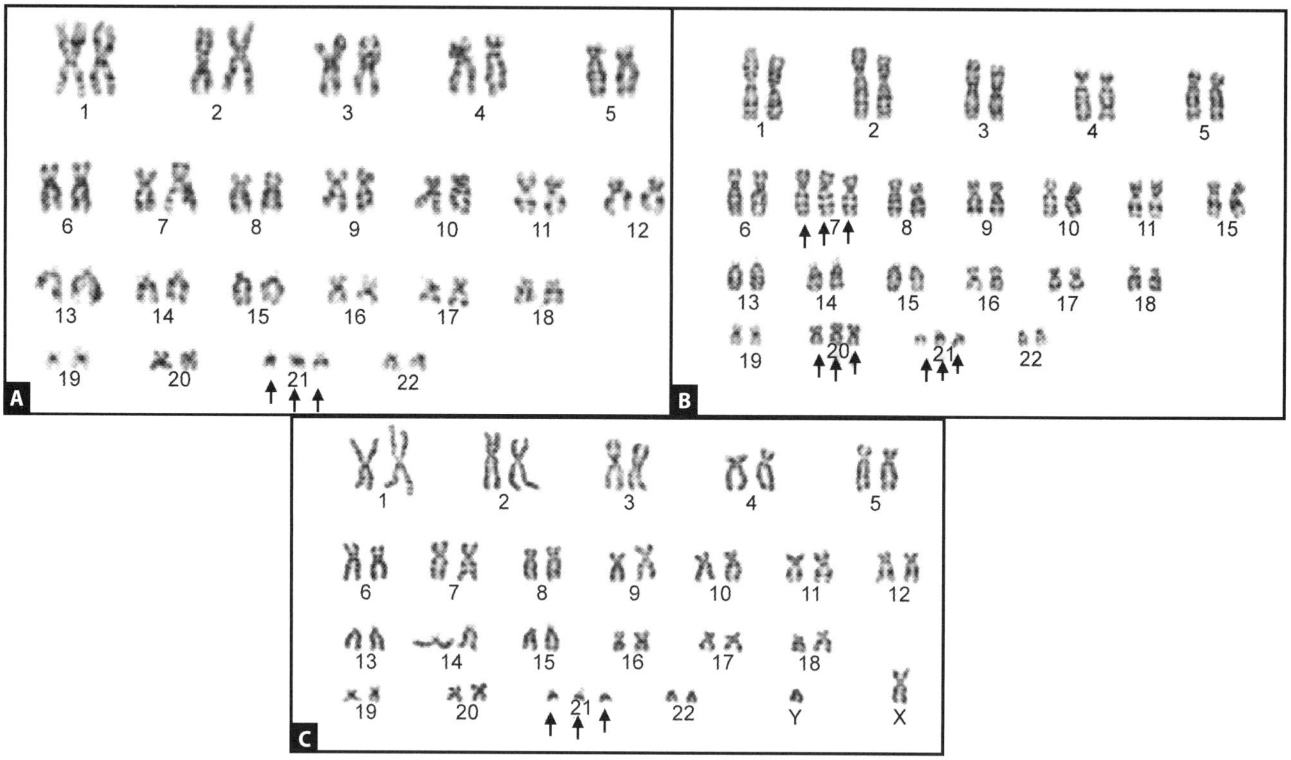

Figs 7.4A to C Mosaicism of a recognized and non-recognized trisomy—CVS karyotype of 28-year-old primi with increased NT, tricuspid regurgitation (Mosaic cell line observed) (A) 47,**, (Sex chromosomal pattern cannot be revealed as per PCPNDT Act), +21[19] (B) 49,**,+7,+20,+21[06]; (C) Products of conception after MTP showed:47, **, +21 (Down syndrome)

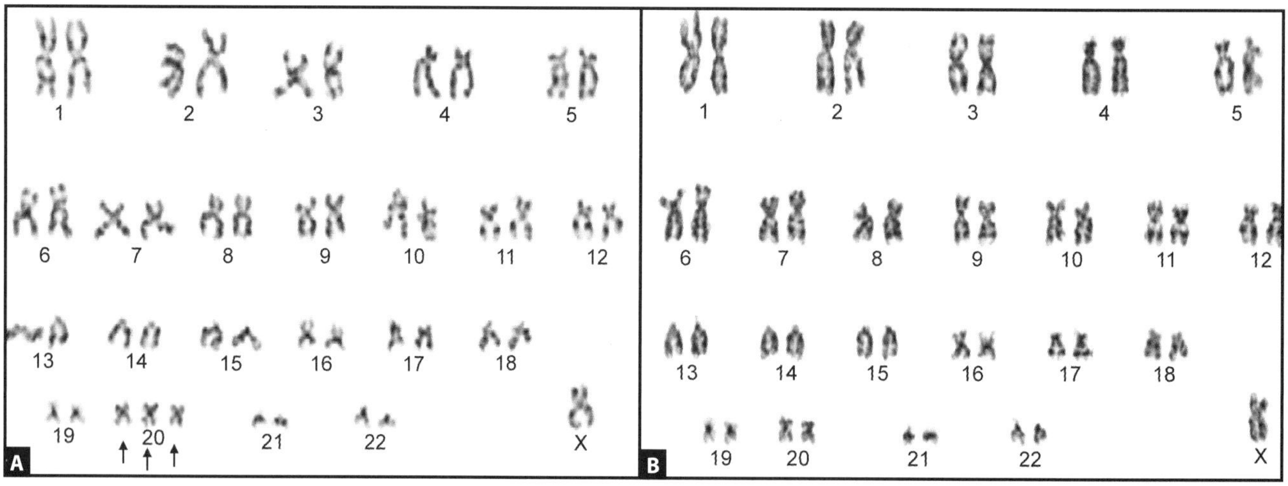

Figs 7.5A and B CVS karyotype from 30 years Gravida 2 with gross hydrops cystic hygroma. (A) Karyotype 46,*, +20; (B) Amniocentesis (in view of cystic hygroma not regressing) karyotype 45, * (Monosomy for sex chromosome)

Sex Chromosomal Aneuploidy and Mosaicism

Sex chromosomal trisomies are compatible with life and symptoms vary from mild to severe hypogonadism and moderately low to normal IQ. They can be seen in mosaic forms as well.

True mosaicism for sex chromosomes exists in patients with sex chromosome abnormalities leading to abnormalities of genitalia or secondary sexual development.[11] In some of the CVS samples this can occur due to maternal cell contamination. It is recommended that the finding can be confirmed by amniotic fluid culture or fetal blood sampling. The common sex chromosome abnormalities seen are intersex, pseudohermaphroditism or Turner's syndrome.

Chromosome Rearrangement

About 0.5% of population is known to have a chromosomal rearrangement where the total genetic material is normal but rearranged.[12] Two types of translocations are known.

Robertsonian Translocation

Male carriers have about 60% chance of transmitting a balanced rearrangement to the pregnancy. There is small chance (1–3%) of having children with unbalanced forms of the translocation. Mothers carrying translocations have 12–15% chance of having a child with an unbalanced translocation leading to pregnancy wastage and congenital malformations in progeny (Fig. 7.6).

Highest known genetic risk for chromosomal disorder in the offspring is for a parent with Robertsonian translocation t(21,21) where there is 100% risk of a pregnancy with Down syndrome.

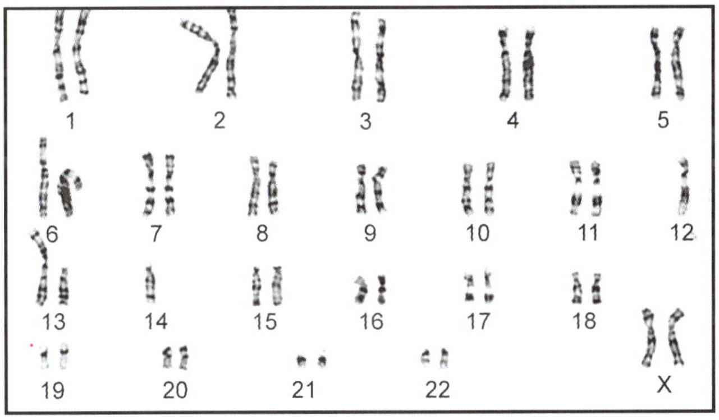

Fig. 7.6 Robertsonian translocation 45,XX,der(13;14)(q10;q10)

Reciprocal Translocations

In reciprocal translocations the risks for paternal and maternal carriers are approximately equal, however, mode of ascertainment remains the determining factor in estimating the risk of inheritance of unbalanced form of translocation or presence of additional material inherited from a parent (Figs 7.7A and B).

Extent of duplication and deficiencies depends on the breakpoints involved as to whether a larger segment is in trisomic or monosomic form. This results into repeated miscarriages, as the unbalanced form of translocation leads to disruptions in genetic material.

If such a karyotype is observed in fetal tissue, following steps are necessary:

- To confirm parental karyotype and check for familial origin of rearrangement (maternal or paternal origin). If similar pattern is seen, the risk to the fetus is low (Figs 7.8A and B).
- Literature survey for mental retardation or dysmorphology syndrome correlation for rare syndromes.
- Confirmation with amniocentesis or fetal blood sampling using high-resolution banding or molecular cytogenetic techniques should be attempted.

SUPERNUMERARY MARKER CHROMOSOME

In supernumerary or marker chromosomes, assessing the prognosis is difficult.[13] This will depend on the size of the marker chromosomes, heterochromatin involvement. The consequences can be mild to serious. FISH can be used to identify the segment involved. Whole chromosome paint is a

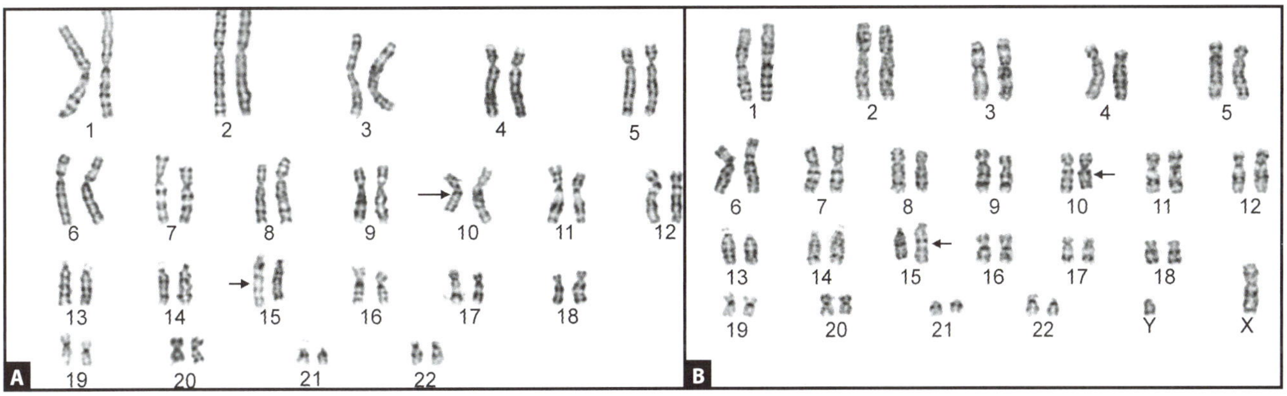

Figs 7.7A and B Reciprocal translocation. (A) Amniotic fluid karyotype showing reciprocal translocation 46, **, t(10;15)(q22;q22); (B) Father had similar karyotype 46,XY, t(10;15)(q22;q22) (Fetus inherited translocation from the father)

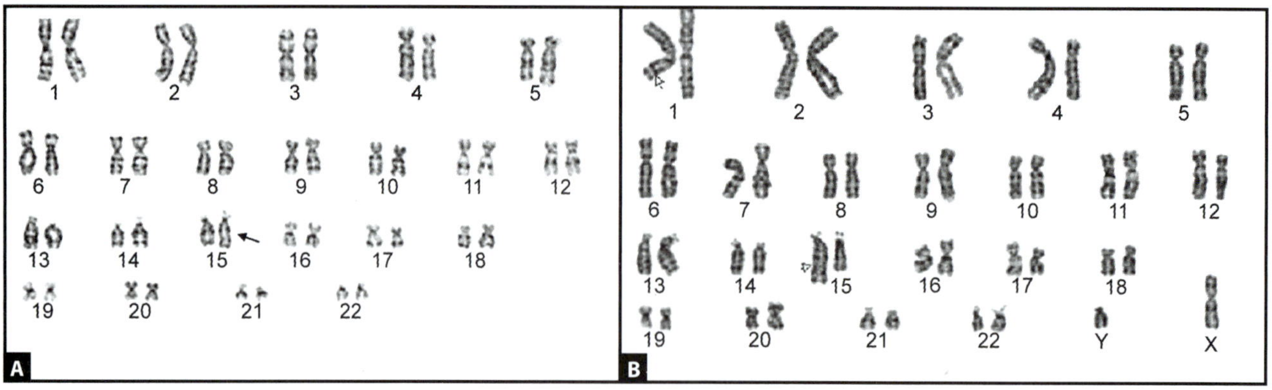

Figs 7.8A and B Progeny of reciprocal translocation. (A) Amniotic fluid karyotype 46, **, add(15)(q26); (B) Father's karyotype: 46,XY,t(1;15)(q32;q24). The additional material on chromosome 15 was thus derived from the father and pathological

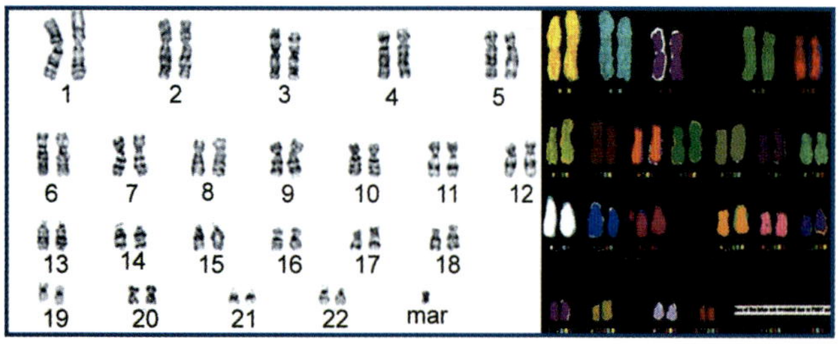

Fig. 7.9 Amniotic fluid culture of 36-year-old with increased risk for Trisomy 21 in TMT and advanced maternal age. (A) 47,**,+mar; (B) Whole chromosome paint : 47,**,+del(15)q21

better option. When a marker chromosome is observed. *The following points need to be considered:*

- Is the marker *de-novo* or of familial origin.
- The percentage of cells having marker chromosomes in the fetus and the parents
- Size of the chromosome compared to the 'G' group of chromosomes.
- Confirmation of composition by AgNOR staining.
- Whole chromosome paint.

Literature survey for risks arising from the presence of a marker chromosome should be reviewed.

However, when seen in the prenatal tissue sample its source from parent need to be confirmed. If the marker is *de novo* in origin, confirmation of its origin by whole chromosome paint is necessary to know the implications in the fetus (Fig. 7.9).

POLYPLOIDY

Polyploidy is known to occur as a postzygotic error can lead to diploid/triploid mosaicism and is seen in the vanishing twin syndrome.[14]

Triploidy is seen commonly in 1st trimester abortions but the pregnancies can even go up to term or end in stillbirth or early neonatal loss. A heteroploid cell can arise due to endoreduplication, i.e. chromosomal replication without subsequent cell division and is mostly a cultural artifact.

Abnormal ultrasound findings are most common indication where rapid karyotyping is requested for management.[15] If the fetus has abnormalities of classical syndromes, e.g. IUGR, choroid plexus cysts, renal or cardiac malformations suggestive of Trisomy 18 on ultrasound scanning, and on placental biopsy, if the karyotype report is normal, this could be a false negative result. In this case, fetal tissue analysis (amniotic fluid or fetal blood) should be done to confirm the karyotypic pattern.

At any time if a chromosomal rearrangement is detected in prenatal diagnostic sample, parental karyotype should be done on an urgent basis (Fig. 7.10).

Vanishing Twin and Mosaicism

It is known that about 7.6% pregnancies are conceived as twin pregnancies of which 6% vanish leading to one healthy twin and the other with an empty sac or remnant of the trophoblastic tissue. In such a pregnancy CVS karyotype can show a mosaic cell line, one of the karyotype will be from a persistent trophoblast of the vanished twin and the other from a healthy fetus. Occasionally in a CVS sample fetal karyotype may represent any one of the fetus. Such a possibility is discussed with a patient at the genetic counseling session.[16]

Normal Chromosomal Variants

Chromosomal variants involve segments of varying size and staining properties, majorly the heterochromatic regions of highly repeated DNA sequences. Mendelian inheritance is usually seen and probably has no influence on phenotype or health.

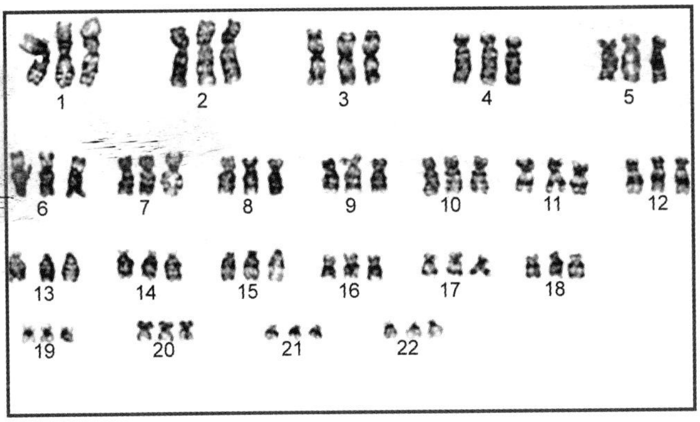

Fig. 7.10 Triploid amniotic fluid karyotype : 69,*** Amniocentesis was done for mild intrauterine growth restriction, oligohydraminos on ultrasound

The variants include large heterochromatic segments of chromosomes 1, 9, 16 and Y. Both size and position are involved in these differences. For example, variants of chromosome 9 are most frequently encountered. Enlarged heterochromatic region are described as 9qh+, small heterochromatic blocks as 9qh.

Parental karyotyping confirmation is required for a familial variant from a parent. In such cases, it should be remember that if a phenotypically normal parent is a carrier of this variant, the prognosis of the fetus is good.[17]

Chromosomal variants are observed in 3–4% of prenatal karyotypes. Such frequency makes the reporting vital for the variants. In such cases, parental karyotype must be requested. The significance of these laboratory tests is well explained to the couples, to avoid unnecessary terminations. This decisions should not be taken without prior investigation of parental karyotypes, which later may reveal a variant identical to that of fetus. Such incidences could be avoided after conducting a careful family studies for each variant. Figure 7.11A shows amniotic fluid karyotype showing 46,**,inv(9)(p11q13). Parental karyotype revealed father having the same variation (Fig. 7.11B) 46,XY,inv(9) (p11q13).

Pericentric Heterochromatic

Chromosomal instability syndrome: Commonly known instability syndromes are—Ataxia telangiectasia, Fanconis anemia, Xeroderma pigmentosum, Bloom's syndrome in at risk cases. Random observation in prenatal diagnostic sample should be carefully considered on the basis of family history. In a known carrier partner of chromosomal instability syndrome prenatal diagnosis can be achieved by studying the chromosomal breakages in cultured cells which are grown in specified media with clastogens.

Origin of chromosomal abnormalities:

- Advanced maternal age and nondisjunctional error at meiosis aneuploidy, e.g. Trisomy 47, +21, 47, +18, 47, +13
- Sex chromosomal abnormalities 47,XXX,47,XXY
- *Supernumerary markers:* Inverted duplication of 15p and cat eye syndrome (partial duplication of 22q)
- Abnormalities (not related to maternal age)possible paternal origin or postzygotic error 47,XYY (error in paternal meiotic nondisjunction at second meiotic division) 45,X (Most are with lost paternal X)
- Rearrangements, deletions, inversions, De novo translocations
- Polyploidy; triploidy—60% cases due to errors at meiosis 1 or 2 in father or dispermy.

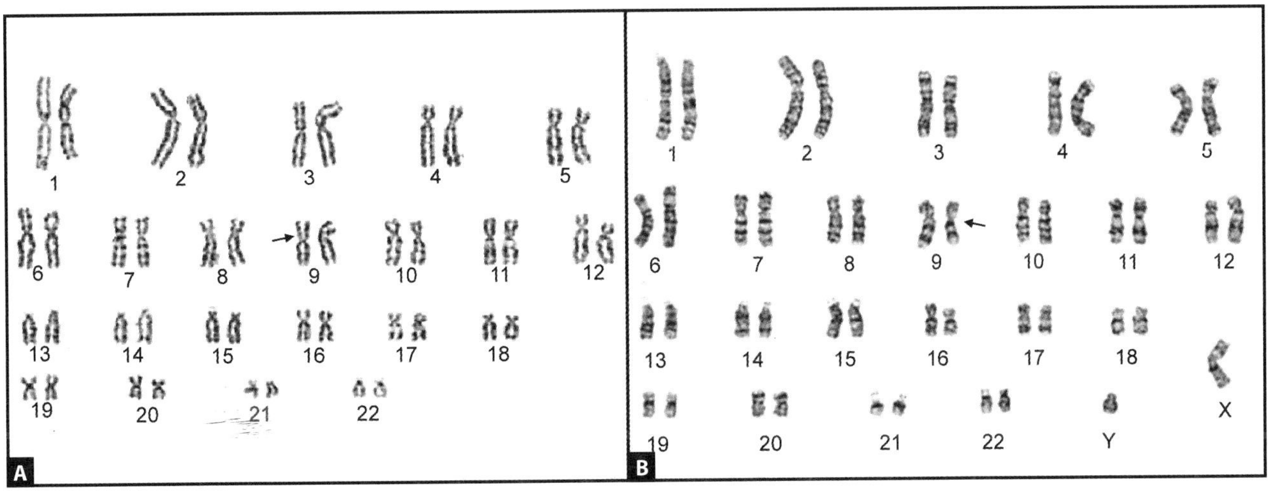

Figs 7.11A and B Amniotic fluid karyotype showing (A) 46,**,inv(9)(p11q13); (B) 46,XY,inv(9)(p11q13)

CONCLUSION

In conclusion, for further pregnancy management in case of all fetal tissue samples, which show abnormal chromosomal pattern, parental karyotyping should be considered to detect the sporadic familial origin of the same. This can help in recurrence or risk estimation and prenatal diagnosis.

REFERENCES

1. Purandarey H. Atlas of Human Chromosomal Disorders. Jaypee Brothers Medical Publishers. 2015.
2. Purandarey H, Fernandes NV, Deshmukh SV, Chavan S. Heterochromatic variations and pregnancy losses in humans. Int J Hum Genet. 2011;11(3):167-75.
3. Luthardt FW, Keitges E. Chromosomal syndromes and genetic disease. Wiley Online Library. 2001.
4. Weijerman ME, Winter de JP. Clinical practice the care of children with down syndrome. European Journal of Pediatrics. 2010;169(12):1445-52.
5. Dorothy W. Aneuploidy: Etiology and Mechanism, 10th edn. USA: Springer, USA; 1985.pp.133-48.
6. Purandarey H, Chakravarty A. Human cytogenetics techniques and clinical applications. Mumbai: Bhalani Publishing House; 2000.pp.183-94.
7. Gosden C1, Nicolaides KH, et al. Fetal blood sampling in investigation of chromosome mosaicism in amniotic fluid cell culture. Lancet. 1988;331:613-7.
8. Bardinger S, Millard C, et al. Prenatal diagnosis of trisomy 20 mosaicism indicating an extra embryonic origin. Prenatal Diagnosis. 1987;4:273-6.
9. Wilkens A, Liu H, et al. Novel clinical manifestations in Pallister-Killian syndrome: comprehensive evaluation of 59 affected individuals and review of previously reported cases. Am J Med Genet A. 2012;158A(12):2981-3214.
10. Theisen A. Rosenfeld JA, et al. aCGH detects partial tetrasomy of 12p in blood from Pallister-Killian syndrome cases without invasive skin biopsy. American Journal of Medical Genetics. 2009;149A:914-8.
11. Brambati B1, Tului L, et al. First-trimester genetic diagnosis in multiple pregnancy: principles and potential pitfalls. Prenatal Diagnosis. 1991;10:767-74.
12. Kaffe S, Perlis TE, Hsu LYF. Amniotic fluid alpha-fetoprotein levels and prenatal diagnosis of autosomal trisomies. Prenatal Diagnosis. 2005;8(3):183-7.
13. Ratcliffe S, Butler G, Jones M. Edinburgh study of growth and development of children with sex chromosome abnormalities. Birth Defects Orig Artic Ser. 1991;26:1-44.
14. Stene J, Stengel-Rutkowski S. Genetic risks of familial reciprocal and Robertsonian translocation carriers, in the cytogenetics of mammalian autosomal rearrangements. Daniel A (Ed.). 1988. pp. 3-72.
15. Benn PA, Hsu LY. Incidence and significance of supernumerary marker chromosomes in prenatal diagnosis. American Journal of Human Genetics. 1984;36(5):1092-102.
16. Hassold TJ, Jacobs PA. Trisomy in man. Annu Rev Genet. 1984;18:69-97.
17. Nicolaides KH, Rodeck CH, Gosden CM. Rapid karyotyping in non-lethal fetal malformations. The Lancet. 1986;327 (8476):283-7.

CHAPTER

8 Preconceptional Counseling and Management

Sharad Gogate

INTRODUCTION

Over the decades, the emphasis has shifted to preventive care in clinical medicine, as it is always better to avoid or diagnose a disease at preclinical stage rather than wait till a full blown stage has reached. This is much more so in field of birth defects and other genetic disorders, though most of these disorders cannot be prevented, but with expanding knowledge and understanding in the field of genetics, embryology, imaging and genetic testing, early, preclinical diagnosis is now possible. Preconception counseling and management of high-risk population is a valuable window of opportunity for seamless management. Unfortunately this window is lost in majority of situations due to lack of awareness, secondly majority of conceptions are unplanned even in high-risk cases!

Pregnancy and child birth are very critical phases in human development, both for the mother and the fetus/neonate with increased mortality and morbidity. Underlying maternal medical, surgical disorders, pregnancy-induced hypertension (PIH), environmental factors, etc. do have significant contribution to maternal fetal morbidity and mortality. Similarly congenital defects, genetic disorders, fetal growth restriction and prematurity are common causes of perinatal mortality and morbidity. Large proportion of these are modifiable by preconception counseling and evaluation.

Goals of advancing preconceptional care (Centers for Disease Control and Prevention, (Johnson et al.).[1]

Improve knowledge, attitude and behavior of men and women related to preconceptional health.

- Assure that all women of childbearing age preconceptional care which will enable them to embark on pregnancy in optimal health
- Reduce the risk of adverse pregnancy outcome in previous pregnancy by interconceptional interventions
- Reduce the disparities in adverse pregnancy outcomes.

WHO NEEDS PRECONCEPTION COUNSELING?

- Ideally every couple embarking on a pregnancy should avail of this facility!
- It will be definitely indicated in following situations:

1. *Maternal Conditions*

- *Maternal exposure*: Alcohol, tobacco, recreational drugs, etc.
- Risk teratogenicity of maternal drugs treatment.
- *Infections*: Cytomegalovirus (CMV), parvovirus, toxoplasma, syphilis, HIV-AIDS, rubella, hepatitis-B, C, exanthematous fevers, etc.
- *Medical disorders*: Diabetes, hypertension, cardiac disorders, renal disorders, hypo/hyperthyroidism, anemia and malnutrition, thrombophilia, epilepsy, psychiatric disorders, obesity, polycystic ovarian disease (PCOD), phenylketonuria (PKU), Marfan syndrome, etc.
- *History of unfavorable pregnancy outcome*: Repeated pregnancy loss, stillbirth, intrauterine growth restriction (IUGR), prematurity, PIH, etc.
- Advanced maternal/paternal age.
- Personal or family history of genetic disorder.
- *Embarking on assisted reproductive technology (ART) program*: IVF-ET, gamete donation, intracytoplasmic sperm injection (ICSI), testicular sperm aspiration (TESA), etc.

2. *Fetal Conditions*

- *Chromosomal disorders*: Aneuploidy, translocation, deletion, etc.
- *Single gene disorders*: Hemoglobinopathies, muscular dystrophy, cystic fibrosis, etc.
- *Multifactorial disorders*: Mental retardation, NTD, coronary heart disease (CHD), deafness, autism, etc.
- Birth defects in previous pregnancies.
  Consanguinity, ethnic history, environmental factors.

Steps of Preconception Counseling

The preconception counseling should be provided by multi-specialty setup, as no one person or specialty can cover all the complex problems involved. Secondly it will help in a seamless management of the pregnancy, childbirth and later management if all the specialties are on board from the beginning. The major steps of involved are as follows (Chitayat D et al).[2]

Information Gathering

- History taking, which should include general medical surgical history, genetic history of the couple, proband, family. A properly designed proforma should be used.
- Prepare a three generation pedigree chart, this helps in understanding the inheritance pattern, risk of recurrence. The pedigree should be three generational and have information on the couple seeking counseling, their first, second and third degree relatives including the existence of birth defects, inherited conditions, mental retardation, multiple miscarriages, stillbirths, infertility, ethnic background, exposure to medication, chronic medical diseases and consanguinity (Jones et al. 1990). Standardized pedigree nomenclature should be used to decrease the chance of wrongly interpreting the family's medical and genetic information (Bennett et al.).[3]
- Gather all information about any underlying medical/ surgical condition, if already identified, to assess its staging, severity, impact on reproductive abilities, risk to mother and fetus, management options, etc.
- Full work-up of previously affected member, family, which will include imaging, mutational analysis, screening test so as to arrive at accurate diagnosis.

Establishing or Verifying Diagnosis

If past medical records are not available and establishing or verifying the diagnosis, either in one member of the couple or a family member is important for providing risk information to the couple, then evaluation, by physical examination, at a clinic visit may be necessary. If a clinical evaluation is recommended for a family member, then that family member or legal guardian needs to provide consent for an evaluation. Often, additional investigations may be ordered as indicated, in order to augment the clinical evaluation in trying to reach a diagnosis.

Risk Assessment

Once the reason for referral, diagnosis of the underlying medical, surgical or genetic condition is established, we have to understand its natural history, staging, short-term, long-term prognosis. The likely impact of the disorder on maternal health as well as fetal health and development as well as that of pregnancy on the underlying condition should be well understood.

Information Giving

Information gathered by the following steps should be shared with patient and family in a frank, nondirectional manner. Likely plan of action if pregnancy is to be embarked upon should be explained in detail along with likely problems, necessary screening, diagnostic tests, ante/postnatal therapy (if required). Options like medical termination of pregnancy (MTP) (if recurrence occurs), Gamete donation, Surrogacy and adoption should be also offered, when so indicated.

Preconception, Periconception Interventions

By the time a conception is confirmed by urinary or serum beta human chorionic gonadotropin (hCG) assay, it is already second/third week post implantation. Organogenesis particularly central nervous system (CNS) development is already underway. Hormonal, immunological and other adjustments in maternal, fetal environment have already being established. Hence, any interventions started at this stage will be suboptimal at it is best! This is the most vital window of opportunity to correct underlying pathology, deficiency so as to improve the chances of more healthy, stable conception and a stable maternal milieu. *More about these measures at a later stage!*

It is not possible to cover all the situations amenable to preconception counseling and management in a small chapter. So, we will take some examples from each of the category.

Maternal Conditions

Maternal exposure to alcohol, tobacco, recreational drugs: With rapid urbanization, changing life styles incidence of alcohol, smoking and recreational drugs is on the rise in adolescence as well as grownups. That includes young women with increasing numbers showing alcohol abuse, addiction. Exposure to alcohol during pregnancy leads to fetal alcohol syndrome (FAS). According to various studies, the worldwide incidence of infants with fetal alcohol syndrome (FAS) ranges from 0.5–3/1000 births and 4.3% among mothers who drink heavily during pregnancy. The incidence of infants with fetal alcohol effects (FAE) is currently estimated to be 2–6/1000 births Sampson et al. 1989). The effects include typical facies, cleft lip/palate, miscarriage, preterm labor, IUGR and IUFD. It has been found that FAS represents only a small part of a much larger clinical and social problem termed fetal alcohol effects (FAE). Although children with FAE have better cognitive abilities than those with FAS, their behavioral functions, especially social adaptability, are similar. The combination of better cognition with poor social adaptability can result in disruptive behavior at school, inappropriate sexual behavior, drug problems, delinquency, dependent living, and unemployment (Stratton et al.).[4] Clinicians should be aware and counsel women contemplating a pregnancy of the clinical and behavioral manifestations of FAS and FAE.

Cigarette smoking: Cigarette smoke contains over 1000 different compounds including nicotine, carbon monoxide, hydrogen cyanide and trace elements such as lead, nickel and cadmium. Cigarette smoking has been associated with a decrease in fertility in males and females. In males, cigarette smoking has been associated with a decrease in sperm motility. In females, cigarette smoking increases the incidence of conception delay and primary and secondary infertility. Furthermore, women who smoke may have a modest increase in risks for ectopic pregnancy and spontaneous abortion. Carbon monoxide has a high affinity to hemoglobin forming carboxyhemoglobin and thus decreasing the hemoglobin ability to carry oxygen, which can lead to fetal hypoxia. Nicotine is known to cross the placenta and can reach levels in the amniotic fluid and fetal blood that exceeds the maternal blood levels (Koren et al.)[5] leading to cardiovascular and central nervous system effects. In addition, nicotine has been shown to be a potent vasoconstrictor and can reduce the blood supply to the uterus and placenta, which may be the reason for the higher incidence of spontaneous abortions among pregnant women who smoke. Cigarette smoking has also been found to be associated with an increased incidence of placenta previa and placental abruption and thus increased perinatal mortality and morbidity.

Diabetes in pregnancy: India going to be a world hotspot for diabetes cases! It is estimated that about 1 in 200 women of childbearing age have type I or type II diabetes before pregnancy (pre-existing diabetes) and another 2–5% develop gestational diabetes. Women with poorly controlled pre-existing diabetes in the early weeks of pregnancy are three to four times more likely than nondiabetic women to have a baby with a major congenital abnormality mainly heart defect or neural tube defect (NTD) as well as being at increased risk of miscarriage and stillbirth. They also have a higher incidence of pregnancy-related high blood pressure, polyhydramnios, preterm delivery and stillbirth. The effect of deranged diabetic control on incidence of major congenital deformities is shown in graph below (Sheffield et al.).[6]

Women with gestational diabetes do not have an increased risk of having a baby with a birth defect. However, poorly controlled gestational diabetes with fasting hyperglycemia has higher risk of congenital anomalies as well as risk of stillbirth. Some of these women may have had unrecognized diabetes that began prior to pregnancy and therefore would be at increased risk of birth defects (Fig. 8.1).

Women with poorly controlled diabetes (gestational or pre-existing) are at increased risk of macrosomia, respiratory

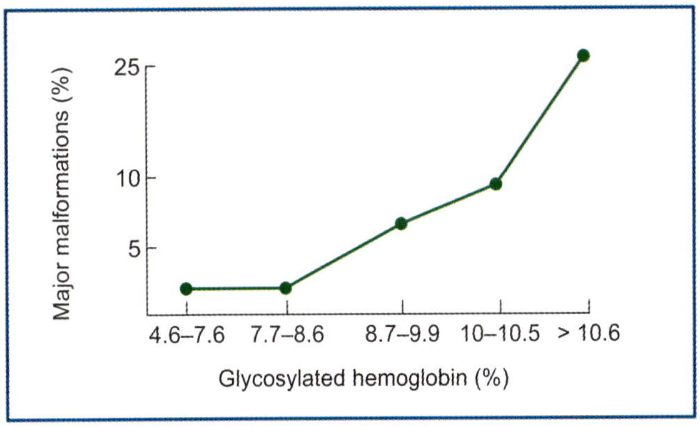

Fig. 8.1 First trimester glycosylated values and congenital malformations in diabetes

distress syndrome hypoglycemia and hyperbilirubinemia. Babies of women with poorly controlled diabetes also may be at increased risk of developing obesity and diabetes as young adults.

A detailed evaluation about severity, duration, possible end organ damage, medication for diabetes should be done before planning for pregnancy. Associated problems like obesity, hypertension should be kept under control.

Hypothyroidism: Thyroid hormones are important regulators of metabolism and development and have effects on many body organs. Thyroid dysfunction is common in the general population. Furthermore, subclinical thyroid dysfunction [defined as serum thyroid-stimulating hormone (TSH) levels outside the normal reference range with normal levels of fT4 and fT3], is even more common. The prevalence of both clinical and subclinical hyper- and hypothyroidism was found to be greater in women and increased with age. Hypothyroidism occurs during pregnancy relatively frequently. A nationwide US survey showed that a raised serum thyrotropin concentration, in excess of 6 µU/mL, has been reported in 2.5% of all pregnant women, with overt hypothyroidism in more than 10% of that group. Untreated hyper and hypothyroidism in women can result in infertility. The developing fetal brain, furthermore, is critically dependent on circulating levels of maternal thyroxine (T4) during the first 12 weeks of pregnancy, before the fetal thyroid begins to produce thyroid hormones (Contempre et al.)[7] Moreover, pregnant patients with hypothyroidism are at increased risk of obstetric complications, such as fetal loss, gestational hypertension, abruptio placentae, and a poor perinatal outcome (Davis et al. 1988). Adequate treatment with thyroid hormones started as soon as pregnancy is diagnosed and properly monitored all through the pregnancy greatly reduces the frequency of these maternal, fetal complications (Glinoer et al.).[8]

Other Maternal Conditions

Certain genetic disorders and concurrent pregnancy can have mutually deleterious effects. Increased risk of thrombophlebitis, embolic episodes is seen during pregnancy and childbirth in homocystinuria (Parris WCV et al.)[9] Ehler-Danlos syndrome and Marfan syndrome have higher risk of aortic/vascular rupture and uterine rupture during pregnancy and childbirth (Lipscomb KJ et al.).[10] Sickle cell, epilepsy, SLE and myotonic muscular dystrophy and untreated maternal Phenylketonuria increase risk of pregnancy losses, birth defects considerably. Elevated maternal phenylalanine levels during pregnancy are teratogenic. Unmonitored and untreated pregnant women with PKU have an increased risk (24%) for spontaneous miscarriage and their offspring have an increased risk for intrauterine growth retardation (40%), microcephaly (73%), psychomotor retardation (92%), and congenital heart defects (10%). Hence proper control of these prior to conception and close monitoring of maternal and fetal health all through the pregnancy is essential.

History of Unfavorable Pregnancy Outcome

Repeated pregnancy loss, stillbirth, IUGR, prematurity, PIH contribute considerably to maternal and fetal mortality, morbidity. The underlying cause, investigative protocol and treatment modalities depend at what period of gestation the event has occurred. It is best to evaluate such cases at preconception stage, identify the underlying cause (which is possible in only 50–60% cases). Etiology is varied genetic, hormonal, anatomical, immunological, and infection, environmental, etc. Complete evaluation and correction of specific cause identified cause is essential before embarking on conception (Gogate SG).[11]

Genetic Disorder in Couple/Family Member/ Previous Conceptions

Although individual genetic disorders are rare, collective incidence is not insignificant (Table 8.1).

Table 8.1 Incidence of various genetic disorders in general population (Baird et al.)[12]

Category	Rate per million livebirths	Percentage of total births
Autosomal-recessive	1395.4	0.14
Autosomal-dominant	1665.3	0.17
X-linked	532.4	0.05
Chromosomal	1845.4	0.18
Multifactorial	46582.6	4.64
Genetic unknown	1164.2	0.12
Total	53175.3	5.32
All congenital anomalies	52808.2	5.28

It is essential to do complete evaluation of the underlying genetic problem at preconception stage. This includes confirmation of the genetic disorder, find out exact mutation/ chromosomal defect in the affected person; mutation studies of the couple, risk of recurrence and various options for prenatal diagnosis should be discussed along with reproductive options with patient and family.

Preconception and Periconception Interventions: Nutritional Status and Physical Fitness

This is most vital as adequate, balanced nutrition of the would be mother is vital for taking on the responsibilities of pregnancy childbirth and nursing of the newborn. We have two extreme scenarios, on one side, majority of the young girls from rural and low socioeconomic sections have chronic malnutrition, moderate to severe anemia, poor physical development resulting in higher risk of infections like STIs, TB, parasitic infections, etc. These girls also have higher risk of pregnancy complications like severe anemia, PIH, prematurity, intrauterine growth restriction (IUGR), antepartum and postpartum blood loss, etc.

On other hand, we have increasing incidence of childhood obesity in the adolescent girls and boys mainly in urban areas due to unbalanced diet and lack of proper exercise, high incidence of PCOD. Hence, it is vital to correct these nutritional disorders prior to conception.

MANAGEMENT OF SPECIFIC DISORDER IDENTIFIED

Any specific factor found during the evaluation should be thoroughly evaluated, brought under reasonable control; medication should be adjusted to achieve good control at minimum effective dose and switching over to safer molecule where ever possible. Good liaison with the relevant clinician before and during pregnancy is essential.

Vaccinations and Immunization

Prophylactic immunization for Rubella, Hepatitis B, C, E, etc. should be done at preconception stage only. Prophylactic and screening for potentially teratogenic maternal infections like TORCH group, HIV-AIDS and other sexually transmitted infections is equally important prior to conception.

Environmental factors like illicit drugs, smoking, and alcohol, exposure to excessive heat and occupational exposure to potential teratogens should be curtailed where ever possible in both partners.

It is also necessary to evaluate the couple from fertility point of view and take care of any problems identified, as the couple is very anxious to conceive and any delay in attaining conception adds to the anxiety.

Table 8.2 The role of various vitamins, micronutrients, and daily requirement deficiency effects

	Metabolic role	Deficiency effect	MDR
Folic acid	Cell metabolism, DNA, CNS	NTD, clefting, BOH, IUGR, PIH, anemia, aneuploidy	500 μg
Vitamin B_{12}	CNS, hematological	NTD, anemia, CNS dysfunction, hyper-homocysteinemia	500 μg
Choline	Metabolism, brain function, transport, lung maturity		450 mg
DHA	Brain, retina, skin	CNS, eye problems	100–300 mg
Iodine	Thyroid function, CNS	Maternal, fetal hypothyroidism	150 μg
Iron	RBCs, muscle protein	Anemia	30–40 mg

Periconception Therapy

Folic acid, B_{12}: Folic acid, methylcobalamin (B_{12}) play vital role during all stages of conception. Incidence of folic acid deficiency is quite high in general population (~7–10%). Incidence of B_{12} deficiency is much more common (almost 30%), particularly in strict vegetarians. The role of various vitamins, micronutrients, deficiency effects and daily requirement are shown in Table 8.2.

Hence preconception therapy with supplementation with folic acid, B_{12}, pyridoxine hydrochloride (vitamin B_6) is recommended. It is necessary to start this at least 2–3 months before conception and to be continued for first 12–14 weeks. As daily replacement only 500 μg of folic acid and B_{12} is adequate. For therapeutic purpose in high risk of BOH, NTD, etc. 1500 μg of folic acid and 1500 μg of B_{12} is enough. Any higher dosing can have toxicity. Active forms of these vitamins are needed only in cases with genetic causes like methylene tetrahydrofolate reductase (MTHFR) deficiency, hyperhomocysteinemia.

Zinc supplementation: Zinc plays very vital role in cell metabolism, embryogenesis. Deficiency of zinc is quite common so it is necessary to supplement it as well.

Low dose aspirin therapy: Low dose aspirin therapy is indicated in patients with h/o PIH, IUGR and antiphospholipids syndrome in past conceptions. 75 mg of enteric coated aspirin should be started preconceptionally and continued during pregnancy. A word of caution about patients with gastric acidity disorders when putting them on this drug.

Low molecular heparin, steroid therapy: This is indicated in unexplained IUGR or stillbirth, thrombophilia disorders and autoimmune disorders like systemic lupus erythematosus (SLE). Any patient on oral Warfarin should be immediately switched to Low molecular heparin as soon as conception is confirmed by rising titres of beta-hCG.

Pure progesterone: It may be indicated cases with early pregnancy losses due to LPD and should be started in second half of the cycle and continued for first 10 weeks.

CONCLUSION

Preconception counseling, evaluation and management forms an integral and vital part of high-risk pregnancy management. It requires a multispecialty approach, it requires to be incorporated in mean corpuscular hemoglobin (MCH) program. The overall benefits to the couple and the society are worth the extra efforts!!

REFERENCES

1. Johnson K, Posner SF, BiermannJ, et al. Recommendations to improve preconception health and healthcare-United States, DRP reconception care Working Group. MMWR Recomm Rep. 2006;55(6):1.
2. Chitayat David, Riyana BH. Preconception genetic counseling. In: Preventive Genetics, Sharad Gogate (Ed), Jaypee Brothers Medical Publishers (P) Ltd. 2006. pp. 78-80.
3. Bennett RL, Steinhaus KA, Uhrich SB, O'Sullivan CK, Resta RG, Lochner-Doyle D, et al. Recommendations for standardized human pedigree nomenclature. Pedigree Standardization Task Force of the National Society of Genetic Counselors. Am J Hum Genet. 1995;56:745-52.
4. Stratton WT. Medical care and the criminal law. Kans Med. 1996;97(1):8-9.
5. Koren G, Gladstone D, Robeson C, Robieux I. The perception of teratogenic risk of cocaine. Teratology. 1992;46:567-71.
6. Sheffield JS, Butler-Koster EJasey BM, et al. Maternal diabetes melitus and infant malformations. Obstet Gynecol. 2002; 100:925.
7. Contempre B, Jauniaux E, Culvo R, Jurkovic D, Campbell S, de Escobar GM. Detection of thyroid hormones in human embryonic cavities during the first trimester of pregnancy. J Clin Endocrinol Metab. 1993;77:1719-22.
8. Glinoer D. Management of hypo- and hyperthyroidism during pregnancy. Growth Horm IGF Res. 2003;13(Suppl A):S45-54.
9. Parris WCV, Quimby CW. Anaesthetic considerations for the patient with Homocystinuria. Anaesth Analg. 1982;61:708.
10. Lipscomb KJ, Smith JC, Clarke B, et al. Outcome of pregnancies in women with Marfan's syndrome. Br J Obstet Gynaecol. 1997;104:201.
11. Gogate SG. Preventive genetics: holistic healthcare. In: Preventive Genetics, Gogate SG (Ed), Jaypee Brothers Medical Publishers (P) Ltd. 2006. pp.10-12.
12. Baird PA, Anderson TW, Newcomb HB, et al. Genetic disorders in children and young adults. Am J Hum Genet. 1988;42:677.

CHAPTER

9 Role of Genetics in Reproductive Failure

Rajendra M Jain

INTRODUCTION

Development of life depends on nature and nurture, i.e. genetic and environment factors. The nuclear integrity of the gametes is essential for gametogenesis to have healthy baby.

This chapter basically covers common genetic conditions which affect the reproductive failure and requires genetic testing to evaluate the infertile couples.[1] Preimplantation genetic diagnosis (PGD) is out of scope for this chapter hence will not be covered. *This chapter is broadly divided into five sections namely:*

1. General considerations of genetic testing and genetic counseling for infertile couple
2. Genetic testing during female infertility work up
3. Genetic testing during male infertility work up
4. Genetic testing for the cases of spontaneous abortions
5. Role of genetics in special situation in fertility practice.

GENERAL CONSIDERATIONS ON GENETIC TESTING

Infertility or subfertility is defined as the inability of a couple to conceive a child for at least one year having regular, unprotected sexual intercourse. In contrast to the WHO criteria, which define the period as two years but one year is more appropriate due to time pressure and increasing age of the patients in current scenario.

As clinician, we commonly address and stress for seminal, cervical, uterine, tubal, peritoneal factors, but hardly give a thought to genetic factor during infertility work up. The unexplained infertility constitutes significant number of patients, hence, it is imperative to diagnose genetic causes for infertility before offering them any ART treatment.

Genetic counseling mainly focuses on an extensive evaluation of the familial history and if necessary, clinical-genetic examinations, which is required in order to decide whether and which further genetic testing is appropriate for the couple and the possible consequences for the carriers and for potentially affected family members.

In the era of assisted reproductive technologies (ART), we realized now that genetic factors play significant role in successful reproductive outcome. The spermatogenesis, oogenesis, fertilization, embryo cleavage, blastocyst formation with paternal gene expression, implantation, these all requires genetic integrity of gametes, hence, it is more relevant to understand the various available genetic tests for infertility work up in each partners.

In female partner, reproductive failure due to premature ovarian failure[2] or early menopause or low ovarian reserve poses great dilemma and some phenotype presentations such as Turner syndrome may offer some clue about genetic abnormalities and genetic counseling for RPL or RIF, POF, Fragile-X and PCOD plays significant role.[3,4] While in male partner, abnormal semen analysis requires explanations and available modalities of treatment. The counseling of these couples usually require support of genetic testing reports. Repeated failures of ART cycles (IUI/IVF) frustrate clinician as well as patients therefore genetic testing is more relevant in present scenario in them and suggest preventive strategies by knowing in advance. The genetic status of couple thus can improve results of treatment or offer them PGD or prenatal genetic diagnosis and therapy.

Traditionally, we categorize genetic causes in four groups which are chromosomal aneuploidies, single gene disorders, multifactorial inheritance and non-Mendelian inheritance of mitochondrial disorder.

Spectrum of chromosome abnormalities:

- Too many or too few chromosomes (aneuploidy)
- Structural alterations
  - Missing piece of a chromosome (deletion)
  - Duplication of a chromosome
  - An upside-down chromosome (inversion)
  - Swapping of chromosome pieces (translocation)
- A change in the gene's DNA sequence (mutation).

Various traditional methodological approaches of genetic analyses are cytogenetic (karyotyping), molecular cytogenetics (FISH technique), molecular (*FMR1* gene[5] and

Y-microdeletion of AZF region). The various highly sensitive and advanced techniques such as array comparative genomic hybridization (aCGH), which is future diagnostic approach and aimed at improving the quality and efficiency of aneuploidy analysis. Next generation sequencing or massively parallel sequencing will be soon the part of molecular diagnostic panel.

Up to now, approximately 300 gene mutations are identified, of which 70 are syndromes,[6] are known to cause reproductive disorders. During risk assessment, consideration is given for genetic hetrogeneity and environment impact and the problems of calculation of risk are mainly due to reduced penetration, delayed age of onset of disorder and use of linked marker for genetic diagnosis. Some external environmental factors which can result in DNA damage of oocytes or sperms are smoking, xenobiotic, radiation, chemotherapy or accumulation of the reactive oxygen species.

Research is going on to identify novel biomarkers (proteomics application) for embryo implantation and maintenance of pregnancy by corpus luteum and oocyte aging may available in near future for female infertility work up.

Genetic Counseling[7] for Infertile Couple

- Genetic counselor's role:
  - Risk assessment by drawing pedigree chart (keeping in the mind about reduced penetration/delayed age of onset of disorder and use of linked marker in laboratory for genetic analysis). The autosomal dominant disorders have vertical pattern of inheritance while autosomal recessive disorders have horizontal pattern of inheritance but sex-linked recessive disorder has male-to-male transmission. It means knights move pattern of inheritance.
  - Interpretation of positive genetic test results is required by genetic counselors.
- Patient's expectation (communication) from genetic counselor:
  - Want to understand the medical facts and genetic diagnosis.
  - Want to know heredity contributes to the genetic disorder.
  - Want to know the risk of recurrence.
  - Able to arrive at their own informed decision about reproductive options and other alternative approaches to conception.
  - Explanation of prenatal diagnostic techniques, their limitations and risks.
- Family member's expectation from genetic counselor:
  - They like to know appropriate diagnosis and require preconception counseling.
- To address their concerns relating to development/ transmission of hereditary disorder and carrier status about such as sickle cell anemia, thalassemia, etc.
- Consideration should be given to consequences of each possible course of action and counselor must be nonjudgmental and nondirective in his opinion.

INVESTIGATION OF GENETIC FACTOR DURING FEMALE INFERTILITY WORK UP

From all infertility cases approximately 3.3–9.8% are attributed by female chromosomal abnormalities.[8,9] Chromosomally abnormal embryos have a low rate of implantation, and often lead to miscarriages or livebirth with physical abnormalities, developmental delay, and mental retardation. The chromosome analysis of the parent identifies inherited genetic problems in less than 5% of couples.

Chromosome Analysis (Cytogenetics)

Aneuploidy karyotype 45X, which causes Turner syndrome is the most common chromosomal abnormality in females and the incidence is 1/2500 live-born girls. The diagnosis is often delayed until pre-school when growth retardation becomes apparent. Adolescents with Turner syndrome are clinically short statured 1.5 mt height, neck webbing, broad chest, wide elbow carrying angle and amenorrhea but 10% attend menarche. Some are only diagnosed when presenting with primary ovarian failure (primary amenorrhea) but patient's intelligence is usually normal. The high incidence of mosaicism in Turner syndrome of 50% is quite remarkable. Mosaicism is defined as the presence of at least two cell lines with different karyotypes, which have developed from a single fertilized egg. The prognosis and therapeutic options of the existence of genetic mosaicism is essential to understand in case of infertility. In some mosaicism, 45X/46XX germ cell formation may be functional, which allows for a normal or only slightly impaired fertility. If the chromosomal abnormalities are detected early, the patient should be told about the high risk of premature ovarian failure and thus be recommended to procreate early in life. The pregnant women with Turner syndrome or Turner mosaicism have an empirical chance of 15% to have children with 45X monosomy. A mosaicism 45X/46XY is associated with a high risk for gonadoblastoma thus gonadectomy should be considered.

The 47XXX karyotype has an incidence of 1 in 1000 and suffer from premature ovarian failure with infertility. The 2/3rd of the carriers has a clinically normal phenotype while 1/3rd has learning difficulties and psychotic disorders. In women with 47XXX karyotype, the risk for the offspring to carry X chromosomal aneuploidy is <1%.

The structural chromosomal abnormalities include translocations, deletions and duplications. Translocation is the most common of these conditions. Parent who carries a translocation is frequently normal, but embryo may receive too much or too less genetic material, and a miscarriage often results. Couples with translocation chromosome defects may be benefitted from preimplantation genetic diagnosis (PGD) in conjunction with in vitro fertilization (IVF).

- Balanced translocations (chromosomal exchange without loss or gain of genetic material)
  - Robertsonian translocations: (incidence 1.35%) in which two acrocentric chromosomes fuses.
  - Classical balanced reciprocal translocations: (incidence 2.0%) It is hampering the normal course of meiosis, and the affected chromosomes form quadrivalents instead of bivalents, which can cause chromosomal segregation problems and germ cell arrest. Amongst all infertility patients, females are less affected by translocations than males. Translocations can very often lead to abortions due to chromosomal imbalances.[10]
- Unbalanced translocations (chromosomal exchange with loss or gain of genetic material)

The loss (deletion) of the short arm of the X chromosome results in the typical clinical picture of Turner syndrome. The chromosomal findings can vary from a simple loss of the short arm (monosomy Xp) to its partial loss or the loss of the short arms due to the fusion of the long arms of the X chromosome at the centromere. The latter results in the karyotype of monosomy Xp combined with trisomy Xq.

Premature ovarian failure is characterized by the loss of normal function of the ovaries before the age of 40 years having incidence of 1:100. It can be caused by autoimmune diseases, but in most of the cases, the exact cause is unknown. Geneticists claim that there is likely to be a genetic basis for the condition in few women, since number of cases occurs within families. Some of chromosome X defects are also attributed for primary ovarian insufficiency such as:

- Turner syndrome (45XO or mosaicism)
- Fragile-X syndrome[11,12] (*FMR1* gene premutation): 14% of those with a family history of POF carry a Fragile-X permutation. Mutations in the *FMR1* (Fragile X Mental Retardation 1) gene located in the long arm of the X chromosome (Xq27.3) are differentiated into full mutations. Premutations and Intermediate alleles depends on numbers of CGG repeat.

A typical *FMR1* gene mutation is caused by expanded CGG repeats[5] in the untranslated region of the first exon. Normal alleles have 5–49 repeats, intermediate alleles 50–58 repeats, premutations 59–200 repeats and full mutations >200 repeats. A full mutation develops due to transmission of a permutation from the mother with the subsequent expansion of CGG repeats.

A full mutation results in the hypermethylation of the surrounding DNA region with a more or less complete transcriptional gene silencing and thus a missing gene product and the prevalence of full mutations is rather low with 1:8000 in women.

A premutations result in an overexpression of the gene. The incidence varies from 1:75 to 1:152, depending on the geographical region. On average, these patients enter menopause five years earlier compared to the general population. During counseling, it should be emphasized that carriers of premutations have an increased risk for male offspring with fragile X syndrome and increased risk for female progeny with learning difficulties or slight mental impairment (late onset progressive neurodegenerative diseases).[13]

Molecular Genetic Testing

Single-gene abnormalities are mutations caused by changes in the DNA sequence of a gene and alters the functioning of cells due to a lack of protein/enzymes. Single-gene disorders usually indicate a family history of a specific genetic disease such as cystic fibrosis (CF) and Tay Sachs.

The Tay Sachs disease is fatal disorder, having feature of harmful quantities of a fatty substance build up in tissues and nerve cells in the brain. These single-gene abnormalities diseases are rare and usually devastating to a family. Although a couple may otherwise have no fertility problems, IVF and PGD can work together to spare couple from problem, where there is a known single-gene family history.

The female partner of the CBAVD patient carrying CFTR mutation should be screened for the mutations in *CFTR* gene before ART procedures. When *both partners are carriers of CFTR mutations*, the prenatal diagnosis (CVS or amniocentesis) for CF should strongly be recommended during genetic counseling as the fetus is at risk of cystic fibrosis disease.[14]

Young women at risk of premature ovarian failure and endometriosis and early menopause may have changes in specific genes. There are a number of genetic modifications that are associated with syndromal or non-syndromal ovarian failure, XX gonadal dysgenesis or other fertility problems. Women with fertility issues and increased FSH levels before the age of 40 with a normal cytogenetic report should undergo genetic counseling and molecular genetic testing of the *FMR1* gene.

Adrenogenital syndrome having polycystic ovaries and approximately 95% of all androgenital syndrome cases are caused by the autosomal recessive transmission of 21-hydroxylase deficiency due to mutation of the gene *CYP21A2* located on chromosome 6. The prevalence of the classic type is 1:10000 to 1:15000 and can already be diagnosed in child or infancy stages. In contrast, late-onset androgenital syndrome (presence of >20% enzymatic activity) has a prevalence of 1 in 1000.

Apart from polycystic ovaries and menstrual disorders (secondary amenorrhea or oligomenorrhea), hirsutism and acne as well as increased DHEAS and 17-OH progesterone blood levels in the follicular phase of the cycle are typical symptoms of late-onset Androgenital syndrome. If there is suspicious late-onset androgenital syndrome then molecular diagnostics should be performed in order to exclude or confirm mutations in the *CYP21A2* gene.

There is currently only one Genome Wide Association Study (GWAS)[15] performed by Knauff et al. 2009 on 99 POF patients with 235 unrelated female controls and one single nucleotide polymorphism (SNP) in the gene *ADAMTS19* (Disintegrin-like and Metalloprotease with thrombospondin type I motif) having a role in normal gonad formation and function. Among the other genes under study are *GDF9* (Growth Differentiation Factor 9) and Bone Morphogenetic Protein 15 (*BMP15*) for diagnosis of POF/POI.

Mitochondrial DNA Disorders (Non-Mendelian Pattern of Inheritance)

Mitochondrial DNA is inherited only from our mothers unlike nuclear genes (oocyte has ~2x 2000 thousand mitochondrial copies). The increased ROS that results in mitochondrial DNA damage and aging of oocytes, patients usually present as unexplained poor ovarian reserve.

Since the identification of first mitochondrial DNA mutation[16-18] in 1988, there has been more and more identification of mitochondria DNA mutations, which are responsible for mitochondrial disorders. Genetic heterogeneity together with heterogeneous clinical picture associated with mitochondrial dysfunction poses a major challenge in management of disorder and effective therapy has remained elusive till date. The impaired oxidative phosphorylation[19] leading to a decrease in cellular energy (ATP) production is the significant cause underlying mitochondrial DNA disorder.

The nuclear and environmental factors may also influence the expression of mitochondrial DNA defect. Due to complexities of mitochondrial DNA transmission and segregation, the prenatal diagnosis of mitochondrial disorders has not been very successful. The results obtained from chorionic villus sampling (CVS) have not been very reliable for prenatal diagnosis due to the difference in the level of mutant mitochondrial DNA in CVS and the fetus. Studies have also shown that the mitochondrial DNA mutants may segregate in the placenta. Therefore, single CVS samples may not represent the mutant level in the complete placenta. Prenatal genetic diagnosis has been successfully employed in a few mitochondrial DNA point mutations, such as T8993G for NARP and A3243G for MELAS[20] mitochondrial disorders.

Screening test for mitochondrial DNA disorders is by pre-implantation genetic diagnosis (PGD)[21,22] (Trophectoderm biopsy) of mitochondrial DNA disorders has been applied to a very limited extent for few common point mutations (3243A>G load is measured).[23,24] PGD generally eliminates the risk of an affected child by selecting an embryo with zero percent mutation.

Treatment is mitochondrial replacement in oocyte or zygote[25,26] is still under research by following methods like the transfer of the metaphase II spindle (nucleus) from the unfertilized oocyte of an affected woman to an enucleated donor oocyte or the nuclear genome from the pronuclear stage zygote of an affected woman is transferred to an enucleated donor 2PN zygote.

INVESTIGATION OF GENETIC FACTORS DURING MALE INFERTILITY WORK UP (TABLE 9.1)[27]

Due to natural selection of sperm during fertilization, a genetic defect cannot be transmitted to the offspring results the maintenance of reproductive fitness of the species.

Table 9.1 Male infertility work up algorithm

Azoospermia	Obstructive	Congenital bilateral or unilateral absence of vas deferens	CFTR mutations sequencing in both partners essential
	Nonobstructive	Y microdeletion (8–18% incidence)	
		Sex chromosome aneuploidy	47XXY, 48XXYY, mosaicism (XO/XY), XX male (SRY +ve on X chromosome)
Oligospermia	Chromosome abnormalities		
	Y microdeletion		
Normal sperm count	Chromosome abnormalities: Balanced translocations, etc.		

The causes of male factor infertility are multifactorial with an estimated 50% contributed by genetic abnormalities. The development of intracytoplasmic sperm injection (ICSI)[28] has completely changed the treatment of severe male infertility (severe spermatogenesis defects) and allowing many men the opportunity to father their own children (Palermo et al. 1992) and bypassing nature's protective mechanisms that were developed during evolution to prevent fertilization by defective sperm is cause of concern to all and the long-term implications for child conceived through ICSI remain largely unknown,[29] hence there may be an increased risk of sex chromosome aneuploidies and birth defects in the children of these men.

The seminal parameters obtained through a conventional semen analysis does not provide complete answer about the fertilizing potential of semen and the ability to lead to a healthy embryo and an on-going pregnancy. Therefore, comprehensive study of male factor is required to determine other parameters, such as sperm aneuploidies, DNA fragmentation index, and Y microdeletion.

Cytogenetic Analysis

In India, burden of genetic defect is high and mainly due to consanguineous marriage. The cytogenetic analysis (karyotyping) and polymerase chain reaction (PCR) testing for Y-chromosome microdeletions are the genetic tests currently recommended by the American Urological Association (AUA) and American Society of Reproductive Medicine (ASRM, 2001) to detect genetic abnormalities in men with a sperm density $\leq 5 \times 10^6$ who are considering IVF.

Karyotyping is conventional cytogenetic analysis tool used widely to study and analyze chromosomes. The structure and number of chromosomes have been linked to various genetic disorders that are classified into different categories, such as aneuploidy (Klienfelters syndrome 47XXY), deletion, duplication (extra copy of chromosome), translocation (reciprocal-swapping of two chromosome pieces or Robertsonian-fusion of two long arms of acrosomic chromosomes and complete loss of short arms).

The most common genetic disorder in male is Klinfelter syndrome,[6,30] karyotyping 47 XXY,[31] not diagnosed until adulthood, patient is azoospermic with small soft testes and gynecomastia. They are under musculine and have normal lifespan with normal intelligence. They may require hormonal replacement with screening for diabetes mellitus and breast cancer. Azoospermia hence no genetic implication in their offspring (AID child) but some opt for Micro-TESE + ICSI and may have child and genetic implication is under study till now but seems lower than expected.

Sperm DNA Fragmentation

A high level of sperm DNA fragmentation in sperm cells[32] may be cause of male infertility that conventional examinations like sperm concentration, motility, and morphology assessment cannot detect but also occurs in men with normal semen parameters in 10% cases. The genetic integrity of the spermatozoa is essential for normal embryo development and in order for spermatozoa to be fertile; the correct decondensation of chromatin after fertilization is must. The abnormal chromatin structure (microdeletions or DNA fragmentation) will all reduce the sperm's ability to produce a viable embryo.

The journal scan shows that regardless of the type of ART used, high level of sperm DNA fragmentation over the critical threshold will significantly compromise the possibility of a successful pregnancy due embryonic implantation failures and miscarriages.

It is observed that high sperm DNA fragmentation does not appear to affect fertilization or the first/second embryo cleavage stages but affect cleavage once the paternal genome is switched on and result in initiation of apoptosis and subsequent blastocyst developmental arrest, miscarriage or abnormalities in offspring.

DNA integrity is due to disulfide cross-link between protamines which cause DNA compaction in sperms. Sperm DNA fragmentation may be due to the protamine deficiency or gene mutation are intrinsic factors which affect compaction, the elevated testicular temperature due to heat/varicocele/radiation/oxidative stress/gonadotoxine exposure/chlamydia or mycoplasma infection are extrinsic factors and other factors include abnormalities in the regulation of apoptosis or defects in topo-isomerase activity.

Direct methods for detection of DNA fragmentation:

- COMET test (Single cell gel electrophoresis assay)
- TUNNEL assay (Terminal deoxynucleotide transferase {duTP} nick end labeling).

Indirect methods for detection of DNA fragmentation:

- *SCSA (Sperm chromatin structure assay)*: This SCSA test is an effective method for measuring thousands of sperm in an ejaculate. The sperms are stained with a fluorescent probe that interacts with the DNA. The fluorescence signal alters when the DNA is fragmented and monitored using a flow cytometer. The results are reported showing 3 statistical categories: Less than 15% DFI = excellent fertility potential; More than 15–30% DFI = good fertility potential; More than 30% DFI = fair to poor fertility potential.

- *High DNA stainability*: Immature chromatin can be measured by increased DNA stainability (HDS) and is associated with asyngamy and poor IVF fertilization rates when it exceeds 15%.

Measuring sperm DNA fragmentation confers clinicians the power to make more informed decisions in their clinical practice and take action based on quantitative results. When sperm DNA fragmentation levels are above 30%, the probability of delivery is significantly reduced from 19.0% to 1.5–2.0% in the IUI cycles, hence, ICSI with testicular sperm results in significant increase in the chance of deliveries rate.

Modification of lifestyle, diet rich in antioxidants and treatment of infection with antibiotics would be expected to reduce DNA fragmentation percentage. Literature data have evidence that varicocele repair may result in improvement of sperm DNA integrity. The swim-up sperm preparation or magnetic-activated cell sorting (MACS) or the electrophoretic separation of spermatozoa decreases SDF percentage and may improve IUI results. Semen can be reassessed by undertaking a second test three months after the first report.

Sperm FISH (Fluorescence *in situ* Hybridization)

Human sperm FISH was introduced to determine aneuploidy in the sperm of oligospermic and aging men (Martin, 2007; Miharu, 1994; Holmes and Martin, 1993).[33-35] It is recommended screening tool to help in counseling the couples with severe male factor infertility having prior repeated in vitro fertilization/ICSI failure, recurrent pregnancy loss and men recovering from gonadotoxic treatment. Sperm FISH[36] allows us to analyze part of the sperm chromosomes (commonly tested chromosomes 13, 18, 21, X and Y), which are involved in miscarriage and fetal malformations. It enables the affected couple to make informed reproductive choices. In normal fertile men the rate of aneuploidy are low (less than 2% of sperms).

Multicolor FISH allows the analysis of thousands of sperms in short time period and increases the statistical power of the analysis. The use of sophisticated image analysis software obviates cytogeneticist to analyze the results.

Other indications of sperm FISH are men with structural sex chromosome abnormalities (XX phenotypic male) to determine whether the sex-determining (SRY) region is present. The patient stained positive (red) for the SRY region at the tail of one of the X chromosomes. Availability of probes for the XPAR1 pseudo-autosomal regions can detect other regions of the Y chromosome for the diagnosis of XX SRY negative males. Some Y-chromosome microdeletions, rearrangements, duplications, and inversions may be better characterized by using FISH along with the routine karyotype and multiplex PCR. FISH is also recommended to confirm mosaicism if less than 10% of cells are mosaic by karyotype, e.g. mosaic Klinefelter's syndrome.

Y Chromosome Microdeletion Testing (AZF Screening)

Nonobstructive azoospermia patients having normal karyotype should be tested for Y-microdeletion. Y-chromosome[37] plays an essential role in the genetic regulation of spermatogenesis and genes are mapped to the proximal long arm of the Y chromosome (Yq11) and are arranged in azoospermia factor (AZF) region. The microdeletions in the Y chromosome have been found frequently in infertile men than in fertile controls but some time the partial microdeletions are also detected in normozoospermic males.

Y chromosome microdeletion is currently diagnosed by using polymerase chain reaction amplification and gel electrophoresis to test whether the DNA sequence corresponding to the selected markers is present in the DNA of Y chromosome.

AZF region includes three subregions[38]—AZFa, AZFb, and AZFc. The Y chromosome deletions include RBM, DAZ, SPGY, and TSPY, which results in reduced fertility due to affected spermatogenesis process. The deletion incidence of AZFa: 3%, AZFb: 9%, AZFc: 79%, AZFb+c: 6%, AZFa+b+c: 3% reported in the literature.

When the deletion of entire subregion AZFa/AZFb there is poor prognosis for sperm retrieval and in case of deletion of AZFc subregion,[39] the TESA with ICSI possible but there is risk for AZF deletion passing to child. The concerns are more obvious for male infertility related to Y chromosome microdeletions because they are good candidates for ICSI[40] and spermatozoa or spermatids suitable for the procedure can be recovered from semen or the testis, therefore all male offspring will invariably inherit the deleted Y chromosome from the father. The Yq microdeletion analysis[41] should be recommended in all patients, who are undergoing IVF/ICSI treatment.

Molecular Genetics (CFTR Analysis) in the Male Partner

Congenital bilateral absence of the vas deferens (CBAVD) is significant cause of obstructive azoospermia in otherwise healthy men. It is approximately present in 95% of men with an autosomal recessive disease so-called cystic fibrosis. Affected CF patients present clinically as a spectrum of genital phenotypes ranging from normal fertility to severely impaired spermatogenesis and CBAVD. Cystic fibrosis with CBAVD is caused by mutations in *CFTR* (cystic fibrosis trans-membrane conductance regulator) gene[42,43] which requires investigation of female partner for carrier status.

GENETIC TESTING IN CASES OF SPONTANEOUS ABORTIONS

Prothrombotic Disorders

Recurrent pregnancy loss (RPL)[44-50] problem with three or more losses affecting 1–2% and two or more losses affecting up to 5% of women at the reproductive age. Congenital thrombophilia and prothrombotic disorders[51] have drawn the interest of gynecologist for its potential link with recurrent miscarriage.

In the meta-analyses of Robertson et al. and Rey et al. Factor V Leiden and FII G20210A were the only thrombophilic mutations associated with recurrent miscarriage. Robertson et al. has observed that the presence of FII G20210A and Factor V Leiden mutation increases the risk for recurrent early pregnancy loss (odds ratios 2.49 for FII G20210A while 2.71 for homozygous and 1.68 for heterozygous FVL), whereas homozygosity for MTHFR C677T has not significantly increasing the risk (odds ratio 1.40, 95% CI 0.77-2.55).[51-54]

Common mutation for the *MTHFR* gene[55] is resulted in a 40% reduction in the activity of the enzyme. Homozygosity of C 677T (TT) results in significant increase in total plasma homocysteine levels, whereas the homocysteine level do not appear significantly elevated with the 1298CC genotype. Although the presence of MTHFR mutations is significantly more common in miscarried embryos, current evidence fails to support an association between these polymorphisms and increased risk for recurrent miscarriage.

Deficiencies of the natural anticoagolant protein S, C and antithrombin occur in less than 1–2% of the population. Alireza Parand et al.[56] found a significant association of RPL with protein S deficiency and a non-significant correlation with protein C deficiency. Anticoagolant protein deficiencies increased the risk of fetal loss in most of studies.

In the majority of women with inherited thrombophilia, pregnancy is uneventful but the risks for miscarriage, IUFD, placental abruption and intrauterine growth restriction are increased in carriers of thrombophilia. Certain women with thrombophilia present with gestational vascular complications[57] (vasculopathy) but cause of miscarriage is still unknown and it may be related to a combined effect with another inherited or acquired prothrombotic risk either systemic or operating locally at the placental level. The EPCOT study showed that the risk for stillbirth (but not miscarriage) is highest in women with combined thrombophilic defects.

Fetal Aneuploidy and Balanced Translocation

Majority of miscarriage before 10th week of gestation are due to fetal aneuploidy or balanced translocation. Cytogenetic analysis (G banding at high resolution) of both the male and female partner is recommended by various guidelines. Couples with balanced reciprocal translocation have a 50% chance of having RSAs and a 20% risk of having children with abnormal genetic makeup. The formation of balanced, unbalanced and normal gametes depends on the basis of the break point and also on the chromosomes involved. Balanced chromosomal translocations may also lead to sequence rearrangements of the functional genes that may result in the reproductive errors accompanied by repeated abortions.

Karyotyping of Product of Conception

The chromosome aneuploidy[58] is found in high frequency in the spontaneous abortions hence chromosomes 13, 21, 16, 18, 22, X, Y study is recommended by FISH technique.

Karyotyping from 'products of conception' (POC) of a spontaneous or missed abortion is carried out by fibroblast culture to rule out a chromosome abnormality but cytogenetic analysis of POC using tissue culture technique has limitations because of longer time for results, culture failure, and maternal cell contamination.[59] To avoid contamination of tissue, the sample of early abortions should be transported in a sterile container with normal saline to which 2–3 drops of sodium heparin and gentamicin are added to prevent bacterial growth. The sac surrounded by chorionic villi is the tissue of choice in early abortions while a small piece of placenta and fetal skin should be collected from 2nd and 3rd trimester abortions. Cord blood 0.5–1 mL should be collected in sodium heparin tube, from 3rd trimester abortions. The samples can be stored in the freeze overnight if required, before transportation at room temperature. Tissue samples should never be put into formalin for karyotyping or FISH.

SNP microarray analysis provides an improved method for POC karyotype evaluation with ability to determine maternal cell contamination, otherwise 43% of results (46,XX) would have been uninformative and could be misinterpreted. Additionally, results are obtained quickly with no failure rate. It is observer that the majority of aneuploidy is of maternal origin but further study on incidence of maternal and paternal source of aneuploidy is needed.

Couple has significant grieving after a miscarriage and knowing the results of the chromosomal analysis of POC[60] may help patients understand the cause of their miscarriage and start planning for future pregnancy attempts.

SPECIAL SITUATION IN INFERTILITY TREATMENT

- *Late marriages or elderly infertile couple:* Trisomy 21 known as Down syndrome due to non-disjunction of chromosome at the time of meiosis is more frequent in children born to elderly mothers. Hence, earlier marriage of females is better than late marriage from the point of view of preventing mongolism.

- *Disputed paternity:* Genetic fingerprinting using 'mini-satellite repeat sequence probes', the pattern of DNA fragments generated by those probes is so highly polymorphic that the restriction map is unique to each individual specific as fingerprints.
- *X-rays or Radiotherapy:* Patients undergoing X-ray examination should be protected against unnecessary exposure of the gonads to radiation and X-ray examination of the pregnant uterus to determine the twins or the lie of the fetus is strongly deprecated.
- *Indian (south Asians) women:* The ovaries age early in Indian population due to ethnic constitutional factor as per various literature data hence fertility should be started at early age. It is observed that Indian are higher risk of obesity with increased risk of infertility and they have extra fat in subcutaneous tissue of abdomen while East Asians have fat in visceral fat in abdomen. It is better to start infertility treatment at an early age than western women.
- Consanguinity and incest:
  - Mental retardation 25%
  - Autosomal recessive disorder 10–15%
  - Congenital malformations 10%
- *Gene signature of endometrial receptivity:* DNA micro-array analysis, molecular tool allows us to diagnose whether the endometrium is receptive or not by analyzing the expression of a group of genes related to endometrial receptivity and endometrial biopsy is performed at P+5 (hormone replacement therapy cycle) or at LH+7 (natural cycle) for gene expression profile. It is proposed that using lavage of the uterine cavity rather than endometrial biopsy could be useful to investigate endometrium proteome particularly secretory proteins to predict implantation outcome in women are under treatment of IVF. At the clinical level, the most important contribution of the ERA test is the objective diagnosis of the window of implantation, thus leading to the creation of the concept of personalized ET (pET).

  Role of Proteomics technique in female reproductive work up to address many molecular biological basis of gametogenesis, fertilization, endometrial receptivity, embryo implantation is under research and may viable in near future for clinical work up.

  The protein expressed by the genome of a tissue so-called proteome could be analyzed by use of gel electrophoresis[61] coupled with mass spectrometry method, which is called proteomic study. Studies[62] have found 76 proteins production of 41 genes which are differently regulated between mid-proliferative and mid-secretory phase of endometrium. Parmar et al. study[63,64] documented 57 spots are up regulated in mid-proliferative phase compared to 104 spots which were down regulated in mid-secretory phase by 2DE gel electrophoresis method. Chen et al. reported Annexin A2 was up regulated and PGRMC1 decreased in receptive endometrium.
- *Genetic screening of gametes donor is based on ethnicity:* Asian, African, and Mediterranean descent gametes donors should undergo a hemoglobin electrophoresis screening test (for sickle cell/thalassemia disorder). French and Canadian descent gamete donors is required to be screened for cystic fibrosis/Tay-Sachs disease. The Caucasian donors are usually tested for cystic fibrosis (CF) mutation.

  Donor of Ashkenazi Jewish origin should be screened for [CF mutation/Tay-Sachs disease, Canavan disease (nuerological disorder) and Gaucher disease (hepatosplenomegaly)].
- Sperm motility proteins and gene therapy

  Centrin (centrosomal protein): There are proximal centriole and distal centriole. In some spermatozoa of the male infertility, centrin protein was located abnormally at the base of flagellum and immunofluorescence labeling antibody staining signals were spread and could not be recognized separately. The lower gene expression of centrin assessed by testicular biopsy subjected for PCR analysis. This low expression affects the ART outcome in terms of fertilization rate, embryo quality and pregnancy rate in asthanospermic patients. The gene therapy in animal study demonstrated poor sperm motility may be treated by replacement of centrosome rather than simply being by passed with ICSI procedure (Schatten et al., 2009).[65,66]

REFERENCES

1. Markus S, Hehr U. Genetic counseling and testing prior to assisted reproduction. J Reproduktionsmed Endokrinol. 2009;6:6 10.
2. The ESHRE Capri Workshop Group. Genetic aspects of female reproduction.Hum Reprod Update. 2008;14:293-307.
3. Jantke A. Unerfüllter Kinderwunsch:Rationale Diagnostik und Therapie. CME Prakt Fortb Gynäkologie, Geburtsmedizin und Gynäkologische Endokrinologie. 2005;1:14-23.
4. Steck T. Sporadische und wiederholte Aborte – Diagnostische Abklärung und Möglichkeiten der Prävention. CME Praktische Fortbildung Gynäkologie, Geburtsmedizin und Gynäkologische Endokrinologie. 2006;1:14-24.
5. Chatterjee S, Maitra A, Kadam S, et al. CGG repeat sizing in the FMR1 gene in Indian women with premature ovarian failure. Reproductive Bio Medicine Online. 2009;19(2):281-6.
6. Hempel M, Buchholz T. Rare syndromes associated with infertility. J Reproduktionsmed Endokrinol. 2009;6:24-6.

7. Hughes V. Geneticists crack the code of infertility. Nat Med 2008;14:1174.
8. Boivin J, Bunting L, Collins JA,Nygren KG. International estimates of infertility prevalence and treatment-seeking: potential need and demand for infertility medical care. Hum Reprod. 2007;22:1506-12.
9. JL Simpson, Genetic factors in common disorders of female infertility. Reproductive Medicine Review. 2000;8:(3):173-202.
10. Dep, Chakravarty S, Charvarty A, Novel balanced chromosomal translocations in females with recurrent spontaneous abortions: Two case studies. J Hum Reproduct Sci. 2015;8;114-7.
11. Martin JR, Arici A. Fragile X and reproduction. Curr Opin Obstet Gynecol. 2008;20:216-20.
12. The Fragile X Premutation: A Cause for Premature Ovarian Failure. Emory University School of Medicine. Department of Human Genetics. Division of Medical Genetics (2006). *http://genetics.emory.edu/pdf/factsheet46.pdf.*
13. Chitayat D, et al. Joint SOGC-CCMG committee opinion: Genetics Committee of the Society of Obstetricians and Gynaecologists of Canada (SOGC); Prenatal Diagnosis Committee of the Canadian College of Medical Geneticists (CCMG). J Obstet Gynaecol Can. 2008;216:837-41.
14. Dequeker E, et al. Best practice guidelines for molecular genetic diagnosis of cystic fibrosis and CFTR-related disorders - updated European recommendations. Eur J Hum Genet. 2009;17:51-65.
15. Knauff EA, Franke L, van Es MA, et al. Genome-wide association study in premature ovarian failure patients suggest ADAMTS19 as a possible candidate gene. Human Reproduction. 2009;24: 2372-8.
16. Chinnery PF, Thorburn DR, Samuels DC, White SL, Dahl HM, Turnbull DM, et al. The inheritance of mitochondrial DNA heteroplasmy: random drift, selection or both? Trends Genet. 2000;16:500-5.
17. Chinnery PF, Howell N, Andrews RM, Turnbull DM. Clinical mitochondrial genetics. J Med Genet. 1999;36:425-36.
18. Naviaux RK. Developing a systematic approach to the diagnosis and classification of mitochondrial disease. Mitochondrion. 2004;4:351-61.
19. Khan NA, Govindaraj P, Meena K, Thangaraj K. Mitochondrial disorders: Challenges in diagnosis and treatment; Indian J Med Res 141. 2015;141:13-26.
20. Bouchet C, Steffann J, Corcos J, Monnot S, Paquis V, Rotig A, et al. Prenatal diagnosis of myopathy, encephalopathy, lactic acidosis, and stroke-like syndrome: contribution to understanding mitochondrial DNA segregation during human embryofetal development. J Med Genet. 2006;43:788-92.
21. Hellebrekers DM, Wolfe R, Hendrickx AT, de Coo IF, de Die CE, Geraedts JP, et al. PGD and heteroplasmic mitochondrial DNA point mutations: a systematic review estimating the chance of healthy offspring. Hum Reprod Update. 2012;18:341-9.
22. Steffann J, Gigarel N, Corcos J, Bonniere M, Encha-Razavi F, Sinico M, et al. Stability of the m.8993T->G mtDNA mutation load during human embryofetal development has implications for the feasibility of prenatal diagnosis in NARP syndrome. J Med Genet. 2007;44:664-9.
23. Kaufmann P, Engelstad K, Wei Y, Kulikova R, Oskoui M, Sproule DM, et al. Natural history of MELAS associated with mitochondrial DNA m.3243A>G genotype. Neurology. 2011;77:1965-71.
24. Poulton J, Chiaratti MR, Meirelles FV, Kennedy S, Wells D, Holt IJ. Transmission of mitochondrial DNA diseases and ways to prevent them. PLoS Genet. 2010;6:pii:e1001066.
25. Marchington D, Malik S, Banerjee A, Turner K, Samuels D, Macaulay V, et al. Information for genetic management of mtDNA disease: sampling pathogenic mtDNA mutants in the human germline and in placenta. J Med Genet. 2010;47:257-61.
26. Poulton J, Kennedy S, Oakeshott P, Wells D. Preventing transmission of maternally inherited mitochondrial DNA diseases. BMJ. 2009;338:b94.
27. Ludwig M, et al. Stellungnahme der Arbeitsgemeinschaft Reproduktionsgenetik der Deutschen Gesellschaft für Reproduktionsmedizin: Empfehlung zur genetischen Diagnostik bei Kinderwunschpaaren. J Reproduktionsmed Endokrinol. 2004;1:190-3.
28. The ESHRE Capri Workshop Group. Optimal use of fertility diagnostic tests and treatments. Hum Reprod Update. 2000;15:723-32.
29. Meschede D, Lemcke B, Behre HM, De Geyter C, Nieschlag E, Horst J. Non-reproductive heritable disorders in infertile couples and their first degree relatives. Hum Reprod. 2000;15:1609-12.
30. Abramsky L, Chapple J. 47,XXY (Klinefelter syndrome) and 47,XYY:Estimated rates of and indication for postnatal diagnosis with implications for prenatal counselling. Prenat Diagn. 1997;17:363-8.
31. Tartaglia N, Davis S, Hench A, Nimishakavi S, Beauregard R, Reynolds A, et al. A new look at XXYY syndrome: medical and psychological features. Am J Med Genet A. 2008;146(A):1509-22.
32. Practice committee of American society for reproductive medicine. The clinical utility of sperm DNA integrity testing. Fertil Steril. 2008;90:S178-80.
33. Holmes JM, Martin RH. Aneuploidy detection in human sperm nuclei using fluorescent in situ hybridization. Hum Genet. 1993;91:20-4.
34. Martin, et al. Defective spermatogenesis. Environ Health Perspect. 2008;116(8):A332.
35. Miharu N, Best RG, Young SR. Numerical chromosome abnormalities in spermatozoa of fertile and infertile men detected by fluorescence in situ hybridization. Hum Genet. 1994;93:5026.
36. O Martınez-Pasarell, C Marquez MD Coll. Analysis of human sperm-derived pronuclei by three-colour fluorescent in-situ hybridization. Human Reproduction. 1997;12(4):641-5.
37. Choi JM, et al. AZF microdeletions of the Y chromosome and in vitro fertilization outcome. Fertil Steril. 2004;81:337-41.
38. Ferlin A, et al. Molecular and clinical characterization of Y chromosome microdeletions in infertile men: A 10-year experience in Italy. J Clin Endocrinol Metab. 2007;92:762-70.

39. Oates RD, Silber S, Brown LG, Page DC. Clinical characterization of 42 oligospermic or azoospermic men with microdeletion of the AZFc region of the Y chromosome, and of 18 children conceived via ICSI. Hum Reprod. 2002;17:2813-24.
40. Kihaile PE, Kisanga RE, Aoki K, Kumasako Y, Misumi J, Utsunomiya T. Embryo outcome in Y-chromosome microdeleted infertile males after ICSI. Mol Reprod Dev. 2004;68:176-81.
41. Simoni M, Bakker E, Krausz C. EAA/EMQN best practice guidelines for molecular diagnosis of Y-chromosomal microdeletions. State of the art 2004. Int J Androl. 2004;27:240-9.
42. Kusic J, Radojkovic D, Maletic V, Brankovic S, Savic A. Mutations and polymorphisms in CFTR genes in infertile men with oligospermia or azoospermia. Srp Arh Celok Lek. 2002; 130(1-2):1-6.
43. Stuhrmann M, Dörk T. CFTR gene mutations and male infertility. Andrologia. 2000;32(2):71-83.
44. Bennett SA, Bagot CN, Arya R. Pregnancy loss and thrombophilia: the elusive link. Br J Haematol. 2012;157(5):529-42.
45. Dossenbach-Glaninger A, van Trotsenburg M, Dossenbach M, Oberkanins C, Moritz A, Krugluger W, et al. Plasminogen activator inhibitor 1 4G/5G polymorphism and coagulation factor XIII Val34Leu polymorphism: impaired fibrinolysis and early pregnancy loss. Clin Chem. 2003;49(7):1081-6.
46. Hoekema L, Castoldi E, Tans G, Girelli D, Gemmati D, Bernardi F, et al. Functional properties of factor V and factor Va encoded by the R2-gene. Thromb Haemost. 2001;85(1):75-81.
47. Hohlagschwandtner M, Unfried G, Heinze G, Huber JC, Nagele F, Tempfer C. Combined thrombophilic polymorphisms in women with idiopathic recurrent miscarriage. Fertil Steril 2003;79(5):1141-8.
48. Inbal A, Muszbek L. Coagulation factor deficiencies and pregnancy loss. Semin Thromb Hemost. 2003;29(2):171–4.
49. Pildner von Steinburg S, Schneider KTM. Recurrent spontaneous abortions – An update on diagnosis and management. J Reproduktionsmed Endokrinol. 2009;6:11-6.
50. Stern JJ, Dorfmann AD, Gutiérrez-Najar AJ, Cerrillo M, Coulam CB. Frequency of abnormal karyotypes among abortuses from women with and without a history of recurrent spontaneous abortion. Fertil Steril. 1996;65(2):250-3.
51. Robertson L, Wu O, Langhorne P, Twaddle S, Clark P, Lowe GD, et al. Thrombophilia in pregnancy: a systematic review. Br J Haematol. 2006;132(2):171-96.
52. Altintas A, Pasa S, Akdeniz N, Cil T, Yurt M, Ayyildiz O, et al. Factor V Leiden and G20210A prothrombin mutations in patients with recurrent pregnancy loss: data from the southeast of Turkey. Ann Hematol. 2007;86(10):727-31.
53. Coulam CB, Jeyendran RS, Fishel LA, Roussev R. Multiple thrombophilic gene mutations rather than specific gene mutations are risk factors for recurrent miscarriage. Am J Reprod Immunol. 2006;55(5):360-8.
54. Resch B, Gallistl S, Kutschera J, Mannhalter C, Muntean W, Mueller WD. Thrombophilic polymorphisms--factor V Leiden, prothrombin G20210A, and methylenetetrahydrofolate reductase C677T mutations--and preterm birth. Wien Klin Wochenschr. 2004;116(17-18):622-6.
55. Haviv YS, Shpichinetsky V, Goldschmidt N, Atta IA, Ben-Yehuda A, Friedman G. The common mutations C677T and A1298C in the human methylenetetrahydrofolate reductase gene are associated with hyperhomocysteinemia and cardiovascular disease in hemodialysis patients. Nephron. 2002;92(1):120-6.
56. Parand A, Zolghadri J, Nezam M, Afrasiabi A, Haghpanah S. Inherited thrombophilia and recurrent pregnancy loss. Iran Red Crescent Med J. 2013;15(12):e13708.
57. Tincani A, Cavazzana I, Ziglioli T, Lojacono A, De Angelis V, Meroni P. Complement activation and pregnancy failure. Clin Rev Allergy Immunol. 2010;39(3):153-9.
58. Ogasawara M, Aoki K,Okada S, Suzumori K. Embryonic karyotype of abortuses in relation to the number of previous miscarriages. Fertil Steril. 2000;73:300-4.
59. RB Lathi, S Sigurjonsson, et al. Informatics-based molecular karyotyping of products of conception (POC) with maternal cell contamination (MCC) detection: report on 344 consecutive analyses; Fertility and sterility. 2011;96(3):S33.
60. Carp H, Toder V, Aviram A, Daniely M, Mashiach S, Barkai G. Karyotype of the abortus in recurrent miscarriage. Fertil Steril. 2001;75:678-82.
61. Mitra A, Mandana BB. Application of gel-based proteomic technique in female reproductive investigation. J Hum Reprod. Sci. 2015;8:18-24.
62. Chen JI, et al. proteomic characterization of midproliferative and midsecretory human endometrium. J Proteom Res. 2009;8: 2032-44.
63. Parmar T, et al. protein profiling of human endometrial tissues in mid secretory and proliferative phases of menstrual cycle. Fertil Steril. 2009;92:1091-103.
64. Palermo G, Joris H, Devroey P, Van Steirteghem AC, Pregnancies after intracytoplasmic injection of single spermatozoon into an oocyte. Lancet. 1992;340(8810):17-8.
65. Bundesärztekammer:(Muster-)Richtlinie zur Durchführung der assistierten Reproduktion – Novelle 2006. Dtsch Arztebl. 2006;103:1392-403.
66. GfH (Deutsche Gesellschaft für Humangenetik e.V.). Leitlinien zur molekulargenetischen Diagnostik: Fragiles-X und Fragiles-X assoziiertes Tremor/Ataxie Syndrom. Medgen. 2009b;21:276-83.

CHAPTER

10 Genetics and Counseling of Female Hereditary Breast and Ovarian Cancers

Shailesh Pande

INTRODUCTION

Breast cancer is a cancer that develops from breast tissue.

Signs

- Lump in the breast
- Alteration in breast shape
- Dimpling of the skin
- Abnormal fluid coming from the nipple
- Red scaly patch of skin
- Constant pain in part of the breast or armpit.

Metastasis

Common sites are bone, liver, lung and brain.

Commonly Associated Symptoms

Bone pain, enlargement of lymph nodes, shortness of breath.

Ovarian cancer is a cancer that begins in an ovary.
Signs and symptoms:

- Painless at early stages signs unless growing mass causes ovarian torsion
- Bloating, abdominal or pelvis pain, irregular menses, postmenopausal vaginal bleeding, pain or bleeding after or during, pain during or after sexual intercourse, loss of appetite, urinary problems, indigestion, and fatigue

ETIOLOGY

Hereditary breast and ovarian cancer (HBOC) syndrome is a condition caused by mutation in *BRCA1* or *BRCA2* genes.

Approximately in 5–10% of breast cancer, there is mutations in the *BRCA1* or *BRCA2* genes .

Individuals already diagnosed with cancer have a significantly increased risk of developing a second cancer in the future.

BRCA1 AND *BRCA2* MUTATIONS

BRCA1 and *BRCA2* are genes present in human beings and they produce tumor suppressor proteins. These proteins helps in repairing damaged DNA and plays an important role in maintaining the stability of the genetic material present in the cell. When there is any mutation in these genes, i.e. if there is any alteration in these genes, the protein product is either not produced or does not function correctly. This does not allow the DNA damage to be repaired efficiently. As a result, cells are more likely to develop additional genetic alterations that can lead to cancer.

Specific inherited mutations in *BRCA1* and *BRCA2* are reported to increase the risk of breast and ovarian cancers and are also reported to have association with increased risks of several additional types of cancer. Together, *BRCA1* and *BRCA2* mutations account for about 20–25% of hereditary breast cancers and about 5–10% of all breast cancers. Also it is reported that mutations in *BRCA1* and *BRCA2* account for around 15% of overall ovarian cancers.

A harmful *BRCA1* or *BRCA2* mutation can be inherited from one generation to another. Parent who carries a mutation in one of these genes has a 50% chance (1 in 2) of inheriting the mutation to their offspring. The effects of mutations in *BRCA1* and *BRCA2* are seen even when a person's second copy of the gene is normal.

Targeted Approach: *BRCA1* or *BRCA2* mutation, if identified in an individual with breast and/or ovarian cancer, then that specific mutation can be tested in other family members to assess their risk.

Ethinicity: Specific *BRCA1* and *BRCA2* mutations are associated with some ethnic groups, such as those of Ashkenazi Jewish descent, and can be used to evaluate the risk of individuals in this group.

Genetic tests are now available to detect *BRCA1* and *BRCA2* mutations.

Since a small proportion of population carries a *BRCA1* or *BRCA2* mutation, genetic testing is not recommended for the general population.

BRCA1 and *BRCA2* testing should be considered for individuals with a family history of a *BRCA1*/*BRCA2* mutation or a personal history of breast or ovarian cancer.

GENETIC TESTING

Approximately 6–8 mL of peripheral blood sample of the patient in EDTA Vacutainer is required for the test. The DNA from blood sample is extracted and mutation study is performed. The sample sent to laboratory should reach preferably within 24–48 hours. Completely filled and signed consent form is must. It usually takes about a month to get the test results.

A comprehensive BRCA analysis consists of two components:

1. *BRCA1/BRCA2 mutation by sequencing:* This involves complete *BRCA1* and *BRCA2* gene mutation testing by Sanger sequencing or next generation sequencing (NGS) (Fig. 10.1). All the coding exons as well as exon-intron boundaries are analyzed in both the genes. All the variations are compared against the database (BIC-Breast Cancer Core) and further classified as Class 1 to Class 5 indicating benign to deleterious nature of the mutation.
2. *BRCA1/2 deletion duplication by MLPA:* The large rearrangements in *BRCA1/2* are detected by multiplex probe ligation assay (MLPA). The frequency of these mutations is very low (Fig. 10.2).

Interpretation of Results

A *positive* test result indicates that a person has inherited and having a known harmful mutation in *BRCA1* or *BRCA2* and therefore is at an increased risk of developing certain cancers. However, a positive test result cannot tell whether or when an individual will actually develop cancer. For example, some women who inherit a harmful *BRCA1* or *BRCA2* mutation will never develop breast or ovarian cancer.

A positive genetic test result may also have important health and social implications for family members, including future generations. Unlike most other medical laboratory tests, genetic tests can reveal information not only about the individual being tested but also about that person's blood relatives (Results not limited to patients but also for family).

- Both men and women, who inherit a harmful *BRCA1* or *BRCA2* mutation, irrespective of whether or not they develop cancer themselves, may pass the mutation on to their sons and daughters. There is 50% chance of inheriting a parent's mutation to next generation.
- If a person learns that he or she has inherited a harmful *BRCA1*or *BRCA2* mutation, this will mean that each of his or her siblings also has 50% chance of having inherited the mutation from the parent.

  A *negative* test result can be more difficult to understand than a positive result because what the result means depends in part on an individual's family history of cancer and whether a *BRCA1* or *BRCA2* mutation has been identified in a blood relative (clinical correlation very important).
- If a close (first-or second-degree) relative of the tested person is known to carry a harmful *BRCA1* or *BRCA2* mutation, a negative test result is clear: it means that person does not carry the harmful mutation that is responsible for the *familial cancer*, and thus cannot pass it on to their children. Such a test result is called a *true negative*. A person with such a test result is currently thought and reported to have the same risk of cancer as someone in the general population.

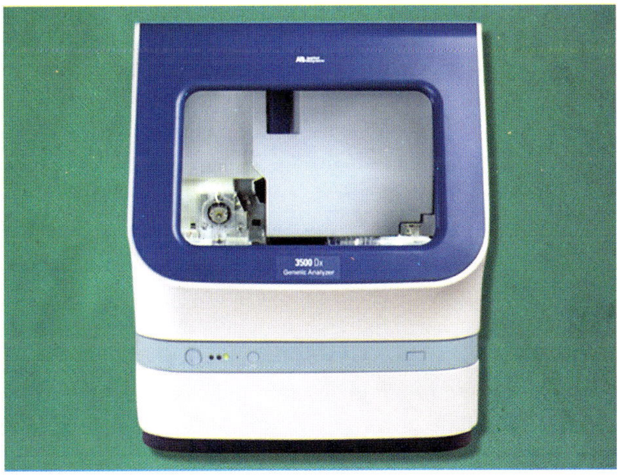

Fig. 10.1 3500Dx Genetic Analyzer (Sanger sequencing)

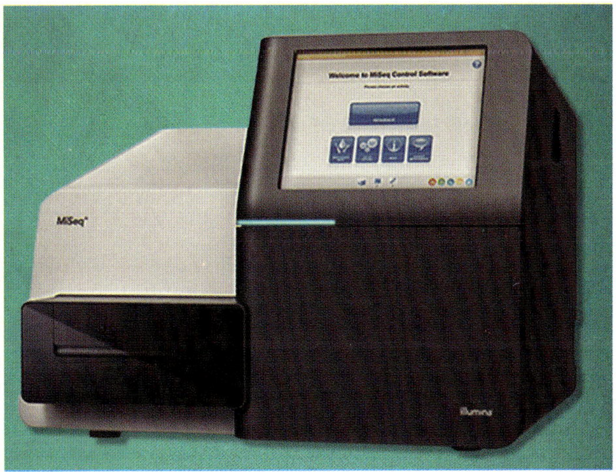

Fig. 10.2 Illumina MiSeq-NGS

- If the tested person has a family history that suggests the possibility of having a harmful mutation in *BRCA1* or *BRCA2* but complete gene testing identifies no such mutation in the family, a negative result is less clear. The likelihood that genetic testing will miss a known harmful *BRCA1* or *BRCA2* mutation though very low, but cannot be neglected and it could happen. Moreover, scientists continue to discover new *BRCA1* and *BRCA2* mutations and have not yet identified all potentially harmful ones. Therefore, it is possible that a person in this scenario with a "negative" test result actually has an as-yet unknown harmful *BRCA1* or *BRCA2* mutation that has not been identified (Follow-up with the center is necessary).
- It is also possible for people to have a mutation in a gene other than *BRCA1* or *BRCA2* that increases their cancer risk but is not detectable by the test used. People considering genetic testing for *BRCA1* and *BRCA2* mutations may/should discuss these potential uncertainties with a *genetic counselor* before undergoing testing.
- Sometimes, a genetic test finds a change in *BRCA1* or *BRCA2* that has not been previously associated with cancer. This type of test result may be described as "ambiguous" (often referred to as a **genetic variant of uncertain significance—VOUS**) because it is not known whether this specific gene change affects a person's risk of developing cancer. As more research is conducted and more people are tested for *BRCA1* and *BRCA2* mutations, scientists will learn more about these changes and cancer risk. Genetic counseling can help a person understand what an ambiguous change in *BRCA1* or *BRCA2* may mean in terms of cancer risk. Over time, additional studies of variants of uncertain significance may result in a specific mutation being re-classified as either harmful or clearly not harmful (Follow-up with the center is necessary).

WHAT IS YOUR RISK? ...PRETEST COUNSELING

Genetic Counseling Session

- Detail personal and family medical history
- Explain differences between sporadic and hereditary cancer
- Transmission of hereditary breast and ovarian cancer.
- Cancer and family risk assessment
- Choosing a right and appropriate genetic test
- Benefits and limitations of genetic testing to help to make an informed decision
- The medical implications of a positive or a negative test result
- Psychosocial assessment and support
- Possible options for cancer risk management including enhanced screening and surgery
- Support services available
- Knowing the potential risk can help them to take more informed decisions about the health before the onset of cancer or development of second cancer.

Whom Should We Offer the Test (HBOC Criteria)?

Individual from a family with a known deleterious *BRCA1*/*BRCA2* mutation

- *Personal history of breast cancer and one or more of the following:*
  - Diagnosed at or <45 years
  - Diagnosed at or <50 years with:
    - An additional breast cancer (Primary)
    - One or more close blood relative with breast cancer at any age
    - One or more close relative with pancreatic cancer
    - One or more relative with prostate cancer (Gleason score 7 or more)

  An unknown or limited family history:
  - Diagnosed at or below 60 years with a triple negative (ER, PR, HER2 Negative) breast cancer
  - *Diagnosed at any age with:*
    - One or more close blood relative with breast cancer diagnosed at or below 50 years
    - Two or more close blood relative with breast cancer at any age
    - One or more close blood relative with invasive ovarian cancer
    - Two or more close blood relative with pancreatic cancer and/or prostate cancer (Gleason score 7 or more) at any age
    - A close male blood relative with breast cancer
    - For an individual of ethnic group (e.g Ashkenazi Jewish) with higher mutation frequency no additional family history may be required
- Personal history of invasive ovarian cancer.
- Personal history of male breast cancer.
- Personal history of Prostate cancer (Gleason score of 7 or more) at any age with one or more close blood relative with breast (at or ≤50 years) and/or invasive ovarian and/or pancreatic or prostate cancer at any age.
- Personal history of pancreatic cancer at any age with one or more close blood relative with breast (≤50 years) and/or invasive ovarian and/or pancreatic cancer.
- Personal history of pancreatic cancer, and Ashkenazi Jewish ancestry.

- *Family history only:*
  - First or second degree blood relative meeting any of the above criteria.
  - Third-degree blood relative who has breast cancer and/ or invasive ovarian cancer and who has ≥ 2 close blood relatives with breast cancer (at least one with breast cancer ≤50 years) and /or invasive ovarian cancer

  "In general, individual with both breast and ovarian cancer and family history of both breast and ovarian cancer are of high clinical suspicion for BRCA mutation."

IF HBOC TESTING CRITERIA ARE MET?

Depending upon Family status following could be plan of action.

1. If deleterious *BRCA1/BRCA2* mutation known (Refer Flow chart 10.1)
2. If deleterious *BRCA1/BRCA2* mutation unknown (Refer Flow chart 10.2).

HBOC SYNDROME MANAGEMENT

Women

- Breast awareness starting at age of 18 years.
- Clinical breast exam every 6–12 month, starting at age 25 years.
- *Breast screening:*
  - Age 25–29 years, annual breast MRI screening (Preferred) or mammogram, if MRI unavailable or individualized based on F/H
  - Age 30–75 years annual mammogram and breast MRI screening
  - Age > 75 years individualized management
  - For women with a BRCA mutation who are treated for breast cancer—Annual mammography and breast MRI should continue.
- Screening for ovarian cancer with transvaginal ultrasound and Tumor marker studies
  - Discuss options of risk-reducing medicine and surgery (Ideally in consultation with a gynecologist/ oncologist) between 35–40 years and upon completion of childbearing and lifestyle modifications.

Men

- Breast self-examination training and education for disease awareness starting at age of 35 years
- Clinical breast examination, every 12 months starting at 35 years of age
- Starting at age of 40 years:
  - Recommend prostate screening for *BRCA2* carriers
  - Consider prostate screening for *BRCA1* carriers

Flow chart 10.1 If deleterious *BRCA1/BRCA2* mutation known

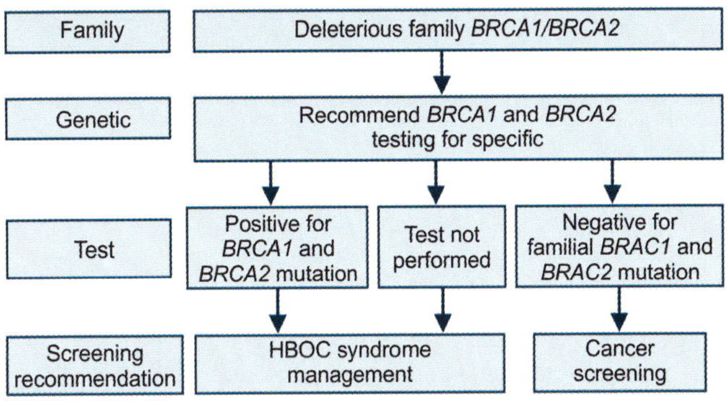

Flow chart 10.2 If deleterious *BRCA1/BRCA2* mutation unknown

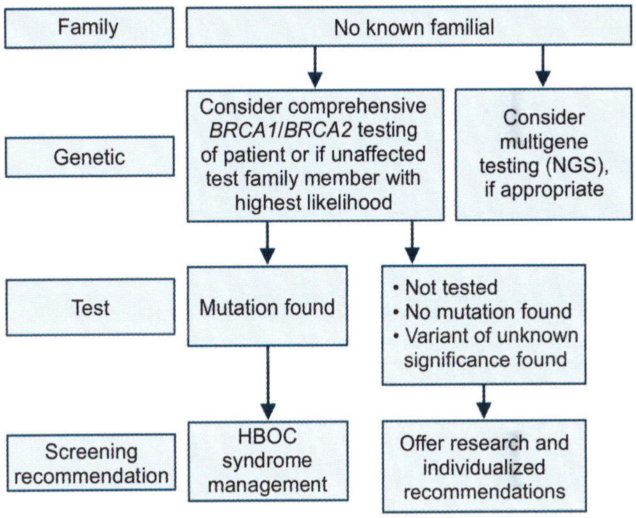

Men and Women

- Education about signs and symptoms of cancer especially those associated with *BRCA* gene mutation
- As no specific screening guidelines exists individualized based familial observation screening for pancreatic cancer and melanoma.

Risk to Relatives

- Advice about possible inherited cancer risk to relatives, options for risk assessment, and management.
- Recommend genetic counseling and consideration of genetic testing for at risk relatives.

Reproductive Options

For patients of reproductive age group advice about options for prenatal diagnosis and ART including PGD also risk associated, limitations and benefits of these technologies.

Some images of BRCA analysis are shown in Figures 10.3 to 10.7.

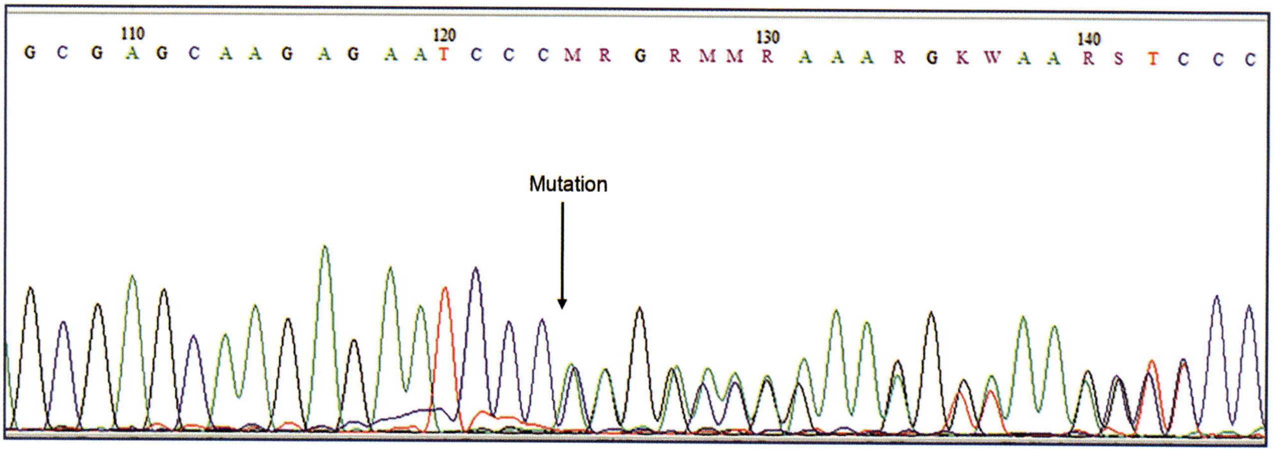

Fig. 10.3 *BRCA1*-Nt 5382 insC (Ex20)—deleterious (Class 5) mutation

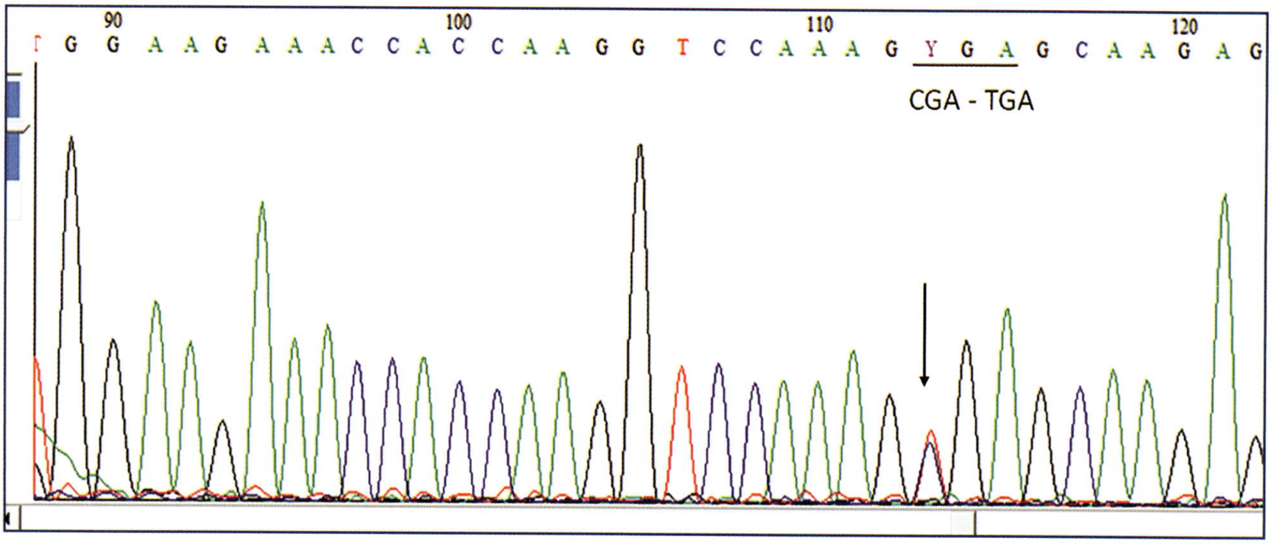

Fig. 10.4 *BRCA1*-Ex 20 Nt 5370 R1751X {c.5251C>T (p.R1751X)}—deleterious (Class 5) mutation

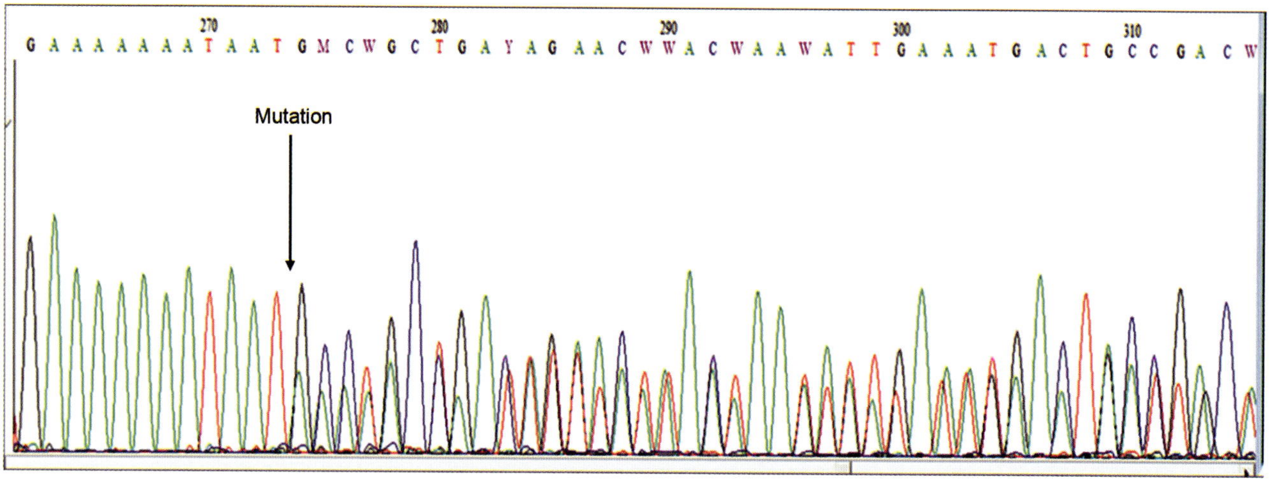

Fig. 10.5 *BRCA2*-Ex11.- Nt 4093 C.3865_3868delAAAT (P.Lys1289Alafs)—deleterious (Class 5) mutation

SECTION

3

Prenatal Screening: Noninvasive

CHAPTER

11

Global Rainbow Healthcare

Neharika Malhotra, Rinoy Sreedharan, Narendra Malhotra

Prenatal screening strategies are undergoing rapid changes owing to the introduction of new testing techniques and has marked a revolution in obstetrics.

The scope of prenatal testing has increased because of increased sensitivity of ultrasound and genome-wide molecular tests. In addition, noninvasive prenatal diagnosis is likely to be our near future for all pregnancies.

Screening is the process of surveying a population, using a specific marker or markers and defined screening cut-off levels, to identify the individuals in the population at higher risk for a particular disorder. Screening is applicable to a population; diagnosis is applied at the individual patient level.[1]

PRENATAL DIAGNOSIS

It is defined as the method of detection of structural or functional abnormalities in the developing fetus including genetic disorders and congenital malformations detected by biochemical markers or by ultrasound.

Indications for prenatal testing:
- A possibly heritable condition in one (or both) of the couple
- A history of longstanding infertility
- History of recurrent pregnancy loss
- A family history of possibly heritable conditions
- Population group with a high frequency of certain genetic diseases (ethnic or geographic region)
- A consanguineous marriage
- Advanced age.

Prenatal diagnosis of aneuploidy and single-gene disorders is usually performed by collecting fetal samples through amniocentesis or chorionic villus sampling. However, these invasive procedures are associated with some degree of risk to the fetus and/or mother. Therefore, in recent years, considerable effort has been made to develop noninvasive prenatal diagnostic procedures.

Aneuploidies are major causes of perinatal death and childhood handicap. Consequently, the detection of chromosomal disorders constitutes the most frequent indication for invasive prenatal diagnosis. Multiple marker screening uses a combination of maternal age and two or more biochemical tests, with or without an ultrasound examination, to produce a single result for risk of Down syndrome, trisomy 18, and open neural tube defects (ONTDs), which is used to offer options for clinical management. A screen is positive when the risk of one or more of the screened disorders falls above a designated risk cut-off. Counseling and further testing options are offered when a screen is positive.

Maternal risk factors:
- Age more than 35 years
- History of congenital malformation in previous pregnancy
- Chromosomal anomaly in previous issue
- Family history of NTDs or familial genetic diseases
- One or both partners is a carrier of chromosomal disorder
- History of recurrent abortions
- Patient belonging to any particular community with prevalence of any certain disease.

Antenatal risk factors in current pregnancy:
- Intake of teratogenic drugs or exposure to environmental teratogens
- Uncontrolled maternal diabetes in periconceptional period or raised glycosylated hemoglobin
- Amniotic fluid abnormalities like oligohydramnios or polyhydramnios
- Severe symmetrical fetal growth restriction
- Decreased fetal activity.

Various Noninvasive Prenatal Diagnostic Methods

- Detailed history, pedigree tree
- Maternal serum biochemistry.
  - Maternal serum alpha fetoprotein (MSAFP): Alpha fetoprotein (AFP) is the main glycoprotein produced by fetal liver which increases steadily in fetal serum and amniotic fluid until 13 weeks after which levels decrease rapidly. Crosses into maternal serum.

Table 11.1 Conditions associated with abnormal MSAFP levels

Elevated levels	Low levels
• Neural tube defects • Abdominal wall defects • Esophageal/ duodenal atresia • Renal anomalies (polycystic kidneys, absent kidneys) • Cystic hygroma, sacrococcygeal teratoma • Multiple pregnancy • Intrauterine death • Low maternal weight	• Trisomy 21 • Trisomy 18 • Overestimated gestational age • High maternal weight • Gestational trophoblastic disease

MSAFP rises steadily throughout pregnancy after 12 weeks (Table 11.1).

Clinical significance

- Measured between 16 and 20 weeks in ng/mL values at 2.5 multiples of the median (MOM) is considered upper limit of normal. Raised levels can detect 90% cases of anencephaly and 80% cases of open spina bifida.[2]

- Human chorionic gonadotropin
  - Secreted by placenta with max levels at 8–10 weeks
  - Raised levels seen in trisomy 21 and Turner's syndrome[3]
  - Low levels seen in Edward's syndrome.
- Unconjugated estriol
  - Produced by fetoplacental unit with levels gradually rising in pregnancy
  - Maternal serum levels are lower[4] in Down's, Turner's and Edward's syndrome.
- Inhibin A levels
  - Produced by syncytiotrophoblast
  - Raised levels seen in Down's syndrome.[5]
- Pregnancy associated plasma protein A (PAPP-A)
  - Secreted by syncytiotrophoblast
  - Levels reduced in Down's syndrome.[6]

FIRST TRIMESTER SCREENING

Uses **PAPP-A** and **free beta hCG** between 11 and 14 weeks. Can detect 62% Down's syndrome pregnancies with 5% false positive rate. Serum markers when combined with nuchal translucency measurement comprise **combined test** which has as detection rate of 79–87% with a 5% false-positive rate for Down's syndrome.[4] Trisomies 18 and 13 can be screened with 90% sensitivity and 1% false-positive rate.[7]

SECOND TRIMESTER SCREENING

- Done between 15 and 20 weeks
- Accurate gestational age is essential

Triple Test—MSAFP, hCG and Unconjugated Estriol (uE3)

- Down's syndrome—uE3 and MSAFP levels are lower and hCG is higher
- Edward's syndrome (trisomy 18)—levels of all three markers are low
- Turner's syndrome—picture similar to Down's syndrome
- Detection rate—60–69%, false positive rate—5%.[6]

Quadruple Test—MSAFP, hCG, Unconjugated Estriol and Inhibin A

- Raised inhibin A is seen in Down's syndrome
- Detection rate—67–81%, false-positive rate—5%.[6]

Risk ratios with a cut off of 1:250 are taken as screen positive requiring amniocentesis for confirmation of diagnosis.

Integrated Screening

Combines results of both the first and second trimester screening tests into a single risk.[8]

- Highest Down's syndrome detection: 94–96%

Stepwise Sequential Screen—First Trimester Screen and Quad Test

- 1% offered diagnostic test after first trimester screen
- 99% proceed to Quad test, results withheld until Quad test completed
- Detection rate: 90–95%

Contingent Sequential Screen

- 1% offered diagnostic test after first trimester screen
- 15% proceed to Quad test, results withheld until Quad test completed
- 84% have no additional test after first-trimester screen
- Detection rate: 88–94%.

Ultrasound

- Basic ultrasonographic examination
- Parameters to be noted
- Number of fetuses, presentation
- Documentation of fetal life (cardiac activity and movements)
- Placental localization
- Condition of internal os, cervical length, internal os diameter

- Detection of uterine mass (e.g. fibroids) or adnexal masses
- Any obvious anomaly like anencephaly, abdominal defect.

Soft Tissue Markers for Down's Syndrome and Other Anomalies

Fetal nuchal translucency: Abnormal accumulation of fluid in fetal neck is seen in Down's syndrome and other chromosomal anomalies. It is the maximum thickness of subcutaneous translucent area between skin and tissue overlying the fetal spine in the sagittal plane measured with ultrasound (Fig. 11.1).[7]

Advantage is that early termination of pregnancy can be done if any abnormality is suspected. NT of more than 3 mm during 10–14 weeks or more than 5 mm after 5 weeks is considered normal (Fig. 11.2).

Detection rate with NT alone[6]—64–70% with 5% false positive rate.

Other ultrasound markers: Echogenic bowel, slightly shortened long bones, absent nasal bone, choroid plexus cyst (Fig. 11.3), pyelectasis, cardiac echogenic foci. Presence of two or more markers raises the chance of having a chromosomal anomaly and the woman may have to undergo amniocentesis for confirmation.

Targeted/Detailed Ultrasound Examination

This is usually done in high risk pregnancies or with previous suspicious ultrasound. First viability and amniotic fluid index and placental location are noted.

Then the following standard views are taken:

- *Transverse sections of the fetal head*: To assess size (biparietal diameter, head circumference) in thalamic or cerebellar view to detect anencephaly, hydrocephalus. To assess shape and internal structures (Fig. 11.4).
- *Fetal abdomen*: Longitudinal and transverse views identifying intra-abdominal organs like stomach, kidneys, bladder, integrity of anterior wall, abdominal circumference is measured at level of stomach and umbilical portion of portal vein (Fig. 11.5).
- *Transverse section of fetal thorax*: Four chamber view of fetal heart to screen for cardiac defects (Fig. 11.6).
- *Limbs*: Identify three long bones in each limb. Femur length is measured.
- *Fetal spine*: Sagittal, coronal and transverse views are taken to rule out spinal bifida (Fig. 11.7).

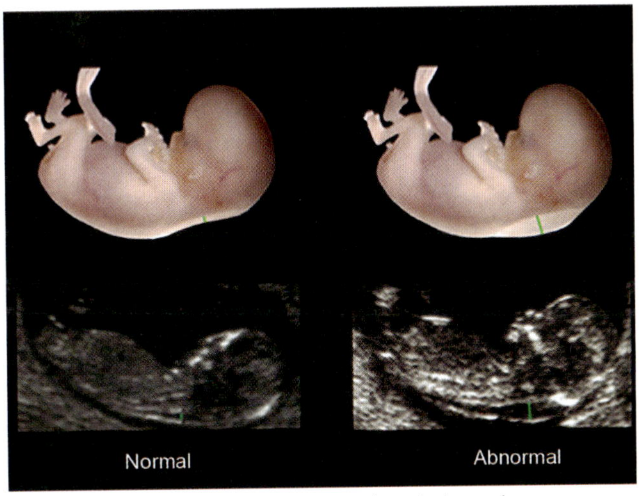

Fig. 11.2 Normal and abnormal nuchal translucency

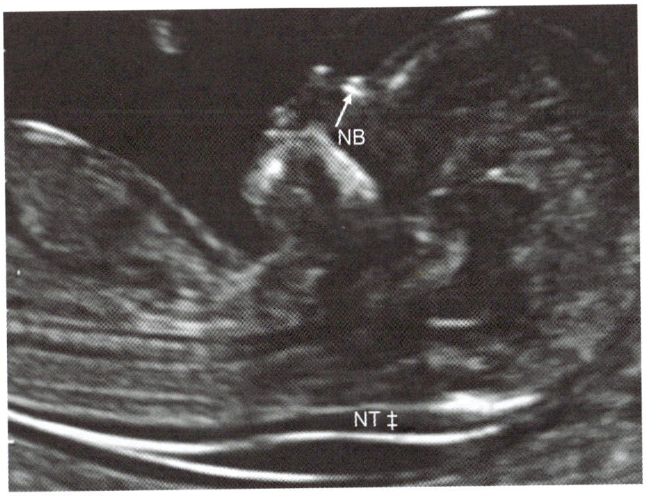

Fig. 11.1 Sagittal view with clear views of fetal nasal bone (NB) and nuchal translucency (NT)

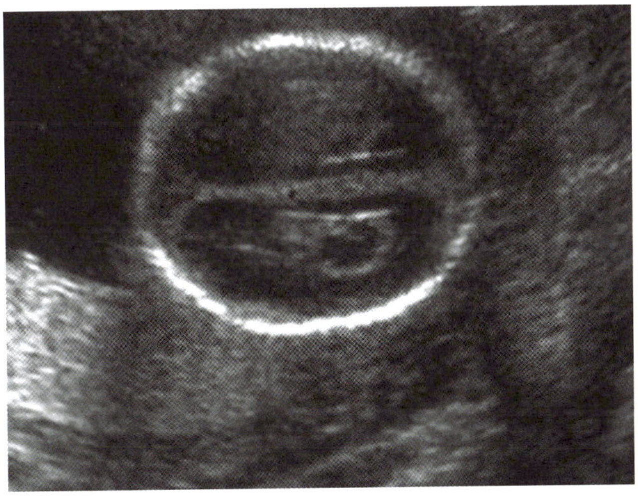

Fig. 11.3 Choroid plexus cyst

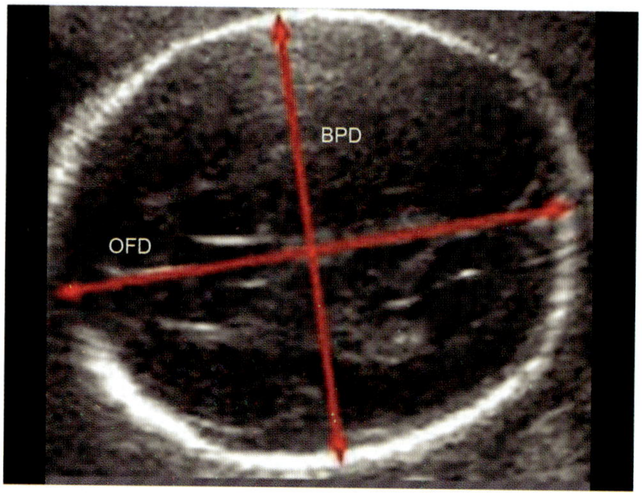

Fig. 11.4 Measurement of biparietal diameter (BPD) and occipitofrontal diameter (OFD)

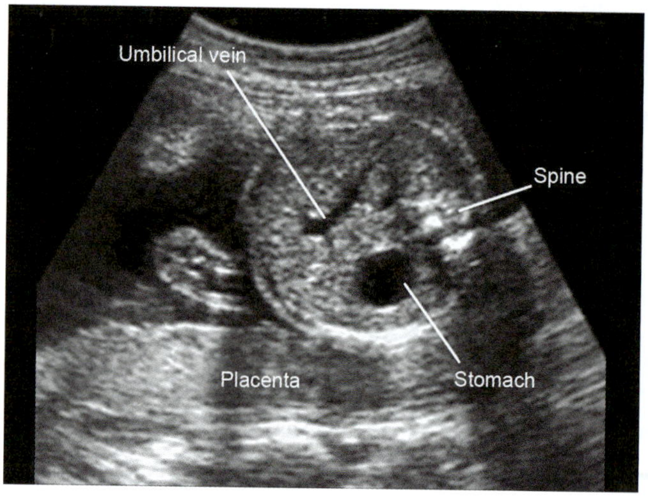

Fig. 11.5 Transabdominal section of fetal abdomen showing stomach, spine and umbilical vein

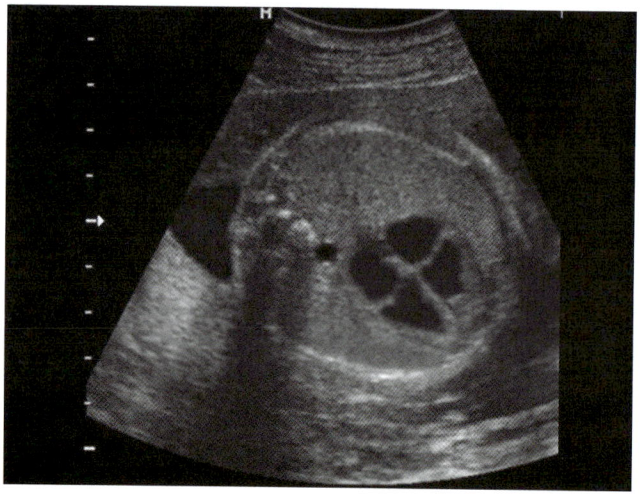

Fig. 11.6 Fetal heart

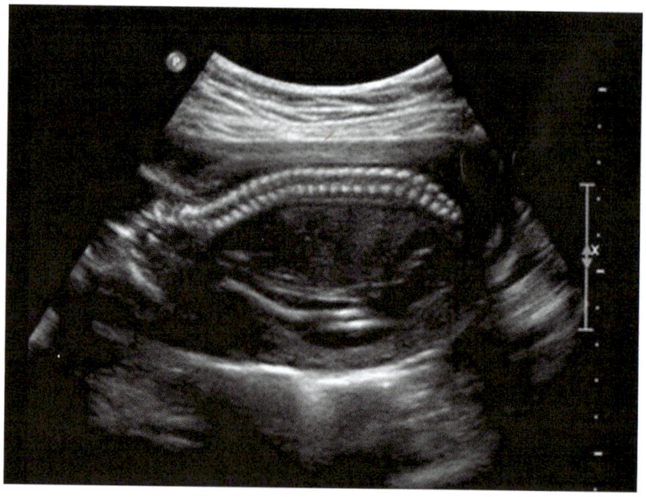

Fig. 11.7 Normal fetal spine—sagittal view

THIRD TRIMESTER (LATE) SCREENING

Certain malformations which are detected in the third trimester by ultrasound are:

- Hydrocephalus
- Neural tube defects—spina bifida
- Diaphragmatic hernia
- Cardiac anomalies
- Omphalocele
- Cleft lip with or without cleft palate
- Renal agenesis—unilateral or bilateral
- Urethral abnormalities
- Posterior urethral valves
- Limb reduction defects
- Osteogenesis imperfecta.

If any abnormality is visualized then one should look for any associated chromosomal or genetic syndrome and other invasive techniques if required.

If a lethal anomaly is detected, a cesarean delivery can be avoided and morbidity can be reduced.

In cases such as diaphragmatic hernia—patient can be referred for corrective surgery.

Screening for Down's Syndrome (Table 11.2)

Newer Noninvasive Methods

- *Fetal cells from maternal circulation:* Fetal cells isolated from maternal blood by density gradient, fluorescence and

Table 11.2 Screening for Down's syndrome

Method	Fetal nuchal translucency (USG)	Fetal NT + First trimester maternal serum screening (USG + Blood Test)	Second trimester maternal serum screening—triple test (blood test)
Timing of test	11–14 weeks	11–14 weeks	15–20 weeks
Detection rate	About 64–70%[6]	About 79–87%[6]	60–70%
False positive	5%	5%	5%
Advantages	Early test Screens for aneuploidy/ cardiac anomalies also	Early test	Relatively cheap
Disadvantages	1. Operator dependent 2. Requires high quality US machine	1. Operator dependent 2. Requires high quality US machine 3. Requires standardization of assay kits 4. Expensive	1. Lab dependent 2. Requires accurate dating 3. Affected by other factors—diabetes, ethnicity

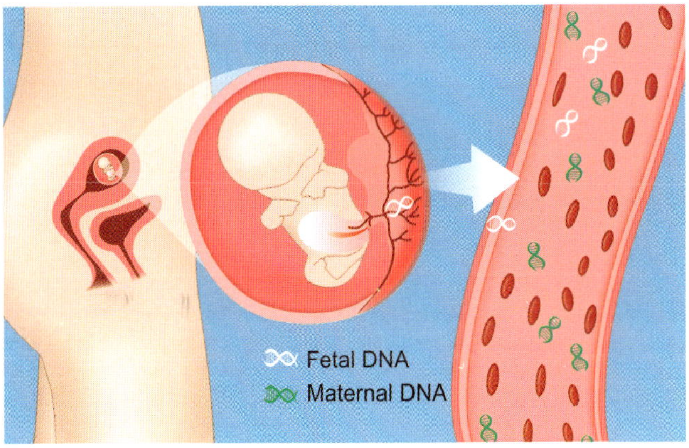

Fig. 11.8 Fetal DNA in mother's blood

other methods. It is useful in screening for aneuploidies because the number of cells in maternal blood increases six fold. Using fluorescence *in situ* hybridization many gene defects can be detected, but this method is still under research (Fig. 11.8).

- *Fetal cells in endocervical mucus:* It can be obtained in upto 50% of cases. However, this method too is under study.
- *Noninvasive prenatal testing (NIPT):* NIPT using maternal plasma DNA is available for several conditions. Obstetricians have used NIPT to guide management of women who are RhD-negative and whose fetuses are at risk of hemolytic disease of the fetus and newborn (HDFN) for many years and guidelines should already reflect this change in practice. Fetal sex determination for clinical indications in pregnancies at high sex-linked genetic risk is also established practice. Testing for aneuploidy and especially Down syndrome by maternal plasma MPS is now available commercially but while the test result is much more accurate than existing screening strategies, it is still not a diagnostic assay. Hence, the term 'noninvasive testing' is currently used.

Fetal genetic testing and aneuploidy diagnosis have until recently both needed invasive diagnostic sampling procedures carrying a small but significant risk of miscarriage. In 1997, the presence of cell-free fetal DNA (cffDNA) in the maternal circulation was reported.[9] Fetal DNA comes from the placenta,[10] can be detected from the first trimester of pregnancy onwards[11] and is rapidly cleared from the maternal circulation after delivery.[12] Maternal blood is therefore a reliable source of material for prenatal diagnosis. However, the cffDNA is mixed with a larger proportion of maternal cell-free DNA and current methodologies do not allow complete separation of fetal from maternal DNA *in vitro*.[13] Therefore, the first applications of this phenomenon focused on the detection, or exclusion of, paternally-inherited fetal DNA sequences that are not present in the mother, such as Y chromosome sequences in pregnancies with a male fetus or rhesus D (RhD) sequences in women who are RhD-negative. Recently, DNA sequencing technologies have allowed very precise relative quantification of DNA fragments and so the detection of the extra material resulting from fetal chromosome trisomy within the maternal plasma DNA can now be performed in a robust manner.

REFERENCES

1. Cuckle HS, Wald N. Tests using single markers. In: Wald N, Leck I (Eds). Antenatal and Neonatal Screening. Oxford: Oxford University Press. 2000. pp. 3-19.
2. Milunsky A, Canick JA. Maternal serum screening for neural tube and other defects. In: Milunsky A (Ed). Genetic Disorders and the Fetus: Diagnosis, Prevention and Treatment, 5th edn.

Baltimore and London the Johns Kopkins University Press. 2004 .p. 719.
3. Wapner R, Thom E, Simpson JL, et al. First trimester screening for trisomies 21 and 18. N Eng J Med. 2003;349(15):1405-13.
4. Haddow JE, Palomaki G, Knight GJ, et al. Screening of maternal serum for fetal Down's syndrome in the first trimester. N Engl J Med. 1998;388:955.
5. Spencer K, Wallace EM, Ritoe S. Second trimester dimeric Inhibin A in Down's syndrome screening. Prenat Diagn. 1996;15:1101.
6. Malone FD, Canick JA, Ball RH, et al. First trimester or second–trimester screening, or both, for Down's syndrome. N Engl J Med. 2005;353(19):2001-11.
7. Nicolaides KH. Nuchal translucency and other first trimester sonographic markers of chromosomal abnormalities. Review article. Am J Obstet Gynecol. 2004;191:45.
8. American College of Obstetricians and Gynaecologists: Screening for fetal chromosomal abnormalities. Practic Bulletin No.77, January 2007b.
9. Lo YM, Corbetta N, Chamberlain PF, Rai V, Sargent IL, Redman CW, et al. Presence of fetal DNA in maternal plasma and serum. Lancet. 1997;350:485-7.
10. Lo YM, Zhang J, Leung TN, Lau TK, Chang AM, Hjelm NM: Rapid clearance of fetal DNA from maternal plasma. Am J Hum Genet. 1999;64:218-24.
11. Alberry M, Maddocks D, Jones M, Abdel Hadi M, Abdel-Fattah S, Avent N, et al. Free fetal DNA in maternal plasma in anembryonic pregnancies: confirmation that the origin is the trophoblast. Prenat Diagn. 2007;27:415-8.
12. Lo YM, Tein MS, Lau TK, Haines CJ, Leung TN, Poon PM, et al. Quantitative analysis of fetal DNA in maternal plasma and serum: implications for noninvasive prenatal diagnosis. Am J Hum Genet. 1998;62:768-75.
13. Finning KM, Martin PG, Soothinll PW, Avent ND. Prediction of fetal D status from maternal plasma: introduction of a new noninvasive fetal RHD genotyping service. Transfusion. 2002;42(8):1079-85.

CHAPTER

12 First Trimester Screening

Geetha Balsarkar

Trisomy 21 popularly called Down's syndrome, affects approximately one in 800 live-born babies. Both Trisomy 21 and trisomy 18 cause significant physical and mental disadvantage and disabilities. With the wide variation in affection of Down's syndrome, from being severely affected to mild problems, there is no way of predicting how badly a particular baby might be affected. They have associated cardiac abnormalities as well requiring surgical intervention and long-term treatment. There is also an increased risk of cancers such as leukemia, and numerous metabolic problems including diabetes and thyroid disease. There is no cure for Down's syndrome, and antenatal diagnosis allows for preparation for the birth and subsequent care of a baby with Down's syndrome, or offer termination of pregnancy.[1]

Screening for fetal chromosomal abnormalities is an essential part of antenatal care in modern obstetrics. Initially, screening was determined only by using maternal age to classify a pregnancy as high or low risk for trisomy 21, as it was known that older women had a higher chance of carrying a baby with Down's syndrome. Antenatal screening is used for several reasons, medical and social. New developments in screening methods have increased the number of options for patients (Table 12.1).[2]

Definitive invasive tests [amniocentesis and chorionic villus sampling (CVS)] exist that allow the diagnosis of Down's syndrome accurately before birth, but carry a risk of miscarriage. Hence they cannot be offered to all patients. Cost of performing these tests is also more, placing a burden on the health system, where these are not covered by insurance. Though karyotyping can conclusively ascertain whether the fetus has trisomy 21, no test can predict the severity of problems a person with Down's syndrome will have.[3]

Noninvasive screening tests based on biochemical analysis of maternal serum or urine, or fetal ultrasound measurements, allow an estimate of the risk of a pregnancy being affected and provide parents with information to

Table 12.1 Key recommendations for practice

Clinical recommendations	Evidence rating	Comment
Pregnant women should be offered screening and invasive diagnostic testing regardless of age	B	Limited or inconsistent evidence
Combined testing is recommended for first-trimester screening	A	Evidence-based practice guidelines
Quadruple screening is recommended for second-trimester screening	A	Evidence-based practice guidelines
Women with isolated nuchal thickening or isolated maternal serum AFP (with normal ultrasonography and normal karyotype) should be followed closely because they are at increased risk of poor pregnancy outcomes	B	Limited or inconsistent evidence
Combined first- and second-trimester screening offers superior detection rates while maintaining low false-positive rates	B	Limited or inconsistent evidence
Genetics counseling and chorionic villus sampling or amniocentesis should be offered to all women with elevated risk, as determined by serum screening	A	Evidence-based practice guidelines
Women who pursue first-trimester screening alone should be offered maternal serum AFP testing in the second trimester to screen for neural tube defects	A	Evidence-based practice guidelines
Nuchal translucency testing and serum screening can be performed in multiple gestations, but they are less sensitive than first-trimester screening in singleton gestations	B	Limited or inconsistent evidence

Abbreviations: AFP, alpha-fetoprotein; *A,* consissstent, good-quality patient-oriented evidence; *B,* inconsistent or limited-quality patient-oriented evidence; *C,* consensus, disease-oriented evidence, usual practice, expert opinion, or case series.

enable them to make choices about definitive testing. Such screening tests are used during the first and second trimester of pregnancy.[2]

In some countries with a defined screening policy like the UK, first trimester screening plays a major role, although usually in combination with first trimester ultrasound scanning. In others however, there may only be a limited range of tests or markers available, often second trimester markers, rather than first trimester markers. The results of this review should be interpreted and applied in the context of test availability and local restrictions, populations or policies.[2]

In India, expectant mothers are given the choice to be screened for Down's syndrome during pregnancy to assist them in making decisions. Ideally all women should have the option of invasive diagnostic testing for fetal aneuploidy by CVS, if available, or amniocentesis. Benefits include diagnosis of all major aneuploidies and large chromosomal rearrangements. For women who do not initially want a invasive diagnostic test, screening for aneuploidy with non-invasive test is an acceptable option. Women should be informed of the adjusted risk for aneuploidy and allowed to make individual decisions.[4]

The First Trimester Screen is a new, optional noninvasive evaluation that combines a maternal blood screening test with an ultrasound evaluation of the fetus to identify risk for specific chromosomal abnormalities, including trisomy 21 and trisomy-18. It is now determined that first trimester screening is the most accurate noninvasive screening method available. In addition to screening for these abnormalities known as the nuchal translucency can assist in identifying other significant fetal abnormalities, such as cardiac disorders.[5,6]

The First Trimester Screen is performed between the 11th and 13+6 weeks of pregnancy (Tables 12.2 and 12.3).[7]

This screening test combines measurements from a nuchal translucency on ultrasound and a blood test, preferably done on the same day, to estimate the chances of a baby having Down syndrome. It then adjusts for the woman's age and gives a numerical estimate of the chance of Down syndrome, such as 1/2000 or 1/8.[8,9]

First trimester nuchal translucency should be interpreted for risk assessment only when measured by sonographers or sonologists trained and accredited for this service. Ultrasound dating should be performed if menstrual or conception dating is unreliable. For any abnormal serum screen calculated on the basis of menstrual dating, an ultrasound should be done to confirm accurate gestational age. Information such as gestational dating, maternal weight, ethnicity, insulin-dependent diabetes mellitus, and use of assisted reproduction technologies should be provided to the laboratory to improve accuracy of testing.[10]

Nuchal translucency (NT) is the sonographic appearance of a collection of fluid under the skin behind the fetal neck in the first-trimester of pregnancy. The term translucency is

Table 12.2 Glossary of terms

Term	Definition
Combined screening	Combination of nuchal translucency testing, serum measurement of PAPP-A and free or total hCG, and maternal age
Contingency screening	Nuchal translucency, PAPP-A, and hCG measurements are used to determine risk; no further testing is recommended in women at low risk of Down syndrome; maternal serum AFP should be performed in the second trimester to assess risk of neural tube defects
hCG	Hormone made from the fetal part of the placenta; elevated levels associated with increased risk of Down syndrome
Inhibin A	Hormone produced by the placenta; high levels associated with increased risk of Down syndrome
Integrated screening	Nuchal translucency testing and measurement of PAPP-A and hCG are integrated with the quadruple screen to produce a single risk result
Maternal serum AFP	Plasma protein found in mother's blood that is produced by the fetal liver; elevated levels associated with open neural tube defects, older than expected fetus (i.e. dating error), or multiple gestations; low levels associated with Down syndrome
Nuchal translucency	Thickness of the fluid under the skin of the fetal neck, measured by ultrasonography
PAPP-A	Zinc-binding protein that acts as an enzyme; low levels associated with increased risk of Down syndrome
Stepwise sequential screening	Nuchal translucency testing and measurement of PAPP-A and hCG are used to determine risk; if at increased risk, proceed directly to invasive testing; if not at increased risk, a second calculation with the addition of the quadruple screen produces another risk determination
Unconjugated estriol	Protein produced by the placenta and the fetal liver; low levels associated with Down syndrome

Abbreviations: AFP, alpha-fetoprotein; hCG, human chorionic gonadotropin; PAPP-A, pregnancy-associated plasma protein-A.

Table 12.3 Available options for antenatal testing

Test	Timing (weeks)	Detection rate of down syndrome (%)	False-positive rate (%)
First trimester			
Chorionic villus sampling	10–13	97.8	1–2
Nuchal translucency	10–4/7 to 13–6/7	70 –71	3.5–5
hCG and PAPP-A	10–12	53– 58	5
hCG, PAPP-A, and nuchal translucency	11–14	78.7–89	Less than 3–5
First and second trimester			
Integrated serum screening (PAPP-A with nuchal translucency)	11–14 and 15–20	94–96	Less than 3–5
Integrated serum screening (PAPP-A without nuchal translucency)	11–14 and 15–20	85–88	Less than 3–5
Stepwise sequential screening (PAPP-A with nuchal translucency)	11–14 and 15–20	95	5
Contingency screening (PAPP-A with nuchal translucency)	11–14 and 15–20	92	5

Abbreviations: AFP, alpha-fetoprotein; hCG, human chorionic gonadotropin; PAPP-A, pregnancy-associated plasma protein A.

used, irrespective of whether it is septated or not and whether it is confined to the neck or envelopes the whole fetus. In fetuses with chromosomal abnormalities, cardiac defects and many genetic syndromes the NT thickness is increased.[11]

Screening by NT alone can detect about 80% of fetuses with trisomy 21 and other major aneuploidies for a false positive rate of 5%. The combination of NT and maternal serum free β-hCG and pregnancy-associated plasma protein (PAPP-A) improves the detection to 90%. There is now evidence that the detection rate can increase to about 95% and the false positive rate can be reduced to 3% by also examining the nasal bone, ductus venosus flow and tricuspid flow.[12] Tests involving two markers in combination with maternal age, specifically PAPP-A, free β-hCG and maternal age are significantly better than those involving single markers with and without age. They detect seven out of 10 Down's syndrome affected pregnancies for a fixed 5% false positive rate (FPR). The addition of further markers (triple tests) has not been shown to be statistically superior; the studies included are small with limited power to detect a difference.

Protocol for measurement in NT:[10]

- The gestational period must be 11–13 weeks and 6 days.
- The fetal crown-rump length should be between 45 and 84 mm.
- The magnification of the image should be such that the fetal head and thorax occupy the whole screen.
- A mid-sagittal view of the face should be obtained. This is defined by the presence of the echogenic tip of the nose and rectangular shape of the palate anteriorly, the translucent diencephalon in the center and the nuchal membrane posteriorly. Minor deviations from the exact midline plane would cause nonvisualization of the tip of the nose and visibility of the zygomatic process of the maxilla.
- The fetus should be in a neutral position, with the head in line with the spine. When the fetal neck is hyperextended the measurement can be falsely increased and when the neck is flexed, the measurement can be falsely decreased.
- Care must be taken to distinguish between fetal skin and amnion.
- The widest part of translucency must always be measured.
- Measurements should be taken with the inner border of the horizontal line of the calipers placed on the line that defines the nuchal translucency thickness—the crossbar of the caliper should be such that it is hardly visible as it merges with the white line of the border, not in the nuchal fluid.
- In magnifying the image (pre or post freeze zoom) it is important to turn the gain down. This avoids the mistake of placing the caliper on the fuzzy edge of the line which causes an underestimate of the nuchal measurement.
- During the scan more than one measurement must be taken and the maximum one that meets all the above criteria should be recorded in the database.
- A new approach for the measurement of NT which improves the accuracy of measurements is with the use of a semi-automated technique. The operator places a box in the nuchal area and the machine automatically selects the best measurement, which uses an algorithm that draws a line through the center of the nuchal membrane and another line at the edge of the soft tissue overlying

the cervical spine. The measurement obtained by this method is similar to that obtained manually and it is therefore applicable to the software of the fetal medicine foundation.

- The umbilical cord may be round the fetal neck in about 5% of cases and this finding may produce a falsely increased NT. In such cases, the measurements of NT above and below the cord are different and, in the calculation of risk, it is more appropriate to use the average of the two measurements.

Absence of the nasal bone can be used as a marker for Down syndrome in the first trimester of pregnancy. Inclusion of the nasal bone in the current first-trimester screening protocol along with nuchal translucency, free β-hCG and PAPP-A can achieve high detection at a very low false-positive rate. Large datasets are needed to confirm whether the measurement of nasal bone length provides additional benefits beyond the assessment of the presence or absence of the nasal bone.[12]

In a high proportion of fetuses with trisomy 21 and other chromosomal abnormalities the nasal bone is hypoplastic or not visible at 11–13 weeks' gestation. Assessment of the nasal bone at 11–13 weeks improves the performance of combined screening for trisomy 21 by maternal age, fetal nuchal translucency (NT) and serum biochemistry. The difficulty is when the gestation is 11 weeks or the beginning of the 12th week and the nasal bone is absent but the NT, the other ultrasound markers and the serum biochemistry are normal. In such cases the scan should be repeated in one week and if there is persistence of absence of the nasal bone then the risk for trisomies is increased.[13]

The combined accuracy rate for the combined screen to detect the chromosomal abnormalities is approximately 85% with a false positive rate of 5%. About one in 20 women (5%) having this test will have a 'high risk' result but most of these women will not be carrying a baby with Down's syndrome. If the test indicates the chance for Down syndrome is greater than 1/350, the result is called screen positive. The test will also indicate a screen positive for Trisomy 18/13 if the chance of chromosome abnormalities Trisomy 18 and Trisomy 13 is greater than 1/100.[14]

For the first 14 weeks of pregnancy, the evidence supports the use of the double blood markers; pregnancy-associated plasma protein A (PAPP-A) and free beta-human chorionic gonadotropin (β-hCG), in combination with the mother's age.[12,14] This test detects around seven out of every 10 (68%) pregnancies affected by Down's syndrome. It is important to realize a positive result does not equate to having an abnormality, but rather serves as a attempt to discuss further testing. The screen should not be confused with screens performed during the second trimester known as the triple marker or quadruple screen.[15]

It is very important to counsel a patient what a screening test is before getting one performed. Counseling must be nondirective and must respect a woman's right to accept or decline any or all of the testing or options offered. Screening test is not a diagnostic test. This will help alleviate some of the anxiety that can accompany test results. Screening tests do not look only at results from the blood test done, but they compare a number of different factors (including age, ethnicity, results from blood tests, etc.) and then estimate what a person's chances are of having an abnormality. The blood tests themselves have no adverse effects for the woman, over and above the risks of a routine blood test. There is a 5% false positive rate for the test. Parents should be counseled of the possibility of receiving abnormal results and then finding, after further testing, the baby is normal.[12]

It is routine to offer amniocentesis or CVS to women with a high risk test result. Because the test is performed early, right in the first trimester, it is often used to determine whether a mother should consider undergoing an early diagnostic test, such as chorionic villus sampling, or second trimester amniocentesis.[16] If a mother is carrying a baby with Down's syndrome, then there is the decision about whether to terminate or continue with the pregnancy. In India, the upper limit of 20 weeks as legal limit for second trimester termination, often compels the obstetrician to look for early result.[17] The information offers parents the opportunity and counseling to plan for life with a Down's syndrome child, if termination cannot be offered, or there has been a late diagnosis. In the first 14 weeks of pregnancy, there is little evidence to support the use of other serum tests made up of more than two blood markers.[15]

However, some women who have a 'high-risk'screening test result, and are given amniocentesis or CVS have a risk of miscarrying a baby unaffected by Down's syndrome. Parents will need to weigh up this risk when deciding whether or not to have an amniocentesis or CVS following a 'high-risk' screening test result. In babies who are at an increased risk for chromosomal abnormalities, increased fluid is often found in the nuchal translucency. Abnormally high or low hCG and PAPP-A levels are also often found. The first trimester screen combines the results from these three measurements (nuchal translucency, hCG, and PAPP-A) with maternal age risk factors and determines an overall risk factor for chromosomal abnormalities.[15]

A disadvantage of first trimester screen in the general literature is that it is less accurate than an integrated prenatal screening which also screens for Down syndrome. 10–15% of pregnancies with Down syndrome screen negative, compared to 10% with integrated prenatal screening (IPS). The false positive rate is also higher with first trimester screening (FTS) at 4–5%, compared to 2–3% with IPS. In addition, another blood test for alpha fetoprotein is required in the 2nd trimester to determine an increased chance of spina bifida.[2]

Some couples may opt not to pursue screening or additional testing for various reasons:

- They are comfortable with the results no matter what the outcome, especially in certain religious communities
- Because of personal, moral, or religious reasons, making a decision about carrying the child to term is not an option
- Some parents choose not to allow any testing that poses any risk of harming the developing baby.

For *in vitro* fertilization (IVF)/intracytoplasmic sperm injection (ICSI) singletons, combined first trimester prenatal screening based on maternal age, nuchal translucency scan and biomarkers is appropriate. However, biomarkers seem to be altered, causing a higher false-positive rate, in IVF/ICSI singleton gestations. Correction factors have been developed and should be used when screening for Down's syndrome in singleton pregnancies.

With regard to IVF/ICSI twin pregnancies, biomarker values seem to be dependent on chorionicity as well as gestational age. Whether the use of a correction factor for mode of conception in the risk calculations for Down's syndrome in twin pregnancies is valid has not been fully elucidated. In vanishing twin pregnancies with a second gestational sac with a dead fetus, first trimester screening should be based solely on the maternal age and the nuchal translucency scan as biomarkers are significantly altered in these cases.

First trimester prenatal screening after IVF/ICSI treatment requires specific precautions in both singleton and twin pregnancies.[14]

Combined first- and second-trimester screening: To improve detection rates of aneuploidy with antenatal screening, combining of existing first- and second-trimester screening has been advocated. With combined testing, detection rates are improved to 92–96%, with false-positive rates of 5%.[18-21]

INTEGRATED SCREENING[21]

Integrated screening involves PAPP-A and nuchal translucency testing in the first trimester and the quadruple screen in the second trimester. After the first trimester tests are completed, the results are held until the quadruple screen is performed. A single risk determination is made using all available data and the patient's age-associated risk. Integrated serum screening uses PAPP-A and quadruple screening without nuchal translucency, if it is unavailable.

STEPWISE SEQUENTIAL SCREENING[21]

Stepwise sequential screening combines PAPP-A and nuchal translucency testing with an age-associated risk to provide a risk determination in the first trimester. If the patient is at increased risk based on results of the first trimester PAPP-A and nuchal translucency testing, she may undergo invasive diagnostic testing or await the triple or quadruple screen in the second trimester for revised risk determination. If the patient chooses to undergo second-trimester serum testing, a second risk determination is made with all available data.

CONTINGENCY SCREENING

Contingency screening also involves PAPP-A and nuchal translucency testing with an age-associated risk to provide a risk determination in the first trimester. However, with contingency testing, the risk determination is stratified. If the risk is above a certain cut-off, invasive diagnostic testing is offered. If the risk is below a second cut-off, the patient is told that no further testing is required. If the patient's risk determination falls between these two cut-offs, then second-trimester maternal serum screening is advised.

First trimester screening, with the use of maternal age, nuchal translucency and the biochemical markers free β-hCG and PAPP-A, dramatically reduces the number of women who will need CVS or amniocentesis for prenatal diagnosis. As a result the cost for prenatal diagnosis of the population and also the risk of iatrogenic missed miscarriages is also significantly lower. Finally, this screening method gives the advantage of early counseling and of diagnosis quite as early as in the first trimester of pregnancy. With the advent of first-trimester options, patients will need to choose early and be comfortable with their choice.

REFERENCES

1. First Trimester Screening for Trisomies 21 and 18. National Down Syndrome Society. N Eng J Med. 2003;349(15):1405-13.
2. ACOG Committee on Practice Bulletins. ACOG Practice Bulletin Number 77: screening for fetal chromosomal abnormalities. Obstet Gynecol. 2007;109:217-27.
3. Tabor A, Philip J, Madsen M, Bang J, Obel EB, Nørgaard-Pedersen B. Randomised controlled trial of genetic amniocentesis in 4606 low-risk women. Lancet. 1986;1(8493):1287-93.
4. Alfirevic Z, Sundberg K, Brigham S. Amniocentesis and chorionic villus sampling for prenatal diagnosis. Cochrane Database Syst Rev. 2003;3:CD003252.
5. Bahado-Singh RO, Wapner R, Thom E, et al. for the First Trimester Maternal Serum Biochemistry and Fetal Nuchal Translucency Screening Study Group. Elevated first-trimester

nuchal translucency increases the risk of congenital heart defects. Am J Obstet Gynecol. 2005;192(5):1357-61.
6. Palomaki GE, Steinort K, Knight GJ, Haddow JE. Comparing three screening strategies for combining first- and second-trimester Down syndrome markers. Obstet Gynecol. 2006;107 (2 pt 1):367-75.
7. Wapner R, Thom E, Simpson JL, et al. For the first trimester maternal serum biochemistry and fetal nuchal translucency screening (BUN) study group. First-trimester screening for trisomies 21 and 18. N Engl J Med. 2003;349(15):1405-13.
8. Nicolaides KH. Nuchal translucency and other first-trimester sonographic markers of chromosomal abnormalities. Am J Obstet Gynecol. 2004;191(1):45-67.
9. Saltvedt S, Almström H, Kublickas M, et al. Screening for Down syndrome based on maternal age or fetal nuchal translucency: a randomized controlled trial in 39,572 pregnancies. Ultrasound Obstet Gynecol. 2005;25(6):537-45.
10. Snijders RJ, Thom EA, Zachary JM, et al. First-trimester trisomy screening: nuchal translucency measurement training and quality assurance to correct and unify technique. Ultrasound Obstet Gynecol. 2002;19(4):353-9.
11. Hyett J, Perdu M, Charland G, Snijders R, Nicolaides KH. Using fetal nuchal translucency to screen for major congenital cardiac defects at 10–14 weeks of gestation: population based cohort study. BMJ. 1999;318(7176):81-5.
12. Whitworth M, BrickerL, Mullan C. Ultrasound for fetal assessment in early pregnancy; Cochrane Database Syst Rev. 2015;7:CD007058.
13. Souka AP, Von Kaisenberg C, Hyett JA, Sonek JD, Nicolaides KH. Increased nuchal translucency with normal karyotype. Am J Obstet Gynecol. 2005;192(4):1005-21.
14. Spencer K, Souter V, Tul N, Snijders R, Nicolaides KH. A screening program for trisomy 21 at 10–14 weeks using fetal nuchal translucency, maternal serum free beta-human chorionic gonadotropin and pregnancy-associated plasma protein-A. Ultrasound Obstet Gynecol. 1999;13(4):231-7.
15. Malone FD, Berkowitz RL, Canick JA, D'Alton ME. First-trimester screening for aneuploidy: research or standard of care? Am J Obstet Gynecol. 2000;182(3):490-6.
16. Caughey AB, Hopkins LM, Norton ME. Chorionic villus sampling compared with amniocentesis and the difference in the rate of pregnancy loss. Obstet Gynecol. 2006;108(3 pt 1): 612-6.
17. Crane JP, LeFevre ML, Winborn RC, et al. A randomized trial of prenatal ultrasonographic screening: impact on the detection, management, and outcome of anomalous fetuses. The RADIUS Study Group. Am J Obstet Gynecol. 1994;171(2):392-9.
18. Cunningham FG, Leveno KL, Bloom SL, Hauth JC, Gilstrap LC III, Wenstrom KD. Williams Obstetrics, 22nd edn. New York, NY: McGraw-Hill. 2005. pp. 328-30.
19. Jenkins TM, Wapner RJ. Prenatal diagnosis of congenital disorders. In: Creasy RK, Resnik R (Eds). Maternal-Fetal Medicine: Principles and Practice, 5th edn. Philadelphia, Pa: WB Saunders. 2004. pp. 263-9.
20. Shipp TD, Benacerraf BR. Second trimester ultrasound screening for chromosomal abnormalities. Prenat Diagn. 2002; 22(4):296-307.
21. Palomaki GE, Steinort K, Knight GJ, Haddow JE. Comparing three screening strategies for combining first- and second-trimester Down syndrome markers. Obstet Gynecol. 2006;107 (2 pt 1):367-75.

CHAPTER

13 Maternal Serum Screening for Chromosomal Abnormalities

Renu Makwana

INTRODUCTION

Birth of babies with congenital defects is the most frustrating experience to the parents.

Prenatal diagnosis is the science of identifying malformations, disruptions, chromosomal abnormalities, and other genetic syndromes in the fetus. It encompasses routine screening tests for aneuploidy and neural-tube defects, invasive diagnostic tests such as chorionic villus sampling and amniocentesis, additional screening and diagnostic tests offered to those at risk for specific genetic disorders, and the diagnosis of structural malformations with specialized sonography and other fetal imaging technique. We cannot use diagnostic tests for entire population, that is why we need screening tests to identify high risk from low risk. Patients with high-risk screening tests will be offered definite diagnostic test. The screening tests help reducing need of costly, potential harmful diagnostic tests, save costs.

Over the last past 40 years, there have been revolutionary changes in the approach to prenatal diagnosis and screening. In the 1960s and 1970s, prenatal diagnosis and screening evolved from merely wishing patients "good luck" to then asking "how old are you?" maternal age was, and still is, a cheap screening test for aneuploidy. However, an emergence of techniques has dramatically changed the statistical performance of screening tests to identify high-risk patients. Biochemical and ultrasound screens have gone through multiple generation with increasing sensitivities and specificities to the point where there has been considerable (and sometimes deliberate) confusion as to the distinction between screening and diagnosis.

CHROMOSOMAL DISORDERS

Chromosomal abnormality screening in an antenatal OPD meant, screening for Down syndrome. Much of the change in attitude has come from improvements in the ability to accurately detect genetic health status of the fetus. Although Down syndrome (DS) represents only a small proportion of the serious genetic disorders observed worldwide (Box 13.1), it continues to be at the forefront of patient concern because that is the name most of us know. Down syndrome has a livebirth incidence of approximately one in 700 and is the single most common cause of mental handicap in school age children. It is associated with a spectrum of mental and physical handicap and in view of this, strategies have been developed to identity those pregnancies. This affords the opportunity for subsequent diagnostic testing and termination of an affected pregnancy, if chosen by the parents. Screening for trisomy 21 is offered routinely as part of antenatal care. All pregnant women should be counseled that both diagnostic and screening tests are available in pregnancy. Usually, all women will choose to have a screening test, as this carries no innate risk to the pregnancy, and will not wish to discuss diagnostic testing in any form but for others, the consequences of having a child affected by aneuploidy are of such enormity that no screening will give sufficient reassurance. If such concerns are expressed, the mother must have ample opportunity to discuss the full range of diagnostic tests that are available. It is for the couple to decide which risk is most acceptable. Screening for trisomy 21 should be performed of an 'opt- in' basis and it is essential that parents who choose to enter a screening program have adequate information about the implications and limitations of the test so that they are not faced with result and decisions for which they are unprepared.

Box 13.1 Worldwide birth defects

- Congenital heart defects: 1,040,835
- Neural tube defects: 323,904
- Hemoglobin disorders: 307,897
- Down syndrome: 217,293
- Glucose-6- phosphate dehydrogenase deficiency: 177,032

Data from global report on birth defects: the hidden toll of dying and disabled children. White plains (NY): March of Dimes Birth Defects Foundation: 2006.

A screening test simply places the individual in a high-risk or a low-risk group. It does not tell us whether or not the condition being screened for is actually present, thus, a woman who has a high-risk screening test result for trisomy 21; would have to undergo a diagnostic test, if she wished to establish whether or not the pregnancy was affected. Similarly, a low-risk result does not exclude the presence of trisomy 21; there is no such thing as no risk on the basis of the screening the result. Appropriate counseling is in therefore paramount to ensure that parents for whom screening is inappropriate do not enter the program. Regardless of age, all women are counseled regarding the differences between screening and diagnostic tests, and they are given the option of invasive diagnostic testing.

DEVELOPMENT OF SCREENING PROGRAMS

Screening programs have advanced from a single marker maternal age to using a combination of markers including biochemical and ultrasound features in addition there has been a drive to offer screening at earlier gestations along with screening involving cell free fetal DNA (NIPT). With the exception of cell-free fetal DNA testing, each first- and/or second-trimester aneuploidy screening test is based on a composite likelihood ratio, and the maternal age-related risk is multiplied by this ratio. This principle also applies to modification of the Down syndrome risk by selected sonographic findings (Box 13.2). Each woman is provided with a specific risk, expressed as a ratio—1:X. However, each screening test has a predetermined value at which it is deemed "positive" or abnormal. For second-trimester tests, this threshold has traditionally been set at the risk for fetal Down syndrome in a woman aged 35 years—approximately 1 in 385 at term. Women with a positive screening test result should be offered a diagnostic test for fetal karyotype by either chorionic villus sampling or amniocentesis (American College of Obstetricians and Gynecologists, 2012a).[1] Detailed counseling is must for couple to make choice.

FIRST BIOCHEMICAL MARKER

In 1984, Merkatz et al. published the association of low maternal serum α-fetoprotein (AFP) with an increased risk of aneuploidy in general and Cuckle et al. confirmed that this holds for Down syndrome. In subsequent years, there was a gradual acceptance of the association, as well as an eventual understanding that the extent of AFP reduction differed according to the type of aneuploidy. For example, trisomy 18 has much lower values on average than Down syndrome.

Since AFP was already widely being used to screen for neural tube defects, at 16–18 weeks' gestation, it was relatively simple to extend the test interpretation to include aneuploidy. This was done by the calculation of a likelihood ratio (proportion of aneuploidy pregnancies divided by proportion of unaffected pregnancies with the given AFP level) and using this to increase or decrease the maternal age-specific risk. The likelihood ratio was derived from a Gaussian model of the AFP distributions in aneuploidy and unaffected pregnancies. In practice, to calculate the risk accurately requires further statistical manipulation, much more than for other tests done in clinical chemistry. Maternal serum AFP screening for aneuploidy was widely adopted and had the potential to increase the detection rate, but it was inefficient. The optimal use of a biochemical or ultrasound marker is to screen all women regardless of age and to define high risk purely on the basis of the screening result.

COMBINED FIRST-TRIMESTER SCREENING

The most commonly used protocol involves measurement of sonographic nuchal translucency and two maternal serum analytes. The goal of first trimester maternal serum screening programs is to identify women at increased risk of having a baby affected with Down syndrome, Patau syndrome, and

Box 13.2 Down syndrome screening protocols over the past 50 years[2-5]

Method	Components	Time frame	Sensitivity %	FPR (%)
Maternal age	Birthday	1960s to present	35	15
Low MSAFP + age	AFP	1980s	50	~5
Double	AFP/hCG	1990s	55	~5
Triple	AFP/hCG/estriol	1990s	60	~5
Quad	AFP/hCG/estriol/inhibin	1990s/2000s	65	~5
NT	US measurements	1990s to present	60	~5
Combined	Free β-hCG/PAPP-A/NT	2000s to present	85	~5
Sequential	Combined + Quad	2000s to present	85–90	~5
Free fetal DNA	Sequence/targeted	Since 2011	98	0.2–1

Abbreviations: FPR, false-positive rate; Free β-hCG, free β-subunit hCG; hCG, human chorionic gonadotropin; inh, dimeric inhibin α; MSAFP, maternal serum alpha-fetoprotein; NT, nuchal translucency; PAPP-A, pregnancy-associated plasma protein–A; uE3, unconjugated estriol.

Flow chart 13.1 Combined first trimester screening[5,9]

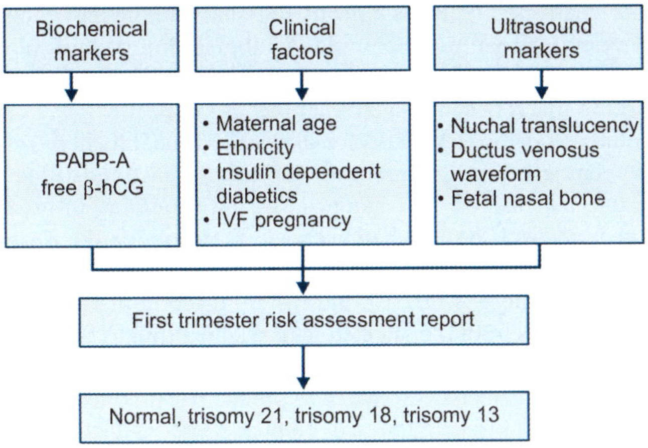

Table 13.1 Detection rate was 89% with 5% false positive[6]

Maternal serum marker (10–14 weeks)	NTD	Down syndrome	Trisomy-18,13	Pattern
PAPP-A		Low	Low	0.45 MoM
Total beta hCG		Normal	Low	1.33 MoM
Free beta hCG		Increased		2.0 MoM

Edward syndrome defects and those that will benefit from the testing (Flow chart 13.1).

This is performed between 11 and 14 weeks' gestation. Two analytes used for first-trimester aneuploidy screening are—4 mL of blood is required and sample to be processed immediately or serum separated or refrigerated. Transporting the sample should be with temperature control.

1. *Pregnancy-associated plasma protein A (PAPP-A):* PAPP-A is a high molecular weight zinc containing metalloglycoprotein. It is produced by the trophoblast and its biological function is still unclear. In addition to being a marker of chromosomal aneuploidy, it is an indicator of early pregnancy failure and complications, Cornelia de Lange syndrome and acute coronary syndrome. PAPP-A and placental growth factor (PlGF) estimation is, a most effective approach to identifying a high proportion of pregnancies at high risk for early onset pre-eclampsia, according to Nicolaides.
2. *Serum free β-hCG:* In cases of fetal Down syndrome, the first-trimester serum free β-hCG level is higher, approximately 2.0 MoM, and the PAPP-A level is lower, approximately 0.5 MoM. With trisomy 18 and trisomy 13, levels of both analytes are lower (Table 13.1).[4,6,7] Similarly, total hCG was found to be a poor marker in the first trimester with an MoM of 1.33, but an adequate marker during the second trimester. Free beta-hCG on the other hand is higher and has a relatively stable MoM from 10 to 18 weeks. Low levels of free β-hCG have been associated with fetal demise.[8]

NUCHAL TRANSLUCENCY

This is the maximum thickness of the subcutaneous translucent area between the skin and soft tissue overlying the fetal spine at the back of the neck. It is measured in the sagittal plane, when the crown-rump length measures between 38 and 84 mm. Specific criteria for nuchal translucency (NT) measurement are there. The NT measurement is expressed as a multiple of the gestational age-specific median, similar to serum markers used for aneuploidy screening. An increased NT thickness itself is not a fetal abnormality, but rather is a marker that confers increased risk. Approximately, one-third of fetuses with increased nuchal translucency thickness will have a chromosome abnormality, nearly half of which are Down syndrome (Snijders, 1998). As an isolated marker, NT detects 64–70% of fetuses with Down syndrome at a false-positive rate of 5%, and it has maximal sensitivity at 11 weeks.[4] The risk conferred by an increased NT thickness is independent of that of serum analytes, and combining NT with serum analyte values results in greatly improved aneuploidy detection.[7] Thus, NT is generally used as an isolated marker only in screening for multifetal gestations, in which serum screening is not as accurate or may not be available (American College of Obstetricians and Gynecologists, 2013c).[10] An exception is that if the NT measurement is increased to 3–4 mm, then the aneuploidy risk is unlikely to be normalized using serum analyte assessment, and invasive testing should be offered (Comstock, 2006). Increased NT thickness is also associated with other aneuploidies, genetic syndromes, and various birth defects, especially fetal cardiac anomalies (Atzei, 2005; Simpson, 2007). Because of this, if the NT measurement is 3.5 mm or greater, the patient should be offered targeted sonography, with or without fetal echocardiography, in addition to fetal karyotyping (American College of Obstetricians and Gynecologists, 2013c).[10] The NT must be imaged and measured with a high degree of precision for aneuploidy detection to be accurate.[11]

Information to be provided by physician as biochemical serum screening depends on many factors:

1. Specimen collection date
2. First or second specimen
3. Date by LMP or gestational age by USG
4. Maternal age and weight
5. Relevant family and obstetric history
6. Presence of maternal diabetes mellitus
7. Maternal race if indicated
8. Whether multiple pregnancies are present/suspected.

Table 13.2 Factors affecting serum analytes[6]

	beta-hCG	PAPP-A	Risk
Age			
Previous Down's	Increase prior risk		
Maternal weight	↓	↑	Variably alters the risk
IDDM	—	↓	
IVF conception		↓	
Smoker	↓	↓	

Proper sample collection and temperature control is very important, collect sample in plain tube and leave for 30 minutes then centrifuge at 1000 rpm for 10–15 minutes. After that, sample can be stored between 2–8°C and transport in thermocol box within 24 hours. Temperature affects analytes—hCG—degradation of hCG is more in whole blood than serum especially at 30°C, at high temperatures and if there is long interval between collection and analysis of the sample (Table 13.2).

PAPP-A levels are stable in serum, 142 days at 2–8°C, 37 days at room temperature and 20 days at 30°C.

Special Circumstances

Patient on injection hCG—Sample to be taken after 5 days of injection—If CRL (crown rump length) at time of scan is >79-rescan to check CRL at the time of blood sample.

In vitro fertilization (IVF)/intracytoplasmic sperm injection (ICSI) pregnancy—ET date to be considered donor embryo transferred—donar age to be used for risk calculation both donor/own eggs transferred !!—avoid screening explaining the same to the patient.

Sample Rejection Criteria-1

- hCG taken <5 days
- EDTA sample
- Clot/lipemic sample.

Sample Rejection Criteria-2

- Triplets, triplet with one empty sac
- CRL >84 mm, CRL < 19 mm.

Reporting

The report should contain

1. MoM (Multiple of median) values for the measured analyte.
2. Down syndrome risk estimate along with risk for NTD or trisomy 18.
3. An interpretation as screen positive or screen negative.

Considerations in Multiple Pregnancies

Chromosomal anomalies in nonidentical (dizygous) twin pregnancies are likely to be discordant. Prenatal diagnosis and selective termination of an affected fetus poses risk to the unaffected fetus. As a result, decision making regarding prenatal screening is complex in the setting of multiple pregnancy. Any form of screening that includes maternal serum markers can only give a pregnancy-specific risk, not a fetus-specific risk. Thus, for dizygotic twins, biochemical screening will not differentiate the risk for each individual fetus. Experience with maternal serum screening in twin pregnancies is limited. On average, the serum markers are twice as high as for singletons of equivalent gestational age. However, there is the risk that where discordant anomaly exists, levels from the affected fetus will be brought closer to the mean by the levels of the unaffected twin. Mathematical models have been constructed to predict risk on the basis of biochemical screening in twin pregnancies. A detection rate of 51% (for a false-positive rate of 5%) using second-trimester beta hCG and AFP has been quoted. However, mathematical modeling may be an oversimplification. It is also recognized that assisted conception, likely to be responsible for a number of multiple premultiple pregnancies, may affect analyte levels. Owing to the paucity of data, biochemical screening is not routinely offered in the majority of centers.

Second Trimester Biochemical Screening Options

- AFP - malformations
- AFP + hCG + uE3 (triple test)
- AFP + hCG + uE3 + inhibin A (Quad test)-preferred one

Alpha-fetoprotein (AFP) was the first serum marker to be used in screening programs for trisomy 21. AFP is a fetal-specific protein that is produced initially by the fetal yolk sac and subsequently by the fetal liver. Pregnancies with fetal Down syndrome are characterized by lower maternal serum AFP levels—approximately 0.7 MoM, higher hCG levels-approximately 2.0 MoM, and lower unconjugated estriol levels—approximately 0.8 MoM.[12] This *triple test* can detect 61–70% of Down syndrome cases as shown in Box 13.2 (Alldred, 2012). Levels of all three markers are decreased in the setting of trisomy 18, with a detection rate similar to that for Down syndrome at a false-positive rate of only 0.5%.[10] Levels of a fourth marker—*dimeric inhibin alpha*—are elevated in Down syndrome, with an average value of 1.8 MoM (Spencer, 1996). The addition of dimeric inhibin to the other three markers is the *quadruple* or *quad test*, which has a trisomy 21 detection rate of approximately 80% at a false-positive rate of 5% (see Box 13.2). As with first-trimester screening, aneuploidy detection rates will be slightly lower in younger women and higher in women older than 35 years at delivery. If second-trimester serum screening is used in twin pregnancies, aneuploidy detection rates are significantly lower.[13]

The quad test is the most commonly used second-trimester serum screening test for aneuploidy. As a stand-alone test, it is generally used if women do not begin care until the second-trimester or if first-trimester screening is not available. As subsequently discussed, combining the quad test with first-trimester screening yields even greater aneuploidy detection rates.

Unexplained Abnormalities of Second-Trimester Analytes

There is a significant association between second-trimester elevation of either hCG or dimeric inhibin alpha levels and adverse pregnancy outcomes. The outcomes reported are similar to those associated with AFP level elevation and include fetal-growth restriction, pre-eclampsia, preterm birth, fetal demise, and stillbirth. Moreover, the likelihood of adverse outcome is increased when multiple marker levels are elevated.[14] However, the sensitivity and positive predictive values of these markers are considered too low to be useful for screening or management.[15]

Low Maternal Serum Estriol Levels

A maternal serum estriol level < 0.25 MoM has been associated with:

- Anencephaly
- Placental steroid sulfatase deficiency
- Aromatase deficiency
- Smith Lemli Opitz syndrome
- 17-Hydroxylase deficiency
- Pituitary ACTH deficiency
- ACTH insensitivity syndromes
- Maternal ingestion of corticosteroids.

Factors Affecting the Level of the Quad Screen Markers

Maternal weight was found to have an inverse relation with the levels of all four markers. Diabetes insulin-dependent (not GDM) AFP was found to be 40% lower than nondiabetics.

Twin pregnancy MSAFP higher than those having single fetus. MoM > 4 significant.

Combined First- and Second-Trimester Screening

Combined screening strategies enhance aneuploidy detection. For this reason, the American College of Obstetricians and Gynecologists (2013c) recommends that a strategy incorporating both first- and second-trimester screening should be offered to women who seek prenatal care in the first trimester.

Three types of screening strategies are available:

1. *Integrated screening:* It combines results of first- and second-trimester tests. This includes a combined measurement of fetal NT and serum analyte levels at 11–14 weeks' gestation plus quadruple markers at 15–20 weeks. An aneuploidy risk is then calculated from these seven parameters. As expected, integrated screening has the highest Down syndrome detection rate—94–96% at a false-positive rate of 5% (see Box 13.2). If NT measurement is not available, *serum integrated screening* includes all six serum markers to calculate risk. This screening, however, is less effective.
2. *Sequential screening:* It discloses the results of first-trimester screening to women at highest risk, who are then offered invasive testing with chorionic villus sampling or amniocentesis (Table 13.3). There are two testing strategies in this category:
   i. *Stepwise sequential screening:* Women with first-trimester screen results that confer risk for Down syndrome above a particular threshold are offered invasive testing, and the remaining women receive second-trimester screening. The threshold is set at approximately 1%, because in a screened population, the 1% at highest risk includes approximately 70% of Down syndrome pregnancies.[3] This method of screening may achieve up to a 95% detection rate (see Box 13.2).
   ii. *Contingent sequential screening*: Women are divided into high-, moderate-, and low-risk groups. Those at highest risk, for example, the top 1%, are offered invasive testing. Women at moderate risk,

Table 13.3 Sequential screening policies: predicted detection rate for a given false-positive rate[3]

First trimester combination with second trimester AFP, Free β-hCG, uE3, and Inhibin	Early detection rate	Second trimester tests	False-positive rate		
			1%	3%	5%
Integrated test					
PAPP-A and NT	0%	100%	85%	91%	93%
Stepwise test					
PAPP-A, free β-hCG, and NT	70%	99%	85%	93%	95%
Contingent test					
PAPP-A, free β-hCG, and NT	70%	15%	85%	92%	94%

Flow chart 13.2 Contingent screening[3]

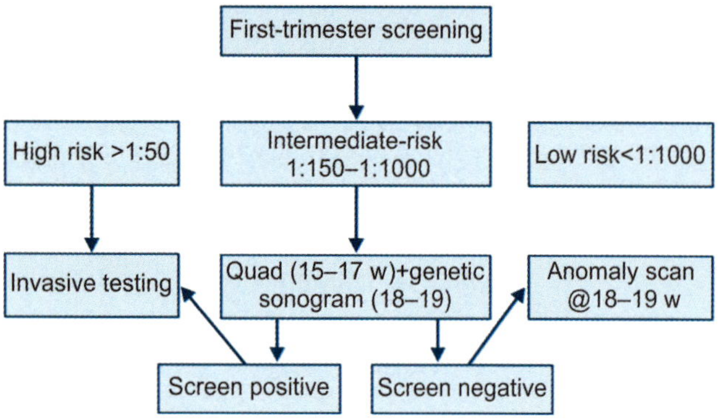

who comprise 15–20% of the population, undergo second trimester screening. The remaining 80–85%, who are at or below a 1:1000 risk, receive negative screening test results and have no further testing (Flow chart 13.2).[3] Thus, most of those screened are provided with results almost immediately while still maintaining a high detection rate. This rate ranges from 88% to 94% (see Box 13.2) This option is also more cost-effective because a second-trimester test is obviated in up to 85% of patients. Integrated and sequential screening strategies require coordination between the provider and laboratory to ensure that the second sample is obtained during the appropriate gestational age window, sent to the same laboratory, and linked to the first-trimester results.[16]

Factor to Consider when Comparing the Three Models of Testing

- Integrated testing achieves the lowest false-positive rate for a given detection rate and is associated with lower procedure-related loss rates of unaffected fetuses.
- Sequential and contingent screening label women as being a high or low risk on the basis of limited information.
- Sequential and contingent screening will identify 66% of affected pregnancies by the end of the first trimester, allowing earlier termination of pregnancy. Some of these first-trimester pregnancies would have miscarried spontaneously, avoiding the distressing decision to opt for pregnancy termination. It has been estimated that approximately 23% of Down syndrome pregnancies miscarry between the time of amniocentesis and term.
- The intermediate positive risk group in the contingent screening program will receive two different risks. A low-risk result from the second-trimester part of the test may not be sufficient to allay the anxiety generated on the basis of all the screening information.
- In contrast to contingent and sequential screening, the integrated screening test treats all women in the same way and a single risk is generated on the basis of all the screening information.

First-Trimester versus Second-Trimester Screening

One of the main reasons for developing first-trimester screening options has been the perceived advantage that earlier detection of chromosomal abnormalities and, hence earlier termination of pregnancy by a surgical method is less emotionally traumatic for the woman. Whether or not this is the case, and obviously individual women will feel differently about this part of their care, certain aspects of first-trimester screening should be considered. There is a natural attrition rate for aneuploid pregnancies as gestation advances and thus first-trimester screening will identify a proportion of pregnancies that were destined to miscarry spontaneously. This criticism obviously also applies to second-trimester programs but the rate of fetal lethality is higher between the time of chronic villus sampling and term (43%) compared with the time of amniocentesis and term (23%). There is evidence to indicate that the fetal lethality in cases of trisomy 21 is higher in those fetuses with the biggest nuchal translucency measurements, demonstrating that is ultrasound marker will detect a number of pregnancies that would otherwise miscarry spontaneously. Thus, the potential advantage of earlier termination pregnancy has to be weighed against the fact that first-trimester screening will 'convert' a proportion of spontaneous miscarriages to pregnancy terminations and the psychological impact of this factor needs to be considered.

Cell-free Fetal DNA Screening

The "holy grail" of prenatal screening was for decades the concept that fetal cells could be obtained from maternal blood, thus avoiding invasive testing. Using massively parallel sequencing or chromosome selective sequencing to isolate cell-free fetal DNA from maternal plasma, fetal Down syndrome and other autosomal trisomies may be detected as early as 10 weeks' gestation. Recent trials of these techniques in high-risk pregnancies have yielded detection rates for trisomies 21, 18, and 13 of approximately 98% at a false-positive rate of 0.5% or less (American College of Obstetricians and Gynecologists, 2012b; Bianchi, 2012; Palomaki, 2011, 2012; Sparks, 2012). This novel technology has recently become clinically available as a screening test, but it is not considered a replacement diagnostic test. So, only a contingent protocol with a few cases "on the bubble" which reflex to NIPS will be cost-effective. Those cases at high risk should go directly to diagnostic procedures rather than just "kicking the can" down the road for more 2 weeks before an answer is then sought. The American College of Obstetricians and Gynecologists (2012b) currently recommends that the test may be offered to the following groups:

- Women 35 years or older at delivery
- Those with sonographic findings indicating increased risk for fetal aneuploidy
- Those with a prior pregnancy complicated by trisomy 21, 18, or 13
- Patient or partner carries a balanced Robertsonian translocation indicating increased risk for fetal trisomy 21 or 13
- Those with an abnormal first-, second-, or combined first- and second-trimester screening test result for aneuploidy.

The College does not recommend offering the test to women with low-risk pregnancies or multifetal gestations (American College of Obstetricians and Gynecologists, 2012b).

TAKE HOME MESSAGE

Over the past 35 years, there has been a steady evolution of biochemical and also biophysical parameters used to adjust the risk that a woman is carrying a fetus with aneuploidy. At every step there has been controversy as to the best methods to employ in this endeavor. Patient counseling is very important and screening should be opt-in procedure, patient should make aware by information brochures, videos and informed consent, discussion and patient decision should be documented.

1. A combined test in the first trimester can yield a very high detection rate for an acceptable false-positive rate;
2. Second trimester multiple marker biochemical screening yields a much lower detection rate and imposes a considerable emotional burden in requiring a woman to be very visibly pregnant, feel the baby moving, and have to undergo second trimester termination methods if an abnormality is found and the woman chooses to end the pregnancy;
3. Sequential screening in both trimesters yields even higher detection rates, and the most efficient method is the contingent test. Centers with appropriate training and experience of newer ultrasound markers such as nasal bone hypoplasia could consider carrying out the contingent test within the first trimester.

Although comprehensive national data are not available, there is a continuing shift towards screening in the first trimester. Only the exact components and timing remain to be determined.

REFERENCES

1. American College of Obstetricians and Gynecologists: Screening for fetal chromosomal abnormalities. Practice Bulletin No. 77, January 2007.
2. Alldred SK, Deeks JJ, Guo B, et al. Second trimester serum tests for Down's syndrome screening. Cochrane Database Syst Rev 2012; 6:CD009925.
3. Cuckle H, Benn P, Wright D. Down syndrome screening in the first and/or second trimester: model predicted performance using meta-analysis parameters. Semin Perinatol. 2005; 29(4):252.
4. Dugoff L, Hobbins JC, Malone FD, et al. Quad screen as a predictor of adverse pregnancy outcome. Obstet Gynecol. 2005;106(2):260.
5. Wapner R, Thom E, Simpson JL, et al. First-trimester screening for trisomies 21 and 18. N Engl J Med. 2003;349(15):1471.
6. Cuckle H. Biochemical screening for Down syndrome. Eur J Obstet Gynecol Reprod Biol. 2000;92(1):97.
7. Spencer K, Souter V, Tul N, et al. A screening program for trisomy 21 at 10–14 weeks using fetal nuchal translucency, maternal serum free beta-human chorionic gonadotropin and pregnancy-associated plasma protein-A. Ultrasound Obstet Gynecol. 1999;13(4):231.
8. Goetzl L, Krantz D, Simpson JL, et al. Pregnancy-associated plasma protein A, free beta-hCG, nuchal translucency, and risk of pregnancy loss. Obstet Gynecol 2004;104(1):30.
9. Nicolaides KH. Nuchal translucency and other first-trimester sonographic markers of chromosomal abnormalities. Am J Obstet Gynecol. 2004;191(1):45.
10. Reaffirmed 2013c, Benn PA, Leo MV, Rodis JF, et al. Maternal serum screening for fetal trisomy 18: a comparison of fixed cutoff and patient-specific risk protocols. Obstet Gynecol. 1999;93(5 Pt 1):707.
11. Nuchal Translucency Quality Review Program: Nasal bone education. 2013. Available at: *https://www.ntqr.org/SM/wfNasalBoneInfo.aspx*. Accessed February 3, 2013.
12. Greene MF, Haddow JE, Palomaki GE, Knight GJ. Maternal serum alpha-fetoprotein levels in diabetic pregnancies. Lancet. 1988;2(8606):345.
13. Lehmann S, Delaby C, Vialaret J, et al. Current and future use of "dried blood spot" analyses in clinical chemistry. Clin Chem Lab Med. 2013; 51(10):1897-909.
14. Dugoff L, Hobbins JC, Malone FD, et al. First-trimester maternal serum PAPP-A and free-beta subunit human chorionic gonadotropic concentrations and nuchal translucency are associated with obstetric complications: a population-based screening study (The FASTER Trial). Am J Obstet Gynecol. 2004;191(6):1446.
15. Dugoff L, Society for Maternal-Fetal Medicine. First- and second-trimester maternal serum markers for aneuploidy and adverse pregnancy outcomes. Obstet Gynecol. 2010;115(5):1052.
16. Greene MF, Haddow JE, Palomaki GE, Malone FD, Canick JA, Ball RH, et al. First-trimester or second-trimester screening, or both, for Down's syndrome. N Engl J Med. 2005;353(19):2001.

CHAPTER

14

Newborn Screening

Saurabh Dani

HISTORY

The idea of Newborn Screening (NBS) was initiated way back in 1960 by the pioneering work of Dr Robert Guthrie in the USA with the screening of Phenylketonuria (PKU). Today NBS is recognized internationally as an essential, preventive public health program for early identification of disorders in newborns that can affect their long-term health.

Newborn screening has expanded from single disorder screening in 1960 to multiple disorders screening as of today. With the introduction of system of collection and transportation of blood samples on filter paper wide scale screening was made possible.

With the introduction of tandem mass spectrometry (TMS) in 1990, there was a move from one test per disorder to one test for multiple disorders. Today in several parts of the world screening is performed universally for as many as 50–60 treatable disorders.

DISORDERS

The NBS can include several disorders ranging from 1 to 60. The list of disorders that should be screened in any population depends on the principles of the Wilson and Jungner classical screening criteria,[2] which has now been updated by WHO as laid down in Table 14.1. Most countries always start with a small list and expand as time goes by. As per guidelines[3] issued by the National Neonatal Forum of India (NNF India), every baby in India should be screened for congenital hypothyroidism (CH), congenital adrenal hyperplasia (CAH) and glucose-6-phosphate dehydrogenase (G6PD) deficiency. It also states that in urban or resource rich settings the babies should be screened for the expanded panel of 50–60 treatable disorders. This list of treatable disorders was the effort of American College on Medical Genetics.[4] All disorders were grouped in three categories based on the screening criteria. Only disorders that fulfilled the screening criteria were included in the list, i.e. 32 core (Table 14.2) and 26 secondary panel (Table 14.3). Any disorders that were not treatable or did not fulfill the screening criteria were excluded.

Table 14.1 Screening criteria[1]

- The screening program should respond to a recognized need
- The objectives of screening should be defined at the outset
- There should be a defined target population
- There should be scientific evidence of screening program effectiveness
- The program should integrate education, testing, clinical services and program management
- There should be quality assurance, with mechanisms to minimize potential risks of screening
- The program should ensure informed choice, confidentiality and respect for autonomy
- The program should promote equity and access to screening for the entire target population
- Program evaluation should be planned from the outset
- The overall benefits of screening should outweigh the harm

Since India does not have any universal screening program/guideline healthcare provider can choose what to offer to the parents. It would be a good practice though to include a minimum of three disorders as advised by NNF to a maximum of 58 as in the current guideline by the US Department of Health and Human Services.[5] Anything outside this list of about 50+ disorders would be inappropriate for now. Algorithm for newborn screening in India can be seen in Flow chart 14.1.

SYMPTOMATOLOGY

In most of the metabolic disorders the child may not have any immediate symptoms or they can be very vague and similar to common diseases, and hence it makes it difficult to detect them clinically. By the time, the parents detect something a miss and the doctor diagnoses the problem valuable time is lost. Table 14.4 lists the common disorders and their effects if untreated.

That is why it is recommended that all the babies be screened irrespective of whether they have any symptoms or not.

Table 14.2 Recommended uniform screening panel: core conditions (as of March 2015)

ACMG code	Core condition	Metabolic disorder: Organic acid condition	Metabolic disorder: Fatty acid oxidation disorders	Metabolic disorder: Amino acid disorders	Endocrine disorder	Hemoglobin disorder	Other disorder
PROP	Propionic acidemia	X					
MUT	Methylmalonic acidemia (methylmalonyl-CoA mutase)	X					
Cbl A,B	Methylmalonic acidemia (cobalamin disorders)	X					
IVA	Isovaleric acidemia	X					
3-MCC	3-Methylcrotonyl-CoA carboxylase deficiency	X					
HMG	3-Hydroxy-3-methylglutaric aciduria	X					
MCD	Holocarboxylase synthase deficiency	X					
βKT	β-Ketothiolase deficiency	X					
GA1	Glutaric acidemia type I	X					
CUD	Carnitine uptake defect/carnitine transport defect		X				
MCAD	Medium-chain acyl-CoA dehydrogenase deficiency		X				
VLCAD	Very long-chain acyl-CoA dehydrogenase deficiency		X				
LCHAD	Long-chain L-3 hydroxyacyl-CoA dehydrogenase deficiency		X				
TFP	Trifunctional protein deficiency		X				
ASA	Argininosuccinic aciduria			X			
CIT	Citrullinemia, type I			X			
MSUD	Maple syrup urine disease			X			
HCY	Homocystinuria			X			
PKU	Classic phenylketonuria			X			
TYR I	Tyrosinemia, type I			X			
CH	Primary congenital hypothyroidism				X		
CAH	Congenital adrenal hyperplasia				X		
HbSS	S,S disease (Sickle cell anemia)					X	
Hb S/βTh	S, βeta-thalassemia					X	
Hb S/C	S,C disease					X	
BIOT	Biotinidase deficiency						X
CCHD	Critical congenital heart disease						X
CF	Cystic fibrosis						X
GALT	Classic galactosemia						X
GSD II	Glycogen Storage Disease Type II (Pompe)						X
HEAR	Hearing loss						X
SCID	Severe combined immunodeficiencies						X

Selection of conditions based upon "Newborn screening: towards a uniform screening panel and system." Genetic Med. 2006;8(5)Suppl: S12-S252" as authored by the American College of Medical Genetics (ACMG) and commissioned by the Health Resources and Services Administration (HRSA).

Since congenital hypothyroidism is a very simple and cheap disorder to manage I have explained, it in detail here. There are several other disorders such as those stated above which are equally simple and cheap to manage but those will not be discussed here.

Congenital hypothyroidism (CH) can cause mental retardation unless thyroid therapy is initiated within two weeks of birth.[6] There is advocacy of screening for CH in the *Rashtriya Bal Swasthya Karyakram* (RBSK). RBSK is a new initiative of the Government of India aiming at early identification and early intervention for children from birth to 18 years to cover 4 'Ds, viz. Defects at birth, Deficiencies, Diseases, Development delays including disability. India is also a signatory to the UN Convention on the Rights of

Table 14.3 Recommended uniform screening panel: secondary conditions (as of March 2015)

ACMG code	Secondary condition	Metabolic disorder			Hemoglobin disorder	Other disorder
		Organic acid condition	Fatty acid oxidation disorders	Amino acid disorders		
Cbl C,D	Methylmalonic acidemia with homocystinuria	X				
MAL	Malonic acidemia	X				
IBG	Isobutyrylglycinuria	X				
2MBG	2-Methylbutyrylglycinuria	X				
3MGA	3-Methylglutaconic aciduria	X				
2M3HBA	2-Methyl-3-hydroxybutyric aciduria	X				
SCAD	Short-chain acyl-CoA dehydrogenase deficiency		X			
M/SCHAD	Medium/short-chain L-3-hydroxyacl-CoA dehydrogenase deficiency		X			
GA2	Glutaric acidemia type II		X			
MCAT	Medium-chain ketoacyl-CoA thiolase deficiency		X			
DE RED	2,4 Dienoyl-CoA reductase deficiency		X			
CPT IA	Carnitine palmitoyltransferase type I deficiency		X			
CPT II	Carnitine palmitoyltransferase type II deficiency		X			
CACT	Carnitine acylcarnitine translocase deficiency		X			
ARG	Argininemia			X		
CIT II	Citrullinemia, type II			X		
MET	Hypermethioninemia			X		
H-PHE	Benign hyperphenylalaninemia			X		
BIOPT (BS)	Biopterin defect in cofactor biosynthesis			X		
BIOPT (REG)	Biopterin defect in cofactor regeneration			X		
TYR II	Tyrosinemia, type II			X		
TYR III	Tyrosinemia, type III			X		
Var Hb	Various other hemoglobinopathies				X	
GALE	Galactoepimerase deficiency					X
GALK	Galactokinase deficiency					X
	T-cell related lymphocyte deficiencies					X

Selection of conditions based upon "Newborn screening: towards a uniform screening panel and system." Genetic Med. 2006;8(5)Suppl: S12-S252" as authored by the American College of Medical Genetics (ACMG) and commissioned by the Health Resources and Services Administration (HRSA).

Flow chart 14.1 Algorithm for newborn screening in India

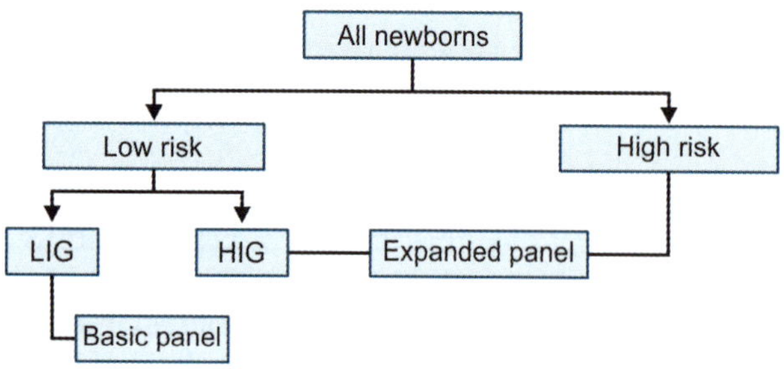

Abbreviations: LIG, low income group; HIG, high income group

Persons with Disabilities adopted on 13 December 2006 during the 61st session of the General Assembly by resolution A/RES/61/106.

Article 25 (b) of the convention clearly states that all the signatory states—one of which is India—should:

"Provide those health services needed by persons with disabilities specifically because of their disabilities, including early identification and intervention as appropriate, and services designed to minimize and prevent further disabilities, including among children and older persons."

It is imperative that all babies be screened for CH. Most infants with CH appear unaffected at birth, probably because

Table 14.4 Symptoms of disorders

Basic disorders	Effect
Congenital hearing impairment	Delayed milestones, poor language and communication skills and lower IQ
Congenital hypothyroidism	Congenital hypothyroidism can lead to intellectual disability and abnormal growth
Congenital adrenal hyperplasia	Babies lose large amounts of sodium in their urine, which can be life-threatening. They can experience poor feeding, weight loss, dehydration, vomiting, and ambiguous genitalia
Galactosemia	Life-threatening complications appear within a few days after birth. Affected infants typically develop feeding difficulties, lethargy, failure to thrive, jaundice, liver damage and bleeding
Glucose-6-phosphate dehydrogenase deficiency	Causes hemolytic anemia which can be triggered by bacterial or viral infections or by certain drugs of foods
Biotinidase deficiency	Children with the more severe form of the condition, often have seizures, weak muscle tone (hypotonia), breathing problems, and delayed development. If left untreated, the disorder can lead to hearing loss, eye abnormalities and loss of vision, problems with movement and balance (ataxia), skin (alopecia), and a fungal infection

of placental transfer of thyroid hormone. Newborns born to mothers who have untreated hypothyroidism have significant impairment of neurointellectual development despite early treatment.

The approach as described in Flow chart 14.2, is the most popular approach in countries having National Newborn Screening programs, is likely to miss central hypothyroidism, thyroid-binding globulin deficiency and hypothyroxinema with delayed elevation of TSH.

Physiology: After birth, the term baby experiences a surge of TSH as a physiological response to cold environment. The TSH concentration rises to 60–80 mU/L within 30–60 minutes after delivery and falls quickly in the first 24 hours to about 20 mU/L, followed by a slower decrease to below 10 mU/L after the first postnatal week. Preterm infants demonstrate a similar but blunted response due to HPT axis immaturity.[7] Perinatal stress factors and mode of delivery significantly impact cord-blood TSH levels, and hence there is limited value of cord blood for newborn screening, especially if we are planning to screen for other disorders along with CH.

Flow chart 14.2 Screening algorithm for congenital hypothyroidism

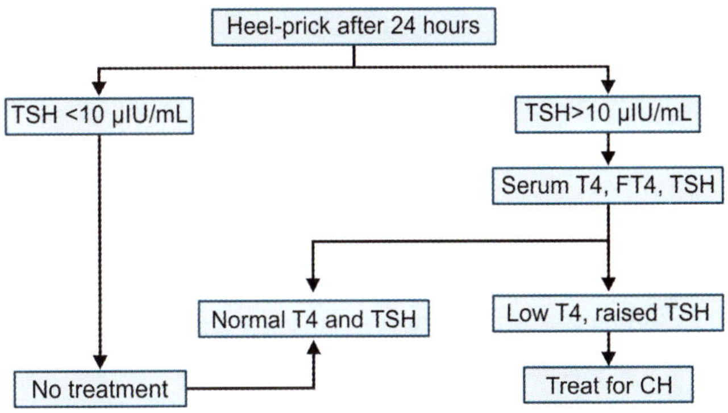

METHOD

The process of screening newborns has been refined over the years to perfection. The salient features are: Collection, Transportation, Technology and Reporting.

- *Collection*: The sample is collected by heel prick using an auto-lancet from the sides as shown by the shaded area in Figures 14.1A and B. *Blood should not be collected within 24 hours of birth.* The sample is directly collected on a Clinical and Laboratory Standards Institute (CLSI) approved filter paper[8] as shown in Figure 14.1C. Umbilical cord blood should not be used for screening as it has limited value and not recommended for comprehensive screening programs.
- *Transportation*: Once the sample has been collected allow it to dry for 2-4 hours. Once dried, it can be shipped to the Newborn Screening Laboratory by post or courier.
- *Technology*: NBS tests are performed using different technologies for different disorders. For CH. CAH. G6PD, galactosemia, biotinidase deficiency and cystic fibrosis biochemical enzyme assay is the preferred. For Hemoglobin variants high-performance liquid chromatography (HPLC) is preferred. For amino acid disorders, organic acid disorders and fatty oxidation disorders tandem mass spectrometry (TMS) is preferred.
- *Reporting*: The results of NBS will mention the following possibilities: Normal, presumptive positive/deficient or request repeat (Table 14.5). Repeat may be requested by the screening lab to reanalyze those samples which are not conclusive or sample is insufficient. Presumptive positive/deficient means that the baby has a high likelihood of a certain disorder and more definitive tests should be done to confirm or disprove the same.

Any screening test is always skewed towards giving false positive than false negative. A false negative test means that an affected baby will be given a clean chit—this is generally

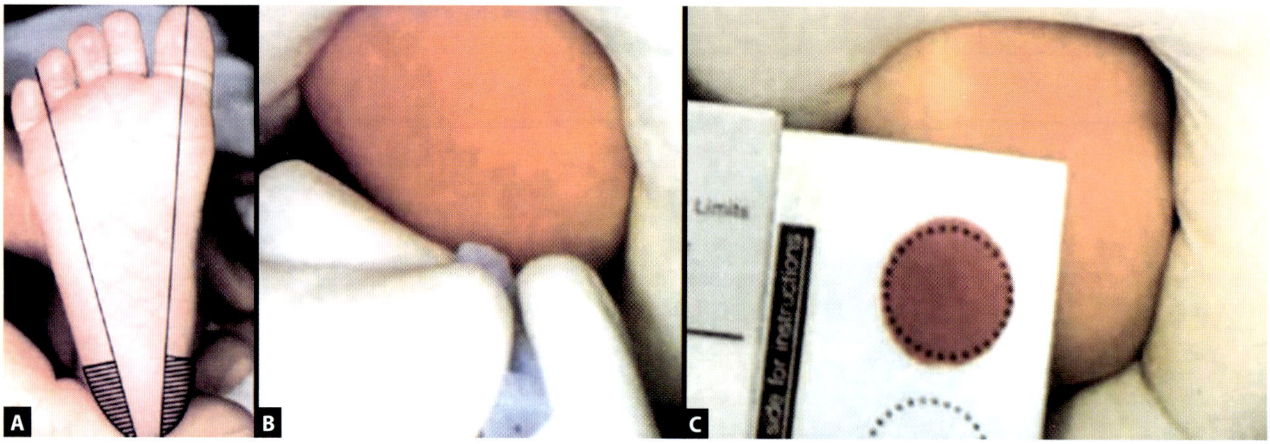

Figs 14.1A to C Collecting a Heel-Prick sample on CLSI approved filterpaper

Table 14.5 Laboratory report for first step[FM] newborn screening test

Test	Result
Acylcarnitine profile Fatty acid oxidation and organic acid disorders	Within normal limits
Amino acid profile Amino acid disorders, urea cycle disorders	Within normal limits
Glucose-6-phosphate dehydrogenase (G6PD) deficiency Glucose-6-phosphate dehydrogenase (G6PD)	Within normal limits
Congenital Adrenal Hyperplasia (CAH) 17-hydroxyprogesterone (17-OHP)	Within normal limits
Cystic fibrosis (CF) Immunoreactive trypsinogen (IRT) *Not valid after 2 months of age	Within normal limits
Galactosemia (GAL) Total galactose (TGAL)	Within normal limits
Congenital hypothyroidism (CH) Thyroid stimulating hormone (TSH)	Within normal limits
Biotinidase deficiency (BIOT) Biotinidase	Within normal limits
Hemoglobinopathies Sickle cell and other hemoglobinopathies *Not valid after 3 months of age	Within normal limits

QNS, quanity not sufficient; *NA*, not applicable; *Specimen*, dried blood spot (DBS); *Panel*, Hb+FS+

Courtesy: NeoGen Labs Pvt. Ltd.

unacceptable but a few can be allowed.[9] The reasons for missed cases are:

- True biologic false negative
- Pre-analytical errors
- Sample mix-ups
- Laboratory errors
- No newborn screening done

Table 14.6 Comparative analysis of incidence of disorders

Disorder	World	India
CH	1:3,000	1:900
CAH	1:7,000	1:2,000
ACMG panel	1:1,350	1:650 ~ 1:1,100

So where do we find the missed cases? They could be found at subspecialty clinics, primary care offices, in birth defects registries, in hospital records, in disease registries or in death certificates.

On the other end, false positive is acceptable, which essentially means that a normal baby is reported as having a problem. The only drawback is that there will be anxiety till the result is disproved and the baby will end up getting more investigations then it would actually require. This happens since there is no ideal screening test as of yet. Dealing with a parent who's baby has been reported as positive will be dealt in the section on counseling.

INCIDENCE

Individually, these disorders may be rare but collectively they are not uncommon. In several studies over the years, we consistently observe that the incidence in India[10,11] is much higher as compared to international statistics as seen in Table 14.6.[12-15] One probable reason could be more number of marriages in India happen within the same caste, unlike the western counterparts.

COUNSELING

Counseling plays a very crucial role for NBS due to the absence of any nationwide NBS program and also since it is still not a very popular advice. Antenatal caregiver or an obstetrician has to play this very important role of counseling the parents. NHS[16] of United Kingdom and ACOG[17] (American College of Obstetricians and Gynecologists) recommend that obstetricians should counsel parents about NBS during the antenatal period. Even in countries like USA and UK where NBS is mandatory obstetricians play a very crucial role. In a study done on focus groups of parents, it was suggested that information on NBS should be incorporated into the prenatal care.[18]

Parents generally do not like the baby to be pricked be it for newborn screening, immunization or blood test. There is a lot of apprehension related to a heel prick. Adequate counseling can help in reducing the anxiety associated with a heel-prick. Things that can be done to reduce the stress and anxiety of the parents are: (i) Collect the sample in the nursery; (ii) Caress the baby and provide skin-to-skin contact; (iii) Feed the baby during the procedure; (iv) Ask some family member or friend to be present along with the mother.

Counseling plays a very important role when parents receive a report from the Newborn Screening Laboratory indicating a possibility of the baby suffering from one of the disorder. Counseling for false positive is all the more difficult. Parents who have had false positive results usually experience five distinct stages: (i) Receiving the news; (ii) Getting the follow-up testing; (iii) Waiting for resolution; (iv) Learning the follow-up test results; and (v) Adapting to life after NBS.[19]

Receiving the news: Because the initial positive NBS result represents a threat to the baby's health, generally all parents experience stress after hearing the news, which would range from mild concern to severe anxiety.

The stress or anxiety would be lesser when informed by their doctor since the doctor would provide some reassurance.

The stress would be higher when informed before weekends or holidays since they cannot immediately visit the doctor or get a follow-up test done.

Getting the follow-up testing: A lot of time re-testing may have to be done at special facilities. The most common stressor was the process of re-testing and multiple tests that baby had to undergo. Financial burden may also add to the stress when not covered by insurance.

Waiting for resolution: Most parents continue with the anxiety they have since the first report till the final report has arrived. It could be a bit nightmarish for some parents. There are several coping methods parents apply: Some read about it on the Internet and are happy to know that their babies are not exhibiting symptoms that are see with those disorders, some use prayer and faith to cope whereas some resolve to be confident and are ready to cope with whatever the result may be. Most parents do not share the initial report with other than spouse or very close family members.

Learning the follow-up test results: On learning that the newborn screening test was false positive, there is a sigh of relief. Generally, all parents move on and leave all the stress and anxiety behind. A few may have questions as to what went wrong the first time or even question the authenticity of the second testing.

Adapting to life after NBS: There is generally no long-term impact. Most parents are happy knowing that their babies are healthy. A few may have lingering anxiety, sometimes triggered by symptoms related to the disease in question. Mostly parents are happy knowing that they choose the right doctor since their doctor has either counseled them properly or adequately reassured or because of the advice given to them about for repeat testing and confirmatory testing to rule out false positive.

Generally, all parents would appreciate appropriate communication and adequate information be provided to them related to the disorder in question, the time it would take for the re-test results and symptoms to watch out.

IMPLEMENTATION

Newborn screening is not just a diagnostic test. It is a screening program. Like any screening test, we need to identify the target population, which in this case is **every newborn**. There are no absolute contraindications to NBS. Relative contraindication is severe prematurity. But, in that situation also NBS may be performed after birth and repeated again after the baby attains maturity. Since there are no government guidelines on NBS it will be the discretion of the individual hospital/doctor to make it mandatory or optional. If mandatory which panel? The choice of panel would depend on the financial status of the parents. It would be wise to make a small basic panel mandatory for all and give option to parents to opt-in for a complete ACMG panel (Table 14.6).

It would save a lot of time, if all parents are counseled together somewhere in the early third trimester. Counseling aids could be used in form of PPT, videos, etc. There are plenty of instruments available for patient education in various languages since NBS is a popular public health program in many countries:

Ontorio NBS program (Hindi)
https://youtu.be/WFWl6HqBvIM
Save Babies Through Screening Foundation (English)
https://youtu.be/G_qjpjO3gFE

Choosing a NBS Laboratory is very important. Choose a laboratory which participates regularly in CDCs NSQAP. NSQAP (Newborn Screening Quality Assurance Program) is a voluntary, non-regulatory program of Centers for Disease Control and Prevention, Atlanta to help laboratories maintain and enhance the quality of test results. The program provides services to newborn screening laboratories in 67 countries. NSQAP has been the only comprehensive source of essential quality assurance services for dried-blood spot testing for more than 33 years. An accreditation like CAP or NABL could be a desirable addition.

It is generally very easy to read and understand a NBS report. The report clearly mentions normal, positive/deficient or repeat. For a normal report, nothing needs to be done. For a positive report a confirmatory test may be needed to confirm the screening test result. For repeat you would be asked to send a second sample to the laboratory. Generally, no expertise is required to decipher the report. In case of a normal report, an obstetrician need not seek help of any other specialist.

CONCLUSION

Every baby should be screened for basic disorders. All parents should be educated and counseled during the antenatal period, preferably in the early third trimester. All parents should be offered NBS after delivery. An opt-out form may be used for parents refusing a NBS test. Heel-prick should be done after 24 hours of birth (not before). A complete ACMG panel should be offered to all affording patients. There is no contraindication of performing a newborn screening test.

REFERENCES

1. Anne Andermann A, Ingeborg Blancquaert B, Sylvie Beauchamp B, Véronique Déry. Revisiting Wilson and Jungner in the genomic age: a review of screening criteria over the past 40 years.
2. Wilson JMG, Jungner G. Principles and practice of screening for disease. Geneva: WHO; 1968.
3. NNF Clinical Practice Guidelines; 2010.pp.289-99.
4. Newborn screening: toward a uniform screening panel and system, 2006;8(5).
5. US Department of Health and Human Services, *https://www.acmg.net/ACMG/Publications/Practice_Guidelines_docs/NBS_report.aspx.*
6. Smith L. Updated AAP Guidelines on Newborn Screening and Therapy for Congenital Hypothyroidism. Am Fam Physician. 2007;76(3):439-44.
7. Brown RS, Huang SA, Fisher DA. The maturation of thyroid function in the perinatal period and during childhood. In: Braverman L, Utiger R, (eds). Werner & Ingbar's The Thyroid: A Fundamental and Clinical Text, 9th edn. Philadelphia, PA: Lippincott Williams & Wilkins. 2005. pp. 1013-28.
8. Clinical and Laboratory Standards Institute. Blood collection on filter paper for newborn screening programs; approved standard - fifth edition. CLSI document. 2007;LA4-A5, 27(20).
9. Chiang SH1, Fan ML, Hsiao KJ. External quality assurance programme for newborn screening of glucose-6-phosphate dehydrogenase deficiency. Ann Acad Med Singapore. 2008; 37(12 Suppl):84-4.
10. High incidence of hypothyroidism in newborns in Chennai: ICMR study; *http://www.thehindu.com/todays-paper/tp-national/high-incidence-of-hypothyroidism-in-newborns-in-chennai-icmr-study/article4517892.ece.*
11. The Goa Newborn Screening Program 3 Year Review 2008–2011; *http://www.dhsgoa.gov.in/documents/new_born.pdf.*
12. Waller DK, Anderson JL, Lorey F, Cunningham GC. Risk factors for congenital hypothyroidism: an investigation of infant's birth weight, ethnicity, and gender in California, 1990–1998. Teratology. 2000;62:36-41.
13. Morreale de Escobar G, Obregon MJ, Escobar del Rey F. Is neuropsychological development related to maternal hypothyroidism or to maternal hypothyroxinemia? J Clin Endocrinol Metab. 2000;85:3975-87.
14. Lubani, MM, Issa ARA, Bushnaq R, Al Saleh QA, Dudin KI, Reavey PC, et al. Prevalence of congenital adrenal hyperplasia in Kuwait. Europ J Pediat. 1990;149:391-2.
15. Virginia Department of Health. Health Practitioner Manual, 2006.
16. Antenatal and newborn screening timeline; *http://cpd.screening.nhs.uk/getdata.php?id=10610.*
17. Committee opinion on newborn screening; Number 481, 2011.
18. Campbell ED(1), Ross LF. Incorporating newborn screening into prenatal care. Am J Obstet Gynecol. 2004;190(4):876-7.
19. Johanna L. Schmidt MPH, et al. The impact of false-positive newborn screening results on families: a qualitative study. Genetics in Medicine. 2002;14:76-80.

CHAPTER

15 Screening and Diagnosis of Inborn Errors of Metabolism

Usha P Dave

Inborn errors of metabolism (IEM) are individually rare, but collectively large numbers of heterogeneous group of single gene disorders wherein loss of function of a single enzyme or cofactor results into abnormal metabolites affecting the normal protein, carbohydrate, lipid and other metabolic pathways. The majority of the IEMs manifests are autosomal recessive disorders meaning the parents are symptomless but carry the 50% of defective genes, and are thus carriers of the metabolic defect. A strong clinical suspicion and the specialized biochemical, metabolic and molecular laboratory tests can confirm the diagnosis in the index case.

Historically, the term Inborn Errors of Metabolism (IEM) was first coined in 1908[1] by Sir Archibald Garrod (1857–1936) who described benign group of disorders like alkaptonuria, benign pentosuria, albinism and cystinuria. He explained these as a result of failure of some steps in metabolism constituting several chemical changes. Each change was benign and transmitted as a recessive trait following Mendel's laws of inheritance. Further experiments on the effects of feeding phenylalanine and its intermediate metabolites, Garrod showed the specific defect in the oxidation of homogentisic acid which is an intermediate in normal phenylalanine and tyrosine metabolism. However, the profound deficiency of homogentisic acid oxidase enzyme was shown 50 years later by La Du in liver biopsy of alkaptonuria patient.[2] Folling in 1934 discovered phenylketonuria (PKU) as a recessively inherited point defect to be 'inborn' in the conversion of phenylalanine to tyrosine but associated with severe mental retardation.[3] Beadle and Tatum offered the concept of one gene–one enzyme.[4] In this theory, an indivisible unit of heredity called a gene was thought to be responsible for the presence and activity of a single enzyme or protein. The discovery of PKU led to search of other clinically relevant and important IEMs well depicted by Charles Scriver and his team in their book *'The Metabolic and Molecular Bases of Inherited Disease.'*[5]

The term "inborn" led IEM as a specialty of pediatricians for a long time. However, several phenotype variants do start in adolescent or adult forms due to different mutant types and degree of enzyme expression, and this concept has yet to reach medical professionals. Neonatal deaths or in-depth family history if available with a clue about IEM should alarm fetal medicine professionals to clinically suspect IEM in a particular family and to further carry out confirmatory diagnostic tests in the index case. Not to mention that severe forms of enzyme/cofactor deficiencies represent early as visible disease in neonates and infants. In the Indian scenario, the confirmed diagnosis is not always available in majority of the index cases. The final diagnosis of the index case either by molecular or biochemical/metabolic tests is a prerequisite for prenatal/fetal diagnosis from chorion villi/amniotic fluid/fetal blood or tissue.

CONCEPT OF INBORN ERRORS OF METABOLISM

Metabolism is the sum total of all chemical reactions constituting the continuing process of breakdown and formation of the body tissues. Enzymes and cofactors play an essential role in conversion of one metabolite into another in generating suitable energy (ATP). However, any block in these steps due to deficiency or genetic defect results into the accumulation of toxic products or deficiency of essential compounds (Fig. 15.1A). Genomic technologies have made clear that there is a spectrum of mild to severe forms of IEM for almost all genetic defects. The biochemical/metabolic phenotype can be due to multiple genetic defects. The mutations may impair the amount or function of enzyme activity, receptor membranes, transport proteins or structural/cellular element with varied degrees. The phenotype-genotype expression and complexity occurs as a result of gene-gene or gene-environmental expression (Fig. 15.1B). Thus, the disease-causing mutations are also influenced by other genes and environmental factors.

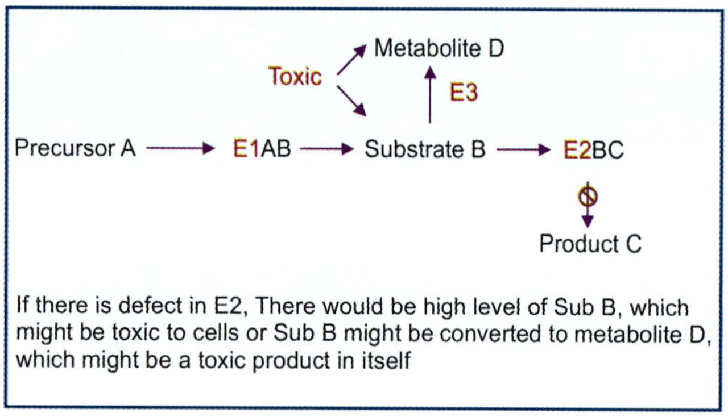

Fig. 15.1A Concept of IEM explaining the mechanism of accumulation of toxic products in body

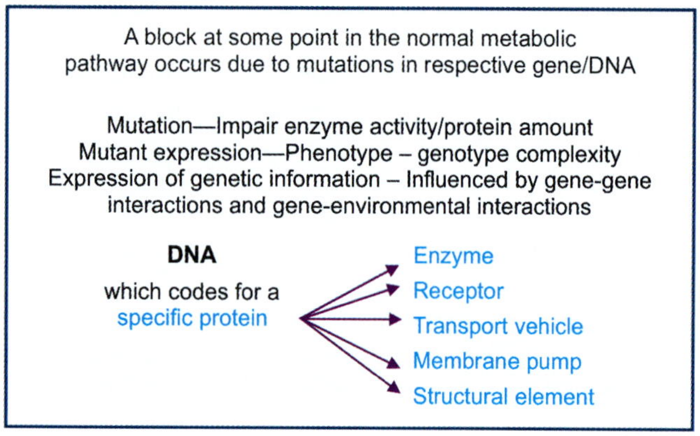

Fig. 15.1B Mechanism of mutation causing phenotype and genotype complexity at DNA level

Classification and Nomenclature of IEMs

Inborn errors of metabolism (IEM) are generally classified in the simplest form based on the characteristic compounds which are involved in the specific metabolic pathway, viz. disorder of proteins, lipid, carbohydrate, fats or mitochondria (Fig. 15.2). From a pathophysiological perspective for better understanding of clinical phenotypes and genotypes the IEMs can be categorized into three groups (Flow chart 15.1). This is based on involvement of cellular organelles (Group 1), acute or chronic accumulation of toxic products as in disorders of amino acids (AA), organic acids (OA), urea cycle disorders (UCD) and carbohydrate disorders (Group 2) and cytoplasmic and mitochondrial energy crisis defects (Group 3). Some of the IEMs still hold the names given after their discovery which may be pertaining to the enzyme involved (e.g. biotinidase deficiency or G6PD) or the gross diagnostic pathological abnormality (e.g. cystic fibrosis or sickle cell anemia) or accumulated metabolic product (e.g. galactosemia) or peculiar chemical abnormality (e.g. phenylketonuria), etc.

- Amino acid metabolism
- Carbohydrate metabolism
- Lipid metabolism
- Protein metabolism
- Pigment metabolism
- Mitochondrial disorders
- Unknown biochemical defects

Fig. 15.2 Classification of IEM according to the type of compounds invoved in IEM

The simple inexpensive biochemical and spectrophotometric tests are used for certain hematologic, endocrinologic and other IEMs (Fig. 15.3). With advancement of analytical techniques coupled with bioinformatics, thousands IEMs are characterized at biochemical and molecular level to precisely pinpoint the metabolic genetic defect, thereby making preconception and prenatal genetic counseling feasible.

Metabolic Screening for IEMs

The significance of preventable and treatable IEMs was realized by Robert Guthrie in 1960s, giving the world ***'Newborn screening' (NBS)*** program. The delay in diagnosis or undiagnosed IEMs can lead to severe mental deterioration and even death.[6] The prompt detection therefore requires vigilance and measurement of biochemical markers with appropriate technology. The successful dietary control of PKU was a remarkable breakthrough in the screening and management of IEM in the neonatal period.[7] The rapid and multicomponent techniques of tandem mass spectrometry (LC/MS-MS) screens about 46 metabolic conditions simultaneously from a single blood spot. Since its first application by Tanaka in 1966 to discover isovaleric acidemia, GC/MS has been used worldwide to diagnose number of IEMs because of its high accuracy, sensitivity and power of analyzing multiple compounds simultaneously. Matsumoto and his research team developed a rapid, practical, noninvasive and simultaneous urinary metabolite analysis in Japan[8] and the author is the first to introduce the same GC/MS method in 1997 in India for ***High-risk screening of IEMs*** using urine filter paper.[9] This was the first study to indicate the common IEMs in Indian neonates and children (Table 15.1). Though individually rare in the population, the collective incidence of IEMs is 1 in 1200–1500.[10]

Three important points of diagnostic confusion of IEM is aptly outlined by Clarke[11] as below:

1. Misdiagnosing IEM in confusion with common non-genetic acquired conditions such as infections, intoxications or nutritional deficiencies. The attending physician fails to consider both types of disorders (IEM and

Flow chart 15.1 Categorization of IEMs according to the organelles and molecules involved

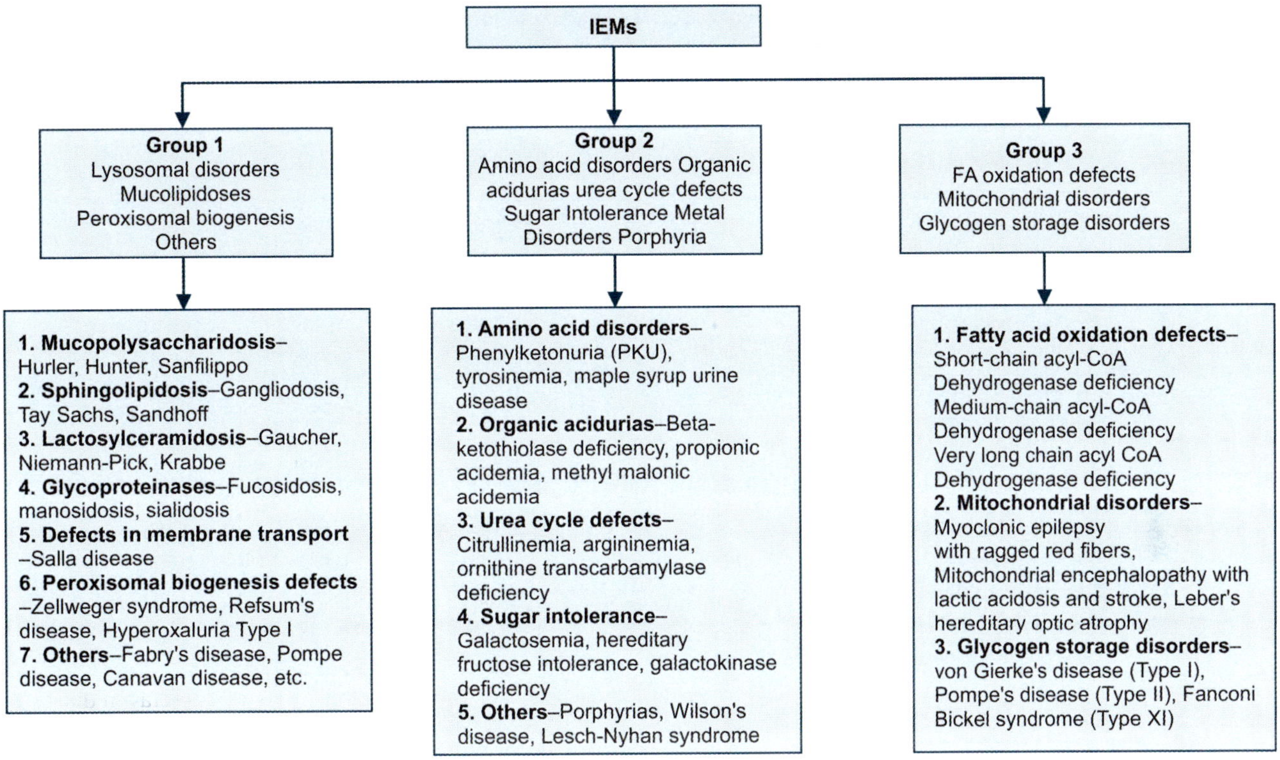

Source: Kothiwale and Varun Kumar, 2013

- Biotinidase deficiency
- Cystic fibrosis
- Congenital adrenal hyperplasia
- Glucose-6-phosphate dehydrogenase deficiency
- Congenital hypothyroidism
- Sickle cell and other hemoglobinopathies
- Galactosemia

Fig. 15.3 The biochemical and hematologic panel of IEMs tested by ELISA, spectrophotometry or radioimmunoassay methods

non-IEM) simultaneously in the acutely ill child, thereby resulting in delay in diagnosis and unnecessary causing further irreversible damage or even death.

2. Intermittent illness often occurs due to an impaired ability to compensate adequately, e.g. intermittent MSUD or fatty acid oxidation defects. This delays the diagnosis of the underlying genetic disorder when the child is described as often sick baby. OR an IEM will often present with an associated infection (*Escherichia coli* sepsis in galactosemia or otitis media in MPS or neutropenia in GSD), misleading the attending physician.
3. Genetic heterogeneity in IEM causes varied phenotypes due to mutation in completely different genes. For example Sanfilippo disease comprises of various defects in different enzymes required to breakdown glycosaminoglycan, heparan sulfate.

CLINICAL MANIFESTATIONS

The IEMs can occur at all ages from neonates, infants, and children to adults and can affect any organ system[12] as explained in Flow chart 15.1. In suspected patient the nonspecific metabolic abnormalities like metabolic acidosis, hyperammonemia, hypoglycemia and abnormal blood-gas and electrolytes provide differential[11] diagnosis. To conclude the specific underlying metabolic defect, consultation with the metabolic expert is required.

In neonates and children, the clinical manifestations of IEM are nonspecific, overlapping and can vary from acute metabolic encephalopathy, failure to thrive, seizures, vomiting, poor feeding to abnormal movements as shown in Figure 15.4. The clue to the fetal medicine expert is that within a few days or weeks after birth, a previously healthy

Table 15.1 Incidence of common IEMs diagnosed by urinary GC/MS profiling (Dave, 2015)

High-risk screening by GC/MS—candidates for NBS (2014)				
S. No.	**IEM disorders (Total = 3341)**	**Incidence of IEM**		
		N = 3341	**Neonates**	**N = 864**
1.	Glutaric aciduria (38)—Type I: 34 and II: 4	1: 90	1: 216 GAII	(4)
2.	Hyperglycinemia (28)	1: 119	1: 432	(2)
3.	Maple syrup urine disease (MSUD) (14)	1: 239	1: 108	(8)
4.	Isovaleric acidemia (4)	1: 835	1: 864	(1)
5.	Multiple carboxylic def. (MCD) (13)	1: 257	1: 432	(2)
6.	Methyl malonic acidemia (MMA) (52)	1: 64	1: 123	(7)
7.	Propionic acidemia (PA) (19)	1: 176	1: 86	(10)
8.	Ornithine trans carbamyl. def. (OTC) (5)	1: 668	1: 288	(3)
9.	Tyrosinemia (6)/hepatic dysfunction (6)	1: 557	1: 173	(5)
10.	Urea cycle disorders (25)	1: 134	1: 72	(12)
11.	Canavan disease (10)	1: 334	1: 864	(1)
12.	3-hydroxy-3-methylglutaryl CoA lyase defi. (6)	1: 557	Not found	
13.	Fructose-1, 6-diphosphatase def. (10)	1: 334	1: 864	(1)
14.	Galactosemia (4)	1: 835	1: 432	(2)
15.	3-ketothiolase deficiency (11)	1: 304	1: 864	(1)
16.	Hyperphenylalaninemia (5)	1: 668	1: 432	(2)
17.	Dihydropyrimidinase deficiency (2)	1: 1671	Not found	

- Poor feeding
- Feeding intolerance
- Failure to thrive
- Seizure
- Vomiting
- Temperature instability
- Tachypnea
- Apnea
- Irritability
- Abnormal movements, etc.

Fig. 15.4 The common signs and symptoms of IEMs raising suspicion

neonate may begin to show the signs of underlying metabolic disorder. Lethargy, tachypnea from acidosis and seizures are the typical signs. With progression in illness there may be abnormalities of tone (hypotonia, hypertonia), posture (fisting) and abnormal movements (lip-smacking, myoclonic jerks) which are enough to initiate metabolic testing. Elevated plasma ammonia, hypoglycemia and metabolic acidosis, if present are sufficient enough for a strong suspicion of IEM.

In addition, the unusual body or urine odor (Table 15.2) is always a first suspect for the clinician.[11,12] The accompanied ketosis causes the sweet odor due to ketone bodies, especially in branched chain ketoaciduria (MSUD). Similarly, unusual urine colors increases the suspicion of certain IEMs (Table 15.2). The history of sibling with similar illness or death (may be reported from sepsis) or sudden infant death syndromes are important in raising clinical suspicion.

Physical Examination

Accumulation of toxic metabolites results into congenital defects. For example, the congenital cataract in galactosemia due to accumulation of galactitol in eye; corneal opacity and cherry red spot in certain lysosomal storage disorders (LSD); erythema and eczema and loss of hair in biotinidase deficiency. Hepatosplenomegaly can occur in carbohydrate disorders (galactosemia, glycogen storage disorder, hereditary fructose intolerance, LSDs). Abnormal brittle hair may be seen in UCDs (argininosuccinic aciduria, citrullinemia), holocarboxylase synthetase deficiency, Menke's syndrome. Cardiomyopathy is invariably associated with mitochondrial disorders.[11]

Dysmorphic Features

The earlier concept of normal phenotype in IEMs no more holds true as consistent pattern of birth defects are reported due to metabolic derangements *in utero* affecting fetal development, e.g. epicanthal folds, large fontanels, Simian crease and renal cysts are features noted in Zellweger

Table 15.2 Characteristic urine odor and unusual color in certain IEMs

S. No.	A. Disorders	Odor	Compound
1.	Phenylketonuria	Musty	Phenyl acetate
2.	Maple syrup urine disease	Maple syrup/burnt sugar	Oxoisocaproic acid Oxomethyl valeric acid
3.	Isovaleric acidema, glutaric acidemia type II	Sweaty feet	Isovaleric acid
4.	Tyrosinemia	Cabbage Rancid butter	Hydroxybutyric acid
5.	Hydroxy methyl glutaric acidurias	Cheesy	Cheesy
6.	Methylmalonic acidemia	Acid smell	Methylmalonic acid
7.	Methylcrotonyl-CoA carboxylase deficiency	Cat urine	Hydroxyisovaleric acid
8.	Multiple carboxylase deficiency	Cat urine	Hydroxyisovaleric acid
9.	Cystinuria	Sulfurous	Hydrogen sulfide
	B. Disorders	**Color**	**Compound**
1.	Hartnup disorder	Blue	Indican
2.	Hyperuricosuria	Light red	Urates
3.	Porphyria	Red	Porphyrins
4.	Alkaptonuria	Blue/brown	Homogentisic acid
5.	Myoglobinuria	Brown	Methemoglobin
6.	Hemoglobinuria	Red/brown	Hemoglobin/methemoglobin
7.	Hematuria	Red	Erythrocytes

syndrome and adrenoleukodystrophy. Similarly, a high forehead, hypertelorism, low set years abdominal wall defects, enlarged kidneys and rocker bottom feet are characteristic of Glutaric aciduria type II (mitochondrial energy involved). Facial dysmorphism in certain peroxisomal disorders can also support the clinical diagnosis, e.g. Smith-Lemli Opitz Syndrome is associated with multiple malformations like congenital heart disease, cleft palate, hypospadias, polydactyly, syndactyly and dysmophic facies.[11] The coarse facial features, hirsuitism are characteristic features of some LSDs and neonatal hydrops. Thus, dysmorphic features in neonates should not exclude the possibility of IEM by the fetal medicine person.

CENTRAL NERVOUS SYSTEM DYSFUNCTION

Majority of IEMs represent developmental delay, mental retardation or neurodegeneration and this may be due to 30% of total human genes being expressed in the brain. Acute life-threatening metabolic encephalopathy often observed in UCDs, organic and amino acidemias is due to accumulation of toxins in the central nervous system (CNS) of neonates. Most of these metabolites cross the placenta and are cleared during the gestation and hence the affected baby is normal at birth. Other signs of CNS dysfunction are seizures, abnormal muscle tone and at times cerebral edema and intracranial hemorrhage.

Vomiting is a striking feature due to protein intolerance in amino acid disorders, and if persistent, points at an underlying IEM. In young children, intermittent or progressive ataxia is seen in many organelle diseases (metachromatic leukodystrophy or Niemann-Pick disease or juvenile Tay-Sachs and Sandhoff disease) and important to differentiate between metabolic ataxia and nonmetabolic hereditary ataxias.[13] Coenzyme Q_{10} (CoQ_{10} deficiency) in young children is a very progressive cerebellar ataxia associated with mental retardation and seizures. Recurrent acute ataxias are common manifestations in patient with UCD, organic acidopathies or MSUD. Stroke is also noticed in some IEMs (e.g. homocystinuria or familial hypercholesterolemia). If occurs in infancy and childhood, it is often associated with metabolic acidosis, psychomotor retardation and failure to thrive. Extrapyramidal movements or muscle weakness is particularly common in certain IEMs.[13] It is important to consider purine and pyrimidine metabolic defects in unexplained neurologic disorders associated with developmental delay, prominent behavioral and language deficits, autistic-like features and seizures.

Consanguinity and Inheritance

As most IEMs are autosomal disorder inheriting the disease in a recessive trait, the recurrence risk is 25% in every pregnancy. A few, like ornithine transcarbamylase deficiency

(OTC) are X-linked disorders and hence a detailed family history and degree of consanguinity is of great importance. The maternal transmission of the disease is very characteristic of mitochondrial disorder as the mitochondria of the ovaries are only transmitted in the fertilized ovum and not from sperms.[11] In specific metabolic disorders maternal illness is very prominent in pregnancy, e.g. in a heterozygous mother having long-chain 3-hydroxyacyl-CoA-dehydrogenase deficiency (LCHAD) acute fatty liver during pregnancy, hypertension, increased liver enzyme, low platelet syndrome (HELLP) may occur.[13] Such information provides clue to monitor pregnancy in the mother of an IEM diagnosed child.

SCREENING AND DIAGNOSTIC INVESTIGATIONS FOR IEM

Although many of the tests can be performed in any laboratory with standard equipment, even the simplest test results may be difficult to interpret without expert knowledge. *The investigations for the clinically suspected IEM case can be grouped into four categories:*

1. Biochemical and metabolic testing
2. Molecular/DNA diagnostic tests
3. Neuroimaging, electrophysiology and radiologic testing
4. Morphological/structural examination in hematologic and biopsy tissue.

Biochemical and Metabolic Testing

The laboratory screening test relevant to fetal expert in infants or children suspected of having an IEM encompasses complete differential blood count, urine analysis, measurement of blood gases, serum electrolytes, blood glucose, plasma ammonia, urine reducing substances, urine ketones, quantitative measurement of plasma and urine amino acids, urine organic acids and plasma lactate.

The '*newborn screening*' test is conducted on the apparently healthy newborns to detect IEM presymptomatically, while '*metabolic screening*' test covers a large group of suspected IEM conditions in a symptomatic case which finally guides the direction of the next confirmatory diagnostic tests.

For example, the metabolic acidosis is the common feature in IEMs and is diagnosed by measurement of blood gases. It is a result of increased bicarbonate or accumulation of acids, e.g. metabolic acidosis with an increased anion gap in organic acidemias is usually persistent with failure to thrive.[11] Additionally, intermittent episodes of acute metabolic decompensation with rapid and deep breathing and respiratory distress may accompany the metabolic acidosis. The biochemical tests for lactic acidosis, increased ketones and combined ketoacidosis are the other metabolic screening tests which pinpoint the abnormality in metabolism of certain organic acids or mitochondrial disorders.

Another important characteristic feature of many IEMs is hypoglycemia and fasting blood glucose forms the baseline metabolic screening test. Hypoglycemia is often noticed in carbohydrate (GSD), fatty acid metabolism defects and mildly in a few organic acid disorders. It is due to the inability of the liver to release glucose from glycogen and is an important feature of galactosemia and fructose intolerance, but hypoketotic hypoglycemia is characteristic of fatty acid disorders, especially in infants and older children.[12]

Furthermore, blood ammonia always offers a clue in differential diagnosis of UCD. Severe hyperammonemia (and no acidosis) after 24 hours should alarm fetal medicine expert to suspect UCD or a few organic acidemias. Transient hyperammonemia of the newborn (THAN) should be kept in mind while differential diagnosis. A high plasma ammonia in any neonate/child with unexplained lethargy, vomiting or encephalopathy is alarming as the degree of developmental delay and neurologic dysfunction noticed subsequently is related to neonatal hyperammonia and coma.[13]

Liver function tests such as SGOT/SGPT, bilirubin will point at hepatic dysfunction and hepatomegaly[11] e.g. galactosemia, alpha-1-antitrypsin deficiency, hereditary tyrosinemia and in some LSDs like Niemann-Pick type C and GSD type-IV (Fig. 15.3); in the latter an abnormal form of glycogen accumulates in liver leading to progressive cirrhosis. A negative dip-stick glucose test with a positive Benedict's reaction test gives a clue for nonreducing glucose in urine and high suspicion of galactosemia.[14] Similarly, urinary succinyl acetone is of diagnostic and therapeutic significance in Tyrosinemia type I along with raised plasma tyrosine, methionine and occasionally generalized aminoaciduria. Hepatocellular dysfunction in terms of persistent hyperbilirubinemia is common in fatty acid oxidation.

CSF Test

A number of IEMs with isolated seizures or progressive encephalopathy and normal routine metabolic screening tests are being reported. Within 48 hours of birth, patient with seizures alone and CSF: plasma glycine ratio more than 0.08 confirms the diagnosis of nonketotic hyperglycinuria in lethargic, hypotonic patients with hiccups and feeding difficulties. The sulfite or xanthine oxidase deficiency either combined or in isolation and secondary to molybdenum cofactor deficiency can be another example of intractable seizures in patients with other biochemical findings normal.[11] Evaluation of CSF total protein (metachromatic leukodystrophy, Krabbe diease, X-linked adrenoleukodystrophy, CMT Dejerine-Sottas disease),

Table 15.3 Qualitative metabolic urine screening test

Test	Result	Compound detected	Disorder
Odor	Muty Maple syrup Sweaty feet Cat urine	Phenylacetate 2-Oxoisocar proate 2-Oxo-3-methyl valerate Isovalerate 3-Hydroxyisovalerate	Phenylketonuria Maple syrup urine disease (MSUD) Isovaleric acidemia 3-Methylcrotonyl glycinuria
Ferric chloride test	Blue-green color Transient blue-green Green-gray Green color	Phenylpyruvate Imidazole pyruvate Xanthurenic acid Homogentisate Branched-chain oxoacids p-Hydroxyphenylpyruvate	Phenylketonuria Histidinemia Xanthuremic aciduria Alkaptonuria MSUD Tyrosinemia, types 1 and 2
Dinitrophenyl hydrazine (DNPH) test	Golden yellow precipitate	Phenylpyruvate 2-Oxoisovalerate 2-Oxoisocaproate 2-Oxo-3-methyl valerate 4-Hydroxyphenylpyruvate Pyruvate	Phenylketonuria MSUD Tyrosinemia, types 1 and 2 Lactic acidosis
Cyanide nitroprusside test	Magenta color	Cystine Homocystine	Cystinuria, hyperarginemia, Homocystinuria
Benedict's test	Brick red precipitate Brown ppt	Glucose Galactose Fructose Xylose 4-Hydroxyphenypyruvate Oxalic acid Homogentisate	Diabetes, Fanconi syndrome Galactosemia Fructose intolerance, Essential fructosuria Pentosuria Tyrosinemias, types 1 and 2 Hyperoxaluria Alkaptonuria
Strip test for ketones (Ketostix)	Positive	Acetone, butanone, acetoacetate, 2-methylacetoacetate	3-Oxothiolase defect, popionic acidemia, methylmalonic acidemia
Berry spot test	Purple ring	Mucopolysaccharides	Mucopolysaccharidoses

Source: Elshaari et al., 2013.

gamma-globulins, glucose (low in De Vivo disease), lactic acid (mitochrondrial encephalomyopathies), and β-crystallin (Alexander disease) from cerebrospinal fluid (CSF) are of great diagnostic value.[13] Elevated CSF GABA (inhibitory CNS neurotransmitter) as a result of 4-aminobutyrate amino-transferase enzyme deficiency is another example of neonatal seizures associated with lethargy, high-pitched cry and hyper-reflexia.[13]

With due consideration of the clinical context, the semi-qualitative 'metabolic urine screening' tests are conducted in most medical centers (Table 15.3) but has *high false positive and negative rate.*[14] The specific tests for copper (Wilson disease), uric acid (Lesch-Nyhan disease), sialic acid (sialic acid storage diseases), N-acetyl aspartic acid (Canavan disease) and sulfathiourea (MLD and multiple sulfatase deficiency) can provide a great diagnostic clue when clinically correlated.

Various methods of chromatography or spectrophotometry are used to detect amino acids, organic acids, sulfatides, mucopolysaccharides, oligosaccharides and purines. The enzyme assays are particularly useful in LSDs to detect specific enzyme deficiency using leukocytes or fibroblast cultures and is an important tool in carrier detection and further prenatal diagnosis. The common IEMs mostly diagnosed by mass spectrometry are given in Table 15.4.

Mass Spectrometry (MS) technology, either Tandem Mass (TMS) for Newborn Screening using DBS or GC/MS urinary metabolic screening for high-risk IEM cases has revolutionized the diagnostic field of IEMs. The mass spectrometry (LC-MS/MS or GC/MS) are used for high-efficiency separation of compounds and identification of the metabolites based on specific mass fragmentation pattern from biological samples. There are no false positive or negative results but the very identification and interpretation of either a precursor ion mass or product after ionization or both requires a special knowledge and expertise to offer specific diagnosis. No doubt, this technology has increased sensitivity, specificity and reliability in IEM diagnosis. Many clinicians

Table 15.4 Various disorders of amino, organic and fatty acid metabolism detected by Tandem mass and GC/MS analysis

S. No.	Primary targets	Secondary targets
	Disorders of amino acid metabolism	
1.	Phenylketonuria	Hyperphenylalaninemia
2.	Maple syrup urine disease	Tyrosinemia type II
3.	Homocystinuria	Tyrosinemia type III
4.	Tyrosinemia type I	Biopterin defects (Bios)
5.	Argininosuccinic acidemia	Biopterin defects (Reg)
6.	Citrullinemia type I	Argininemia
7.		Hypermethioninemia
8.		Citrullinemia type II
	Disorders of organic acid metabolism	
1.	Isovaleric acidemia	Methylmalonic acidemia (Cbl C,D)
2.	Glutaric acidemia type I	2-CH_3 3-OH butyryl-CoA dehydrogenase deficiency
3.	3-OH_3-CH_3 glutaryl-CoA lyase deficiency	Isobutyryl-CoA dehydrogenase deficiency
4.	3-methylcrotonyl-CoA carboxylase deficiency	2-methylbutyryl-CoA dehydrogenase deficiency
5.	β-ketothiolase deficiency	3-Methyl glutaconyl CoA hydratase deficiency
6.	Multiple carboxylase deficiency	Malonic acidemia
7.	Methylmalonic acidemia (mut)	
8.	Methylmalonic acidemia (Cbl A,B)	
9.	Propionic acidemia	
	Disorders of fatty acid metabolism	
1.	Medium-chain acyl-CoA dehydrogenase deficiency	Medium/short-chain L-3-OH acyl-CoA dehydrogenase deficiency
2.	Very long-chain acyl-CoA dehydrogenase deficiency	Short-chain acyl-CoA dehydrogenase deficiency
3.	Long-chain L-3-OH acyl-CoA dehydrogenase deficiency	Medium-chain 3-ketoacyl-CoA thiolase deficiency
4.	Trifunctional protein deficiency	Carnitine palmitoyl-CoA transferase I deficiency
5.	Carnitine uptake defect	Glutaric Acidemia type II
6.		Carnitine acylcarnitine translocase deficiency
7.		2,4 Dienoyl-CoA reductase deficiency
8		Carnitine palmitoyl-CoA transferase I deficiency

recommend TMS screening in strongly suspected IEMs of amino, organic and fatty acids to get the idea about next confirmatory test. As shown in Figure 15.5, acylcarnitine-C3 detected by TMS will give result as organic acidemia. However, further differential diagnosis is confirmed on the basis of specific biomarkers such as methylmalonic acid in MMA. Many intermediate metabolites detected during TMS and GC/MS analysis are elevated in number of different disorders, and hence proficiency in sample preparation and operating systems is critical in interpretation of data and reporting. It is advisable to request a single test which covers a large spectrum of IEM conditions when strong suspicion of a specific IEM is clinically difficult. Urinary metabolic screening by GC/MS is both an IEM screening and diagnostic test in the hands of a competent metabolic expert having knowledge of both laboratory and clinical aspects who can help the referring doctor in arriving at a reliable diagnosis.

Molecular/DNA Diagnostic Tests

Discoveries of new mutations in IEMs is described with astonishing pace and their implications in practice are significant in genetic counseling while making families and relatives aware about the prevention, recurrence risk and explaining the complexities of test results. The fetal medicine expert should be familiar with hereditary transmission such as imprinting, unstable repeats in dynamic mutation, gonadal and somatic mosaicism, etc. because many different mutations can be associated with the same disease (*locus heterogeneity*) and apparently identical mutation may give rise to different clinical phenotypes *(pleiotropy)*.

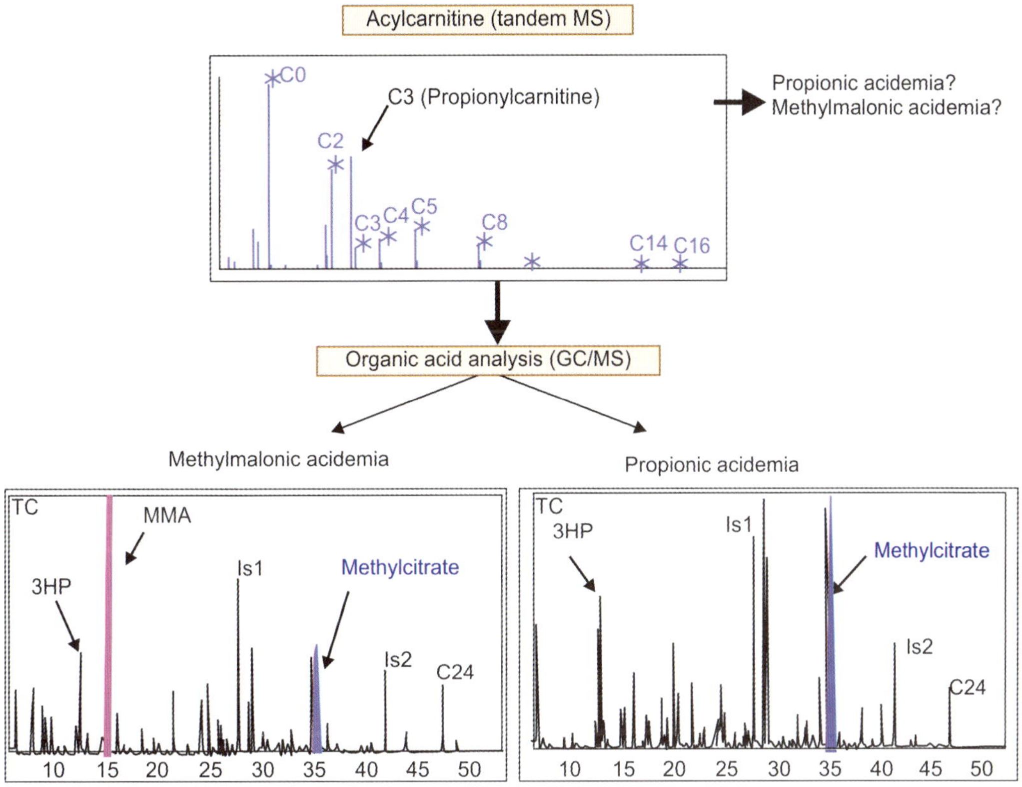

Fig. 15.5 Metabolic profiling showing difference in screening by TMS and confirmatory diagnosis by GC/MS

The one IEM case, *beta-Ketothiolase deficiency* (or *mitochondrial acetoacetyl-CoA thiolase deficiency)* is illustrated below to show how the detection of marker DNA mutation allowed further prenatal diagnosis.

"The female patient born of second degree consanguinity was admitted thrice during past 3 episodes of lethargy and breathlessness at 7 months, 11 months and at 2 yrs 5 months. The lethargy, breathlessness, weak pulse, tachypnea +, acidotic breathing +, and refusal to eat were clinical signs and symptoms along with infection as cough and cold. The normal chest X-ray with urine ketones ++, blood lactate ++ and normal NH_3 *were other findings. During 3rd episode, the urinary GC/MS metabolic profiling revealed abnormally high increase in markers such as 2-methyl-3-hydroxybutyric acids, tiglylglycine, and lactate indicating beta-Ketothiolase deficiency, involving ketone body metabolism and isoleucine catabolism. The referring doctor was immediately contacted for therapy and, intervention; the patient was stable and discharged. The genetic counseling was done. The mutational analysis using Sanger sequencing method confirmed the patient with homozygous c.1124A>G mutation in exon 11 of ACAT1 gene related to aberrant splicing. The parents were confirmed by familial analysis to be heterozygotes at c.1124A>G* (Fig. 15.6)".

Neuroimaging, Radiologic and Electrophysiology Testing

The brain MRI is useful as a supportive tool in diagnosis of few IEMs where cortical atrophy, white matter degeneration, malformations, calcification, agenesis or secondary effects of metabolic error in demyelination or myelin degradation is seen,[11,13] e.g. characteristic basal ganglia involvement (Leigh disease), cerebellar atrophy (CoQ_{10} deficiency), white matter degeneration in leukodystrophies (Canavan disease, Alexander disease, Zellweger syndrome), myelin abnormalities in aminoacidopathies, or subcortical and cerebral cortex in mitochondrial (MELAS and MERRF) and progressive metabolic encephalopathies.[11] Agenesis of corpus callosum is seen in PDH deficiency and nonketotic hyperglycinemia. The characteristic bone alterations of thorax (cardiomyopathy in Pompe disease), skeletal changes (LSDs like MPS and Gaucher disease) or hand X-rays typical in Hurler syndrome are important radiological findings. Ultrasonography is less expensive tool to detect organ defects

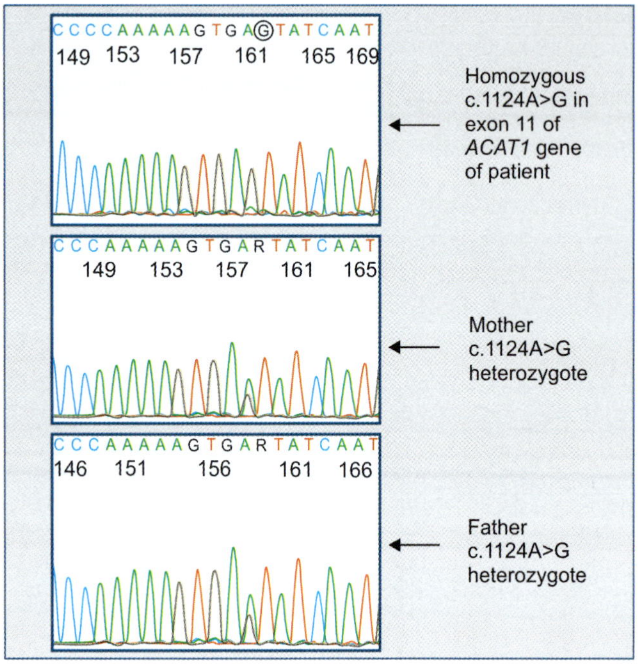

Fig. 15.6 Electropherogram showing mutation in *ACAT1 gene* in beta-ketothiolase deficiency in a patient (homozygous) and parents (heterozygous)

in many metabolic disorders, e.g. cardiomegaly, liver and spleen enlargement, cystic changes of the kidney. Prenatal ultrasound to detect fetal developmental anomalies and brain lesions are useful in minority of metabolic conditions but not before 23–24 weeks of gestation.[13]

The EEG has little role in diagnosing IEMs but information by EMG, nerve conduction velocity, auditory and visual evoked potentials, etc. are used to verify lesional topography of a metabolic condition.

Morphological/Structural Examination in Hematologic and Biopsy Tissue

The observation of accumulated products in blood and bone marrow cells or biopsy of muscle, nerve, liver and skin by histology or electronmicroscopy proves to complement final diagnosis in majority of the LSDs, e.g. intracytoplasmic membraneous inclusions in MPS-IV, or ceroid lipofuscin in fibroblasts and other cell in neuronal ceroid lipofuscinosis or globoid cells in Krabbe disease or sulfatide deposits in MLD, or Gaucher cells in bone marrow in Gaucher disease, or sea blue color histiocytes in Niemann-Pick disease.[15,16] Thus, clinical and biochemical features though essential for diagnosis, the morphologic characteristics play a significant role in differential diagnosis of certain IEMs.

TAKE HOME MESSAGE

Every attending physician appreciates that laboratory test results will never have full meaning unless considered in a clinical perspective. Hence, the competent fetal medicine experts must have knowledge of the laboratory IEM tests as well as the laboratories that provide these tests to the patients/doctors, their competency, reliability, validity and cost. The variable phenotype expression of IEMs is challenging to arrive at the accurate diagnosis, and immediate steps must be taken with a team approach to evaluate the neonate and recommend the appropriate tests by coordinating with a metabolic expert. A detailed knowledge of biochemical pathways is not essential while treating the IEM but the delayed diagnosis or misdiagnosis is a common mistake. Early and presymptomatic detection, precise diagnosis, timely intervention with special diet and therapy management offers the good prognosis in majority of the IEMs. Even with untreatable IEM, it is important to establish diagnosis in the index case so as to offer prenatal diagnosis in subsequent pregnancies.

NORMAL REFERENCE RANGES OF METABOLIC COMPOUNDS

Method

- Liquid chromatography, mass spectrometry (LC/MS)
- *Analytical sensitivity:* 0.02 µmol/L-4.5 µmol/L, depending on analyte
- *Analytical specificity:* No known cross-reaction with other substances
- *Reportable range:* 1.0 µmol/L-25,000 µmol/L.

Age-specific Reference Range

Reference ranges are provided in Table 15.5 for plasma, amino acids and other metabolic compounds.

Method

Chromatography.

Normal Results

All measurements are in micromole per liter (µmol/L). Normal values may vary between different laboratories. Talk to your doctor about your specific test results.

- Alanine
  - *Children:* 200–450
  - *Adults:* 230–510
- Alpha-aminoadipic acid
  - *Children:* Not measured
  - *Adults:* Not measured

Table 15.5 Plasma amino acid age-specific reference ranges (μmol/L)

Amino acid	<1 month	1–23 months	2–17 years	Adults (≥18 years)
Aspartic acid	2–20	2–14	1–8	1–4
Glutamic acid	51–277	32–185	9–109	10–97
Hydroxyproline	13–72	7–63	6–32	4–27
Serine	87–241	83–212	85–185	65–138
Asparagine	12–70	20–77	23–70	31–64
α-Aminoadipic acid	≤3	≤4	≤2	≤2
Glycine	133–409	103–386	138–349	122–322
Glutamine	240–1194	303–1459	405–923	428–747
Sarcosine	≤5	≤4	≤4	≤4
β-Alanine	≤8	≤8	≤5	≤5
Taurine	29–161	26–130	32–114	31–102
Histidine	40–143	42–125	54–113	60–109
Citrulline	3–35	4–50	9–52	16–51
Arginine	14–135	30–147	38–122	43–407
Threonine	56–392	40–428	59–195	67–198
Alanine	83–447	119–523	157–481	200–483
1-Methylhistidine	≤4	≤9	≤27	≤47
γ-Aminobutyric acid	<1	<1	≤2	≤3
3-Methylhistidine	≤10	≤8	1–6	2–9
β-Aminoisobutyric acid	≤9	≤8	≤6	<1
Proline	87–375	104–348	99–351	104–383
Ethanolamine	8–106	5–19	5–15	5–13
α-Aminobutyric acid	1–20	4–30	6–30	7–32
Tyrosine	33–160	24–125	31–108	38–96
Valine	57–250	84–354	130–307	132–313
Methionine	13–45	12–50	14–37	16–34
Cystathionine	<1	<1	<1	<1
Isoleucine	12–92	10–109	33–97	34–98
Leucine	23–172	43–181	65–179	73–182
Homocystine	<1	<1	<1	<1
Phenylalanine	30–79	31–92	38–86	40–74
Tryptophan	17–85	16–92	30–94	40–91
Ornithine	29–168	19–139	33–103	27–83
Lysine	66–226	70–258	98–231	119–233
Alloisoleucine	<1	<1	<1	<1

- Alpha-amino-N-butyric acid
  - *Children:* 8–37
  - *Adults:* 15–41
- Arginine
  - *Children:* 44–120
  - *Adults:* 13–64
- Asparagine
  - *Children:* 15–40
  - *Adults:* 45–130
- Aspartic acid
  - *Children:* 0–26
  - *Adults:* 0–6
- Beta-alanine
  - *Children:* 0–49
  - *Adults:* 0–29
- Beta-amino-isobutyric acid
  - *Children:* Not measured
  - *Adults:* Not measured
- Carnosine
  - *Children:* Not measured
  - *Adults:* Not measured
- Citrulline
  - *Children:* 16–32
  - *Adults:* 16–55
- Cystine
  - *Children:* 19–47
  - *Adults:* 30–65
- Glutamic acid
  - *Children:* 32–140
  - *Adults:* 18–98
- Glutamine
  - *Children:* 420–730
  - *Adults:* 390–650
- Glycine
  - *Children:* 110–240
  - *Adults:* 170–330
- Histidine
  - *Children:* 68–120
  - *Adults:* 26–120
- Hydroxyproline
  - *Children:* 0–5
  - *Adults:* Not measured
- Isoleucine
  - *Children:* 37–140
  - *Adults:* 42–100
- Leucine
  - *Children:* 70–170
  - *Adults:* 66–170
- Lysine
  - *Children:* 120–290
  - *Adults:* 150–220
- Methionine
  - *Children:* 13–30
  - *Adults:* 16–30
- 1-methylhistidine
  - *Children:* Not measured
  - *Adults:* Not measured
- 3-methylhistidine
  - *Children:* 0–52
  - *Adults:* 0–64
- Ornithine
  - *Children:* 44–90
  - *Adults:* 27–80
- Phenylalanine
  - *Children:* 26–86
  - *Adults:* 41–68
- Phosphoserine
  - *Children:* 0–12
  - *Adults:* 0–12
- Phosphoethanolamine
  - *Children:* 0–12
  - *Adults:* 0–55
- Proline
  - *Children:* 130–290
  - *Adults:* 110–360
- Serine
  - *Children:* 93–150
  - *Adults:* 56–140
- Taurine
  - *Children:* 11–120
  - *Adults:* 45–130
- Threonine
  - *Children:* 67–150
  - *Adults:* 92–240
- Tyrosine
  - *Children:* 26–110
  - *Adults:* 45–74
- Valine
  - *Children:* 160–350
  - *Adults:* 150–310

ACKNOWLEDGMENTS

I thank Ms Priyankka Damani for her assistance while writing the manuscript. My sincere thanks to all the doctors and patients who supported me to conduct this work.

REFERENCES

1. Garrod AG. Inborn Errors of Metabolism. Oxford: Oxford University Press; 1909.
2. Du L, Zannoni BN, Laster VG, et al. The nature of the defect in tyrosine metabolism in alcaptonuria. Journal of Biological Chemistry. 1958;230:251-60.
3. Folling A. The excretion of phenylpyruvic acid in the urine, an anomaly of metabolism in connection with imbecility. Zeitschrift fur Physiologische Chemie. 1934;227:169-76.
4. Beadle GW, Tatum EL. Genetic control of biochemical reactions in neurospora. PNAS. 1941;27:499-506.
5. Scriver CR, Beaudet AL, Sly WS, Valle D. The Metabolic and Molecular Bases of Inherited Disease, 8th edn, New York: McGraw-Hill; 2001.
6. Guthrie R. Blood screening for phenylketonuria. JAMA. 1961; 178(8):863.
7. Bickel H, Gerrad J, Hickmans EM. Influence of phenylalanine intake on phenylketonuria. Lancet. 1953;265(6790):812-3.
8. Matsumoto I, Kuhara T. A new chemical diagnostic method for inborn errors of metabolism by mass spectrometry: Rapid, practical and simultaneous urinary metabolites analysis. Mass Spectrometry Reviews. 1996;15(1):43-57.
9. Dave UP, Das BR. Newborn screening: From 'Guthrie age to genomic age.' J Obstet Gynecol India. 2010;60(3):210-20.
10. Raghuveer TS, Garg U, Graf WD. Inborn errors of metabolism in infancy and early childhood: An update. Am Fam Physician. 2006;73:1981-90.
11. Clarke JTR. A Clinical Guide to Inherited Metabolic Diseases, 3rd edn, New York: University Press, Cambridge; 2006.
12. Kothiwale VA, Varun Kumar B. Inborn errors of metabolism: Disorder of adults? Section 18 metabolic disorders; http:// *www.apiindia.org/medicine_update_2013/chap135.pdf*
13. Lyon G, Kolodny EH, Pastores GM. Neurology of Hereditary Metabolic Diseases of Children, 3rd edn. McGraw-Hill; 2006.
14. Elshaari FA, Sheriff DS, Agela AE, Alshaari AA, Muftah SS. Screening for inborn errors of metabolism. International Journal of BioMedicine. 2013;3(3):211-4.
15. Goebel HH. Extracerebral biopsies in neurodegenerative diseases of childhood. Brain Dev. 1999;21(7):435-43.
16. Dave UP. Screening and diagnosis of inborn errors of metabolism (IEM) by mass spectrometry: 15 Years' experience-issues and challenges in India. Invited lecture at Asian Congress of Inherited Metabolic Disorders (ACIMD), Abstract. Taipei, 19-22nd, March 2015.

CHAPTER

16

11 to 13^{+6} Weeks Scan: A Window to Fetal Abnormalities

Vandana Bansal, Hema Purandarey

INTRODUCTION

Changing Trends in Obstetric Management: Inversion of the Pyramid of Care

Traditionally most obstetric books for time immemorial have been recommending one antenatal visit in the first trimester, monthly visits between 12 and 28 weeks, fortnightly till 36 weeks and weekly thereafter till delivery. More frequent antenatal check-ups in the last trimester implied more complications were expected in late pregnancy and adverse outcomes were unpredictable or preventable in the first and second trimester. This pyramid of obstetric care has undergone an inversion in the last 20 years with the advent of the 11–13^{+6} weeks scan for aneuploidy, early malformation and uterine artery Doppler (Figs 16.1A and B).[1] More than 90% of all aneuploidies can be identified, 70–80% of major structural anomalies can be detected and a other pregnancy complications such as miscarriage, stillbirth, pre-eclampsia, macrosomia, fetal growth restriction, preterm delivery and complications due to twin-to-twin transfusion can be predicted.

Screening in the first trimester has an advantage of early reassurance of normalcy or an early definitive prenatal diagnosis can be initiated. Detection of structural malformation and/or aneuploidy can help early, less physically and emotionally traumatic termination of pregnancy, if deemed necessary. Early prediction of patient specific risk for pregnancy complications may help triage pregnant population into high-risk and low-risk group so that individualized care, more frequent antenatal visits, close surveillance under specialist care and more resources can be allocated to the high-risk pregnant group. In addition, any preventive action may be initiated early in gestation for better impact.

NUCHAL TRANSLUCENCY

Nuchal translucency (NT) is an objective evaluation on ultrasound of subcutaneous fluid behind the fetal head, neck and torso in the first trimester of pregnancy.

Langdon Downs first noted in 1866 that individuals with trisomy 21 characteristically have skin deficient in elasticity

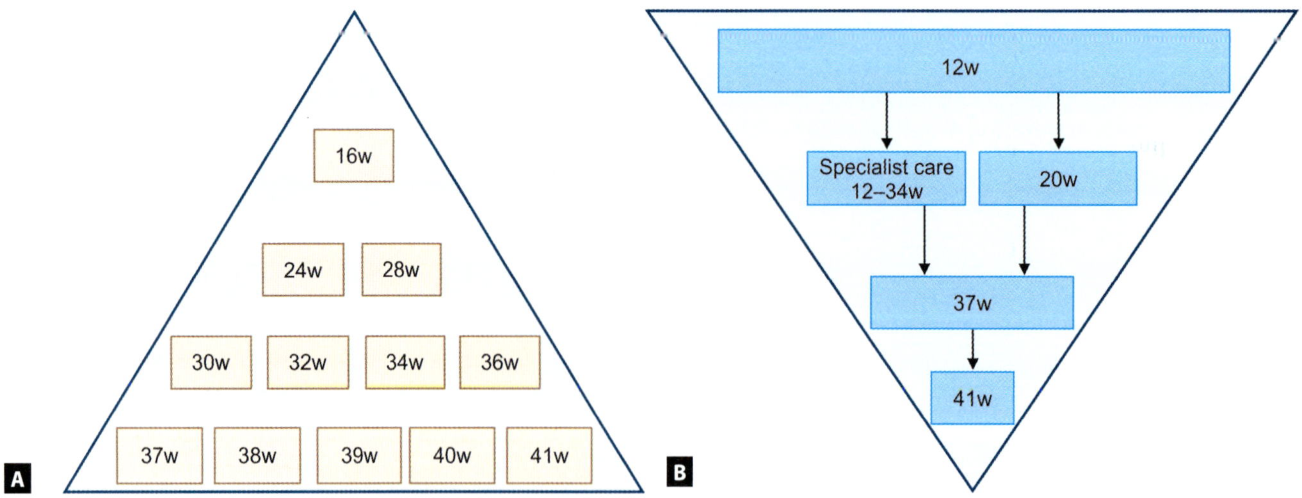

Figs 16.1A and B (A) Pyramid of prenatal care; (B) Inverted pyramid of care

giving appearance of thick loose skin, being too large for the body, with flat faces and small nose.[2] These characteristics have been visualized on ultrasound as increased nuchal translucency and absent nasal bone in intrauterine life between 11 and 13^{+6} weeks. About 75% of fetuses with trisomy 21 have increased nuchal translucency.[3]

Pathophysiology

Since this increased in nuchal translucency, is associated with multiple apparently unrelated fetal conditions, the pathophysiology may also be diverse. Postulated mechanism of increased fluid includes:

- Cardiac dysfunction, decreased myocardial compliance (Reversed a wave), ventricular dilatation (tricuspid regurgitation) as in aneuploidy and cardiac defects.
- Aortic narrowing seen in Down's syndrome and Turner syndrome associated with increased blood flow to the head and neck.
- Venous congestion of the head and neck (Compression of intrathoracic organs as in congenital diaphragmatic hernia, skeletal dysplasia).
- Altered composition of extracellular matrix: Many protein component in extracellular matrix have their code on chromosome 13 and 21 and its abnormality may alter production of hyaluronic acid leading to increased subcutaneous fluid.
- Failure of lymphatic drainage due to delayed or deficient development of lymphatic system (Noonan syndrome) or impaired fetal movement (akinesia deformation syndrome, myotonic dystrophy).
- Fetal infection (Parvovirus B19), fetal anemia (or hypoproteinemia (Congenital nephrotic syndrome).

Technique

It is extremely important that the nuchal translucency measurement is taken in a standardized manner. The Fetal Medicine Foundation has established criteria for proper NT scan and adherence to a well-defined technique will help achieve uniformity of results (Figs 16.2A and B).[3]

Nuchal Translucency Scan: Aneuploidy Screening

Nuchal translucency (NT) measurement is the single most effective screening test for fetal aneuploidy (Table 16.1). Maternal age combined with fetal nuchal translucency at 11–13^{+6} weeks provides detection rates of 75% for fetus affected by trisomy 21 for a false positive rate of 5%. Using a combination of maternal age and NT, similar detection rates are achieved for trisomy 13 and 18, 90% for monosomy X and 60% for triploidy.[4]

Detection rate is improved to 85–90% when maternal serum biochemical markers (free human chorionic gonadotropin (hCG) and Pregnancy Associated Plasma Protein -A) are included. Maternal serum concentration of free hCG is higher (2MoM) and PAPP-A is lower (0.5MoM) in fetuses with trisomy 21. In trisomies 13 and 18, both free hCG and PAPP-A are decreased. In sex chromosomal anomalies, only PAPP-A is low with normal free hCG.

Addition of other first trimester markers (Nasal bone/ Ductus venosus waveform/tricuspid regurgitation) increase detection rate for trisomy 21 to more than 95% for a false positive rate of 2.5% and 95% with false positive rate of 0.1% for trisomy 13 and 18.[5]

In a women with previous history of fetus or infant with Down's syndrome, risk of recurrence in subsequent pregnancy

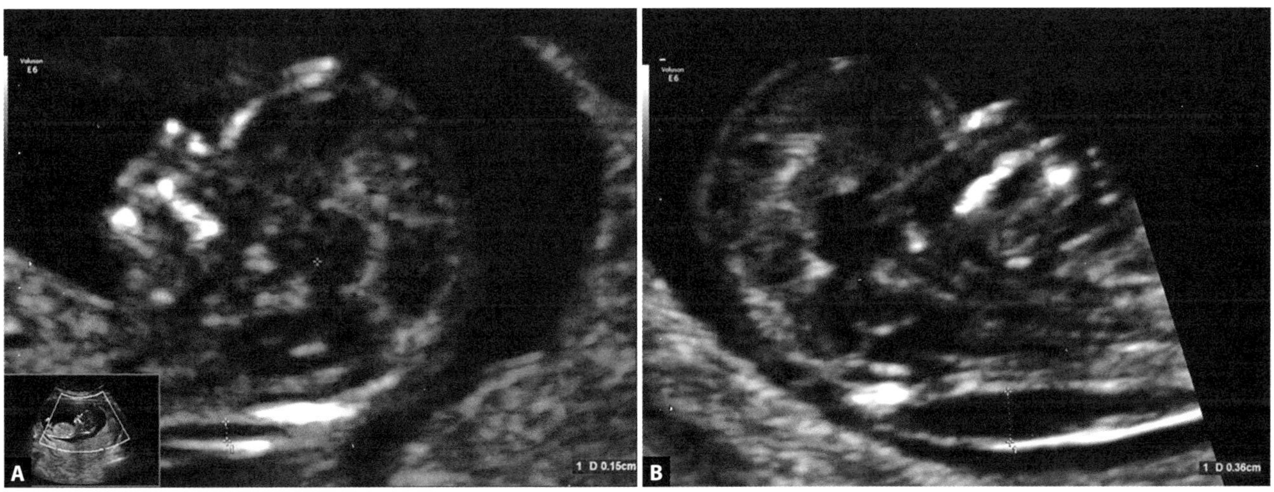

Figs 16.2A and B (A) USG image of normal nuchal translucency measurement; (B) USG image of increased nuchal translucency

Table 16.1 Standard technique for measurement of nuchal translucency

USG machine	High resolution with a video-loop and caliper that provides measurement to one decimal point
Gestational age	11^{+0} weeks to 13^{+6} weeks
Crown rump length	45–84 mm
Magnification	Fetal head and Torso occupy 75% of image
Position	Midsagittal view of fetus with fetus facing towards transducer Neutral position, neither hyperextended nor hyperflexed
Anatomical landmarks	• Tip of the nose • Hard palate is trapezoid in shape • Absence of frontal process of maxilla (Zygoma) • Rounded hypoechoic structure within the centre of the intracranial cavity representing the thalamus • Amniotic membrane to be differentiated from nuchal skin by waiting for spontaneous fetal movement or by tapping the mothers abdomen or coughing to make the fetus jump.
Caliper placement	Horizontal cross-hatch of the caliper should be flushed with the inner aspect of the line bordering the NT
Measurement	• Perform 3 measurement and largest measurement are take for risk assessment • If nuchal cord is present NT is measured below and above the cord and average of the two is taken • Reduce gain before measurement to reduce fuzzy edge of the line
Appearance	It is the amount of fluid accumulation (NT thickness) and not its appearance (presence or absence of septation/fluid accumulation confined to neck or enveloping the whole fetus) that determine risk

increases by 0.75% over and above the risk calculated by maternal age (a priori risk) or risk calculate from combined first trimester screen.

Increased Nuchal Translucency in Euploid Fetus: A Marker for Structural Defects

There is ample evidence that fetuses with thickened nuchal translucency with normal karyotype are at increased risk for other structural anomalies, especially cardiac defects, genetic and nongenetic syndromes. Once fetal karyotype on chorionic villus sampling/amniocentesis comes normal, still reassurance cannot be given. These fetuses with increased nuchal translucency must undergo detailed second trimester malformation scan and fetal ECHO.

Prevalence of fetal anomalies increases exponentially once nuchal translucency is >3.5 mm or >99 centile for gestational age. Structural anomalies and syndromes whose prevalence is substantially higher in fetuses with increased NT are:

- Cardiac defects
- Congenital diaphragmatic hernia
- Omphalocele
- Body stalk anomaly
- Skeletal dysplasia (Achondrogenesis, achondroplasia, camptomelic dysplasia, thanatophoric dysplasia)
- Megacystis
- Fetal akinesia deformation syndrome (FADS)
- Asphyxiating thoracic dystrophy (Jeune syndrome)
- Joubert's syndrome
- Noonan's syndrome
- Smith-Lemli Opitz syndrome
- Jarcho-Levin Syndrome
- Robert's syndrome
- Fryn's syndrome.

Counseling in Fetus with Increased Nuchal Translucency, Euploid Fetus with Normal Anatomy

Long-term outcomes of fetuses with increased NT, normal karyotype and normal anomaly scan in the second trimester have not found any increased neonatal or long-term adverse outcome or neurodevelopmental delay.[6]

Additional First Trimester Ultrasound Markers for Aneuploidy

Additional soft markers have been assessed which increase the detection rate for aneuploidy. About 75% of trisomy 21 fetuses have increased NT and 60–70% of them have absent nasal bone at the $11–13^{+6}$ weeks scan. Nasal bone may not be visualized in 2% of chromosomally normal fetuses. Abnormality of ductus venosus waveform are observed in 80% of trisomy 21 fetuses and 5% of euploid fetus. Tricuspid regurgitation is seen in 55% of trisomy 21 fetuses but also in 1% of normal fetuses.

Biochemical testing in first trimester along with increased nuchal translucency, absent nasal bone, ductus venosus reverse a wave and tricuspid regurgitation together improve detection rate for trisomy 21–95% with a false positive of 2.5%. Similar detection rate is achieved with a false positive of 0.1% for trisomies 13 and 18.[5]

Absent Nasal Bone

In the first trimester checking whether nasal bone is present or absent is a good screening marker. Measurement of size of nasal bone in the first trimester does not provide additional information. However, in the second trimester hypoplastic nasal bone or absent nasal bone are both useful screen for trisomy 21.[7]

In about 60–70% of fetuses with trisomy 21, 50% of trisomy 18, 45% of trisomy 13 and in 2% of euploid fetuses, nasal bone is not visualized/ossified at 11–13 weeks. Absent nasal bone is affected by ethinicity and is higher in black and Asian population and least in Caucasians. Presence or absence of nasal bone in the first trimester is a marker which improves the performance of first trimester screening for trisomy 21.

Technique

Nasal bone is evaluated in the same standard plane as for nuchal translucency during the same 11 to 13^{+6} weeks. Transducer should be such that it is parallel to the long axis of nasal bone. Nasal bone is located in the substance of the nasal bridge beneath the skin of the nasal bridge. So, it is seen as two echogenic lines roughly parallel to each other (equal sign). Nasal bone should be at least as echogenic as the skin. Less echogenic line may be seen representing the cartilage, if the nasal bone is absent (Fig. 16.3).

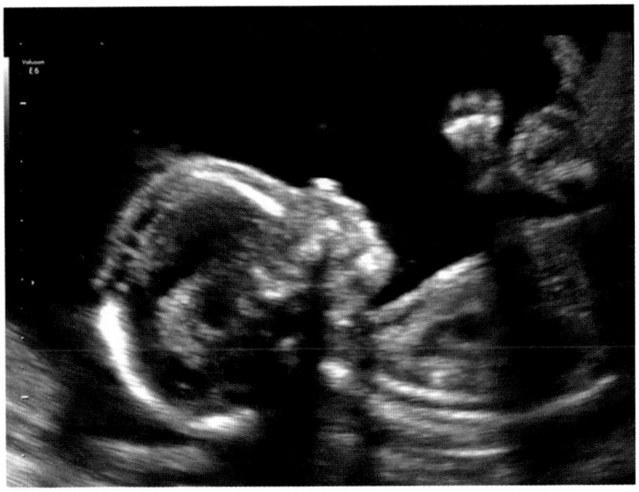

Fig. 16.3 USG image of absent nasal bone

Reversed a-Wave in Ductus Venosus

Ductus venosus is a small fetal venous system which connects hepatic portion of umbilical vein with inferior vena cava and sends 50% of oxygenated blood from the placenta to the right atria and then to left atria via the foramen ovale.

Normal wave form is an M-shape biphasic pattern with a forward flow throughout the cycle and characteristically corresponds to the cardiac cycle. Reversed a-wave during atrial contraction is observed in 3% of euploid fetus and in about 66% of fetuses with trisomy 21, 55% of trisomy 13 and 18 and 75% of fetuses with monosomy X (Figs 16.4A and B).[8]

Potential pathophysiology may be poor right ventricular compliance causing increase filling pressure generated in the right atria which is transmitted backward into the venous system as reversal of flow or secondary to a cardiac anomaly.

Standard Technique (Table 16.2)

Assessment of ductus venosus during first trimester scan improves performance of combine screen for aneuploidy by increasing the detection rate to 95% and reducing false positive to 2.5%. In addition, it has an advantage of identifying pregnancy at risk for cardiac defect and fetal death.

In fetuses with normal karyotype, ductus venosus has a sensitivity of 50% and specificity of 93% in detection of congenital heart defect. Sensitivity of reverse a-wave in ductus venosus is much higher in fetuses with increased nuchal translucency (83%).[9]

Table 16.2 Standard technique for measurement of ductus venosus

Position	Right parasagittal view of fetal upper abdomen
Magnification	Abdomen and thorax occupying majority of the image
Identifying DV	On color Doppler aliasing seen in vessel connecting hepatic portion of umbilical vein with inferior vena cava is the ductus venosus
Sample gate	Small sample gate (0.5–1 mm) in order to avoid contamination with hepatic veins and artery
Angle of insonation	$<30°$

Tricuspid Regurgitation (Table 16.3)

Blood flow across tricuspid valve is a biphasic waveform with first wave due to forward flow in ventricular diastole and second larger wave due to atrial systole. Tricuspid valve regurgitation is seen in 55% of trisomy 21, 30–38% in trisomy 13, 18 and monosomy X (Figs 16.5A and B).[10]

Probable pathophysiology is due to cardiac dysfunction, right ventricular dilatation causing tricuspid valve annulus to stretch with resultant regurgitation. Tricuspid regurgitation may also be seen in 1% of normal fetuses.

11–13^{+6} Weeks Scan for Cardiac Assessment

With the shift in screening for aneuploidy to the first trimester, early screening and detection of congenital heart defects at 11–13^{+6} weeks by early fetal ECHO has become possible. However, assessment of fetal heart at so early gestation requires high level of expertise and equipment (Figs 16.6A and B).

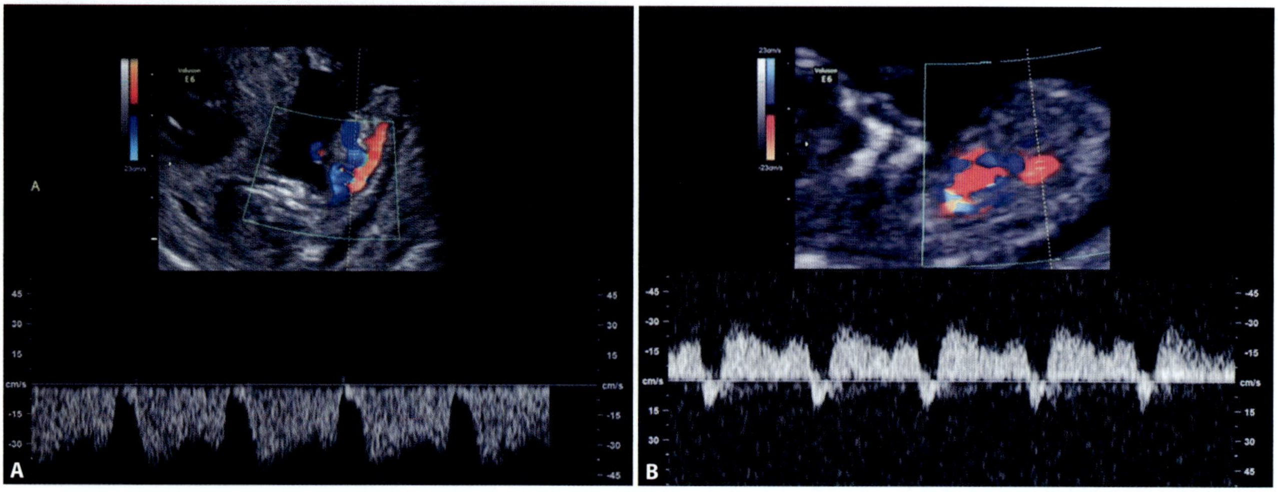

Figs 16.4A and B (A) USG image of normal ductus venosus flow; (B) USG image of reversed a-wave in ductus venosus

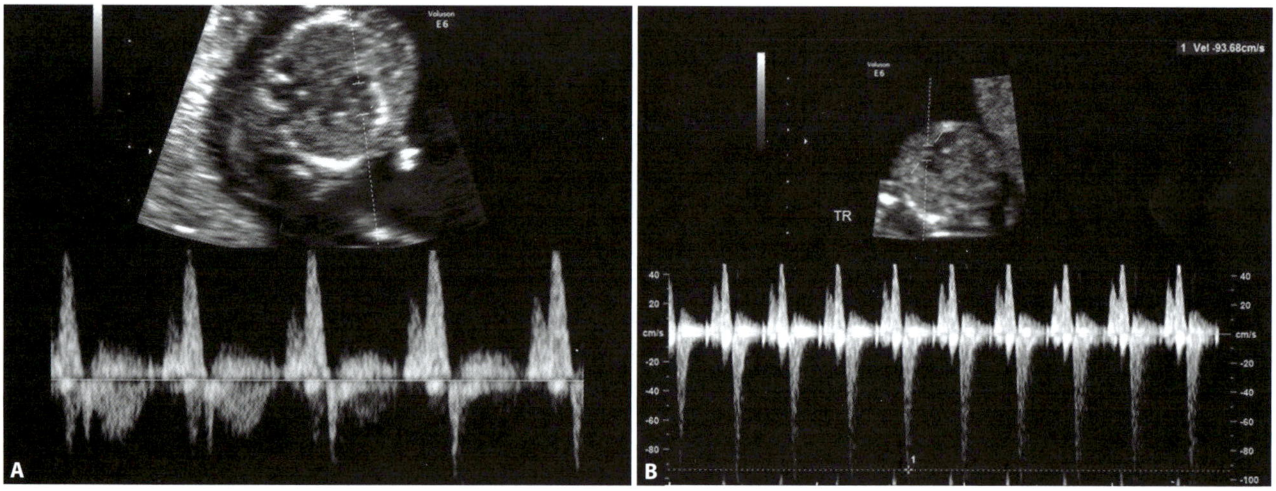

Figs 16.5A and B (A) USG image of normal tricuspid flow waveform; (B) USG image of tricuspid regurgitation

Table 16.3 Standard technique for measurement of tricuspid regurgitation	
Position	Transverse 4-chamber heart
Magnification	Chest occupies 75% of the image
Doppler sample	Doppler gate placed across tricuspid valve Large sample size used (2–3 mm)
Angle of insonation	≤30%
Normal waveform	Biphasic waveform with first wave due to forward flow during diastole and second larger wave due to atrial systole
Tricuspid regurgitation	During ventricular systole, any backward flow across tricuspid valve is considered regurgitation if the peak velocity of the regurgitant jet is more than 60 cm/s and should remains for at least 30% of ventricular systole

Detection rate varies according to the type of cardiac anomalies (50% for hypoplastic left heart syndrome to 18% for Fallot's tetralogy, transposition of great arteries and coarctation). Pooled detection rate of cardiac defects in the first trimester has been reported to be between 17–29% in different studies.[11]

Detection of major congenital heart defects at 11–13 weeks scan can be improved by their association with first trimester soft markers which are easily detectable, like increased nuchal translucency, absent or reversed a wave in ductus venosus or a tricuspid regurgitation.

Increased nuchal translucency >95th centile predicts 37–44% of major cardiac defects. NT > 99th centile is associated with more than 20 times increased risk of major heart defects. In chromosomally normal fetus, increased NT

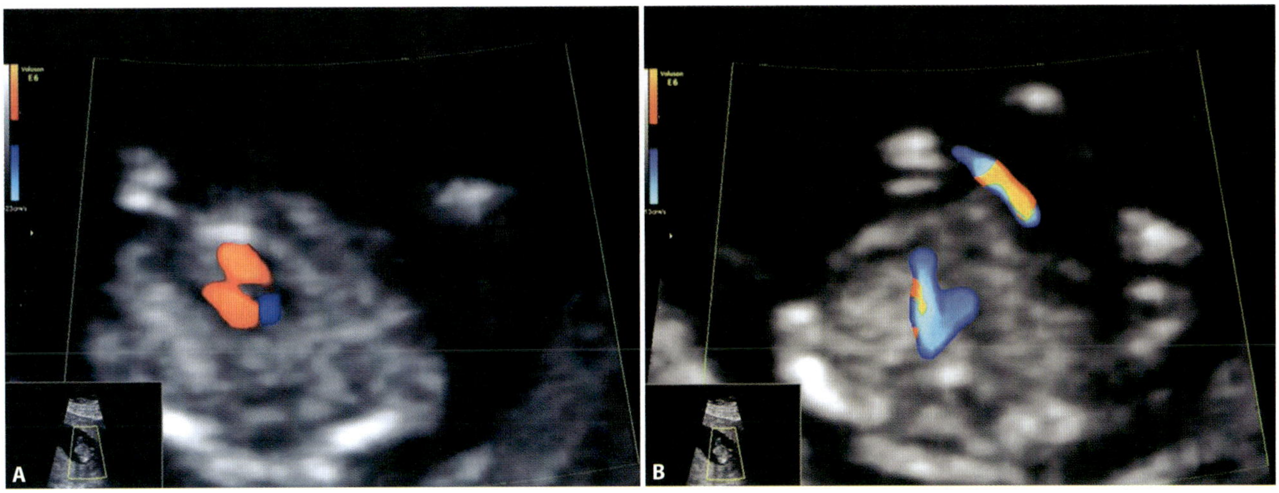

Figs 16.6A and B (A) Early fetal ECHO 4-chamber view on color Doppler; (B) Early fetal ECHO outflow tracts on color Doppler (tick sign)

combined with absent or reverse a-wave in ductus venosus is associated with three-fold increase likelihood of major cardiac defects. Tricuspid regurgitation is a frequent finding in 1/3rd of euploid fetuses with heart defects.

11–13^{+6} Weeks Scan for Early Anomaly Assessment

Detailed structural assessment by ultrasound has a potential for detection of fetal abnormalities in the first trimester. However, the reported efficacy for anomaly detection has considerable variation ranging from as low as 12.5% to high detection rate of 83.7%. This variance is mainly attributed to different population studied, different level of expertise and anatomical checklist used. Detection may also be dependent on the natural history of the disorder, the time of onset, the systems involved and the severity of the disease.[12]

Anomalies in the first trimester can be classified into:

- *Always detectable:* Anencephaly, body stalk anomaly, alobar holoprosencephaly.
- *Potentially detectable:* Congenital diaphragmatic hernia, cardiac defects.
- *Not detectable:* Microcephaly, hydrocephalus, echogenic lung lesions, agenesis of corpus callosum.

Although second trimester scan remains the gold standard to rule out anomalies, early detection of anomalies can be achieved by meticulous scanning in the first trimester with a structured protocol.

11–13^{+6} Weeks Scan for Screening for Spina Bifida

Diagnosis of open spinal defect in the second trimester by typical intracranial findings due to Chiari Type II malformation and scalloping of frontal bones is well known. Obliteration of intracranial translucency during the 11–13^{+6} weeks scan as a marker for open neural tube defect was first reported by Chaoui et al. in 2008. Presence of intracranial translucency between 11–13^{+6} weeks can confidently exclude open spina bifida (Fig. 16.7).[13]

In the sagittal view of the head in the standard 11–13 weeks NT scan, hypoechoic structure within the intracranial cavity is the developing brainstem. It is bracketed anteriorly by the sphenoid bone and floor of the fourth ventricle posteriorly. Another hypoechoic structure seen posteriorly represents the fourth ventricle which has been defined as the intracranial translucency (IT). Additional thin hypoechoic area between the cerebellum and the occipital bone represent the cisterna magna. Obliteration of intracranial translucency in the first trimester suggests open neural tube defect.

11–13^{+6} Weeks Scan in Multiple Gestation

In addition to determining the number of fetuses and viability in multiple pregnancy, chorionicity is best assessed during the 11–13^{+6} weeks scan (Fig. 16.8).

Maternal serum biochemistry for aneuploidy alone does not perform well in multiple pregnancy both in the first or second trimester. Ultrasound screen by nuchal translucency and additional markers are more useful to determine risk and identify abnormal fetus. Combined screen using ultrasound markers and serum biochemistry perform almost similarly in multiple pregnancy as in singleton. In MCDA twins, (Monozygotic) risk for aneuploidy is pregnancy-specific and is calculated by an average of NT measurement of both fetuses. However in a DCDA, risk assigned is fetus-specific and two separate risks are given depending on individual nuchal translucency (Fig. 16.9).[14]

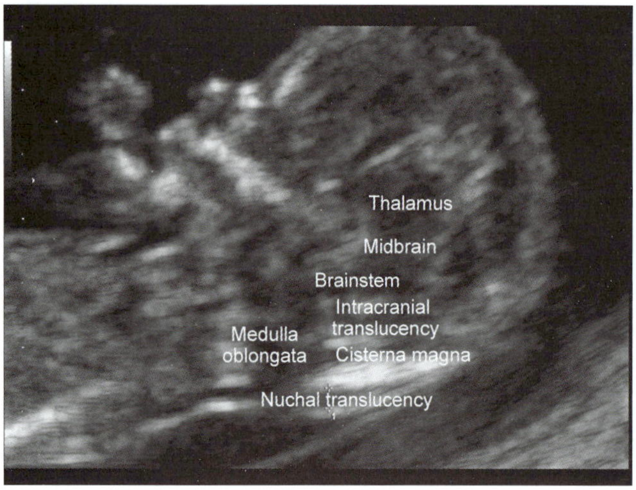

Fig. 16.7 Intracranial translucency

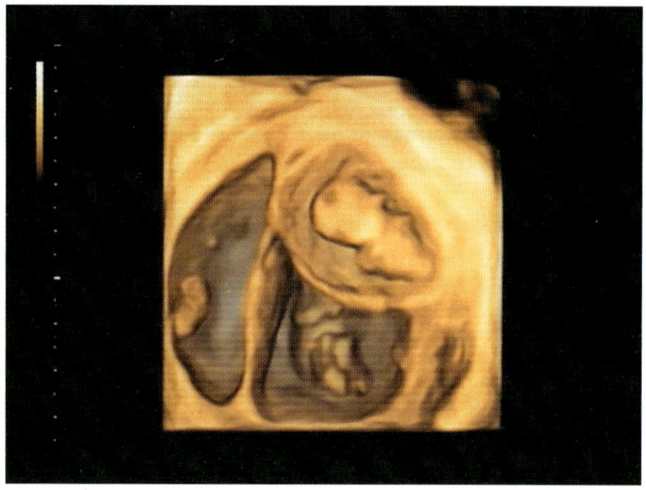

Fig. 16.8 Multiple pregnancy chorionicity determination

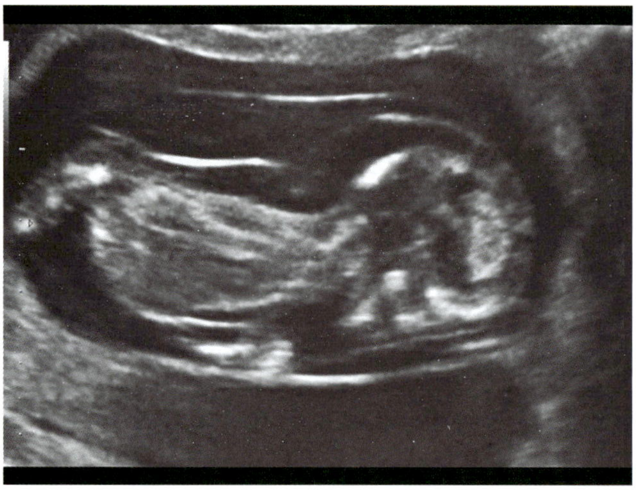

Fig. 16.9 USG image with discordant NT in twin fetus

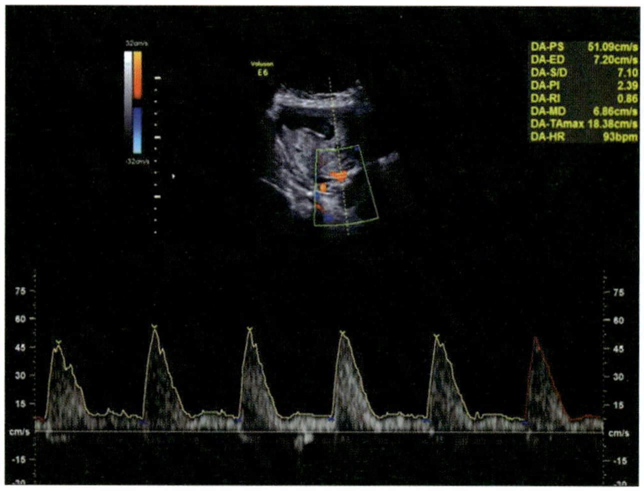

Fig. 16.10 First trimester screening uterine artery flow

In addition, discrepancy in NT between two fetuses in MCDA twins may be an early marker for twin-to-twin transfusion syndrome.

11–13^{+6} Weeks for Screening for Pre-eclampsia and Fetal Growth Restriction

As a consequence of shift in aneuploidy screening from second to the first trimester of pregnancy, extensive research is being done for predicting faulty placentation as early as possible. Early identification of women at risk for pre-eclampsia and fetal growth restriction would facilitate targeted antenatal surveillance and prevention by administration of low dose aspirin before 16 weeks.

Effective screening for pre-eclampsia can be achieved by measurement of uterine artery pulsatility index (PI) at 11–13 weeks NT scan, combined with maternal history, mean arterial blood pressure, serum pregnancy associated plasma protein-A and placental growth factors. This combined method of screening in the first trimester can predict 90% of cases of early onset pre-eclampsia, 45% of case of late onset pre-eclampsia at a false positive rate of 10% (Fig. 16.10).[15]

Until the mid-eighties, first trimester scan was done primarily for confirmation of intra- or extrauterine pregnancy, viability, dating and determining number of fetuses. However with the advent of high resolution ultrasound, better training and expertise and improved understanding of fetal development, the 11–13^{+6} weeks scan provides much more information and has become a window for detection of aneuploidy, anomalies, cardiac defects, genetic and non-genetic syndromes and pregnancy complications.

However, to maintain high level of quality in these screening method, adherence to strict standardized technique and extensive training and auditing cannot be overstated.

Genetic Evaluation after Detecting a Sonography Marker or Anomaly

The sole purpose of ultrasound screening is for ensuring the normalcy of the fetus, however, if any parameters of the fetal development are not met for the said gestation, evaluation of the fetus to ascertain the cause is recommended. The cause of fetal abnormality is commonly associated with aneuploidy of chromosomes. Once the anomaly is detected, the patients are more interested in prognosis than diagnosis. The patients are counseled for the same and confirmation by cytogenetic tests by chorion villus biopsy (11–14 weeks) and amniotic fluid studies (15–17 weeks) is offered.

In single gene disorders, the confirmation by biochemical or molecular test is needed. In order to ascertain the inheritance pattern and environmental insult, pedigree charting, family medical history, teratogenic exposure is looked into. If the karyotype report comes normal and teratogenic factors and contributory family history are ruled out, further evaluation by microarray testing by using fetal DNA is suggested. In cases for risks of aneuploidy, patients who are not willing for invasive testing, high end screening by NIPT can be suggested. However, in positive NIPT results, confirmation by invasive procedures is mandatory before any irreversible action is taken.

Once the results of laboratory tests/karyotype are obtained, couple is counseled again with interpretation of the result (Ref Chapter 7). Certain follow-up tests may be required in case of structural fetal anomalies and normal karyotypes to see the additional associated defects of late origin. Once the diagnosis is made, in case of abnormal result, the continuation or termination of pregnancy is entirely couple's decision.

The results of genetic diagnostic tests, not only applies to the patient for reproductive decision making for next pregnancy. Genetic work-up of the couple is necessary for the same. The test determines recurrence risk estimation, early diagnosis and risk for immediate blood relatives.

Today, reproductive options to the couple in adverse cases are easily available through *in vitro* fertilization evaluating your own fetus or fetus through sperm, egg or embryo donation. Preimplantation genetic diagnosis is also available for certain genetic disorders and is always discussed in conjunction with an IVF expert.

CONCLUSION

Genetic screening and diagnostic testing are of great help to the couples for reassurance and early intervention when needed. Confirmation of the affected by related diagnosis is the key to ascertain the cause and further evaluation and follow-up for next pregnancy.

REFERENCES

1. Nicolaides KH. Turning the pyramid of prenatal care. Fetal Diagn Ther. 2011;29(3):183-96.
2. Downs LJ. Observations on an ethnic classification of idiots. Clin Lectures and Reports, London Hospital. 1866;3:259-62.
3. Nicolaides KH. The 11-13^{+6} weeks scan: In Fetal Medicine Foundation, London 2004.
4. Nicolaides KH. Screening for chromosomal defects. Ultrasound Obstet Gynecol. 2003;21:313-21.
5. Retzke JD, Sonek JD. First trimester screening and diagnosis of fetal defects. In: Current Progress in Obstetrics and Gynecology. Studd J, Tan SL, Chervenak FA (Eds). Tree Life Media, India. 2011. pp. 13-36.
6. Sotiriadis A, Papatheodorou S, Makrydimas G. Neurodevelopmental outcome of fetuses with increased nuchal translucency and apparently normal prenatal and/or postnatal assessment: a systematic review. Ultrasound Obstet Gynecol. 2012;39:10-9.
7. Sonek JD. Nasal bone in screening for trisomy 21: defining hypoplasia. Am J Obstet Gynecol. 2007;197:335-6.
8. Nicolaides KH. Screening for fetal aneuploidies at 11 to 13 weeks. Prenat Diagn. 2011;31:7-15
9. Maiz N, Plasencia W, Dagklis T, Faros E, Nicolaides K. Ductus venosus Doppler in fetuses with cardiac defects and increased nuchal translucency thickness. Ultrasound Obstet Gynecol. 2008;31:256-60.
10. Kagan KO, Valencia C, Livanos P, Wright D, Nicolaides KH. Tricuspid regurgitation in screening for trisomies 21, 18 and 13 and Turner syndrome at 11^{+0} to 13^{+6} weeks of gestation. Ultrasound Obstet Gynecol. 2009;33:18-22.
11. Khalil A, Nicolaides KH. Fetal heart defects: potential and pitfalls of first-trimester detection. Seminars in Fetal and Neonatal Medicine. 2013;18:251-60.
12. Iliescu D, Tudorache S, Comanescu P, et al. Improved detection rate of structural abnormalities in the first trimester using an extended examination protocol. Ultrasound Obstet Gynecol. 2013;42:300-9.
13. Chaoui R, Nicolaides KH. From nuchal translucency to intracranial translucency: towards early detection of spina bifida. Ultrasound Obstet Gynecol. 2010;35:133-8.
14. Sebire NJ, Snijder RJM, Hughes K, et al. Screening for trisomy 21 in twin pregnancies by maternal age and fetal nuchal translucency thickness at 10–14 weeks of gestation. Br J Obstet Gynecol. 1996;103:999-1003.
15. Akolekar R, Syngelaki A, Sarquis R, Zvanca M, Nicolaides KH. Prediction of early, intermediate and late pre-eclampsia from maternal factors, biophysical and biochemical markers at 11–13 weeks. Prenat Diagn. 2011;31:66-74.

CHAPTER

17 Fetal Anomaly Scan

Geeta Shah, Arati Joshi, Sonali Gandhi

A fetal anomaly scan is a detailed, systematic and meticulous fetal survey usually done in the 2nd trimester between 18 and 22 weeks to detect major fetal abnormalities. It is now offered to all pregnant women, as it is found that most anomalies occur sporadically in low-risk pregnant women and is now an essential part of obstetric screening. It can detect major fetal malformations with reasonable accuracy and a normal scan is very reassuring to the parents and the obstetrician.[1] It also provides important information regarding other aspects of pregnancy such as placental abnormalities, umbilical cord, amniotic fluid, cervix, fibroids and uterine artery circulation. This can have a huge impact on management.[2]

The timing of the fetal anomaly scan varies among centers. Later scans provide better anatomic detail and greater sensitivity for structural defects, earlier scans can detect major malformations earlier and also give information about the risk of fetal chromosomal abnormality. At our center, we usually perform a NT scan at 11–14 weeks and an anomaly scan at 18–20 weeks. We also include a follow-up survey, especially for heart between 24–26 weeks, as chamber asymmetry and some other abnormalities such as kidneys, agenesis of corpus callosum sometimes manifests later.

There are several limitations in detection of fetal anomalies such as equipment quality, expertise of the sonologist, length of time spent on the study, maternal obesity, fetal position where the osseous structures may obscure soft tissue anatomy especially in late gestation. Oligohydramnios often compresses fetal parts making identification of some structures difficult and certain measurements inaccurate.

GUIDELINES OF FETAL ANATOMIC SURVEY

Many organizations have published guidelines[3] for a complete obstetric ultrasound which have the following components:

- Establish gestational age to evaluate fetal growth and assess the size of certain structures. Detailed measurements such as transcerebellar diameter, binocular diameter, clavicles, all the long bones, etc. also should be done as and when required.
- Extrafetal survey such as evaluation of the amniotic fluid, umbilical cord, placenta, cervix, fibroids, uterine artery Doppler should also be done.
- Specific anatomic landmarks within organ systems of the entire fetal body is surveyed from head to toe for presence of major anomalies. Highest frequency probe possible should be used to maximize resolution of targeted anatomy, even transvaginal sonography can be done for evaluation of the fetal brain when in a cephalic presentation.

Detection of any abnormality requires a thorough familiarity with normal fetal anatomy, sonographic landmarks and normal variants so that deviation from normal can be easily identified.

ULTRASOUND FEATURES OF FETAL ANEUPLOIDY

A detailed anomaly scan in the 2nd trimester also aids in the diagnosis of fetal aneuploidies and is also known as a "Genetic Sonogram". All pregnancies are theoretically at risk for aneuploidies.[4] The other risk factors are advanced maternal age, gestational diabetes, abnormal biochemical screening, history of chromosomal abnormality, known genetic defects in one of the parents and abnormalities visualized on prenatal ultrasound. The sonographic features are as follows:[5]

- Minor or soft markers which are variations in normal anatomy. They are unlikely to be clinically significant, if not associated with aneuploidies (especially trisomy 21). They are usually transient and nonspecific findings which can also occur in normal fetuses unlike structural abnormalities or major markers.
- The most common ultrasound markers seen in the 2nd trimester are nuchal fold thickening, mild ventriculomegaly, echogenic intracardiac focus, shortened long bones, hyperechoic bowel, renal pelvicaliectasis, choroid plexus cysts, clinodactyly, hypoplastic or absent nasal bone and the more recent aberrant right subclavian

artery (ARSA), which is more common in fetuses with chromosomal abnormality especially trisomy 21, where it was 29% as compared to euploid fetuses.[6] As the number of markers increase, the risk of chromosomal abnormalities also rises.

- Structural abnormalities or major markers include central nervous system, facial abnormalities, cystic hygroma, diaphragmatic hernia, cardiac defects, gastrointestinal and genitourinary abnormalities, nonimmune hydrops and limb abnormalities.
- Many fetuses with trisomy 18 and 13 have multiple major structural anomalies (See Figs 17.14A to H), however, only 25% of Trisomy 21 fetuses have sonographically detectable major congenital anomalies.[7]

Patterns of Anomalies Seen in Certain Common Fetal Aneuploidies

The type of abnormalities seen on sonography in aneuploidy fetuses may vary from one fetus to another, however, certain patterns are noted (Tables 17.1 to 17.3).[8,9]

Table 17.1 Trisomy 21

Markers	Structural abnormalities
• Nuchal thickening ventriculomegaly • Brachycephaly echogenic intracardiac focus • Pyelectasis • Hypoplastic/absent nasal bone • Clinodactyly • Hyperechoic bowel • Sandal gap • Short limbs • Wide iliac angle	• Cardiac anomalies • Hydrocephalus • Esophageal atresia • Duodenal atresia • Omphalocele • Aberrant right subclavian artery (ARSA)

Table 17.2 Trisomy 18

Markers	Structural abnormalities
• Choroid plexus cysts • Clenched hands • Small omphalocele • Single umbilical artery (SUA) • Club feet • Short limbs • Small low set ears • Strawberry-shaped head	• Cardiac defects • Cystic hygromas • CNS anomalies (agenesis of corpus callosum, hydrocephalus, Dandy-Walker malformation, NTD) • Micrognanthia • Hydronephrosis IUGR, nonimmune hydrops

Table 17.3 Trisomy 13

Markers	Structural abnormalities
• Small low set ears • Ventricular dilatation • Polydactyly • SUA • Club/rocker bottom feet • EIF • Nuchal thickening	• CNS-microcephaly, holoprosencephaly • Facial–Micrognathia, Cleft lip/palate, ocular anomalies • Cardiac defects • Cystic hygromas • Radial aplasia • GU-hydronephrosis, echogenic kidneys • IUGR, polyhydramnios
Turner's syndrome • Cystic hygroma • Cardiac defects—coarctation of aorta • Short limbs • Horse-shoe kidneys • Broad chest • Ovarian dysgenesis	
Triploidy • CNS anomalies—hydrocephalus • Facial abnormalities • Syndactyly, SUA	• Renal anomalies • Cardiac defects • Low set ears

Fetal Anatomic Survey at 18–22 Weeks

We now briefly describe the technique of fetal anatomic survey that is routinely evaluated. A few, examples of common abnormalities in each organ system with images are also included that can be seen as a deviation from the normal anatomy. A few, three-dimensional ultrasound images are also incorporated as it is a part of our routine anomaly scan, especially when an abnormality is detected for better delineation. This is modified from guidelines for the performance of the antenatal obstetrical ultrasound examination, American Institute of Ultrasound in Medicine (AIUM), Bethesda, MD, 1994.[3,10]

Head and Brain

Calvaria: Shape.

Brain: Thalami, lateral ventricles, cerebellum, vermis, cisterna magna and cavum septum pellucidum to be documented. They are obtained in the transthalamic, transventricular and transcerebellar views (Figs 17.1A to F). Minor markers for fetal aneuploidy are also seen (Figs 17.2A to C).

Anomalies detected in these views are: anencephaly, holoprosencephaly, hydrocephalus, posterior fossa abnormalities such as Dandy-Walker syndrome, vermian agenesis, etc. (Figs 17.3A to K).

Face/Neck

Face: Lips, anterior maxilla (premaxillary triangle, PMT), nose, orbits and profile views for mandible (Figs 17.4A to E).

Neck: Nuchal fold and thyroid.

Anomalies detected in these views are cleft lip/palate, hypo/hypertelorism, micrognathia (Figs 17.5A to E).

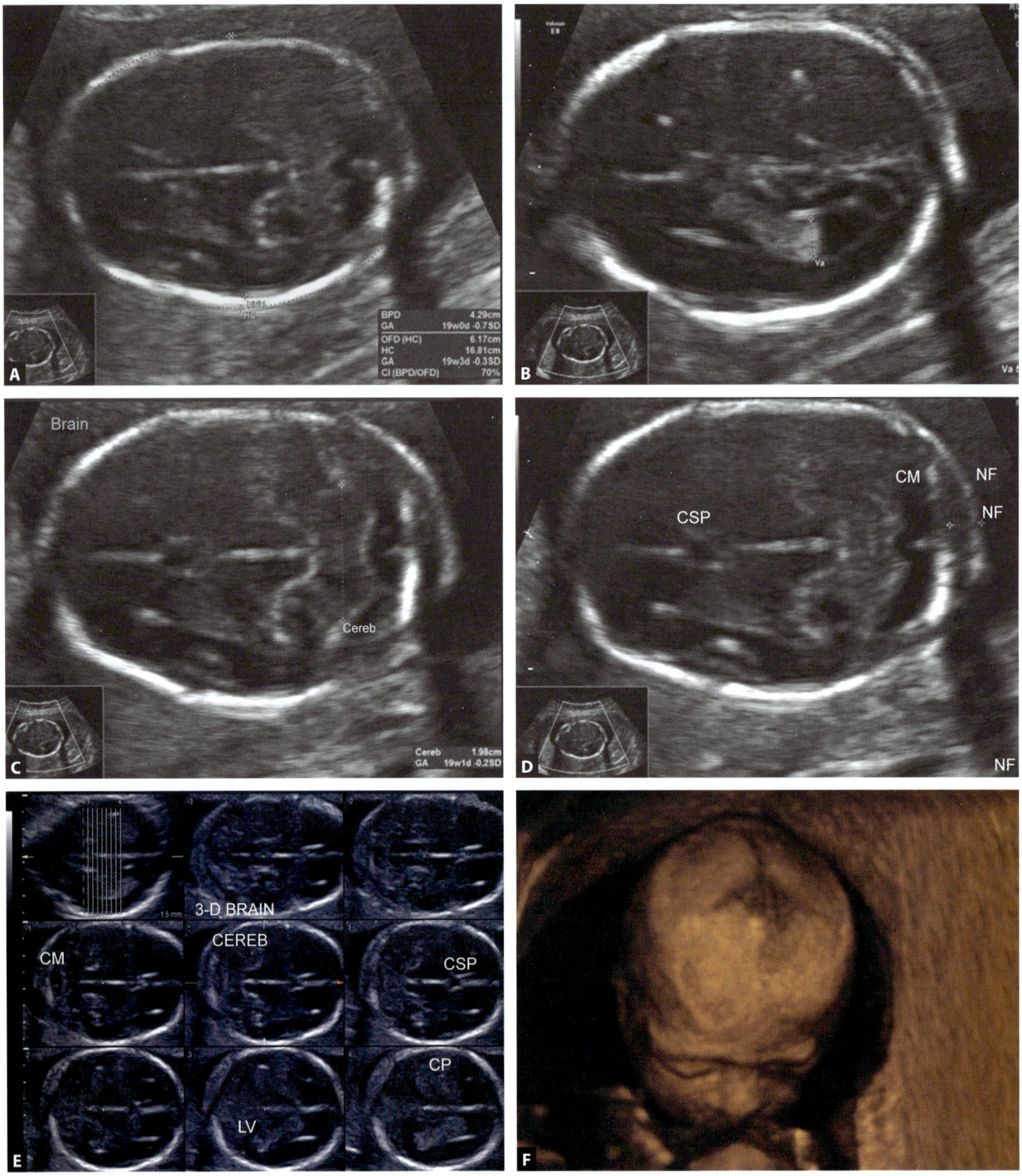

Figs 17.1A to F Brain. (A) Axial image of brain showing hypoechoic thalami, interhemispheric fissure/midline falx and cavum; (B) Lateral ventricles showing the echogenic choroid plexus and CSF. Look for hydrocephalus and choroid plexus cysts in this view; (C) Transcerebellar diameter, cisterna magna. Abnormalities seen are Dandy-Walker syndrome and posterior fossa cysts; (D) Nuchal fold thickness (normal is less than 5 mm); (E) Tomographic ultrasound imaging of brain showing the various structures in three-dimensional planes; (F) Cranial sutures seen on three-dimensional examination, which is useful in diagnosis of craniosynostosis

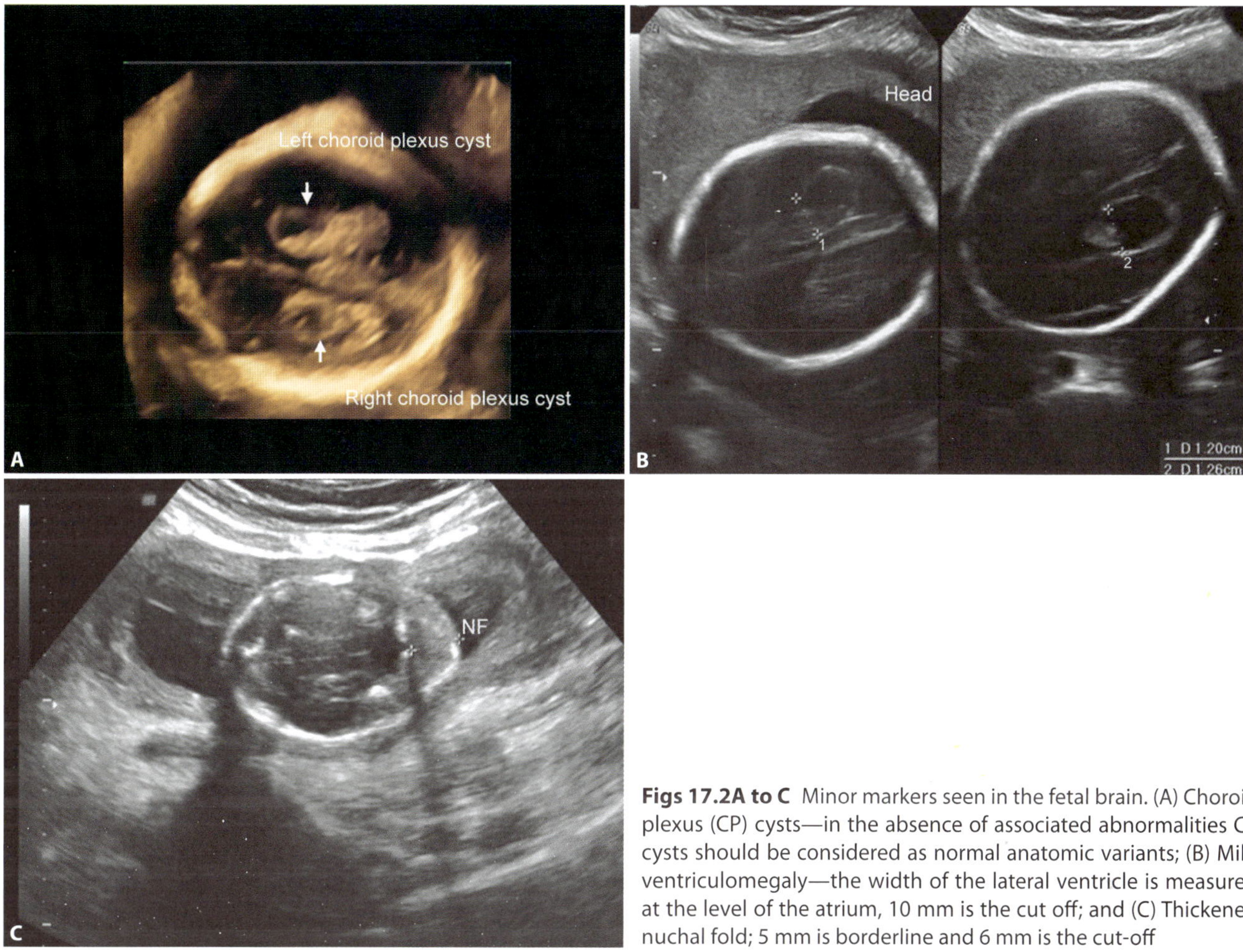

Figs 17.2A to C Minor markers seen in the fetal brain. (A) Choroid plexus (CP) cysts—in the absence of associated abnormalities CP cysts should be considered as normal anatomic variants; (B) Mild ventriculomegaly—the width of the lateral ventricle is measured at the level of the atrium, 10 mm is the cut off; and (C) Thickened nuchal fold; 5 mm is borderline and 6 mm is the cut-off

Spine

Longitudinal, transverse and coronal views. Three-dimensional imaging of the spine gives more information about the defects and is very useful for subtle defects (Figs 17.6A to G).

Abnormalities detected are neural tube defects, kyphoscoliosis, diastematomyelia (Figs 17.6A to G).

Thorax

Heart: Four chamber view, outflow tracts, three vessel view, ductal and aortic arches and the "Hammock view" for IVC and SVC (Figs 17.7A to F).

Abnormalities detected in the heart in these views are atrioventricular septal defects, hypoplastic right heart and left heart, outflow tract abnormalities such as tetralogy of Fallot, truncus arteriosus (Figs 17.7G to N).

Lungs

Abnormalities detected in the lungs are cystic adenomatoid malformations, pleural effusion (Figs 17.8A and B).

Abdomen

Stomach: Presence, situs and size. Liver, gallbladder, spleen, Intestine, large and small, Anterior abdominal wall (Figs 17.9A to G).

Abnormalities detected: Tracheoesophageal atresia, duodenal atresia, calcifications in the liver seen in uterine infections, echogenic bowel more than the bones as a marker for chromosomal abnormality, meconium cysts, ascites, omphalocele (Figs 17.10A to D), gastroschisis, single umbilical artery (Figs 17.11A and B) as a soft marker for chromosomal abnormality, etc.

Genitourinary Tract

Kidneys, adrenals, urinary bladder (Figs 17.12A to F).

Abnormalities detected: Bilateral pelvicaliectasis which is a soft marker for chromosomal abnormality, hydronephrosis, renal cysts, dysplastic kidney, renal agenesis, urogenital sinus abnormalities, posterior urethral valves with a thick-walled urinary bladder, cloacal exstrophy (Figs 17.12A to F).

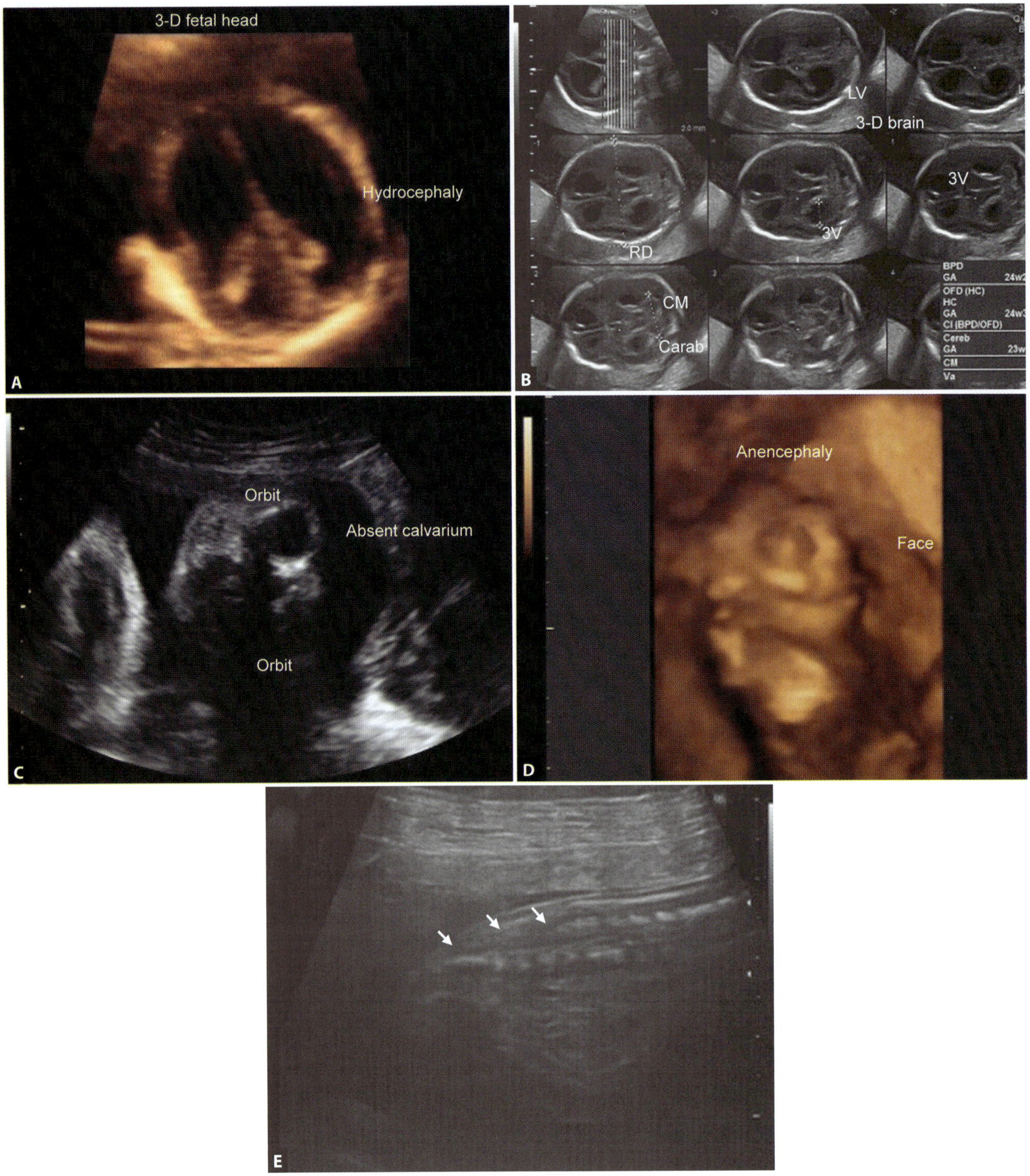

Figs 17.3A to E (A and B) Hydrocephalus, better evaluated on three-dimensional tomographic imaging; (C to E) Anencephaly with absent calvarium and neural tube defect

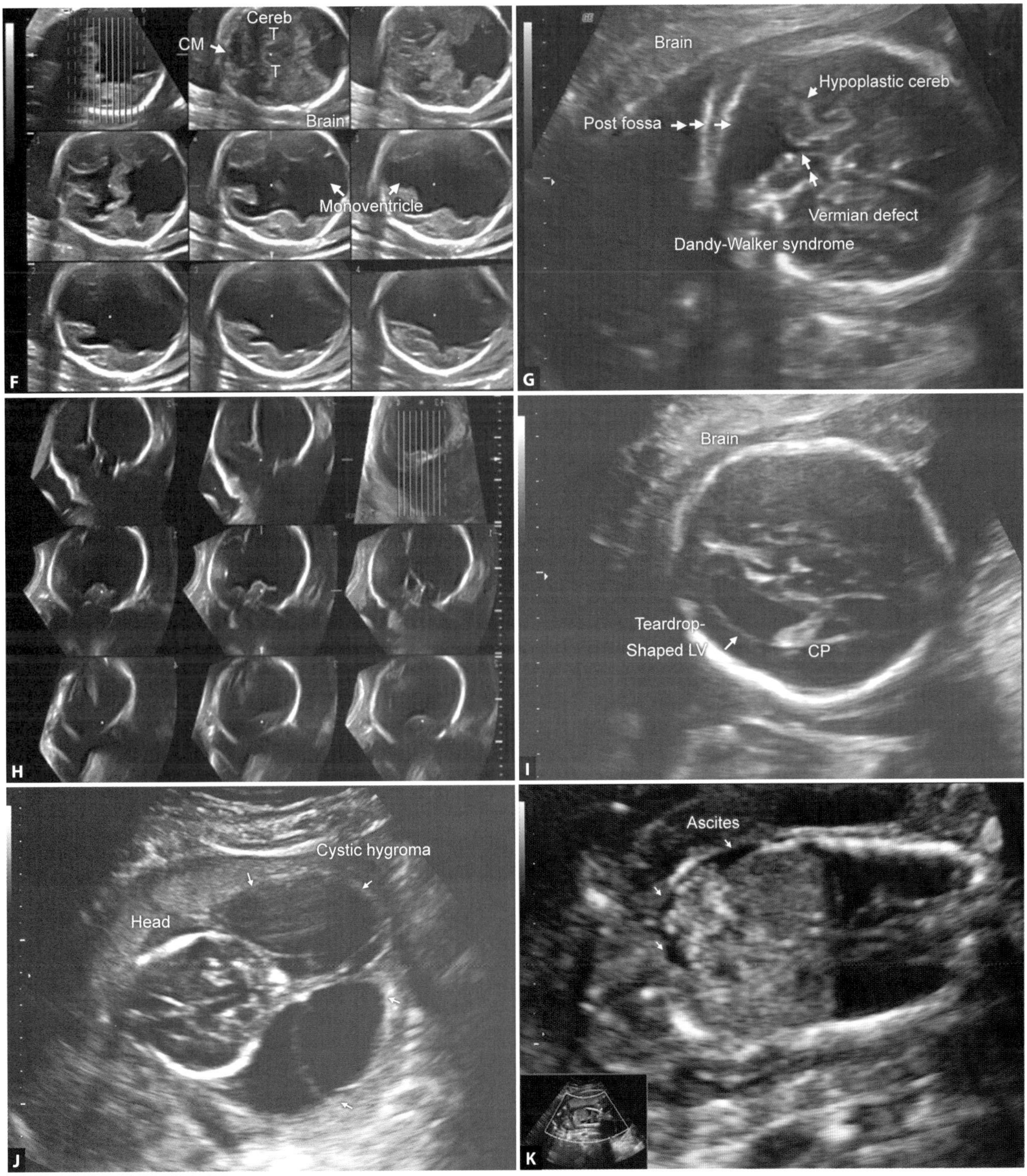

Figs 17.3F to K (F and H) Alobar holoprocencephaly with a monoventricle and absent interhemispheric fissure in axial and coronal planes, better evaluated on three-dimensional tomographic imaging; (I) Colpocephaly or tear-shaped lateral ventricles seen in agenesis of corpus callosum; (G) Vermian defect with cerebellar hypoplasia and posterior fossa cyst suggestive of Dandy-Walker syndrome; (J and K) Multiseptate cystic structure seen below head, in neck region suggestive of cystic hygroma (Abnormality of lymphatic drainage, mainly seen in association with chromosomal abnormalities) with bilateral pleural effusion and ascites suggestive of hydrops fetalis

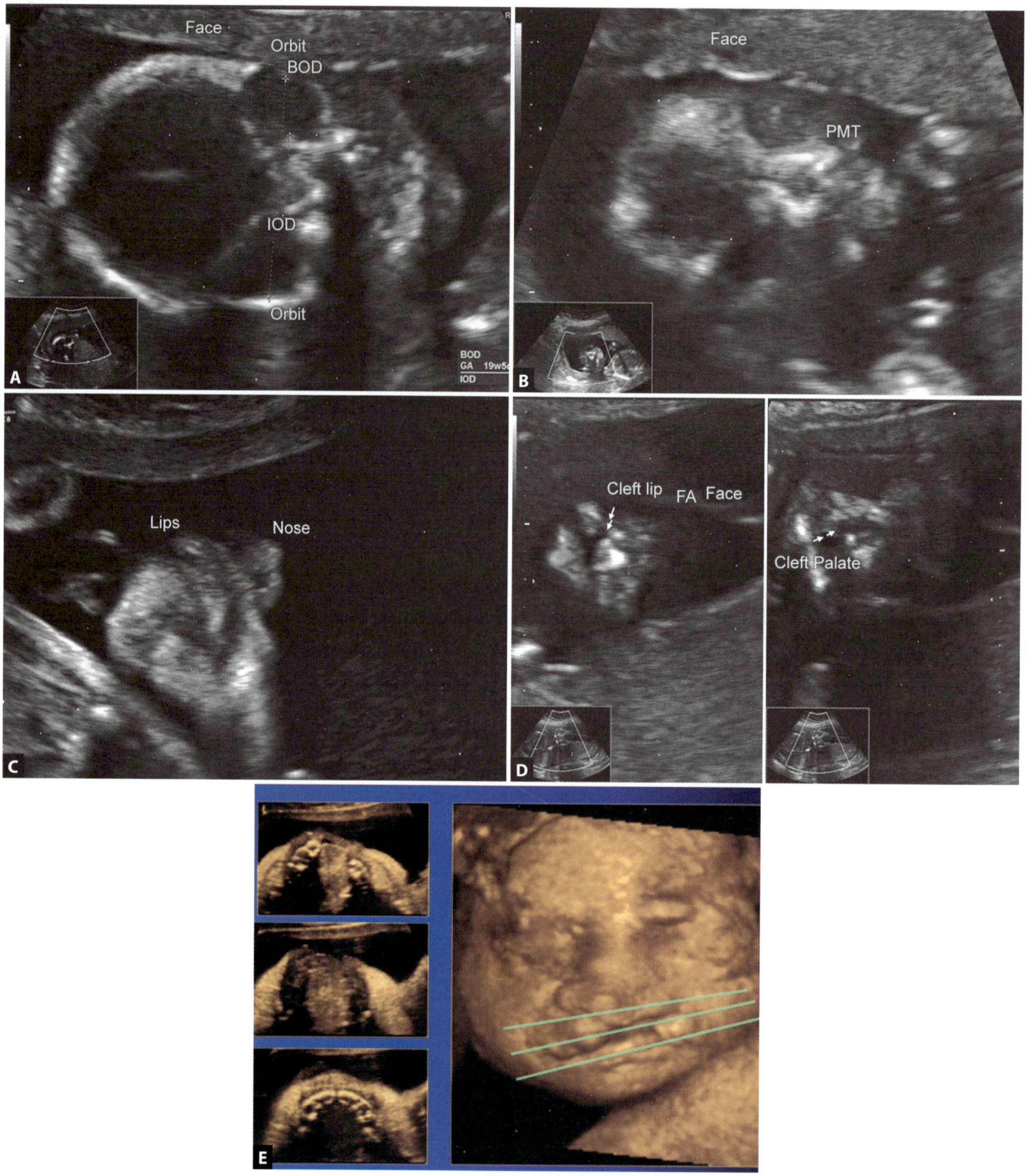

Figs 17.4A to E Face. (A) Axial image of face showing both orbits. The biorbital and interorbital distance is measured in this view to rule out hypo-/hypertelorism; (B and C) Coronal view of face showing premaxillary triangle and soft tissues of lips and nose; (D) Cleft lip and palate in coronal view; (E) Three-dimensional imaging helps in detailed evaluation of cleft lip and palate

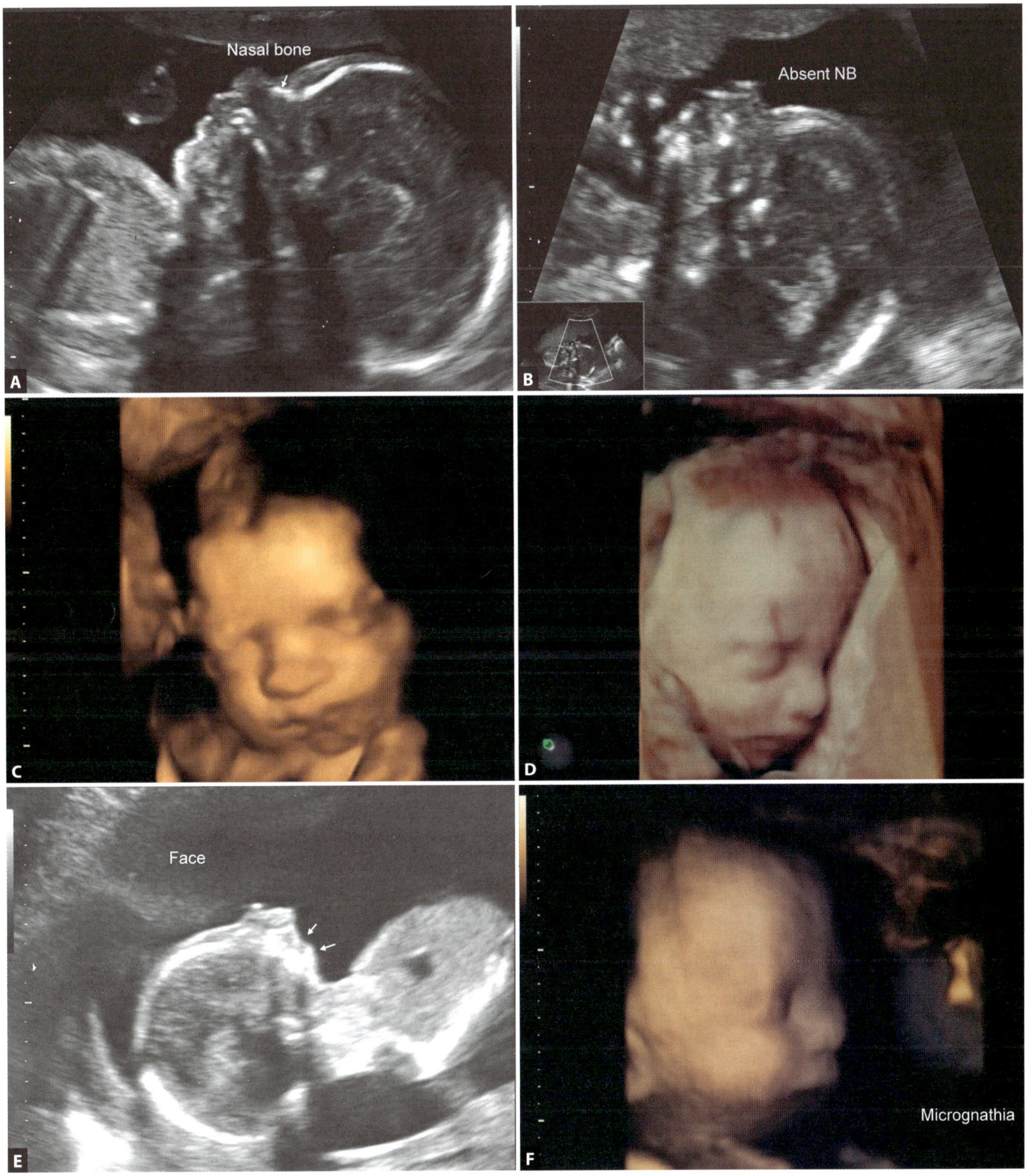

Figs 17.5A to F (A) Midline sagittal view showing the presence of nasal bone; (B) Absent nasal bone in a fetus with Down's syndrome; (C and D) are 3D images of normal face; (E and F) Micrognathia in 2D and 3D (Known case of Pierre-Robin syndrome)

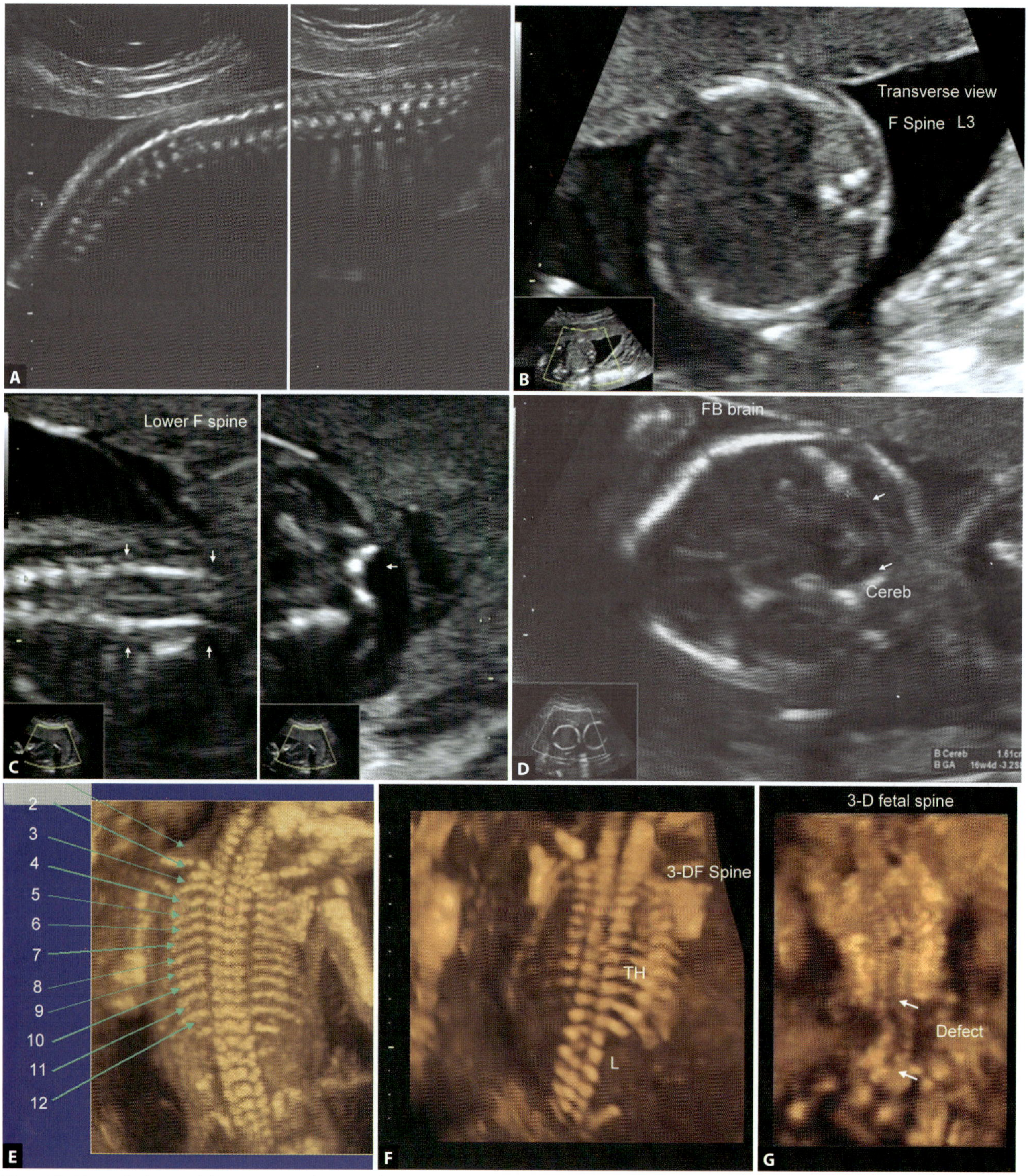

Figs 17.6A to G Spine. (A) Parasagittal view of spine showing the paired parallel ossification centers formed by vertebral bodies and posterior elements; (B) Transverse scan showing the 3 ossification centers. The echogenic skin continuity should be checked to look for subtle neural tube defects; (C and D) Absent skin and widening of posterior ossification centers is suggestive of an early NTD without meningomyelocele. Look for concomitant brain abnormality for associated Arnold-Chiari malformation (lemon-shaped skull, obliteration of cisterna magna and distortion of cerebellum forming banana sign); (E and F) Three-dimensional ultrasound with better delineation of the vertebrae, ribs, scapula and clavicles; (G) Three-dimensional view of kyphoscoliotic deformity of thoracolumbar spine

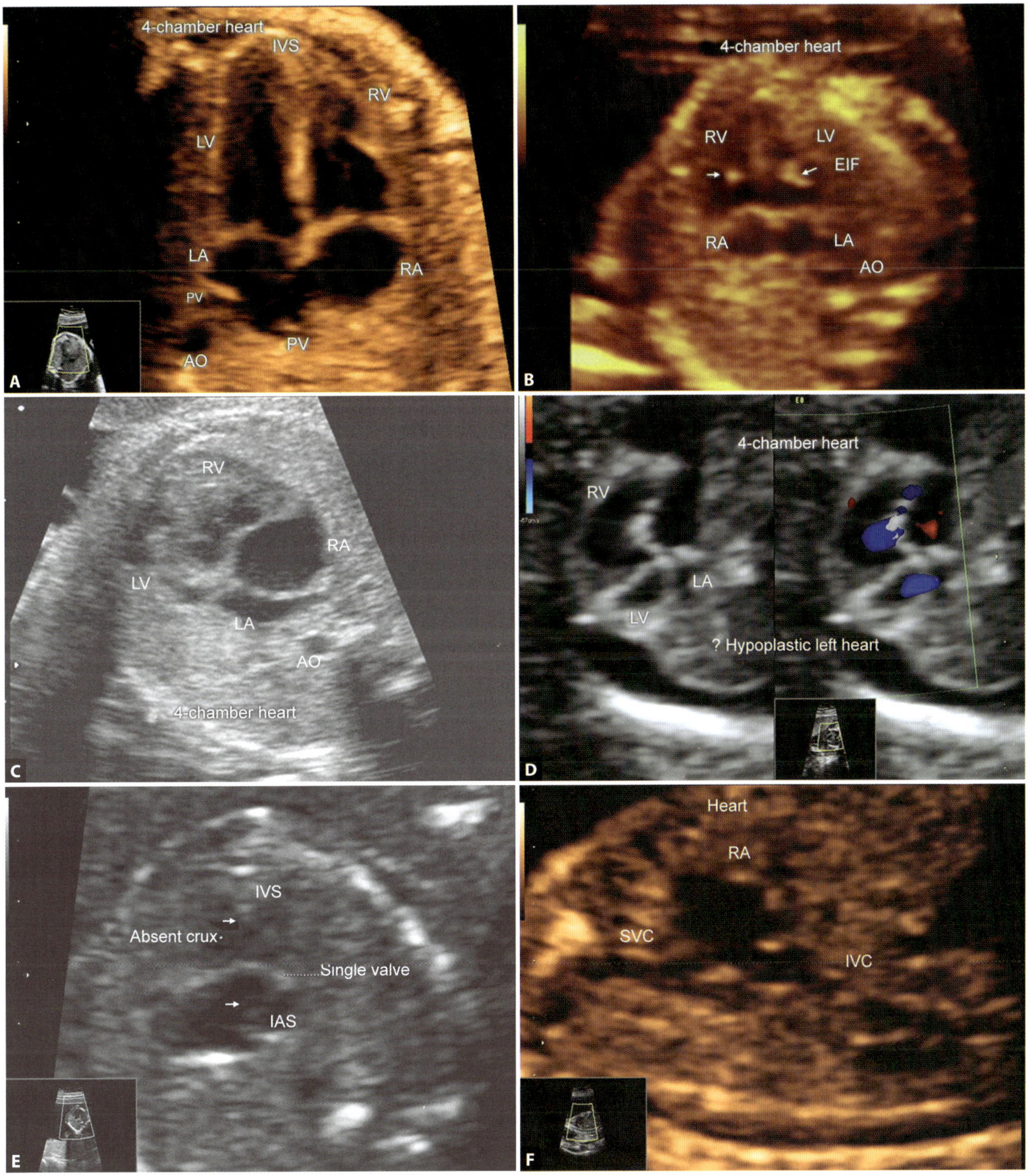

Figs 17.7A to F Heart. (A) The four-chamber view of heart showing equal sized atria and ventricles with the apex seen directed to left (normal angle is 45–60°); (B) Echogenic intracardiac focus (EIF) is commonly seen in 3–4% of normal Asian population and as an isolated finding is of no clinical significance; (C and D) Abnormal 4 chamber view showing small left-sided chambers with hardly any flow across mitral valve on color Doppler examination, suggestive of hypoplastic left heart syndrome; (E) Absent crux in 4 chamber view with a single AV valve seen, suggestive of atrioventricular septal defect (AVSD); (F) Hammock view showing the IVC and SVC draining into right atrium

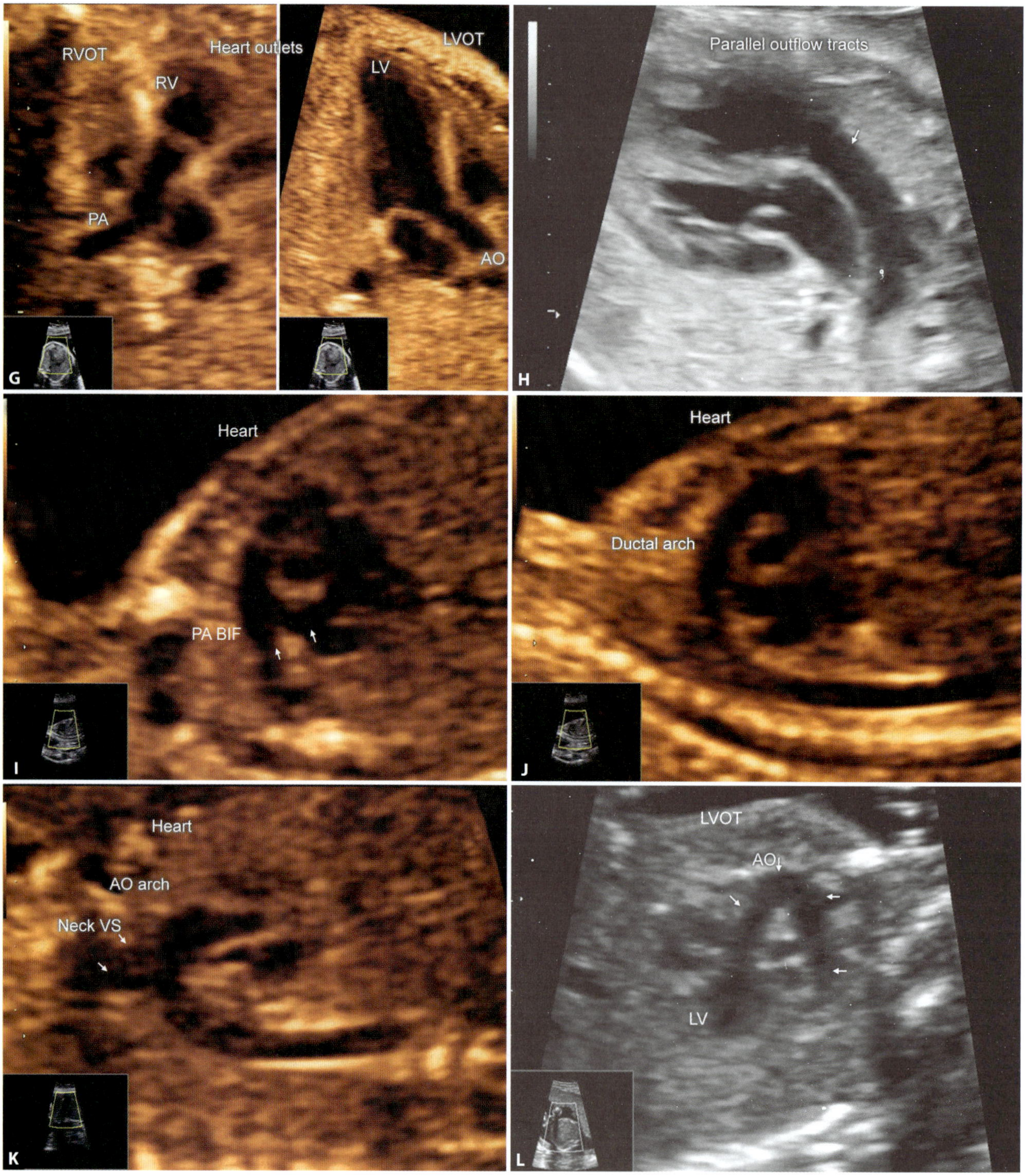

Figs 17.7G to L (G) Right ventricular outflow tract is contiguous with pulmonary artery which is seen bifurcating into two branches. The left ventricular outflow tract is contiguous with aorta. Both outflow tracts are seen crossing each other; (H) Parallel outflow tracts seen and the vessel arising from left ventricle is showing bifurcation, the artery arising from right ventricle is giving rise to neck vessels, suggestive of transposition of great arteries; (I and J) Pulmonary artery bifurcation and ductal arch view; (K) Aortic arch with neck vessels seen arising from it; (L) Right-sided aortic arch

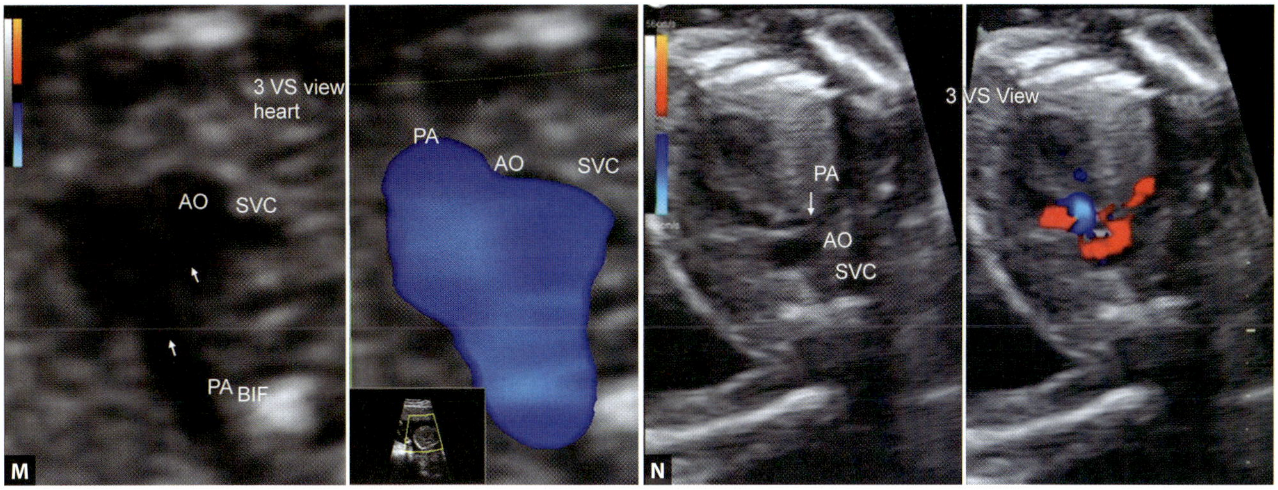

Figs 17.7M and N (M) Three vessel view and three vessel trachea view show the pulmonary artery, aorta and SVC from left to right in decreasing order of AP diameter; (N) Abnormal 3 vessel view with small pulmonary artery seen, suggestive of pulmonary stenosis in tetralogy of Fallot

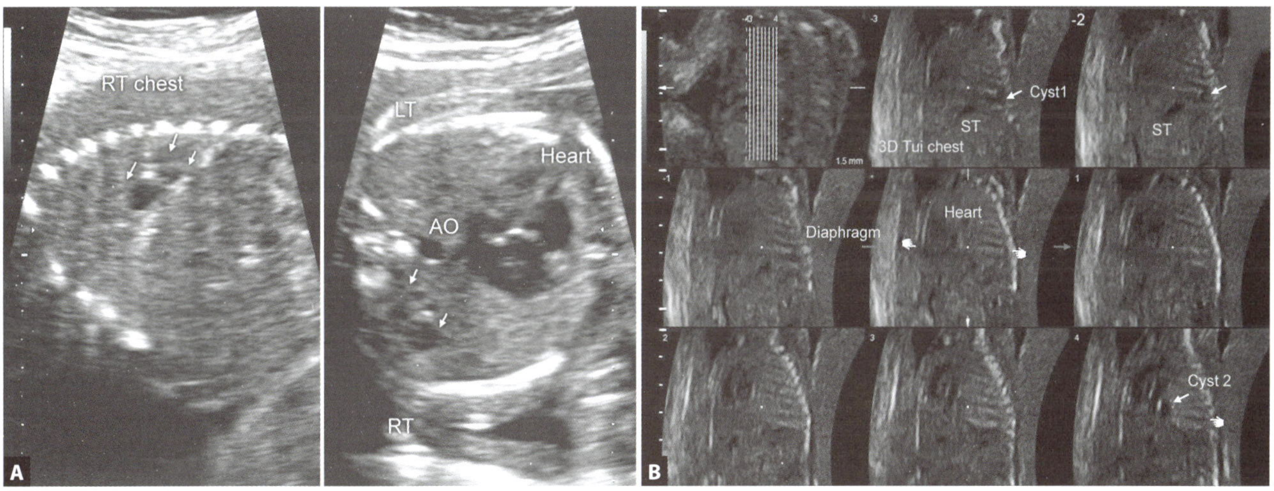

Figs 17.8A and B Lung. (A and B) shows tiny cysts in right lung base with an intact diaphragm, suggestive of cystic adenomatoid malformation

Extremities

Upper extremities including both hands and Lower extremities including both feet (Figs 17.13A to K).

Abnormalities detected: Short femur in Down's syndrome, shortening in skeletal dysplasia, bowing and fractures in osteogenesis imperfecta, arthrogryposis, talipes equinovarus deformity, syndactyly and polydactyly (Figs 17.13A to K).

Umbilical Cord

Umbilical cord insertion and number of vessels in umbilical cord. Single umbilical artery and a two-vessel cord is picked up in this view of cord insertion (Figs 17.11A and B).

Any abnormality detected on the basic examination necessitates a comprehensive and a targeted survey to seek further information on the nature of underlying abnormalities. This includes patients with an abnormal triple marker screening test, abnormal amniotic fluid volume, family history of a syndrome or heritable disorder. Additional components that might be included on a targeted examination are as follows:

Skull: Configuration, mineralization, contiguity.

Brain: Cerebral hemispheres, third ventricle, fourth ventricle, transcerebellar diameter.

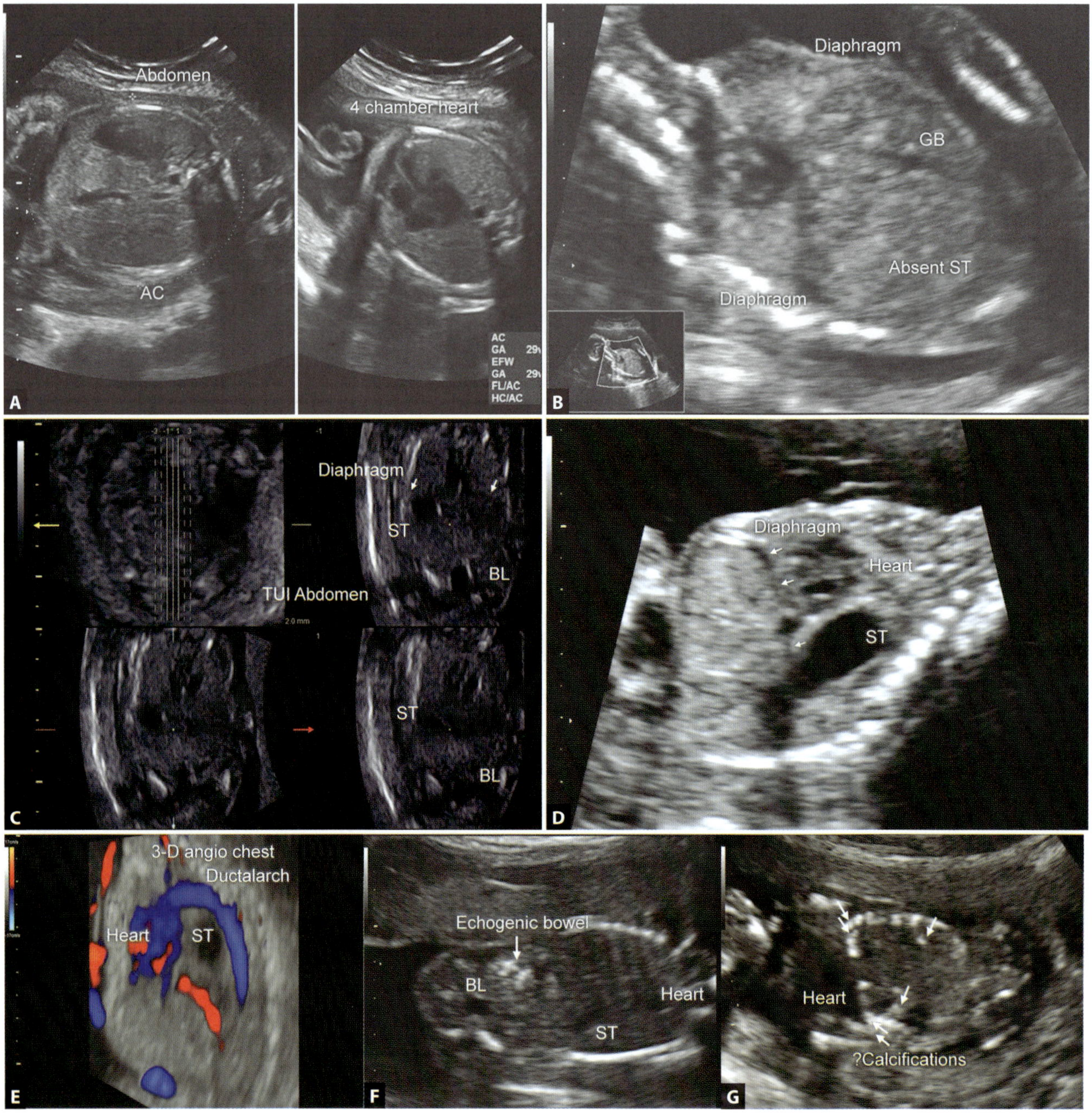

Figs 17.9A to G Abdomen. (A) Abdominal circumference taken at level where umbilical vein joins the portal vein in axial plane, for evaluation of situs as well; (B) Failure to visualize stomach indicates tracheoesophageal fistula; (C) Three-dimensional tomographic imaging of abdomen showing intact diaphragm separating chest and abdomen. Stomach and bladder are seen in abdomen; (D) Stomach is seen in chest, posterior to the heart, suggestive of congenital diaphragmatic hernia; (E) Three-dimensional color Doppler is useful in better visualization of pathology; (F) Echogenic bowel loops in abdomen, is a marker for chromosomal abnormalities but can be seen in cystic fibrosis and meconium peritonitis; (G) Calcifications in liver, commonly seen in TORCH infections

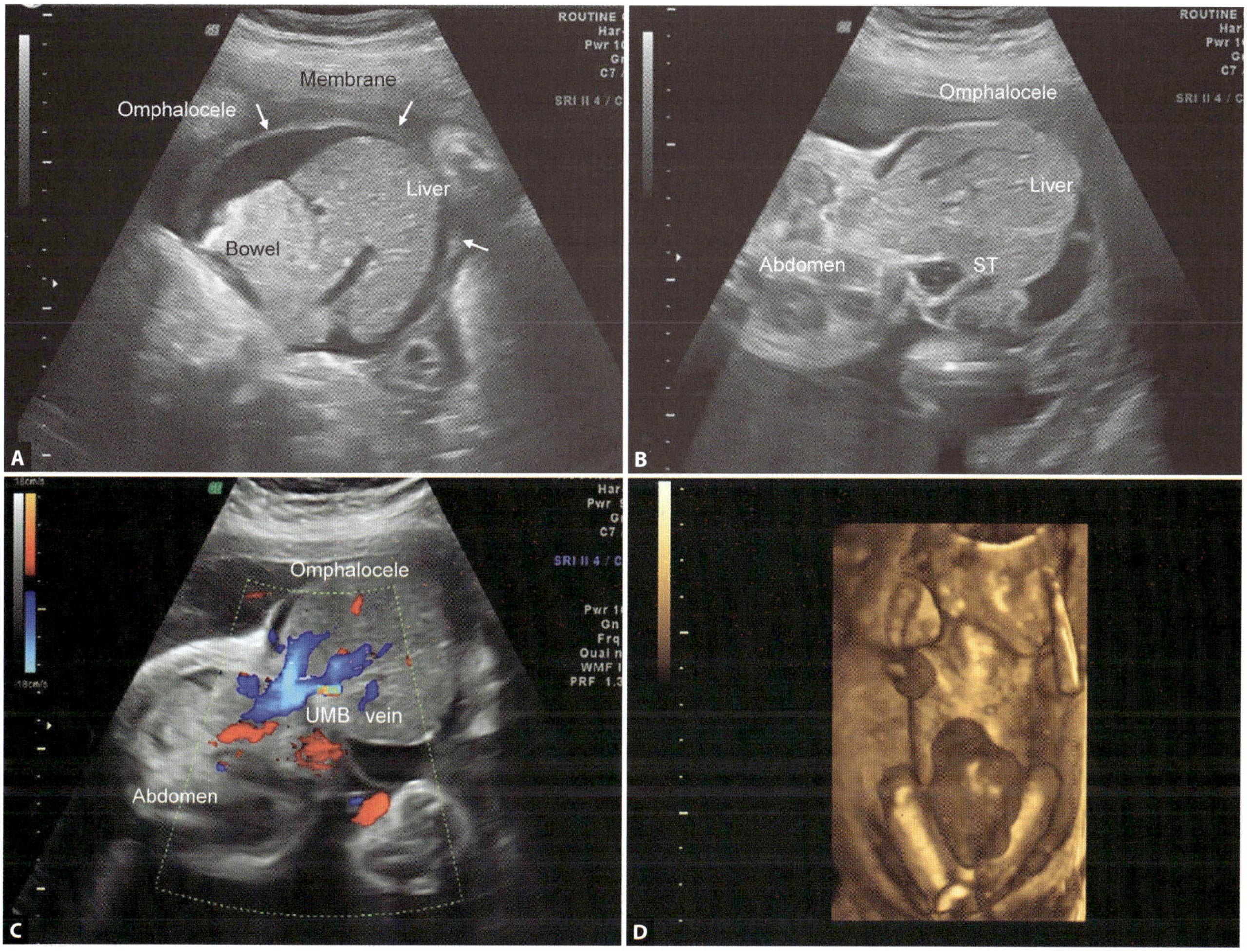

Figs 17.10A to D Ventral wall abnormality—omphalocele with liver within it. (A to C) Defect in the anterior abdominal wall with liver and stomach seen outside the abdomen suggestive of omphalocele; (D) Three-dimensional visualization of the defect

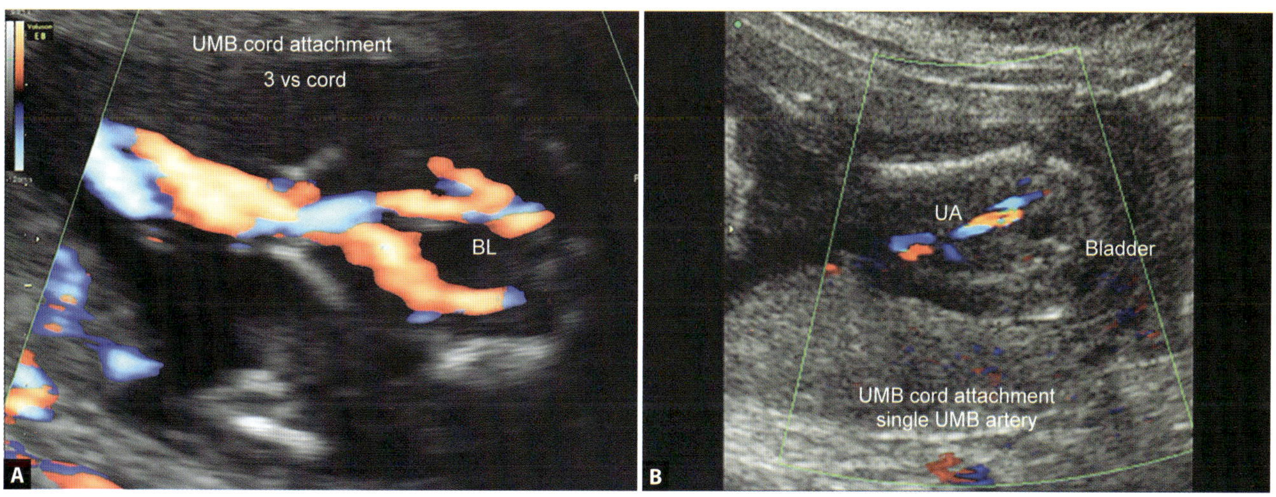

Figs 17.11A and B Umbilical cord attachment. (A) Normal umbilical cord insertion shows two arteries and one vein (3 vessel cord); (B) Single umbilical artery (SUA)/2 vessel cord may be associated with IUGR also is a marker for chromosomal abnormalities

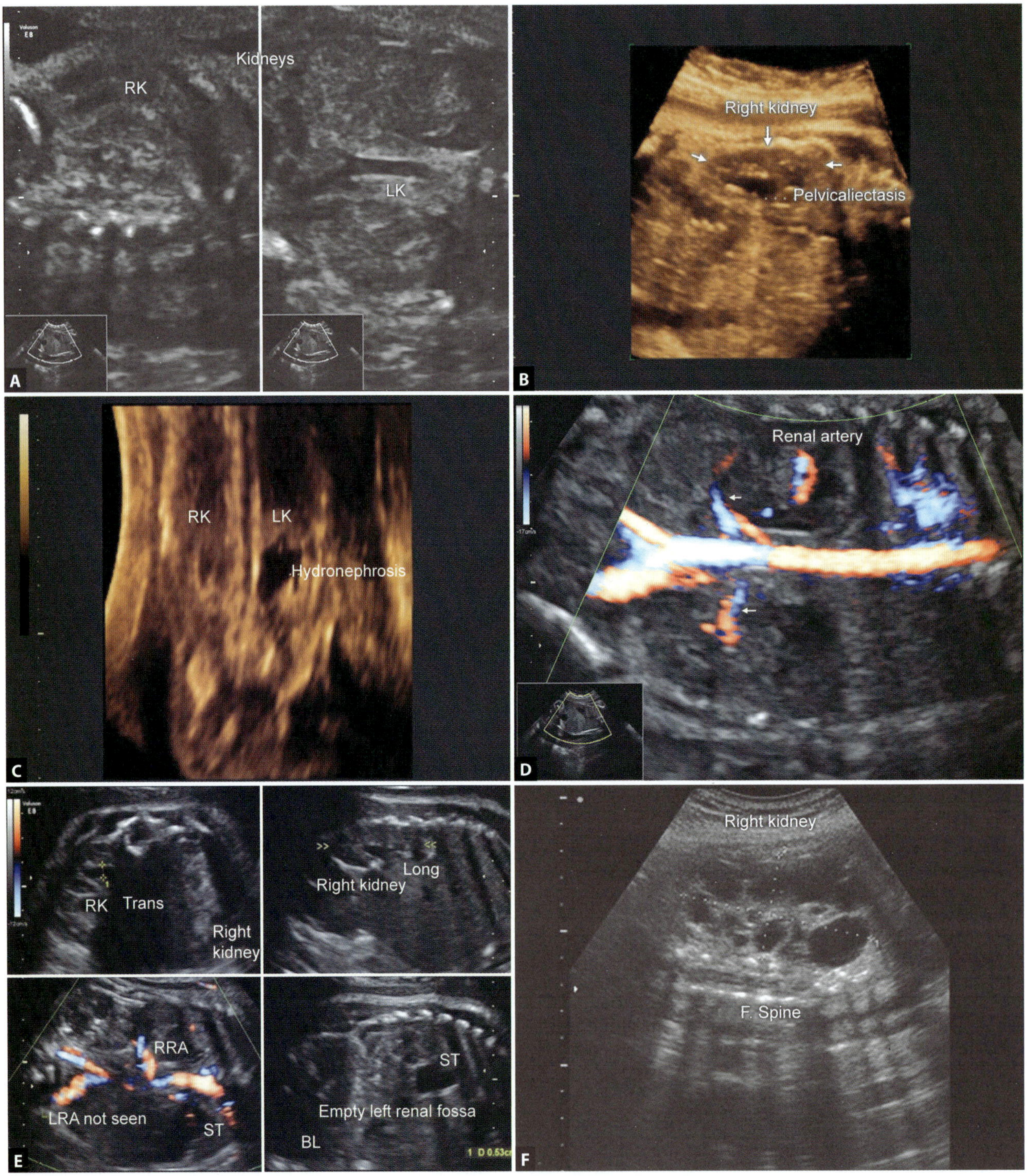

Figs 17.12A to F Kidneys. (A) Kidneys are seen as paraspinal hypoechoic structures with echogenic central sinus and minimal fluid; (B and C) pyelectasis and hydronephrosis; width of renal pelvis in axial view (more than 7 mm is significant and needs further evaluation after birth); (D) Both renal arteries arising from aorta on color Doppler examination of abdomen; (E) Failure of visualization of renal artery raises doubt of dysplastic/absent kidney; (F) Multicystic dysplastic kidney

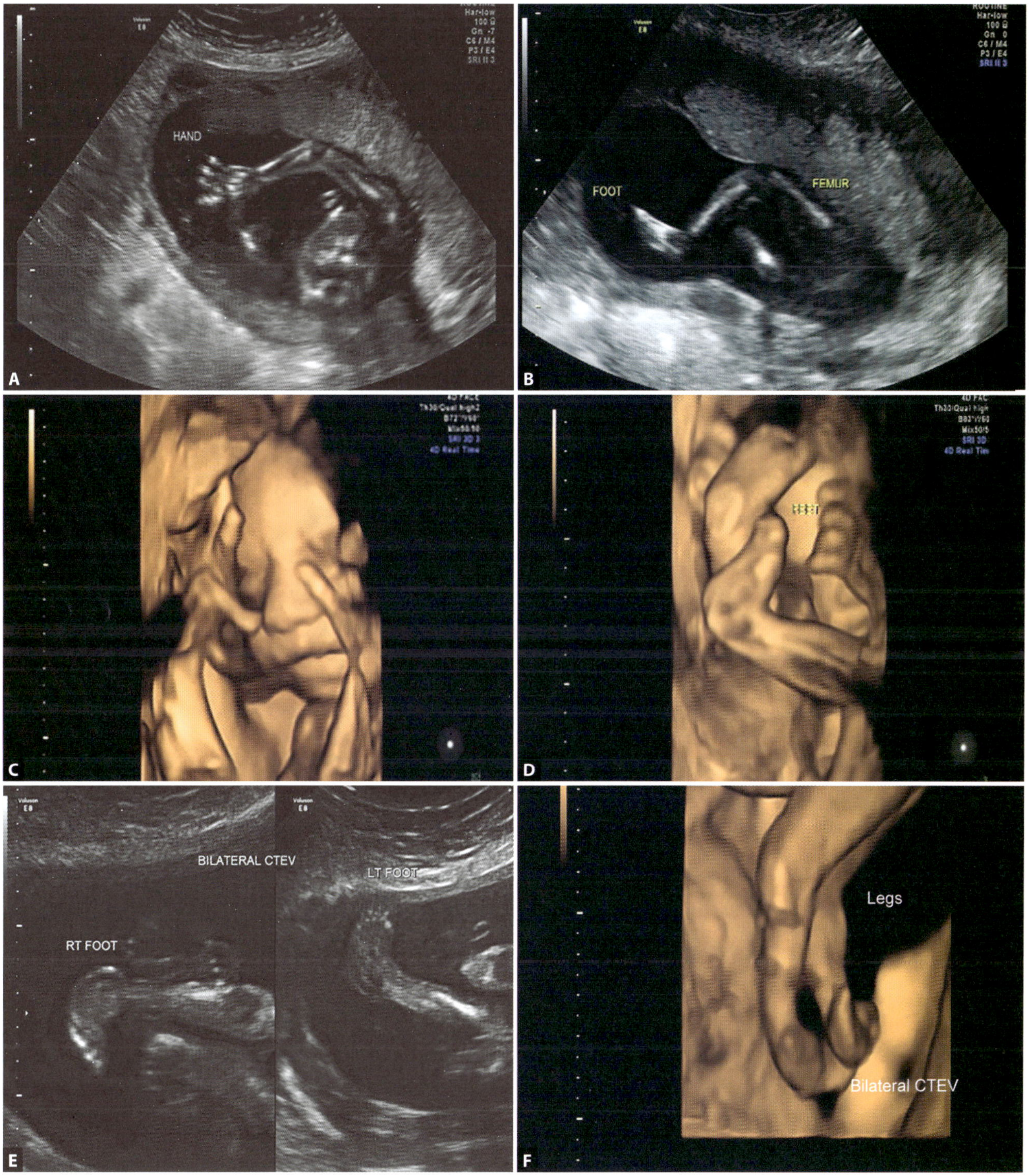

Figs 17.13A to F Extremities. (A to D) Normal hands and legs in 2D and 3D; (E and F) Medial deviation of both feet which are seen in the same plane as tibia-fibula, suggestive of congenital talipus equinovarus deformity (CTEV), in 2D and 3D. Association with trisomies 13 and 18 is known

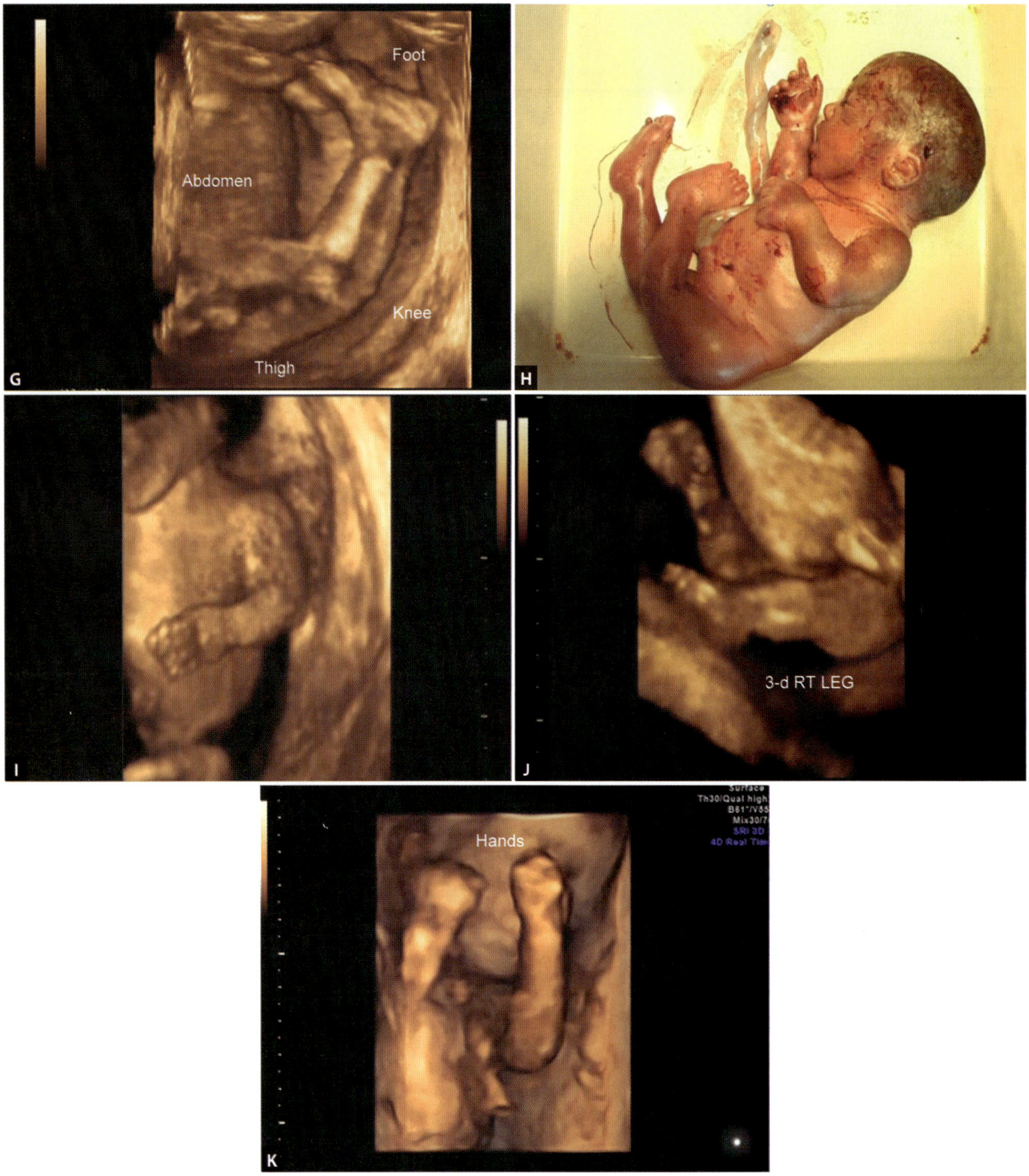

Figs 17.13G to K (G and H) Abnormal and rigid position of legs seen in arthrogyposis/fetal akinesia sequence (3D imaging and subsequent post-termination fetus image); (I and J) Short limb skeletal dysplasia mostly lethal form of thanatophoric type of dwarfism; (K) Persistently seen clenched fists as seen in a case of trisomy 18

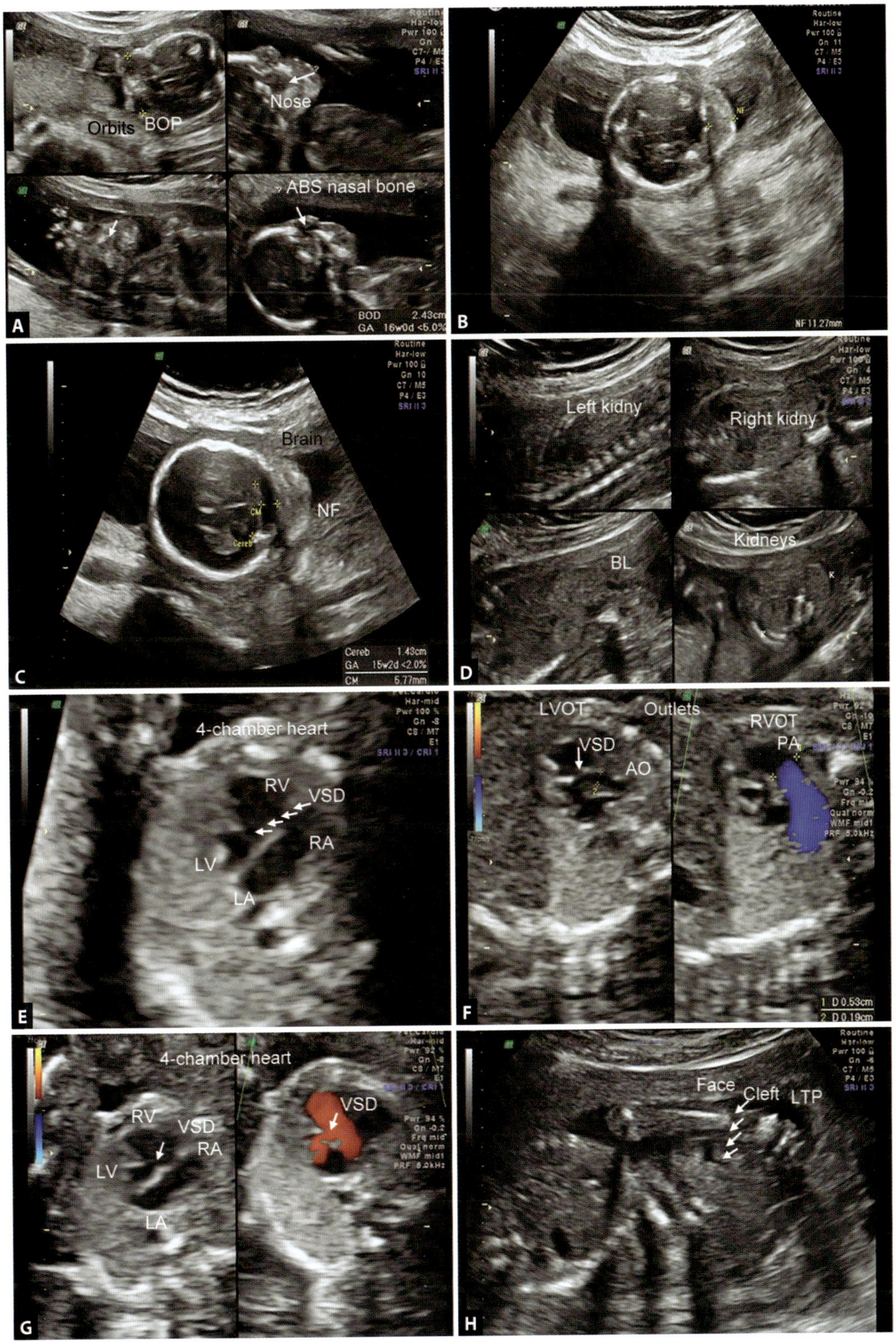

Figs 17.14A to H Multiple abnormalities seen during a routine anomaly scan. Fetal karyotyping confirmed this to be trisomy 13

Face: Nasal bridge, oral cavity/tongue, ears, outer orbital diameter.

Neck: Soft tissues and external contours.

Thorax: Configuration of bony thorax.

Heart: Orthogonal views of four-chamber heart, dynamic views of atrioventricular valves and atrioventricular septa.

Abdominal cavity/bowel/liver/spleen: Any mass or calcification, dilatation.

Long bone lengths: Severity and distribution of shortening, clavicles.

Extremities: Exhaustive survey for limb reductions, malalignment, demineralization, extra digits, deformations.

A CASE STUDY OF MULTIPLE ABNORMALITIES

A 26-year-old female came for routine anomaly scan which showed multisystemic abnormalities as follows (Figs 17.14A to H):

- *Symmetric IUGR:* Fetal growth parameters were 2 weeks less as compared to period of amenorrhea.
- *Brain:* Brachycephaly with strawberry-shaped skull seen. Cerebellar hemispheres are small with a prominent cisterna magna and cavum septum pellucidum (CSP) is not well seen, suggestive of Dandy-Walker variant with? partial agenesis of corpus callosum.
- Markedly thickened nuchal fold seen measuring 11 mm (less than 6 mm is normal).
- *Facial abnormalities:* Absent nasal bone, large midline cleft lip/palate with hypotelorism.
- *Cardiac abnormalities:* Hypoplastic left heart with a large ventricular septal defect (VSD), large pulmonary artery and over-riding of aorta over VSD noted.
- *Renal anomaly:* Bilateral enlarged and echogenic kidneys with tiny cysts, suggestive of ?Dysplastic kidneys with mild oligohydramnios.

CONCLUSION

A systematically performed second trimester anomaly scan and a meticulous targeted or a genetic sonogram can enable us to detect many congenital anomalies as well as fetal aneuploidies, which can give reassurance to the pregnant woman, especially the woman with high risk and has a huge impact on further management of the pregnancy. With the emergence of 1st trimester screening (ultrasound and dual marker), this can give additional information which can be incorporated in the second trimester anomaly scan to give individualized risks for Down's syndrome and better selection of patients for invasive diagnostic testing.

REFERENCES

1. Grandjean H, et al. The performance of routine ultrasonographic screening of pregnancies in the Euro – fetus Study. Am J Obstet Gynecol. 1999;181(2):446-54.
2. David Nyberg, et al. Diagnostic Imaging of Fetal Anomalies; Normal Fetal Anatomic Survey. Lippincott Williams & Wilkins. 2003.
3. Guidelines for Performance of the Antepartum Obstetrical Ultrasound Examination. American Institute of Ultrasound in Medicine, Laurel, Maryland, 1994.
4. Yeo L, Vintzileos AM. The second trimester genetic sonogram. In: Callen, 5th edn. 2008.
5. Stoll C, Dott B, Alembik Y, Roth MP. Evaluation of routine prenatal ultrasound examination in detecting fetal chromosomal abnormalities in low risk population. Hum Genet. 1993;91:37-41.
6. Borenstein M, Minekawa R, Zidere V, Nicolaides K, Allan LD. Aberrant right Subclavian artery at 16 to 23^{+6} weeks of gestation: a marker for chromosomal abnormality. Ultrasound Obstet Gynecol. 2010;36:548-52.
7. Vintzileos AM, Egan JF. Adjusting the risk for trisomy 21 on the basis of second trimester ultrasonography. Am J Obst Gynecol. 1995;172:837.
8. Nyberg DA, Kramer D, Resta RG, et al. Prenatal sonographic findings in of trisomy 18: Review of 4 cases. J Ultrasound Med. 1993;2:103.
9. Lehman CD, Nyberg DA, Winter TC, et al. Trisomy 13 syndrome: Prenatal ultrasound findings in a review of 33 cases. Radiology. 1995;194:217.
10. Bowerman RA. Atlas of Normal Fetal Ultrasonographic Anatomy. Chicago: Year Book Medical Publishers, 1992.

CHAPTER

18

Fetal Growth Restriction

Shantala Vadeyar

Fetal growth restriction (FGR) or earlier called intrauterine growth retardation (IUGR) is defined reduced growth of the fetus *in utero*. Fetal growth is a culmination of a variety of factors—its own genetic growth potential, fetal health, maternal nutrition and placental transfer of these nutrients to the fetus. Hence, a number of reasons that will affect these four factors can result in reduced fetal growth. Table 18.1 outlines various etiological factors in fetal growth restriction.[1]

DEFINITIONS

Small for Gestational Age

This term was used by neonatologists to describe babies/neonates with a birth weight less than 10th percentile for their gestational age. This differentiates neonates that are small because they are born early (preterm), as previously a cut-off of 2.5 kg was universally used as a definition of a "small" baby.

However, small for gestational age (SGA) newborns could be "constitutionally small" due to ethnicity, parental characteristics, altitude, etc., so they may be "small but healthy". On the other hand, SGA newborns could be small because they were unable to reach their growth potential due to uterine, maternal or placental factors that reduced their "nutrition" *in utero*. These form the group that is "growth restricted".

Fetal Growth Restriction

The fetuses that had reduced growth *in utero* were called as IUGR (intrauterine growth retardation). These were diagnosed by ultrasound as fetuses whose estimated weight was less than 10th percentile for that gestational age. However, the term IUGR has now been changed to fetal growth restriction (FGR) although some of the fetuses could be small due to a reduced growth potential (genetic syndromes or chromosomal abnormalities) and hence, strictly not "growth restricted".

However, in general, the terms FGR are used for *in utero* diagnosis of a less than 10th centile fetus, whilst SGA is used for a less than 10th centile newborn.

Classification of Fetal Growth Restriction

FGR was also classified as Types I and II.

Type I FGR or symmetric IUGR was denoted for fetuses who had a small head circumference (HC) and abdomen circumference (AC) and often, also small femur length (FL), hence the ratio of H/A and F/A ratios were normal.

Type II FGR or asymmetric IUGR was denoted when the fetus has a smaller AC compared to the HC and the FL, hence the H/A and F/A ratios are higher than normal.

Type III FGR denotes fetuses that were initially symmetrically small but later became asymmetric.

Table 18.1 Etiological factors in fetal growth restriction

Fetal factors	Maternal factors	Placental factors	Uterine factors
Chromosomal abnormalities	Cardiorespiratory disease	Poor vascularization, thrombosis, infarction	Reduced uteroplacental blood flow
Genetic syndromes IEM	Renal disease, pre-eclampsia, DM	Deciduitis	Atherosclerosis of decidual spiral arteries
Infection	Anemia, fever	Abruption placentae	Large multiple fibroids
Congenital anomalies	Drugs (DES, anticancer drugs)	Placental cysts, chorioangioma	Uterine morphological anomalies
Skeletal dysplasias	Smoking, alcohol, drug abuse	Placentitis, vasculitis, edema	Fibromyoma
Cardiac anomalies	Connective tissue disorders	Placenta previa	
Multiple gestation	Chronic hypertension		

The difficulty with this classification is that it does not offer clarity on the etiopathogenesis and hence, the management. Both type I and type II can have normal as well as pathologic types of growth abnormalities.

PLACENTAL INSUFFICIENCY AS A CAUSE OF FETAL GROWTH RESTRICTION

Normal Placentation

Trophoblastic villi from the pregnancy invade the decidua and also the spiral arteries in the myometrium, destroying the elastic and muscular layers and replacing them with fibrinoid material. This invasion of the spiral arteries is completed by 16 weeks, but in many cases the changes may continue till 22 weeks. Thus, the vessels get transformed into sinusoids that accommodate the increased uteroplacental flow and facilitate nutrient and oxygen transfer to the fetus. The transformed arteries are also not affected by maternal vasoregulatory mechanisms.

Abnormal Placentation

Trophoblastic invasion is largely confined to the decidual layer with absent or incomplete invasion of the myometrial portion of the spiral arteries. Thus, the vascular resistance within these vessels persists and there is lesser blood flowing in the intervillous space. This will reduce the nutrient and oxygen transfer to the fetus. These vessels with intact muscle layer will also remain responsive to vasoactive hormones or substances in the mother's blood, thus predisposing to hypertension. This accounts for the overlap between fetal growth restriction and hypertensive disorders of pregnancy (pre-eclampsia, eclampsia, HELLP, etc).

Placental Thrombosis and Fetal Growth Restriction

Thrombosis in the spiral arteries or intervillous spaces results in poor perfusion and placental infarcts. This in turn, reduces the number of functioning villi and reduces the delivery of oxygen and nutrients to the fetus. Hypercoagulation in the maternal circulation could be the result of congenital or acquired thrombophilias. Congenital thrombophilias include deficiency of protein C, protein S or antithrombin III, factor V Leiden mutation, methylenetetrahydrofolate reductase (MTHFR) mutation and prothrombin 20210A mutation. Antiphospholipid syndrome is the most common acquired thrombophilia and a common cause of placental insufficiency.

The placenta in these cases often shows perivillous fibrin deposition so that the villi within such deposits are non-functional. Some cases show massive infarcts and these again will reduce transfer of oxygen and nutrients to the fetus.

Placentae in multiple pregnancies often show differences in the two placentae, with abnormal placentation in one and not the other. This accounts for discordant growth.

FETAL AND NEONATAL COMPLICATIONS OF FETAL GROWTH RESTRICTION

There are numerous complications of fetal growth restriction as detailed below. Timely delivery would reduce these complications and improve outcomes.

Fetal Hypoxia: Acidosis

Due to poor nutritional support from the placenta, prenatal and intrapartum hypoxia is commonly encountered in FGR fetuses. Early diagnosis and surveillance helps to monitor these fetuses and plan timely delivery. FHR recordings will detect hypoxia by the presence of late or atypical variable decelerations with reduced baseline variability.

Intrauterine Death

Severe FGR can result in fetal death *in utero* or during labor as a consequence of severe hypoxia and acidosis. Timely delivery, often by cesarean section, can prevent this event.

Oligoamnios

Fetal hypoxia results in increased blood supply to the fetal brain and reduced blood supply to organs like the kidney and gut. This results in reduced fetal urine production and oligoamnios.

Respiratory Distress Syndrome

Preterm FGR infants are more likely to suffer RDS than the appropriately grown infants.[2] This is contrary to the previous general thinking that the FGR fetuses are "stressed *in utero*" and this accelerated their lung maturation. It is possible that lungs of preterm FGR infants are also more susceptible to damage due to intrauterine hypoxia and ischemia.

Meconium Aspiration Syndrome

The passage of meconium is seen in fetal hypoxia as happens in growth restriction. This meconium combined with oligoamnios is the major cause of meconium aspiration syndrome, which can lead to considerable neonatal morbidity. Amnioinfusion has been proposed as a method to prevent this, but clinical trials have failed to demonstrate benefit.[3]

Persistent Fetal Circulation

Persistent patent ductus arteriosus is seen as a consequence of intrauterine and intrapartum hypoxia. This usually settles once the extrauterine environment improves for the infant.

Intraventricular Hemorrhage and Periventricular Leukomalacia

Grade III and IV intraventricular hemorrhage (IVH) and periventricular leukomalacia (PVL) are more common in preterm FGR infants than AGA infants.[4] The incidence can be reduced by the use of antenatal steroids. More recent studies have shown a great benefit of the use of magnesium sulfate in the reduction of IVH in preterm infants.[5]

Neonatal Encephalopathy

Neonatal seizures, irritability, apnea, twitching, etc. may be seen after perinatal asphyxia, especially related to FGR.

Hypoglycemia

Intrauterine restriction of nutrients necessitates the use of glycogen stores in the liver by the fetus, thus leaving the FGR neonate extremely susceptible to hypoglycemia. Early feeding is advised, though in severe FGR cases, the reduced blood supply to the gut also increases the risk of necrotizing enterocolitis, hence intravenous total parenteral nutrition is used until the neonate is a few days old.

Hypocalcemia

There is a very high incidence of hypocalcemia which presents with twitching, jitteriness and apnea. All preterm FGR neonates will need calcium supplementation.

Hypothermia

There is a very high-risk of hypothermia due to a reduction in the subcutaneous fat stored in the FGR neonate.

Long-term Poor Growth

Many preterm FGR infants and children continue to exhibit poor long-term growth with or without developmental and neurological sequelae. Some FGR infants do exhibit "catch-up" growth and reach their growth potential within 6–12 months of age. It is possible that if the FGR is early in onset, the risk of poor postnatal growth is higher than if the FGR is of late onset type.

Cerebral Palsy

Preterm FGR infants are at a high-risk of cerebral palsy as reflected by delayed neurological and cognitive development. Minor dysfunction by means of decreased attention span, learning difficulties and poor coordination are also seen in FGR infants and children.

IDENTIFICATION OF FETUSES AT RISK OF FETAL GROWTH RESTRICTION

History

All the factors listed in Table 18.1 are at high-risk. These should be counseled and prophylactic low dose aspirin (75–150 mg/day) should be administered from the first trimester. Serial growth scans with Doppler assessment would be indicated for early diagnosis of FGR.

First Trimester PAPP-A, Free Beta-hCG

A low pregnancy-assisted plasma protein A (PAPP-A) and high free beta-hCG level at the first trimester screening test signifies a high-risk of FGR.[6] If the chromosomal testing is normal (as these values would also likely constitute a high-risk chromosomal abnormality screening result), these mothers could be started on low dose aspirin and serial follow-up with growth scans.

Uterine Artery Doppler

Uterine artery Doppler studies could be used as a screening tool in the first and early second trimester. Increased resistance (>95th centile) in this vessel could be an indicator of FGR to follow. It also has a very good negative predictive value (97–99%), so a low resistance in the uterine artery has a very high probability that FGR will not develop in that pregnancy.

DIAGNOSIS OF FETAL GROWTH RESTRICTION

Accurate Dating of the Pregnancy

This is vital as any diagnosis of the lag/reduction in growth is based on the exact determination of gestational age. Accurate dating should be done in the first or early second trimester and once the dates have been fixed, there should be no change or "redating" done with every subsequent scan.

First Trimester Screening

The determination of PAPP-A and free beta-hCG will be helpful in the prediction of FGR. A low PAPP-A and high free beta-hCG are both predictive of FGR.[7] Indeed, if the PAPP-A is lower than 0.3 MoMs, low dose aspirin may be commenced as a preventative strategy to improve placentation. There is evidence to show that low dose aspirin started before 16 weeks of gestation is more effective in reducing or preventing the onset of FGR than when it is started after 16 weeks of gestational age.

A high NT combined with a smallish CRL (as compared to dates), low PAPP-A and low free beta-hCG may point towards trisomy 18.

Determination of Normal Anatomy

Anomaly screening at 18–20 weeks is vital and demonstration of a normal anatomy excluded genetic causes of FGR. On the other hand, multiple soft markers with a small fetus point towards a genetic syndrome.

Serial Growth Scans with Doppler and Amniotic Fluid Index

Growth restriction is diagnosed on serial scan plotted on a growth chart. This is an important method of assessing "growth trajectory" as this is more important than mere determination of "size". Estimation of the amniotic fluid index (AFI) and assessment of the umbilical and middle cerebral artery (MCA) Doppler is crucial in the diagnosis of FGR.

Thus, a fetus that has had accurate dating, normal screening and anatomy scans, is growing along a centile which may be less than the 50th centile, has normal AFI and umbilical a Doppler, is a "constitutionally small" fetus. Whereas, another fetus that shows a falling growth trajectory with oligoamnios and raised resistance ratios in the umbilical artery with reduced resistance in the MCA circulation has pathological FGR.

BIOPHYSICAL PROFILE SCORE

This was described by manning as a means of assessing fetal health. The fetal tone, movements, breathing movements, AFI and NST (nonstress test) are used in combination to generate a score out of 10. However, since the assessment of fetal tone and breathing may take almost 30 minutes in some cases, this test may take too long in practice. Hence, a modified biophysical profile score (BPS) has been proposed, in which, only the fetal movements with AFI and NST are used.

MANAGEMENT

The crux of the management is dependent on optimal maternal and fetal surveillance with timely delivery so as to reduce prematurity but also avoid *in utero* compromise of the fetus. A balance between all these factors forms the key to good decisions and optimal outcome.

TIMING OF DELIVERY

Maternal monitoring by means of BP control in HDP (hypertensive disorders of pregnancy), renal, liver function tests, coagulation profile, glycemic control in diabetics, etc. is vital. Maternal destabilization is the first important pointer towards deciding the timing of the delivery.

Fetal surveillance by means of serial ultrasound is vital. The parameters for fetal surveillance are discussed turther under different headings.

Fetal Growth

The biometry should be plotted on charts, which would help in an understanding of the growth trajectory, not just the size.

Amniotic Fluid Index and Biophysical Profile Score

Doppler Assessments

Umbilical artery Doppler is the first and most basic of the Doppler assessments in FGR. Initially, there may be a raised PI, followed by intermittent absent end-diastolic flow, followed by reverse end-diastolic flow. The middle cerebral artery (MCA) shows reduced resistance, increased flow patterns. Also, the PSVs may show a low velocity indicative of polycythemia, which is reactive to hypoxia. The Ductus venosus Doppler is helpful in aiding the timing of delivery in very preterm FGR. Thus, when the "a" wave is reverse or absent, it indicates a worse prognosis. The waveforms in the various vessels in FGR and their progression for aiding timing of delivery are shown in Figures 18.1 to 18.11.

Fetal Heart Rate Monitoring

The NST (nonstress test) or a recording of the fetal heart rate (FHR) is a way of determining fetal health. It is a sensitive indicator of fetal hypoxia and acidosis, but lacks specificity. There are some important parameters to be assessed in the FHR recording.

The baseline variability (BLV) is the most sensitive indicator of fetal brain hypoxia. The BLV is determined by the intact autonomous nervous system of the fetal brain. Any hypoxia immediately affects this control of the FHR and this reflects as a reduced BLV.

TREATMENT OF FETAL GROWTH RESTRICTION

There are no evidence-based effective therapeutic interventions for FGR. Most therapies are empiric, but have been used by most clinicians. The best treatment remains early delivery and "feeding" the neonate *ex utero*.

Bed Rest

Increased rest in the left lateral position is considered to improve blood flows to the uterus and hence, may help in FGR. However, randomized clinical trials have failed to show any benefit of bed rest in FGR.[8]

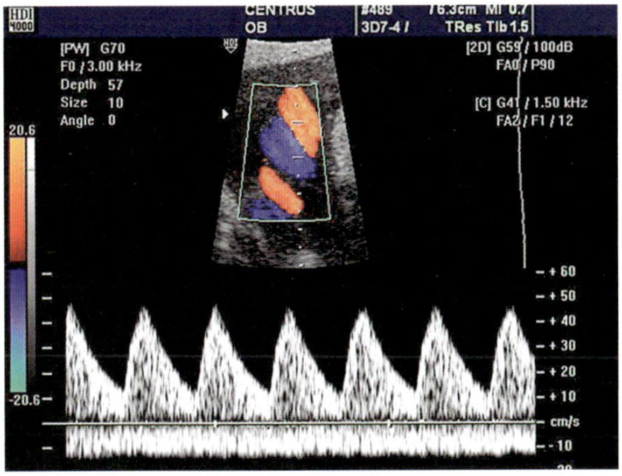

Fig. 18.1 Umbilical artery Doppler: Normal waveform in third trimester

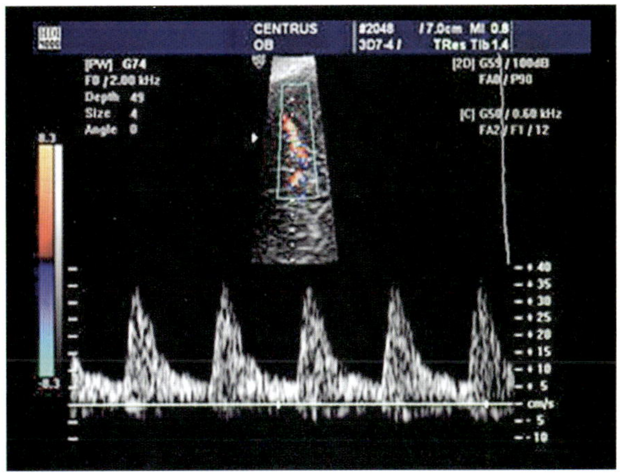

Fig. 18.2 Normal middle cerebral artery Doppler waveform

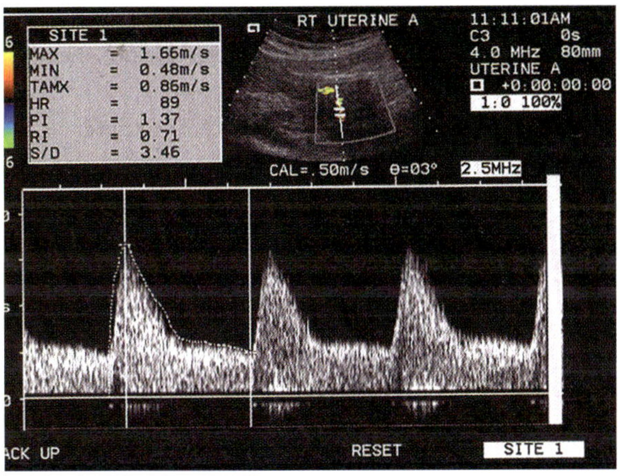

Fig. 18.3 Normal uterine artery Doppler waveform

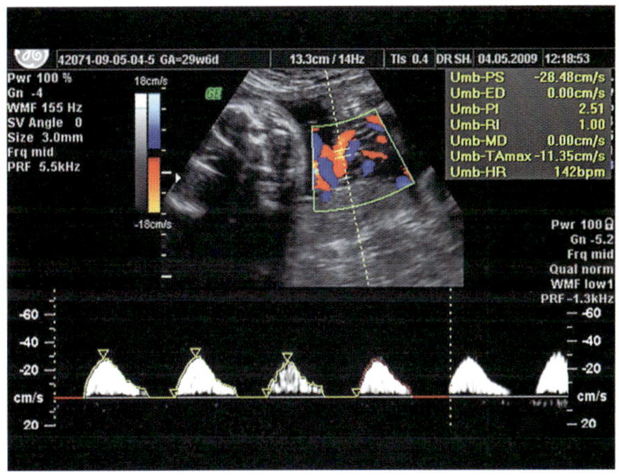

Fig. 18.4 Umbilical artery Doppler in FGR: Absent end-diastolic flow

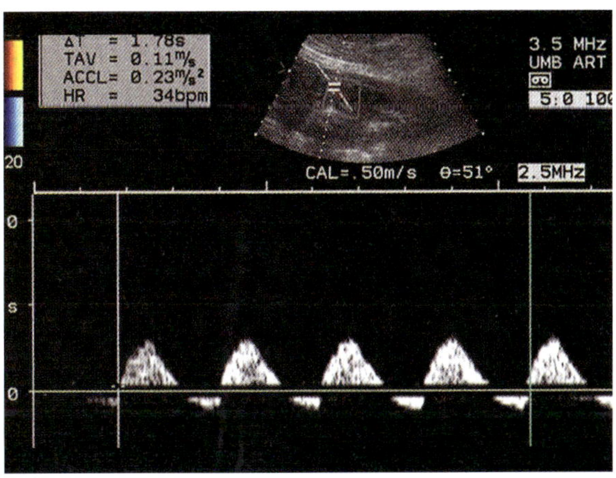

Fig. 18.5 Umbilical artery Doppler in FGR: Reverse end-diastolic flow

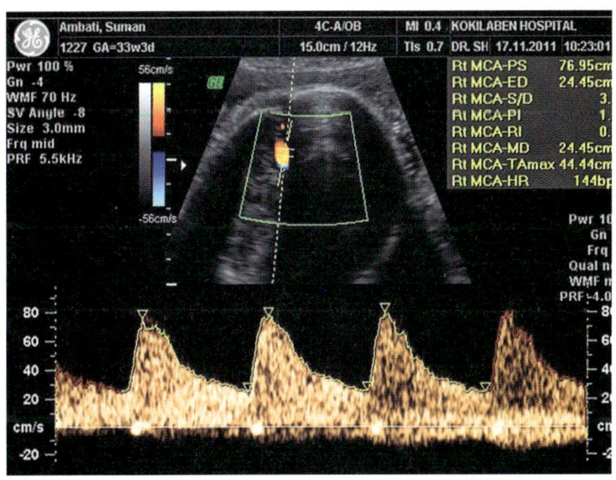

Fig. 18.6 Middle cerebral artery Doppler showing increased end-diastolic flow in fetal growth restriction (redistribution of blood flow towards the fetal brain)

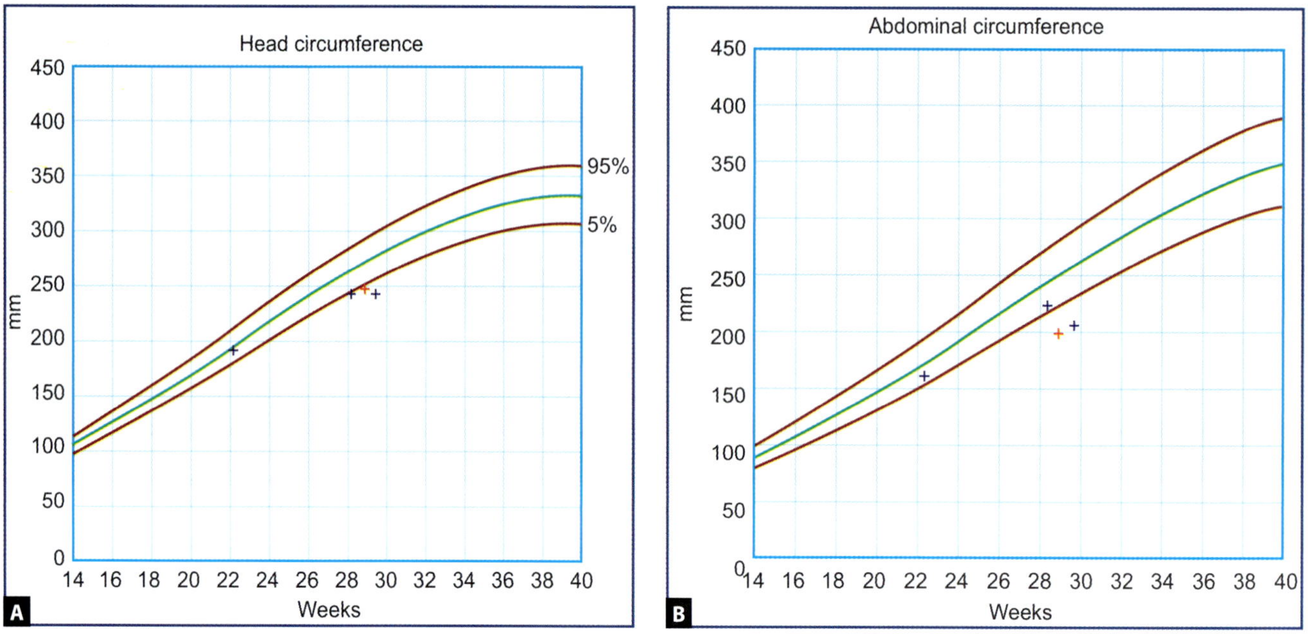

Figs 18.7A and B Fetal growth restriction: Head and abdominal circumference plots show growth below the 5th centile
Source: Snijders RJM, Nicolaides KH. Fetal biometry at 14–40 weeks gestation. Ultrasould Obstet Gynecol. 1994;4:34-48.

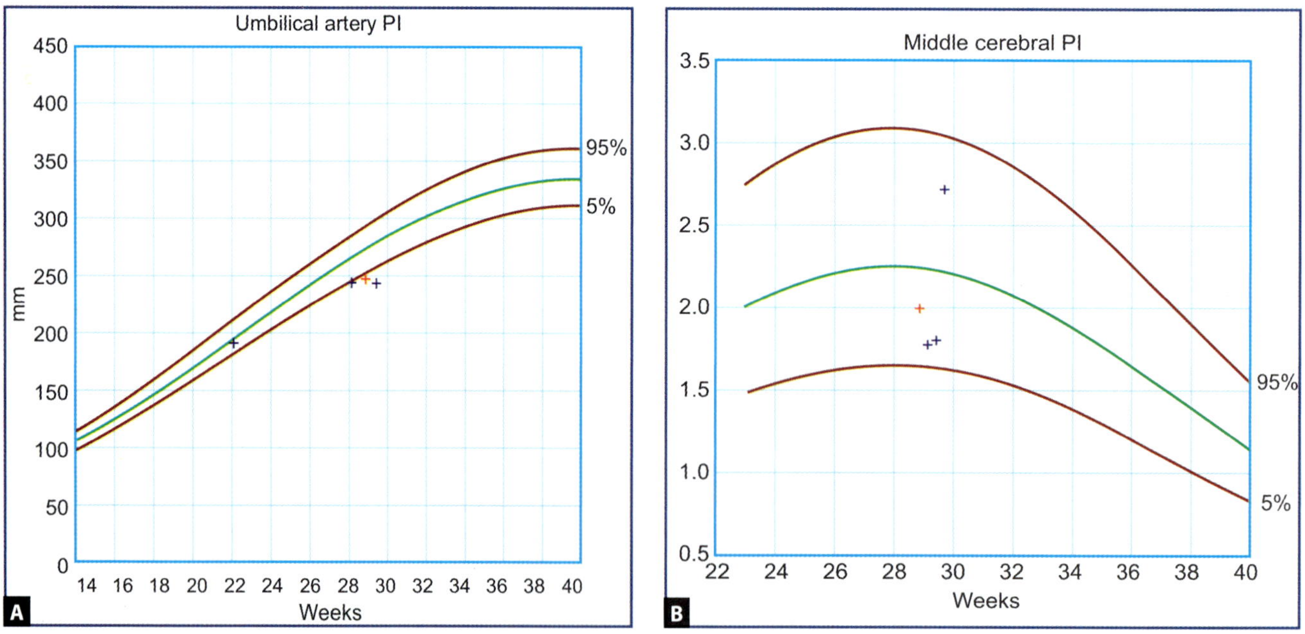

Figs 18.8A and B Fetal growth restriction: Umblical artery Doppler PI shows increased PI and MCA Doppler shows reduced PI
Source: Parra-cordero, et al. Fetal arterial and venous Doppler pulsatility index and time averaged velocity normal ranges. Prenat Diagn. 2007;27(13):1251-7.

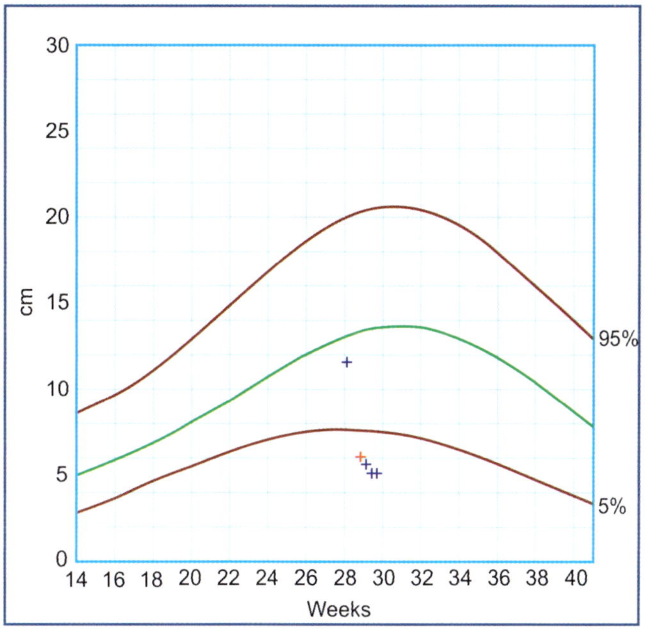

Fig. 18.9 Amniotic fluid index showing oligoamnios in fetal growth restriction (FGR)

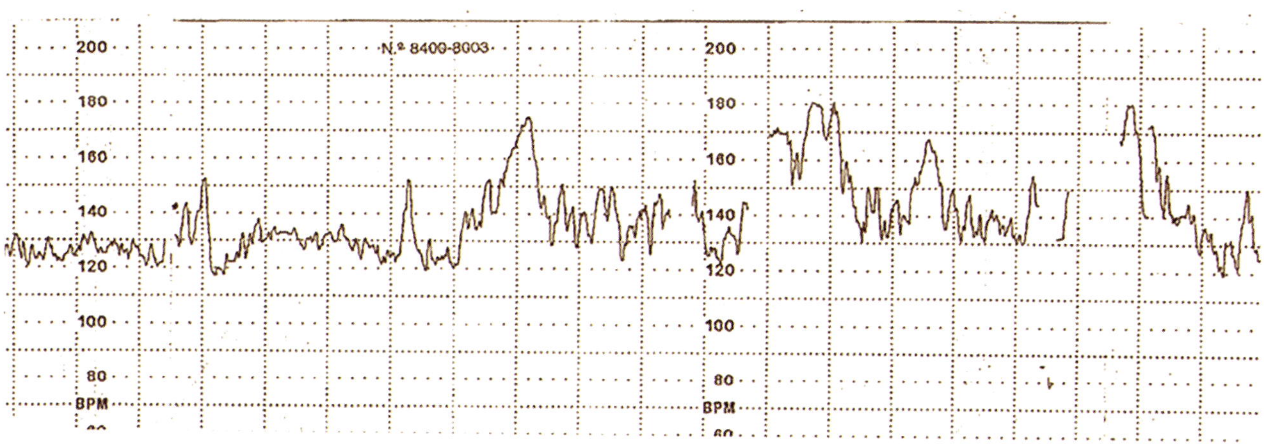

Fig. 18.10 Nonstress test in a normally oxygenated fetus showing good baseline variability and accelerations with fetal movements—Reactive nonstress test (NST)

Amino Acid Infusions

Some Indian data exists to show that IV infusion of amino acids and fluids can help to improve fetal growth in FGR.[9] The amino acid drip was given as 100 mL twice a day for 2 weeks with 5% dextrose fluids.

Oxygen Therapy

Nicolaides et al. (1987) found decreased fetal mortality in cases of severe IUGR when the mothers were given oxygen supplementation (8 L/min by face mask, continuously). No further RCTs have been conducted.[10]

Aspirin

Aspirin in low doses (1–2 mg/kg/day) inhibits the production of thromboxane A2 by the platelets and changes the thromboxane to prostacyclin ratio. This results in vasodilatation in the uteroplacental circulation, which improves placental blood flow. However, the therapy has to be started before the onset of FGR and studies have shown that aspirin therapy started before 16 weeks of gestation is more effective than that started after 16 weeks.[11]

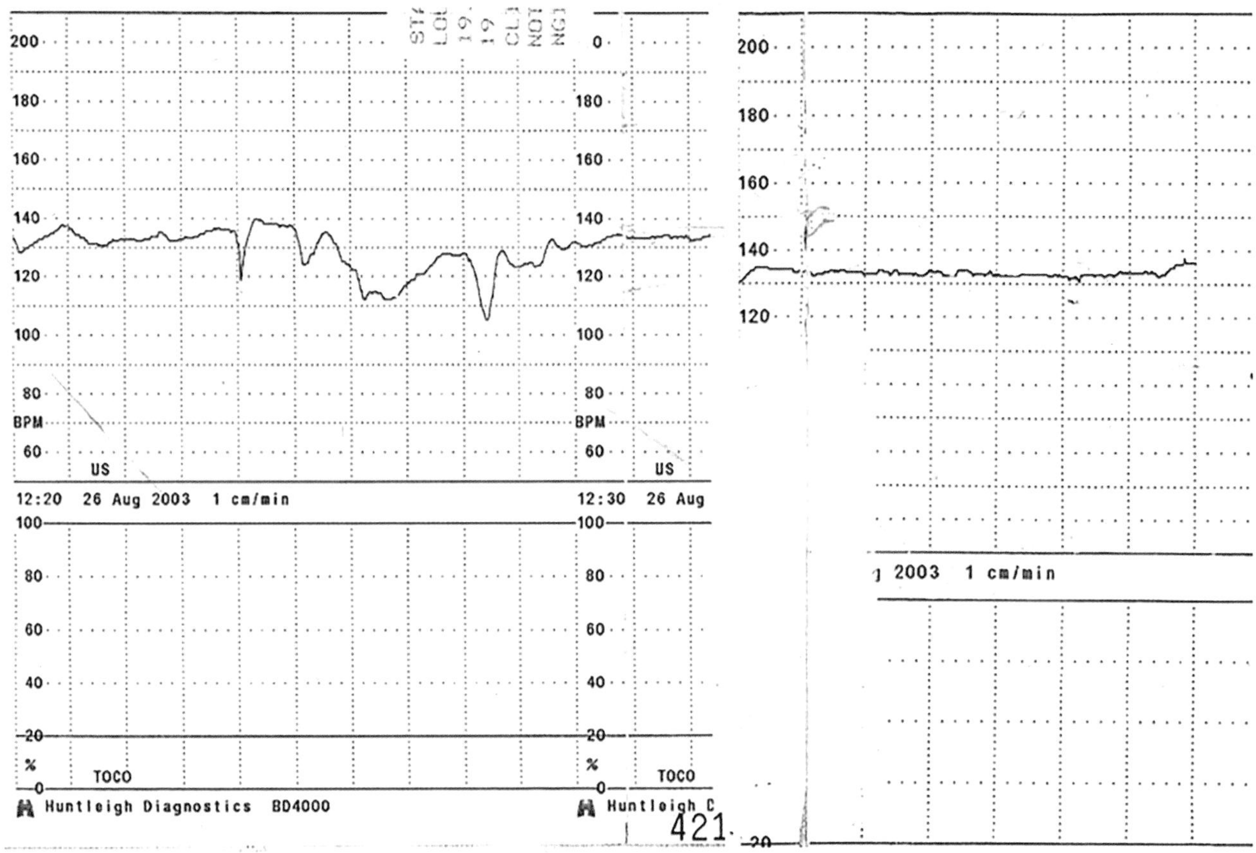

Fig. 18.11 Nonreactive NST: Very poor baseline variability and unprovoked decelerations seen in a fetus at 32 weeks with no fetal movements and severe FGR

Sildenafil Citrate Therapy

Sildenafil citrate vasodilates the myometrial arteries and helps improve blood supply to the uteroplacental unit. It can be used in the dose of 25 mg three times a day for early onset severe FGR with normal chromosomes and after excluding other genetic syndromes that cause early onset FGR.[12] More RCTs are needed as evidence to use this therapy. The STRIDER (Sildenafil therapy in dismal prognosis early-onset intrauterine growth restriction) multicenter trial is ongoing since 2014 in this regard.[13]

Hydrotherapy

Water immersion below the chest for 5–6 hours per day can help FGR and oligoamnios. The water immersion changes the hydrostatic pressures improving blood flows and this can help placental function. Improvement of the AFI has been documented, but there are no RCTs to prove this concept.

PLACE OF DELIVERY

Preterm FGR babies need to be delivered in a tertiary care set-up with excellent neonatal intensive care unit (NICU) facilities. Ideally, such an *in utero* transfer is much preferable to transporting extremely small preterm babies from a small set-up into a NICU. Also, many maternal medical conditions that lead to severe FGR, like severe pre-eclampsia, need a tertiary maternal high dependency unit (HDU) or intensive care unit (ICU) facilities as well.

MODE OF DELIVERY

Most preterm FGR babies will be delivered by cesarean section either for maternal causes (e.g. severe PET) or fetal concern for potential intrapartum asphyxia. Indeed, a fetus with minimal reserves is unable to stand the "stress" of labor and will show signs of "fetal distress". A cesarean section ensures that this stress is minimized.

LONG-TERM FOLLOW-UP

All preterm FGR babies should be followed up in a high-risk neonatal/infant OPD. In these clinics, the growth, feeding, eye check for ROP, hearing, developmental milestones and cognitive development is checked. This ensures a specialized care and improved outcomes.

TAKE HOME MESSAGES

- Screen all pregnancies for "risk factors" that might contribute or lead to FGR.
- Accurate dating is the key in the correct diagnosis of FGR.
- First trimester low PAPP-A and high free beta-hCG increase risk of FGR.
- Uterine artery screening in first and second trimesters can be used as a screening tool for FGR.
- Positive first and/or second trimester screens should initiate therapy with low dose aspirin (75–100 mg/day).
- Anomaly scans, genetic sonograms and if needed, chromosomal and infection testing should be performed in early onset FGR.
- Serial growth scans with AFI, Doppler and BPS assessments are vital in fetal surveillance.
- Maternal surveillance and management of medical conditions appropriately is also important.
- Timely delivery will improve perinatal survival and health.
- Preterm FGR babies will need a tertiary care NICU set-up and are best transferred "*in utero*" for delivery in such a set-up.
- Antenatal steroids and magnesium sulfate will improve neonatal outcomes.
- The placentae of all FGR babies should be examined carefully to determine pathology.

REFERENCES

1. Baschat A. Fetal growth disorders. In: James DK, Steer P, Weiner C, Gonik B (Eds). High-risk Pregnancy: Management Options. Elsevier, 2006.
2. Ley D, Wide-Swensson D, Lindroth M, et al. Respiratory distress syndrome in infants with impaired intrauterine growth. Acta Paediatr. 1997;85:1090-6.
3. Fraser WD, Hofmeyer J, Lede R, et al. Amnioinfusion for the prevention of meconium aspiration syndrome. N Engl J Med. 2005;353:909-17.
4. Spinillo A, Capuzzo E, Piazzi G, et al. Significance of low birth weight for gestational age among very preterm infants. Br J Obstet Gynaecol. 1997;104:668-73.
5. Heyborne K, Bowes WA. The use of antenatal magnesium sulphate for neuroprotection for infants born prematurely. F1000 Medicine Reports. 2010;2:78-89.
6. Habayeb O, Daemen A, Timmerman D, et al. The relationship between first trimester fetal growth, pregnancy-associated plasma protein A levels and birthweight. Prenat Diagn. 2010;10:1002.
7. Spencer K, Cowans NJ, Avgidou F, et al. First-trimester biochemical markers of aneuploidy and the prediction of small-for-gestational age fetuses. Ultrasound Obstet Gynecol. 2008;31(1):15-9.
8. Laurin J, Person PH. The effect of bed rest in hospital on fetal outcome in pregnancies complicated by intrauterine growth restriction. Acta Obstet Gynecol Scand. 1987;66:407-11.
9. Shivkumar PV, Tayade SA, Kumar P, et al. The role of intravenous hydration and amnio influsion in intrauterine growth restriction and oligohydramnios. Int J Biol Med Res. 2011;2(4):1078-83.
10. Nicolaides KH, Campbell S, Bradley RJ, et al. Maternal oxygen therapy for intrauterine growth retardation. Lancet. 1987;1:942-5.
11. Low dose aspirin in the prevention and treatment of intrauterine growth retardation and pregnancy-induced hypertension. Italian study of aspirin in pregnancy. Lancet. 1993;341:396-400.
12. Von Dadelszen P, Dwinell S, Magee LA, et al. Sildenafil citrate therapy for severe early-onset intrauterine growth restriction. BJOG. 2011;118:624-8.
13. Ganzevoort W, Alfirevic Z, von Dadelszen P, et al. STRIDER: sidenafit therapy in dismal prognosis early-onset intrauterine growth restriction—a protocol for a systematic review with individual participant data and aggregate data meta-analysis and trial sequential analysis. Syst Rev. 2014;3:23.

CHAPTER

19

Color Doppler in Fetal Growth Restriction

Chander Lulla

INTRODUCTION

Fetal growth restriction (FGR) is a term used to describe the fetus with a birth weight at or below the 10th percentile for gestational age and sex. The FGR fetus is a fetus that does not reach its growth potential.[1]

To facilitate normal growth in pregnancy, remarkable changes occur in the maternal, placental and fetal vasculatures.[2] When this mechanism fails, abnormal placental vascular resistance patterns develop which lead to compromise of fetal well-being with a 6–10 times higher risk of perinatal mortality, morbidity, and impaired neurodevelopment.[3]

Color Doppler is an excellent tool for repetitive, noninvasive, hemodynamic monitoring in pregnancy. Doppler has proved to be more sensitive in detecting fetal compromise early and aids in the guiding and making of decisions regarding the appropriate timing of delivery.[4,5] The Doppler patterns follow a longitudinal trend with early changes in the middle cerebral artery and umbilical artery followed by other peripheral arteries. There is seen redistribution of blood flow in growth restricted fetuses and these caution us to closely monitor the fetus and intervene before the situation becomes unsalvageable. If adequate measures are not taken at this point, venous changes appear in the severely compromised fetus. These are strong predictors of poor perinatal outcome and indicate impending irreversible damage.

Doppler reveals changes of hypoxia at least a week before the nonstress test or the biophysical profile. It has therefore become the gold standard in the management of the growth-restricted fetus.[6-8]

HEMODYNAMICS IN FETAL GROWTH RESTRICTION

Fetal growth restriction in a majority of the cases is secondary to uteroplacental insufficiency. Flow changes can be observed in both the arterial and venous system of the fetus and in the uterine arteries.

CHANGES IN THE ARTERIAL CIRCULATION

Uterine Circulation

Uterine artery Doppler correlates well with hemodynamic changes in the placental circulation. As gestational age advances, there is an increase in the number of tertiary stem villi and hence the impedance in the uterine artery decreases. The prediastolic notch gradually disappears and a diastolic component in the uterine artery flow velocity waveform appears during the early second trimester, i.e. at 14 weeks' gestation, and progressively increases up to 20–24 weeks (Fig. 19.1).

Pregnancies that show persistent high-resistance waveforms in the uterine artery (Figs 19.2 and 19.3) are at risk of preterm delivery from pre-eclampsia, abruption, fetal growth restriction and overall higher morbidity as well as mortality.[9]

Umbilical Artery

The umbilical artery (UA) is the signature vessel and a direct reflection of the flow within the placenta (Fig. 19.4).[10]

In the normal fetus, the pulsatility index (PI) decreases with advancing gestation. In fetuses with FGR, there is an increase in placental resistance and PI secondary to the decrease, absence or reversal of end-diastolic flow (Figs 19.5 to 19.7). The absent or reversed end-diastolic flows are strongly associated with a higher incidence of perinatal complications, when compared to FGR fetuses with presence of end-diastolic flow (Tables 19.1 and 19.2).[11]

Tables 19.1 and 19.2 show that the prevalence of perinatal death in fetuses with absent or reversed end-diastolic flow velocity used to be over 40% and 60% respectively. Yoon et al. as well as several others demonstrated in their study that absent and diastolic flow (AEDF) is a strong and independent predictor of adverse perinatal outcome.[12] However, the perinatal mortality has shown a progressive downward trend due to efficient monitoring of growth restricted fetuses and timely intervention.

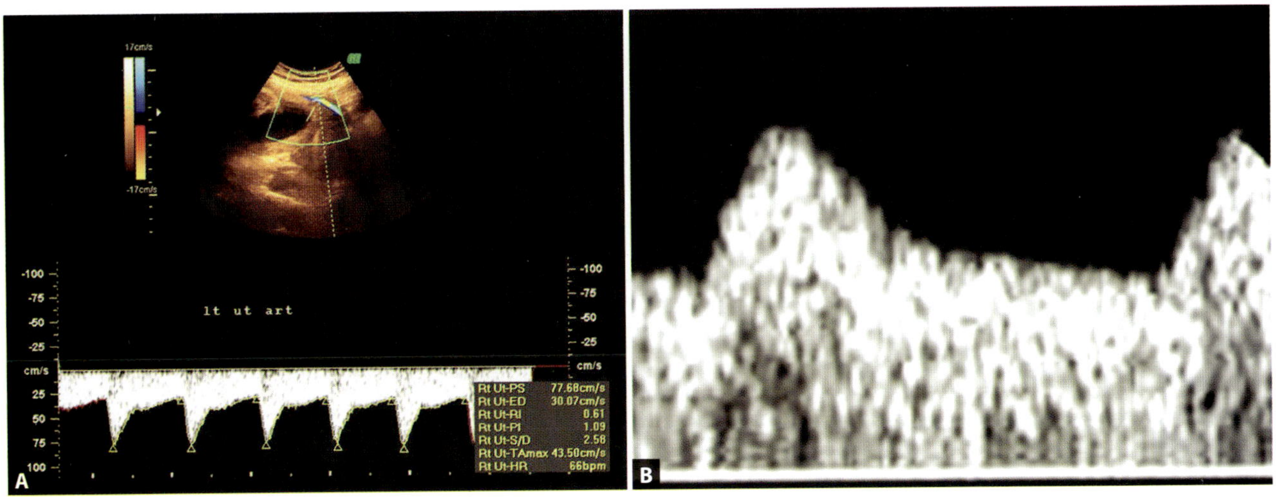

Figs 19.1A and B Uterine artery: The normal first trimester showing high diastolic flow

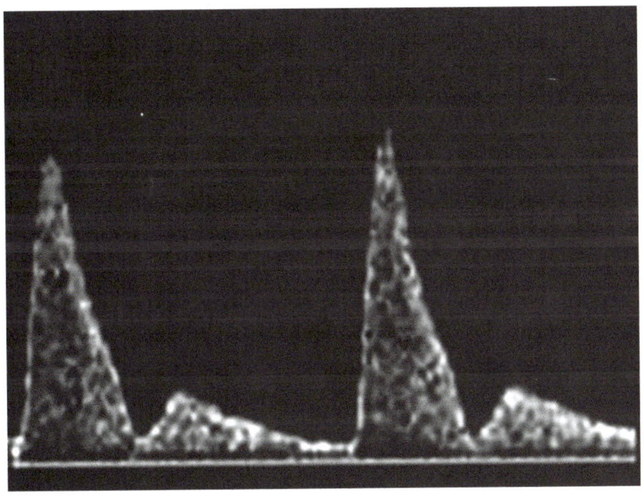

Fig. 19.2 Abnormal uterine artery waveform seen in pre-eclampsia showing high resistance flow (PI > 1.5)

Some fetuses have decreased diastolic flow that remains constant with advancing gestation and never becomes absent or reversed which may be due to a milder form of placental insufficiency.

In some FGR fetuses, the fetus maintains a normal diastolic flow velocity in the umbilical artery by altering the fetal cardiac output in an attempt to conserve placental oxygenation and hence function. This suggests that the umbilical artery functions as a shunt to maintain placental oxygenation.

Although the umbilical artery waveform is a good reflector of placental resistance it does not give any information as to how the fetus is coping with the compromised blood supply and hence does not help to determine optimum time of delivery.

Fetal Cerebral Circulation

The middle cerebral artery (MCA) is the vessel of choice to assess fetal hypoxia. During normal pregnancy, the MCA shows high resistance with continuous forward flow throughout the cardiac cycle (Fig. 19.8).

In presence of progressive fetal hypoxia, a phenomenon known as "brain sparing effect" which provides increased blood flow to the brain at the expense of other organs. Doppler depicts an increase in diastolic flow with decreased pulsatility index (Fig. 19.9), indicating a compromised fetus.[13] In pregnancies with chronic fetal hypoxia, the blood volume in the fetal circulation is redistributed in favor of vitally important organs, i.e. the heart, kidneys and brain.[2] With continuing hypoxia, the overstressed fetus loses the brain sparing effect, brain edema becomes severe, absence or reversal of diastolic flow may be seen due to the raised intracranial tension, which suggests grave and irreversible fetal neurological outcome.[14]

Fetal Aorta

The fetal aorta provides a direct reflection of the cardiac output and the peripheral resistance of the systemic circulation. It gives the summation of blood flow information to the kidneys, abdominal organs, lower limbs and placenta.

Normal blood flow in the fetal descending aorta is highly pulsatile with a minimal end-diastolic component (Fig. 19.10). In the hypoxic fetus with redistribution of flow to the brain, there is peripheral vasoconstrictions, which is reflected in the rising RI and PI values. In presence of severe hypoxia, the diastolic flow reverses and this strongly correlates with gross acidemia and impending neonatal necrotizing enterocolitis due to severe mesenteric ischemia (Fig. 19.11).[15]

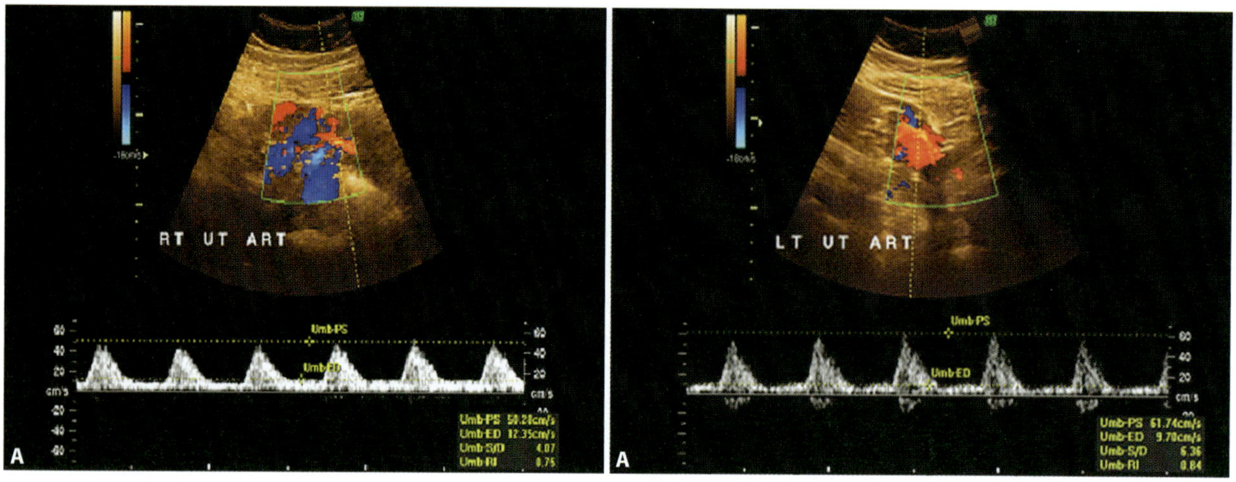

Figs 19.3A and B Increased resistance waveform pattern in bilateral uterine arteries seen in uteroplacental insufficiency with average PI > 2.3

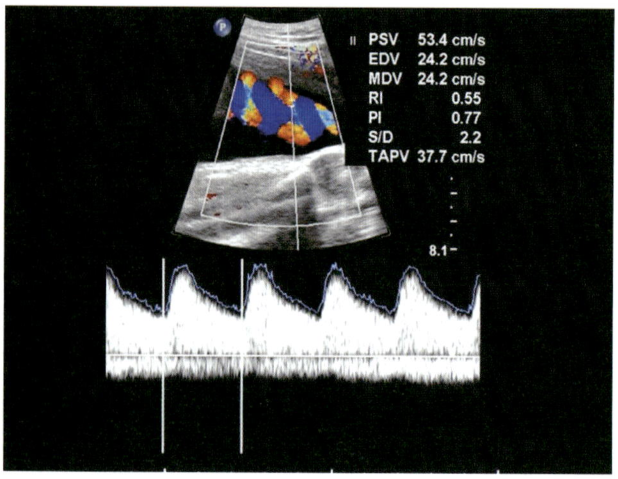

Fig. 19.4 Normal umbilical artery flow pattern

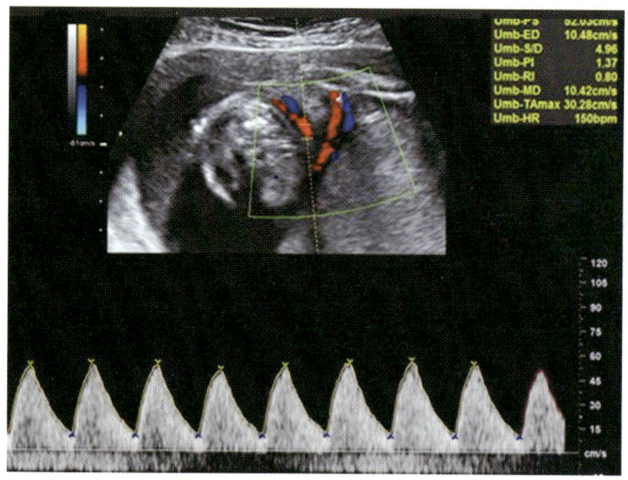

Fig. 19.5 Umbilical artery: Decreased end-diastolic flow with PI and S/D ratio

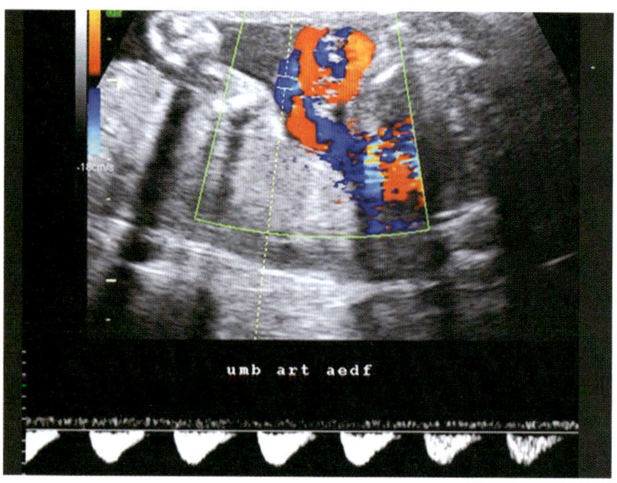

Fig. 19.6 Absent end-diastolic flow in umbilical artery

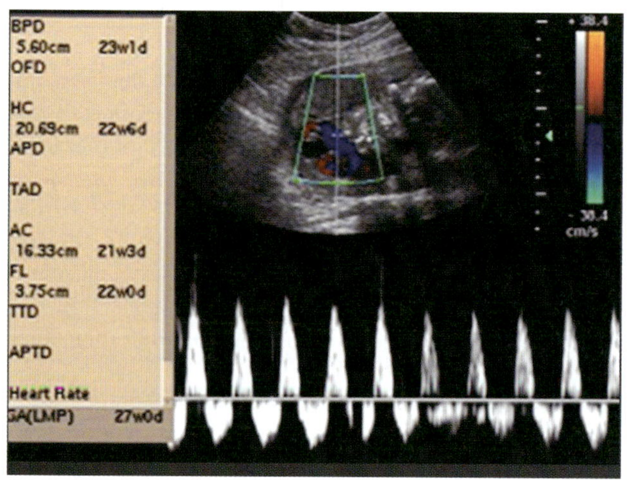

Fig. 19.7 Reversal of diastolic flow in umbilical artery

Table 19.1 Perinatal mortality associated with absent end-diastolic flow (AEDF) velocities in the umbilical artery

Study	AEDF	
	N	%
Rochelson et al. 1987	4/11	40
Pattinson et al. 1991	9/13	69
Erronen et al. 1993	7/23	30
Karsdop et al. 1994	73/178	41
Yoon et al. 1994	13/37	35
McCowan et al. 2000	6/77	8
AEDF and PNM		37.2

Table 19.2 Perinatal mortality associated with reversed end diastolic flow (REDF) velocities in the umbilical artery

Study	REDF		SB	NND
	N	%	N	N
Karsdop et al. 1994	50/67	74.6	16	34
Montenegro et al. 1998	14/22	63.6	10	4
Zelop et al. 1996	8/24	33.3	3	5
Kurkinen-Raty et al. 1997	—	35.7	—	—
Brar et al. 1998	6/12	50.0	—	—
Wang et al. 1998	15/30	50.0	3	12
Brodszki et al. 2002	26/44	59.0	19	7
REDF and PNM		52.3		

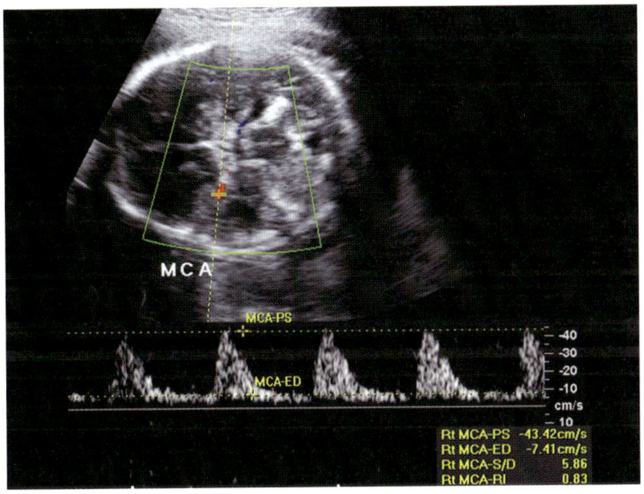

Fig. 19.8 Normal MCA Doppler high resistance waveform

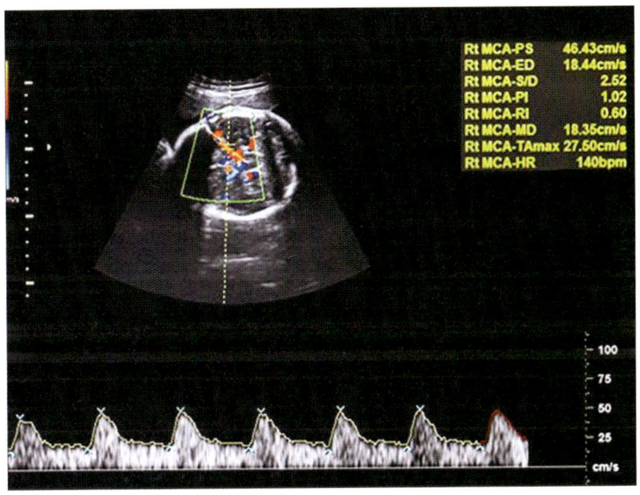

Fig. 19.9 Brain-sparing effect seen in MCA—increased end diastolic flow and decreased PI

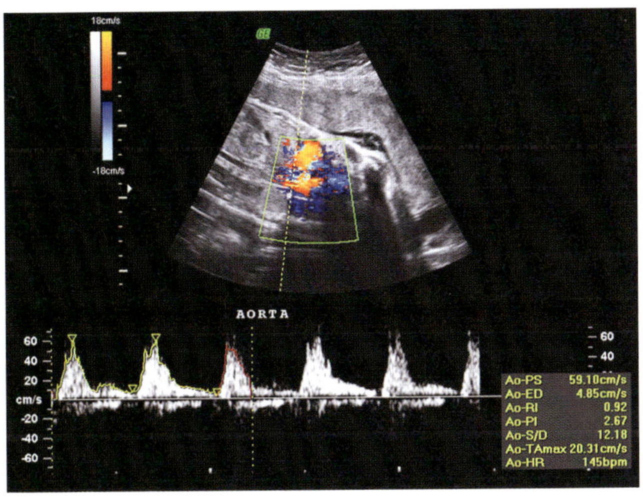

Fig. 19.10 Normal Doppler waveform in the fetal aorta of high resistance pattern

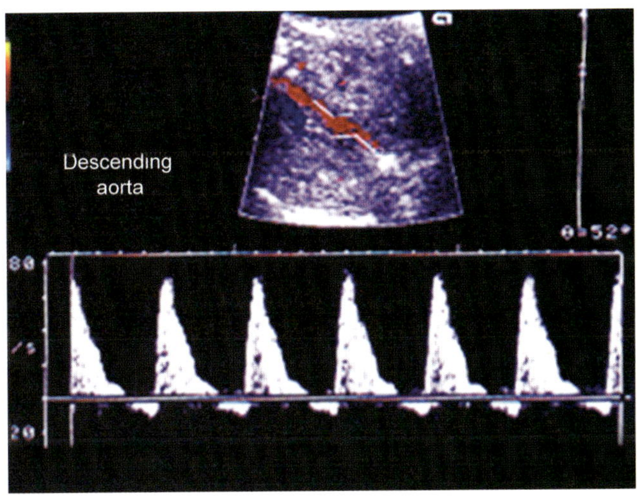

Fig. 19.11 Reversal of diastolic flow in the aorta suggestive of severe hypoxia, predictor of academia and neonatal necrotizing enterocolitis

CHANGES IN THE VENOUS CIRCULATION

Doppler waveforms obtained from the central venous system. Ductus venosus (DV), umbilical vein (UV), inferior vena cava (IVC) of the fetus reflect the physiologic status of the right ventricle giving specific information regarding the ventricular preload, myocardial compliance and right ventricular end-diastolic pressure.

The normal ductus waveform is 'M shaped' (Fig. 19.12). In FGR when there is progressive hypoxia and worsening contractility of the ventricles and atria secondary to myocardial ischemia, the DV shows a progressive decrease in 'a' wave due to increasing pressure gradient in the right atrium (Fig. 19.13). In such cases, tricuspid regurgitation (TR) causes a reversal of flow in the inferior vena cava, which eventually leads to a reversed "a" wave in the DV (Figs 19.14A and B). These abnormalities have been associated with worsening fetal hypoxemia and acidemia, and may precede abnormalities in the fetal heart rate.[16] Gonzalez et al. observed 5 fetuses with reversed 'a' wave and all died *in utero*. In 18 other fetuses with abnormal umbilical and middle cerebral artery waveforms, but without reverse 'a' wave, no deaths occurred.[6]

The umbilical vein is probably one of the last vessels to change its flow pattern in the setting of fetal hypoxia.

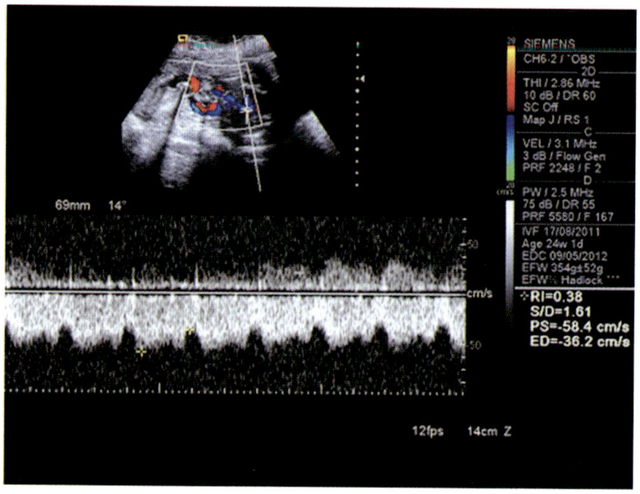

Fig. 19.12 The normal ductus venosus waveform: Reversed M (W)shaped pattern of flow with continuous forward flow in atrial systole

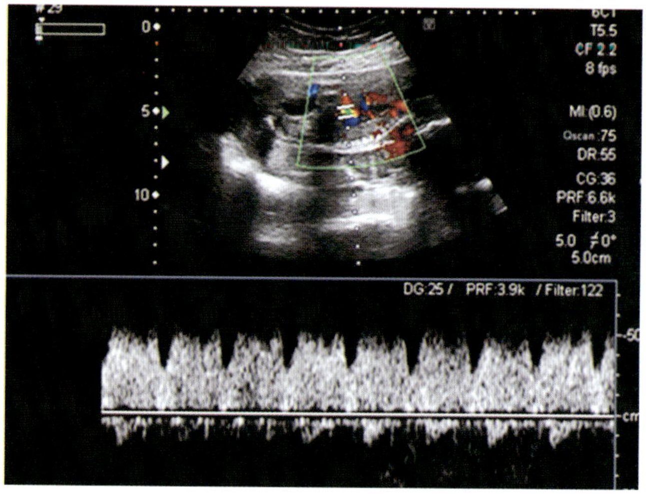

Fig. 19.13 Increased resistance in the ductus venosus due to progressive decrease in the forward flow. This occurs due to rising pressure gradient in the right atrium and is a strong indicator of impending reversal

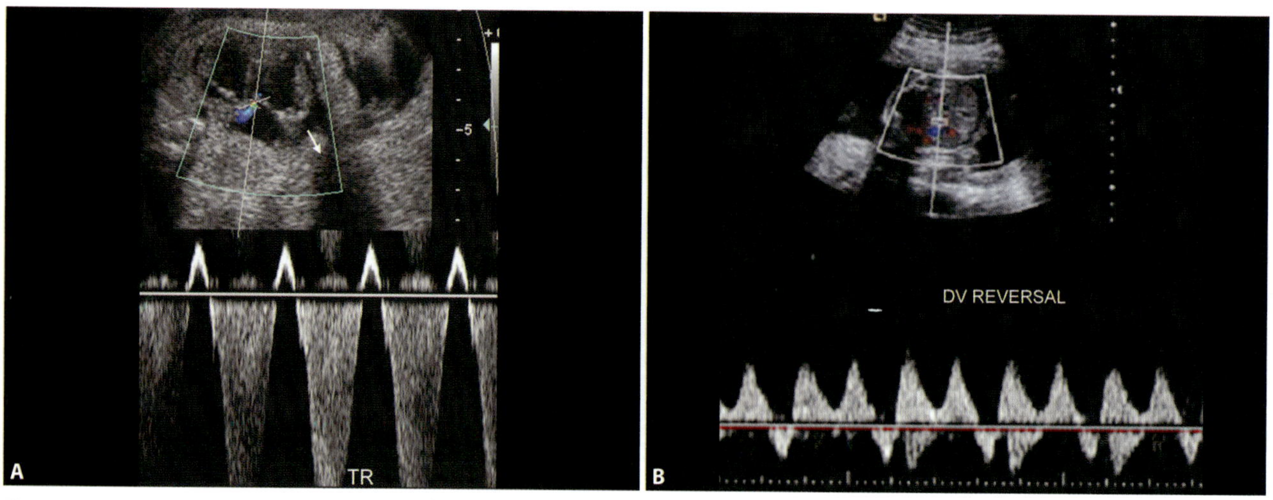

Figs 19.14A and B High pressure gradient in the right atrium causing tricuspid regurgitation (A) followed by flow reversal in ductus venosus (B) due to right heart failure

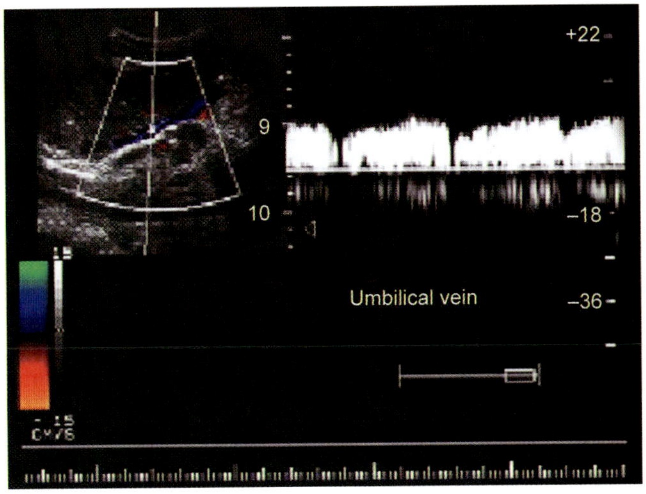

Fig. 19.15 Pulsatile waveform in the umbilical vein seen in right heart failure

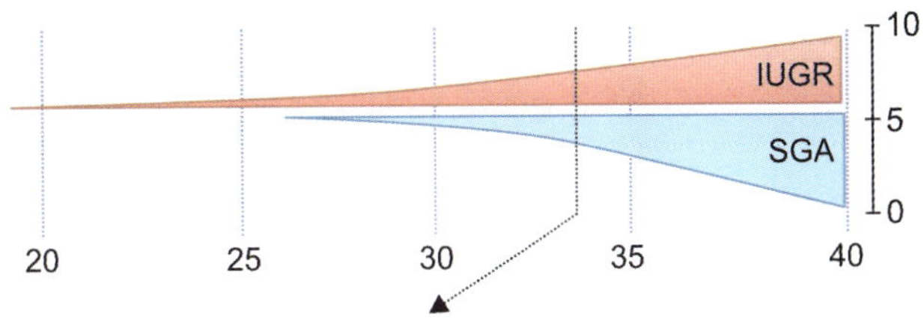

Early IUGR	Late IUGR
Problem : Management	*Problem : Diagnosis*
Degree placental disease: High	Degree placental disease: Low
Frank hypoxia	Subtle hypoxia
Tolerance to hypoxia. Natural history	Low tolerance

Fig. 19.16 Early IUGR versus late IUGR

Table 19.3 Several Doppler pattern

Doppler pattern	Umbilical artery pulsality index (PI)	Middle cerebral circulation pulsatility index	Doppler based management to identify further progression
1	Normal	Normal or Abnormal	Close monitoring with bed rest at home.
2	Abnormal	Normal or Abnormal	Close monitoring with bed rest at home or in the hospital and oxygen therapy
3	Abnormal	Abnormal	Fetus likely to deteriorate, chance of delivery at term term is remote. Biophysical profile and nonstress test twice weekly, Doppler monitoring every 7–10 days ↓ Deliver urgently if absent or reversed end-diastolic flow noted in the umbilical artery and/or ductus venosus (Figs 19.17A and B)

In severe cases, when there is reversal of flow in the IVC and ductus venosus due to right heart failure, a pulsatile flow pattern begins to appear due to the high resistance to forward flow (Fig. 19.15). The presence of umbilical vein pulsations is associated with an increased risk of adverse perinatal outcome.

DOPPLER BASED MANAGEMENT IN FETAL GROWTH RESTRICTION

The management of growth restricted fetuses is largely governed by the timing of onset of the growth restriction. If FGR occurs before the 34th week of gestation, it is called early FGR while late FGR occurs after the 34th week (Fig. 19.16).

Early Onset FGR/Severe Uteroplacental Insufficiency

A. In a small fetus at 22–24 weeks gestation, several Doppler patterns may occur (Tables 19.3 and 19.4). Guidelines to fetal monitoring are based on these early patterns obtained from data based on several longitudinal studies that have proved the efficacy of these methods.
B. The PI of the UA may increase while that of the MCA may decrease popularly known as the brain sparing effect indicating the onset of fetal hypoxia. The fetus starts to show signs of FGR. The biophysical profile may still be normal. The cerebroplacental Doppler ratio (CPR) described by Gramellini et al. in 1992 has facilitated the recognition of these early changes in the fetus. This is the ratio of the PI of the MCA and UA. A ratio below 1.08 can be considered as centralization of cardiac output towards the fetal brain and increasing placental resistance (Fig. 19.18)

At this time, the lack of fetal growth and/or the development of pre-eclampsia/eclampsia, or a persistent abnormal biophysical profile may interrupt the process with delivery of the fetus.

If the fetus is not delivered, the hypoxic environment continues.

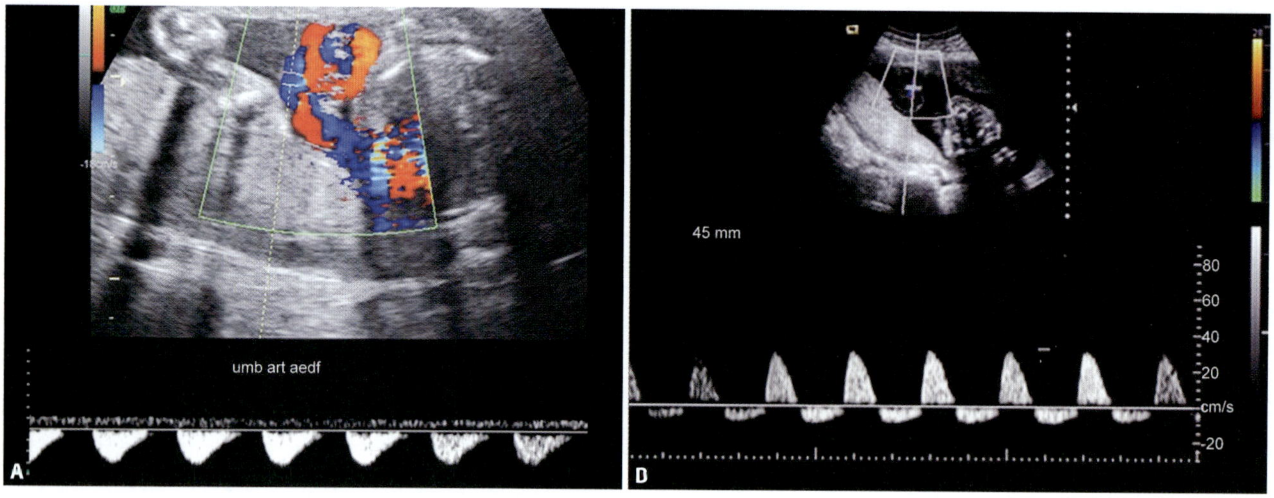

Figs 19.17A and B Absent end-diastolic flow (A) Subsequently leading to reversal of flow in the umbilical artery; (B) Both these are indicators of urgent delivery

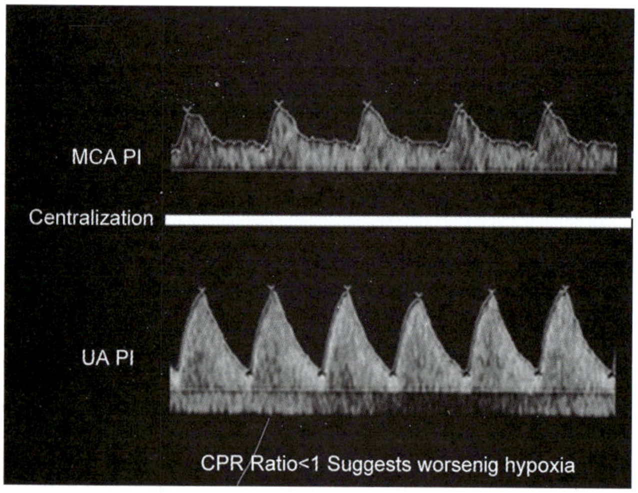

Fig. 19.18 Cerebroplacental ratio (CPR) normal ratio >1

C. At this time TR may appear, DV reversed flow and UV pulsations may be present intermittently. The biophysical profile may still appear normal.[17]
D. DV absent or reversed 'a' wave and UV pulsations are present continuously. The fetus starts to lose the brain sparing effect. The biophysical profile becomes abnormal.[18]
E. *Fetal demise:* The time interval between D and E is variable (from 6 hours to 12 hours to 2 weeks).

Oligohydramnios may appear at any stage of the above process.

In severe early onset FGR the full Doppler spectrum of changes as mentioned above may be observed while waiting for appropriate fetal maturity to ne achieved.

A balance has to be maintained between appropriate time of delivery, so as to avoid irreversible hypoxic changes and the hazards of neonatal immaturity in consultation with the neonatologist.

Late Onset FGR/Mild Uteroplacental Insufficiency

In mild uteroplacental insufficiency no effect may be seen on Doppler and growth until 30–34 weeks gestation. The main challenge in such patients is timely diagnosis as the fetus does not adapt well to hypoxia and therefore continues to have low tolerance if hypoxic conditions continue. Sudden fetal death is the most feared complication of this adverse clinical scenario. Such growth restricted fetuses usually only show arterial changes in their Doppler waveforms while the venous system continues to remain unaffected.[19] The main goal of Doppler monitoring in these patients is to prevent the occurrence of AEDF/REDF in the UA and to prolong the pregnancy as far as possible until complete fetal maturity is achieved. Management guidelines have been suggested based on Doppler findings in these patient.

CONCLUSION

Placental insufficiency is the most common cause of FGR and pregnancy induced hypertension (PIH). It is an important obstetric problem on account of the high associated perinatal mortality and morbidity. Uterine artery Doppler has an important role to play in predicting the onset of PIH and IUGR at the 11–14 and 20–24 weeks. There seems to be a need to recognize placental insufficiency early so that its hazards can be reduced, if not averted. The preventive role of uterine artery Doppler has hence shifted to the first trimester.[20]

Table 19.4 Color Doppler guidelines in practice

S.No.	Doppler findings	Follow-up protocol	Outcome
1.	Mildly abnormal UA/MCA	Aggressive Doppler monitoring every week with bed rest at home	Usually no further deterioration in Doppler findings noted. Deliver at term[22]
2.	CPR worsens/Uterine artery notching appears	Aggressive Doppler monitoring every week with bed rest at home Look for AEDF/REDF	Deliver after 37 weeks when fetal maturity is achieved in a center with good neonatal care
3.	AEDF/REDF	No further follow-up	Urgent delivery (Fig. 19.18)

Fetuses with FGR show evident modifications of Doppler parameters in the uteroplacental and fetal circulation. Sequential studies enable us to determine the condition of these fetuses by observing the Doppler changes in different vascular territories. The delivery of the sick fetus can therefore be appropriately timed to prevent the associated complications.[21,22]

In the past the focus has been to reduce near term mortality and morbidity, but recent studies have documented adverse long-term neurological sequelae even in those fetuses subjected to hypoxia for a short duration.[23] Hence, the role of Doppler has shifted from a curative to a preventive one with truly informed and meaningful brain-oriented fetal care becoming a clinical reality.[24]

The three main questions that need to be answered while evaluating an FGR pregnancy are:

1. Does the small fetus have a circulatory abnormality?
2. What is the ability of the fetus to cope with the altered circulation?
3. When is the correct time to intervene in order to reduce the morbidity and mortality in the growth restricted fetus?

REFERENCES

1. Mandruzzato G. Intrauterine growth restriction (IUGR). J Perinatal Medicine. 2008;36(4):277-81.
2. Adré J du Plessis. Cerebral blood flow and metabolism in the developing fetus. J Obstet Gynaecol India. 2010;60(4):301-11.
3. Scifres CM, Stamilio D, Macones GA, Odibo AO. Predicting perinatal mortality in preterm intrauterine growth restriction. Am J Perinatol. 2009;26(10):723-8.
4. Kingdom JC, Burrell SJ, Kaufmann P. Pathology and clinical implications of abnormal umbilical artery Doppler waveforms. Ultrasound Obstet Gynecol. 1997;9(4):271-86.
5. Mari G, Piconi J. Doppler vascular changes in IUGR. Seminars in Perinatology. 2008;32(3):182-9.
6. Gonzalez JM, Stamilio DM, Ural S, Macones GA, Odibo AO. Relationship between abnormal fetal testing and adverse perinatal outcomes in intrauterine growth restriction. Am J Obstet Gynecol. 2007;196(5):348-51.
7. Padmagirison R, Rai L. Fetal Doppler versus NST as predictors of adverse perinatal outcome in severe preeclampsia and fetal growth restriction. J Obstet Gynecol. 2006;56:134-8.
8. Trudinger BJ. Doppler ultrasonography and fetal well being. In: Reece EA, Hobbins JC, Mahoney M (Eds): Medicine of the Fetus and the Mother. Philadelphia, JB Lippincott Co.; 1992.
9. Zhang J, Merialdi M, Platt LD, Kramer MS. Defining normal and abnormal fetal growth: promises and challenges. Am J Obstet Gynecol. 2010;202(6):522-8.
10. Fleischer A, Schulman H, Farmakides G, Bracero L, Blattner P, Randolph G. Umbilical artery flow velocity waveforms and intrauterine growth retardation. Am J Obstet Gynecol. 1985;151:502-5.
11. Chauhan SP, Gupta LM, Hendrix NW, et al. Intrauterine growth restriction: comparison of American College of Obstetricians and Gynecologists practice bulletin with other national guidelines. Am J Obstet Gynecol. 2009;200:409.e1-409.e6.
12. Yoon BH, Romero R, Roh CR, Kim SH, Ager JW, Syn HC, et al. Relationship between the fetal biophysical profile score, umbilical artery Doppler velocimetry, and fetal blood acid-base status determined by cordocentesis. Am J Obstet Gynecol. 1993;169:1586-94.
13. Scherjon SA, Kok JH, Oosting H, Zondervan HA. Intra-observer and inter-observer reliability of the pulsatility index calculated from pulsed Doppler flow velocity waveforms in three fetal vessels. BJOG: An International Journal of Obstetrics and Gynaecology. 1993;100:134-8.
14. Martinez R, Figueras F, Oros D, et al. Cerebral blood perfusion and neurobehavioral performance in full-term small-for-gestational-age fetuses. Am J Obstet Gynecol. 2009;201:474.e1-7.
15. Manogura AC, Turan O, Kush ML, et al. Predictors of necrotizing enterocolitis in preterm growth-restricted neonates. Am J Obstet Gynecol. 2008;198:638.e1-638.e5.
16. Ozcan T, Sbracia M, d'Ancona RL, Copel JA, Mari G. Arterial and venous Doppler velocimetry in the severely growth restricted fetus and associations with adverse perinatal outcome. Ultrasound Obstet Gynecol. 1998;12:39-44.
17. Ghidini A. Doppler of the ductus venosus in severe preterm growth restriction. A test in search of a purpose? Obstet Gynecol. 2007;109:250-1.
18. Picconi JL. The transitional phase of ductus venosus reversed flow in severely premature IUGR fetuses. Am J Perinatology. 2008;25(4):199-203.

19. Piper JM, Xenakis EMJ, McFarland M. Do growth retarded premature infants have different rates of perinatal morbidity and mortality than appropriately grown premature infants? Obstet Gynaecol; 1996;87(2):169-74.
20. Walid MS. The IUGR prognostic scale. Arch Gynecol Obstet. 2007;276(6):633-40.
21. Rang S, Gert A van Montfrans, Wolf H. Serial hemodynamic measurement in normal pregnancy, preeclampsia, and intrauterine growth restriction. Am J Obstet Gynecol. 2008;198(5):e1-e9.
22. Grivell RM, Wong L, Bhatia V. Regimens of fetal surveillance for impaired fetal growth. Cochrane Database Syst Rev. 2009;CD007113.
23. Tideman E, Marsal K, Ley D. Cognitive function in young adults following intrauterine growth restriction with abnormal fetal aortic blood flow. Ultrasound Obstet Gynecol. 2007;29:614-8.
24. Chander L, Sonal G. Colour Doppler in Intrauterine growth restriction- Where are we and where do we go? J Obstet Gynaecol India. 2010;60(4):301-11.

SECTION 4

Diagnostic Techniques: Invasive

CHAPTER

20 General Principles of Prenatal Diagnosis: Invasive Prenatal Diagnosis

Raju R Sahetya

INTRODUCTION

Invasive prenatal diagnosis techniques include chorionic villus sampling (CVS), amniocentesis, cordocentesis or percutaneous umbilical blood sampling (PUBS), fetal tissue sampling, as well as embryoscopy and fetoscopy (Table 20.1). Some diagnostic results may be obtained by more than one technique: for example, fetal karyotype can be obtained from cells from amniocentesis, chorionic villus sampling or fetal blood sampling.

AMNIOCENTESIS

Amniocentesis is an ultrasound-guided invasive prenatal diagnosis procedure usually performed after 14 weeks gestational age for determination of fetal karyotype, molecular, and biochemical abnormalities. Other genetic diagnoses can be made from cultured amniocytes or by measurement of specific substances in the amniotic fluid. Results can generally be obtained prior to 20 weeks gestational age. The fetal karyotype will usually take 1-3 weeks from the time of amniocentesis, depending on the cytogenetic laboratory. The major disadvantage of amniocentesis is that results of the prenatal diagnosis are not available until 17-20 weeks gestational age. If genetic abnormalities are identified and the patient requests termination of pregnancy, the techniques of pregnancy termination carry a greater emotional and physical risk to the woman than a first trimester termination.

The two most common tests performed on the amniotic fluid are the fetal karyotype from fetal and membrane cells in the amniotic fluid after tissue culturing or direct fluorescent *in situ* hybridization (FISH) techniques, and direct measurement of amniotic fluid α-fetoprotein (AFAFP). Other genetic diagnoses can be obtained by biochemical or molecular techniques after discussion with the local prenatal diagnosis center.

Removal of the amniotic fluid generally takes less than one minute. About 15-30 mL of fluid is drawn, depending on gestational age and the tests required. The patient may experience some mild uterine cramping and pressure sensation. The amniotic fluid is generally similar in appearance to white wine. Occasionally blood tinged amniotic fluid may be obtained, generally due to maternal bleeding into the

Table 20.1 Summary of amniocentesis and chorionic villus sampling (CVS) information

	Amniocentesis	CVS
Procedure	Amniotic fluid removed by needle and syringe	Chorionic villi removed by transcervical (TC) catheter and syringe or transabdominal (TA) needle insertion
Timing	15–17 weeks	10 to 11-6/7 weeks (greater than 12 weeks TA CVS only)
Added risk of miscarriage due to procedure	0.5–1.0%	TA 1.2% TC 2.6%
Fetal malformation risks	—	1 in 3000 vascular limb malformation (suggested but not proven)
Chance of successful sampling	Approximately 99%	Approximately 99%. IF unsuccessful, can follow with amniocentesis
Time required for cytogenetic diagnosis	1–3 weeks (FISH may be available)	2–3 weeks (rapid direct technique may be considered in specific situations)
Accuracy (chromosomes) aneuploidy and major structural rearrangement	Highly accurate	Highly accurate
Mosaicism	Level 3—rare	Confined placental—1.0–2.0%
Open neural tube defects	AFP in amniotic fluid detects approximately 95% on NTDs	Other tests required for detection

amniotic cavity at the time of the procedure. If the patient has previously had a history of antepartum bleeding, the amniotic fluid may be brown or dark red in color due to blood pigments being absorbed across the chorio-amnion membranes. The presence of discolored fluid on amniocentesis is associated with an increased risk of pregnancy loss.[1]

No more than two uterine needle insertions into or through the uterine wall are recommended. If the procedure is unsuccessful, further attempts can be made with a delay of at least 24 hours.

Freshly blood-stained amniotic fluid should be separately analyzed by a Kleihauer test and cell count to determine whether the new blood is maternal or fetal. If the blood is fetal, the AFAFP value may be elevated without a congenital anomaly as the etiology.

DISADVANTAGES AND RISKS OF AMNIOCENTESIS

Fetal Loss

Fetal loss after amniocentesis is estimated to be one in every 100–200 procedures above the background loss rate.[2-4]

Infection

The risk of infection introduced at the time of the amniocentesis is estimated to be 1–2 in 3000 procedures. Recent information indicates that approximately 10–50% of postamniocentesis losses have evidence of low grade infections at the time of the procedure with increased cytokine levels in the amniotic fluid.[5,6]

Fetal Injury

Serious fetal injuries at the time of amniocentesis are rare with or without continuous ultrasound guidance. Small skin dimpling lesions have been reported following contact of the fetus with the needle, but these are generally minimal and the specific anatomic location may be the only consideration.[7] Patients are generally requested to have limited activity for 12–24 hours following the amniocentesis procedure but this has not been well studied.

Minor Complications

Minor complications without fetal loss following amniocentesis include continued leakage of amniotic fluid, bleeding, and uterine irritability. These minor complications are estimated to occur in 1–5% of procedures.[8,9] These complications are generally self-limited. Recommendations may include bedrest and additional serial ultrasound monitoring if continued amniotic fluid leakage is present. The benefit of antibiotic use with amniotic fluid leakage has not been evaluated.

TWIN PREGNANCY

The risk of pregnancy loss following twin amniocentesis is estimated to be 1–2%.[10] It is necessary to define placental location and presence or absence of separating membranes. Good descriptive localization of twin A or B (right- or left-sided twin with placental location) is necessary, especially when an abnormality is identified in only one twin.

EARLY AMNIOCENTESIS

Comparing early amniocentesis (11–12 weeks 6 days) and mid-trimester amniocentesis (15–16 weeks 6 days).[11] Significant differences for early amniocentesis compared with mid-trimester amniocentesis were found for:

- Total fetal losses, including pre-procedure, post-procedure, stillbirth and neonatal death (7.6% for early amniocentesis vs. 5.95% for mid-trimester amniocentesis).
- Newborn clubfoot (incidence of 1.3% in early group compared with the background 0.1% for the mid-trimester group).
- Post-procedural amniotic fluid leakage (3.7% for the early group compared to 1.5% for the mid-trimester group).
- Cytogenetic culture failures were also more likely in the early amniocentesis group (1.8% for early amniocentesis vs. 0.2% for mid-trimester amniocentesis).
- Requiring additional invasive prenatal diagnosis techniques for these women if further diagnosis was requested.

Early amniocentesis does not appear to be appropriate for routine prenatal diagnosis at gestational ages of 11–12 weeks 6 days gestation. The exact safety of amniocentesis for gestational ages 13 and 14 weeks has not been established.

CHORIONIC VILLUS SAMPLING

Chorionic villus sampling (CVS) is the most common first trimester invasive prenatal diagnosis technique for evaluation of fetal karyotype, molecular, and biochemical abnormalities. CVS is an ultrasound-guided technique that is usually performed in the first trimester between 10 and 11 weeks 6 days gestation. Although the procedure was initially developed as a transcervical technique, both transcervical and transabdominal techniques have recently become available. The upper gestational age of 12 weeks is generally considered for the transcervical technique but as more experience is gained with transabdominal CVS, the procedure may be undertaken at a gestational age of 10 weeks gestation or greater.

Procedure

The transcervical chorionic villus sampling technique uses a flexible plastic catheter with a plastic or metal obtruder whose shape can be moulded to allow the catheter to pass, under continuous ultrasound guidance, through the cervix and into the placental tissue. Prior to insertion of the catheter, a speculum is placed in the vagina and the cervix and vaginal walls are cleansed with antiseptic solution. In the majority of cases, further manipulation of the uterus and cervix by a tenaculum is not necessary. The transabdominal chorionic villus sampling technique generally utilizes a freehand technique with continuous ultrasound guidance, similar to amniocentesis or cordocentesis. A 19 or 20 gauge spinal needle is used for the transabdominal technique; other needle options include a two needle set with an outer gauge of 18.

Both the transcervical and transabdominal technique usually obtain 5–25 mg of chorionic tissue which is aspirated into the catheter or needle by applying negative pressure to a 10–20 cc syringe attached to the end of the catheter or needle. The catheter is withdrawn through the placental tissue or the needle is moved back and forth (5–10 movements) in the placental tissue to obtain the specimen with negative pressure by the syringe for both techniques. The transcervical technique is used for the majority of the posterior placental locations, while the transabdominal technique is better suited for the fundal and anterior placental locations. An adequate amount of chorionic villus tissue is generally obtained with one aspiration but two attempts do not increase the risk of post-procedure loss.

Both transabdominal and transcervical chorionic villus sampling have similar accuracy. The transcervical technique is associated with a greater risk of post-procedural spotting or minimal bleeding (10–20%) while the transabdominal technique has increased uterine discomfort and cramps.[12] Infection has not been identified as a significant factor in the large number of patients having transcervical procedures.[13]

Some genetic centers will use CVS techniques for both singleton and twin pregnancies. The safety and accuracy of CVS and twins is reported by a small number of centers.[14] Rh disease prophylaxis should be done similarly to the method described for amniocentesis; however, the optimum schedule is not known.

Advantages of CVS

The major advantage of CVS is the earlier gestational age at sampling, affording earlier results. If a chromosomal or DNA abnormality is detected and pregnancy termination is requested, emotional stresses of pregnancy termination may be less than when termination follows amniocentesis at a later gestational age. A second advantage is related to specific molecular diagnoses with DNA extracted directly from the villi, allowing an earlier result with no cell culturing for these genetic disorders. A third advantage is that direct chromosomal analysis may be used in certain situations for rapid results in less than 24 hours by either cytogenetic or FISH techniques.

Disadvantages and Risks of CVS

Confined Placental Mosaicism

Confined placental mosaicism, a discrepancy between the chromosomes in the chorionic and fetal tissues, is a biologic placental factor which is present in 1–2% of pregnancies.[15] Although this finding is usually limited to the placental tissue and is not usually present in the fetus, additional amniocentesis should be offered for further evaluation. The additional procedure may increase pregnancy risks. Clinical effects of the confined placental mosaicism can vary depending on the specific chromosome involved. The concerns that need to be considered in this situation are uniparental disomy and risks of placental dysfunction with intrauterine growth restriction and fetal death.

Maternal Contamination

Contamination by maternal decidual tissue is possible, but this potential problem can be minimized with very careful attention to cleaning or stripping of the chorionic villi of maternal decidual cells under the dissecting microscope prior to tissue culturing. This has not been a significant problem in most cytogenetic laboratories with long-term experience in CVS.

Pregnancy Loss

The background risk of spontaneous pregnancy loss in the advanced maternal age group, after ultrasound has confirmed a viable pregnancy at 10 weeks gestational age when no procedure is undertaken, is estimated at 2–3%.[16] The CVS procedure adds approximately 1–2% above the background in comparison to the 0.5–1.0% risk for amniocentesis.[4,17,18] Vaginal bleeding occurring prior to the procedure increases the risk of pregnancy loss following CVS by either route. The risk of pregnancy loss increases with the number of attempts needed to obtain the chorionic tissue and should be limited to two attempts. Uterine and placental location may alter procedural risk factors depending on the CVS technique used. Uterine fibroids may cause some additional risks of technique success and pregnancy loss. Transcervical and transabdominal CVS techniques differ in the postprocedure loss rate risk. Risks are approximately doubled with transcervical technique (3–6%).[17]

Limb or Facial Anomalies

The risk of limb or facial anomalies is higher if CVS is done at a gestational age earlier than nine weeks. CVS is generally restricted to greater than or equal to 10 weeks gestational age in most centers. The incidence of transverse limb (minor or major) in the general population is estimated at nine in 10,000 livebirths. One-third of these anomalies may be due to a vascular disruption sequence such as CVS. The risk of a limb or facial abnormality related to the CVS procedure could be as high as one in 3000 fetuses.[19-21] A recent report from the World Health Organization (WHO) registry concluded that CVS is not associated with an increased risks for fetal loss or anomalies.[22]

CORDOCENTESIS

Cordocentesis or percutaneous umbilical blood sampling (PUBS) can be used to obtain fetal blood from as early as 12 weeks gestational age until term, but is usually used after 16 weeks.[23] Indications for cordocentesis include: fetal karyotyping when congenital malformations or intrauterine growth retardation are identified by ultrasound, viral infections, hematological abnormalites including Rh or other immune hemolytic disease, maternal or fetal platelet disorders, and inborn errors of metabolism. In addition, physiological assessment of the fetus can be evaluated by measuring components such as fetal blood gases, glucose, and lactate. The procedure can be used for fetal therapy when intravascular transfusions are required, as well as for the introduction of medications for fetal treatment and in the future for fetal therapy protocols.

Procedure

Cordocentesis is an ultrasound-guided freehand or needle guide technique which allows insertion of a 22 gauge spinal needle into the umbilical cord vessels at its insertion on placenta. Fetal chromosomes can usually be obtained within 48–72 hours by culturing fetal white blood cells. The technique will vary depending on the placental position as well as fetal position and activity. Fetal paralysis (pancuronium) is sometimes required. Fetal blood specimens can usually be obtained in less than 5–10 minutes. Depending on the indications for the test and the gestational age of the fetus, 1–3 mL of blood are removed for analysis. Confirmation of fetal blood is required and can be done by an initial Apt test (a bedside test for differentiating fetal from maternal hemoglobin) followed by laboratory confirmation of fetal hemoglobin (Kleihauer). The reported success rates for cordocentesis range from 93.7% to 98.5%.[24]

Advantages of Cordocentesis

The major advantage of cordocentesis is that it allows direct access to the fetus, not only for diagnostic but also for therapeutic management.

Disadvantages and Risks of Cordocentesis

Pregnancy Loss

Procedure-related pregnancy loss following cordocentesis has been linked to several factors, including procedure indication, fetal distress (bradycardia), and prolonged cord bleeding.[25] The procedure indication greatly increases the risk of procedure-related pregnancy loss. The procedure-related pregnancy loss risk with fetal anomalies or intrauterine growth restriction is approximately 3.2% compared to 1.25% in a group of fetuses with normal growth and anatomy.[26] The incidence of post-cordocentesis pregnancy loss with normal fetal structures, abnormal fetal structures, fetal physiological assessment (IUGR), and nonimmune hydrops, excluding therapeutic abortions, was reported to be 1%, 7%, 14% and 25% respectively.[27] Other reported factors increasing the risk of fetal loss include longer procedures (more than 14 minutes) and placental position (anterior placenta increased over posterior placenta).[24,28]

Fetal Bradycardia

Fetal bradycardia (fetal distress) at or following the procedure may result in fetal morbidity and mortality. The risk of fetal bradycardia is variable but can be estimated at five to 10%. The risk of bradycardia is greater when the umbilical artery is punctured (17%) compared with venous puncture (2%).[29]

Bleeding

Bleeding from the cord puncture site varies from 10% to 40% but in the majority of cases the duration is less than 90 seconds.[28,29]

OTHER FETAL TISSUE SAMPLING

Techniques to obtain tissue from fetal skin and liver or fluid from the fetal urinary tract, abdomen, thorax or cystic hygroma are similar to freehand ultrasound-guided techniques, such as amniocentesis and cordocentesis.

Needle insertion into specific fetal areas requires appropriate fetal positioning. Fetal paralysis may be required. Protocols for fetal paralysis may vary from center to center.[23,24] Risks and complications of the procedures are similar to those quoted for cordocentesis, with the risks of fetal death being increased if major congenital malformations and growth retardation are present.

The accuracy of the test is dependent on the tissue being obtained and the specific analysis required. For urinary tract evaluation, urinary specimens for osmolality, electrolytes, and other urinary factors can be obtained by bladder aspiration. Thoracic and abdominal fluids can be evaluated for cell and protein content, as in a chylothorax. Lymphatic fluid from cystic hygroma can be used for chromosome analysis. Liver, muscle, and skin have been sampled for evidence of specific genetic syndromes.[24] These procedures are rare and should be discussed with regional genetic and perinatal consultants.

FETOSCOPY/EMBRYOSCOPY

There are few indications as yet for fetoscopy in prenatal diagnosis or treatment. The technique allows direct visualization of external fetal features or structures not appreciated by ultrasound, which may assist in non-chromosomal genetic diagnosis. The risks of fetoscopy are greater than the risks of other invasive prenatal diagnosis procedures.[30]

Embryoscopy at present is a research technique and may allow early visualization of the embryo by inserting a rigid scope through the cervix and into the space between the amnion and chorion. Since vaginal ultrasound is able to give similar embryonic and early fetal detail, it is unlikely that this invasive procedure will have any significant indications.

GENERAL PRINCIPLES FOR PRENATAL DIAGNOSIS PROGRAMS

- All patients considering prenatal diagnosis should have access to professionals who are knowledgeable in the field and skilled in the procedures.
- Entire range of services is available to each patient. Innovations in telemedicine technology promise to offer options for distance face-to-face counseling and interpretation.
- A suggested minimum caseload of 50 invasive procedures per year is recommended per practitioner in order to maintain an appropriate level of competence in the provision of invasive procedures.
- In order to maintain a high standard of efficiency, a cytogenetic laboratory should have a minimum workload of 100 prenatal specimens.
- Each patient should have an appropriate assessment of family history and genetic counseling prior to undergoing invasive prenatal diagnosis.
- Counseling should be given in a nondirective manner in order to allow an informed choice by the couple.
- The distinction between screening and diagnostic investigations should be clarified, including the frequency of abnormal results, false-positive, and false-negative tests. Accuracy of results, frequency of need for repeat testing, and risk of pregnancy loss are of particular relevance with invasive prenatal diagnosis procedures. The couple should be reminded that normal test results do not rule out every genetic or structural abnormality in their fetus.
- Prior to embarking on prenatal diagnosis testing, couples should be made aware of the full range of options when confronted with an abnormal test result. Prior commitment to termination of pregnancy following the diagnosis of fetal abnormality is not a prerequisite for prenatal diagnosis.
- Determination of fetal sex for the purpose of sex selection procedures on a nonmedical basis is inappropriate and not allowed under the PCPNDT Act.

SUMMARY OF MAJOR RECOMMENDATIONS

- It is recommended that women at increased risk for having a child with a chromosomal anomaly be identified based on maternal age.
- It is recommended that maternal serum screening be used to identify women at increased risk for having a child with a chromosomal anomaly. Maternal serum screening can be used to modify a woman's age-related risks.
- It is recommended that maternal serum AFP screening be used to identify women at increased risk for having a child with a neural tube defect.
- It is recommended that an amniocentesis be offered to women at increased risk of having a child with a chromosome anomaly.
- It is recommended that CVS be offered to women as an alternative to amniocentesis where resources exist and patients presenting in first trimester.
- Cordocentesis may be offered to high-risk women under certain circumstances and when diagnosis un-conclusive by other methods.

REFERENCES

1. Hess LW, Anderson RL, Golbus MS. Significance of opaque discolored amniotic fluid at second trimester amniocentesis. Obstet Gynecol. 1986;67(suppl):44-6.
2. National Institute of Child Health and Human Development, National Registry for Amniocentesis Study Group. Mid-trimester amniocentesis for prenatal diagnosis: Safety and accuracy. J Am Med Assoc. 1976;236:1471-76.

3. Medical Research Council of Canada. Diagnosis of Genetic Disease by Amniocentesis During the Second Trimester of Pregnancy. Report No. 5. Ottawa: Medical Research Council of Canada, 1977.
4. Canadian Collaborative CVS-Amniocentesis Clinical Trial Group. Multicentre randomised clinical trial of chorion villus sampling and amniocentesis. First Report. Lancet 1989;1(8628): 1-6.
5. Romero R, Munoz H, Gomez R, et al. Two-thirds of spontaneous abortion/fetal deaths after genetic midtrimester amniocentesis are the result of a pre-existing subclinical inflammatory process of the amniotic cavity (abstract). Am J Obstet Gynecol. 1995;172:261.
6. Wenstrom KD, Andrews WW, Tamura T, Du Bard MB, Johnston KE, Hemstreet GP. Elevated amniotic fluid interleukin-6 levels at genetic amniocentesis predict subsequent pregnancy loss. Am J Obstet Gynecol. 1996;175:830-3.
7. Petrikovsky BM, Kaplan GP. Fetal response stoin advertent contact with the needle during amniocentesis. Fetal Diagn Ther. 1995;10:83-5.
8. Wilson RD, Johnson J, Windrim R, Dansereau J, Singer J, Winsor EJT, et al. The early amniocentesis study: a randomized clinical trial of early amniocentesis and midtrimester amniocentesis. II. Evaluation of procedure details and neonatal congenital anomalies. Fetal Diagn Ther. 1997;12:97-101.
9. Sundberg K, Bang J, Smidt-Jensen S, Brocks V, Lundsteen C, Parner J, et al. Randomized study of risk of fetal loss related to early amniocentesis versus chorionic villus sampling. Lancet. 1997;350(9079):697-703.
10. Wilson RD, Kent NE, Johnson J, Bebbington M. Twingestation: evidence-based outcome analysis and literature review for chromosomal aneuploidy, congenital malformations, and pregnancy loss. J Soc Obstet Gynecol Can. 1997;19:1189-200.
11. Winsor EJ, Tomkins DJ, Kalousek D, Farrell S, Wyatt P, Fan YS, et al. Cytogenetic aspects of the Canadian early and mid-trimester amniotic fluid trial (CEMAT). Prenat Diagn. 1999;19:620-7.
12. Wilson RD, Cho K, McGillivrary B, Kalousek D, Shaw D, Baldwin V. Chorionic villus sampling; analysis of fetal losses to delivery, placental pathology and cervical microbiology. Prenat Diagn. 1991;11:539-50.
13. Wilson RD. Chorionic villus sampling: a risk benefit break down. Can J Diagn. 1996;13(2):43-61.
14. DeCatte L, Liebaers I, Foulon W, Bonduelle M, Van Assche E. First trimester chorionic villus sampling in twin gestations. Am J Perinatol. 1996;13:413-7.
15. Kalousek DK, Dill FJ, Pantzar T, McGillivray BC, Yong SL, Wilson RD. Confined chorionic mosaicism in prenatal diagnosis. Hum Genet. 1987;77:163-7
16. Wilson RD, Kendrick V, Wittmann BK, McGillivray B. Spontaneous abortion and pregnancy outcome following normal first trimester ultrasound. Obstet Gynecol. 1986;67: 352-5.
17. Rhoades GG, Jackson LG, Schlesselman SE, et al. The safety and efficacy of chorionic villus sampling for early prenatal diagnosis of cytogenetic abnormalities. N Eng J Med. 1989;320:609-63.
18. Medical Research Council Working Party on the Evaluation of Chorion Villus Sampling, Medical Research Council European trial of chorion villus sampling 1991. Lancet. 1994;337:1491-9.
19. Firth HV, Boyd PA, Chamberlain P, MacKenzie IZ, Lindenbaum RH, Huson SM. Severe limb abnormalities after chorion villus sampling at 56-66 days' gestation. Lancet. 1991;337:762-3.
20. Burton BK, Schultz CJ, Burd LI. Limb abnormalities associated with chorionic villus sampling. Obstet Gynecol. 1992;79:726-30.
21. Froster UG, Jackson L. Limb defects and chorionic villus sampling: results from an international registry, 1992-94. Lancet. 1996;347(9000):489-94 .
22. WHO/PAHO Consultation on CVS. Evaluation of chorionic villus sampling safety. Prenat Diagn. 1999;19:97-9.
23. Hobbins JC, Grannum PA, Romero R, Reece EA, Mahoney MJ. Percutaneous umbilical blood sampling. Am J Obstet Gynecol. 1985;152:1-6.
24. Hickok DE, Mills M. Percutaneous umbilical blood sampling: results from a multicenter collaborative registry. The Western Collaborative Perinatal Group. Am J Obstet Gynecol. 1992;166: 1614-8.
25. Antsaklis A, Daskalakis G, Papantoniou N, Michalas S. Fetal blood sampling: indication-related losses. Prenat Diagn. 1998; 18:934-40.
26. Daffos F, Capella-Pavlovsky M, Forestier F. Fetal blood sampling during pregnancy with use of a needle guided by ultrasound: a study of 606 consecutive cases. Am J Obstet Gynecol. 1985;153:655-60.
27. Maxwell DJ, Johnson P, Hurley P, Neales K, Allan L, Knott P. Fetal blood sampling and pregnancy loss in relation to indication. Br J Obstet Gynaecol. 1991;98:892-7.
28. Orlandi F, Damiani G, Jakil C, Lauricella S, Bertolino O, Maggio A. The risks of early cordocentesis (12-21 weeks): analysis of 500 procedures. Prenat Diagn. 1990;10:425-8.
29. Jauniaux E, Donner C, Simon P, Vanesse M, Hustin J, Rodesch F. Pathologic aspects of the umbilical cord after percutaneous umbilical blood sampling. Obstet Gynecol. 1989;73:215-8.
30. Montemagno R. Soothill P. Invasive Procedures. In: Fisk NM, Moise KJ Jr. (Eds). Fetal Therapy: Invasive and Transplacental. Cambridge: Cambridge UP, 1997;pp.9-26.

CHAPTER

21 Chorionic Villus Sampling

Raju R Sahetya, Ankesh R Sahetya

DEFINITION

1. *Chorionic villus sampling (CVS)*: An invasive procedure performed for first trimester prenatal diagnosis. CVS is typically performed between 70 and 91 days after the first day of last menstrual cycle. In the procedure, tissue withdrawn chorion villi, a part of the chorion frondosum.
2. *Chorion frondosum*: The cellular, outer most extra-embryonic membrane, composed of trophoblastic cells, and develops villi, and forms the fetal component of the placenta.

INTRODUCTION

Sonographically guided chorionic villus sampling (CVS) has been available since the early 1980s and has offered couples at genetic risk an early and rapid prenatal diagnosis.[1] The procedure, which can be performed as early as 10 weeks of menstrual age, provides preliminary cytogenetic results within 48 hours and final culture results within 7 days. In contrast, genetic amniocentesis is not routinely performed until approximately 16 weeks of menstrual age with an additional 7–10 days required to culture the amniotic fluid cells. Thus, the pregnancy is nearly half completed before a definitive diagnosis can be established with amniocentesis. If a significant fetal abnormality is identified, the prospective parents must make a difficult choice of whether to continue or terminate the pregnancy. In addition, the pregnancy is public knowledge, thereby precluding an element of privacy in decision making.

HISTORY

First-trimester prenatal diagnosis is not a new concept. The ability to sample and analyze villus tissue was demonstrated more than 40 years ago by the Chinese who, in an attempt to develop a technique for fetal sex determination.

In 1968, Hahnemann and Mohr attempted blind transcervical (TC) trophoblast biopsy.[2] Although successful tissue culture was obtained, half of these subjects subsequently aborted. In 1973, Kullander and Sandahl used a 5 mm diameter fiberoptic endocervoscope with biopsy forceps to perform TC-CVS in patients requesting pregnancy termination.

In 1974, Hahnemann described further experience with first-trimester prenatal diagnosis using a 2.5 mm hysteroscope and cylindrical biopsy knife.

By this time, the safety of mid-trimester genetic amniocentesis had become well established, and further attempts at first-trimester prenatal diagnosis were temporarily abandoned in the Western hemisphere.

Two technological advances occurred in the early 1980s to allow reintroduction of CVS. The first of these was the development of real-time sonography, making continuous guidance possible. At the same time, sampling instruments were miniaturized and refined. In 1982, Kazy et al. reported the first TC CVS performed with real-time ultrasonography.

CONCEPTS

For years, prenatal diagnosis has relied on the analysis of amniotic fluid fibroblasts as an indirect reflection of the fetal genetic makeup. Similarly, chorionic villi are fetal in origin, and as such are also an appropriate and useful source of tissue for the evaluation of fetal genetic disease. Their cytogenetic, molecular, and biochemical properties reflect those of the fetus. In addition, the villi are partly composed of cytotrophoblast cells, which are an actively dividing source of spontaneous mitoses that can be used to obtain a rapid chromosomal analysis.

INDICATIONS

The major indications are listed below:

- Advanced maternal age (older than 35 years) is the most common indication, accounting for 90% of procedures.[3]
- Previously had a child with a chromosomal abnormality.
- Couples who are carriers of autosomal recessive disease.
- Women who are carriers of a sex linked disease.
- Positive first trimester screen test for trisomies 21, 18 or 13.

PROCEDURE RELATED ANATOMY (FIGS 21.1A AND B)

Between 9 and 12 weeks after the last menstrual period, the developing gestation does not yet fill the uterine cavity. The sac is surrounded by the thick leathery chorionic membranes within which are both the amniotic cavity and the extraembryonic coelom. The amniotic cavity contains the embryo and is enclosed by the thin, whispy, freely mobile amniotic membrane. The extraembryonic coelom is located between the amniotic and chorionic membranes, contains a tenacious mucoid-like substance, and disappears as the amniotic sac grows toward the chorion and the 2 membranes become juxtaposed.

Sampling Techniques

Sampling by CVS is generally performed by transcervial or transabdominal approach, between 70 and 91 days after the first day of last menstrual period. This window is chosen to minimize the background spontaneous miscarriage rate that is higher in early pregnancy, yet still allows sufficient time for results to be available within the first trimester. The chorion frondosum is easily localized by ultrasound as a hyperechoic homogeneous area by this gestational age. In addition, fusion of the amnion and chorion has not yet occurred, thereby decreasing the risk of amnion rupture during the procedure. Sampling significantly earlier in gestation may be associated with an increased risk of fetal abnormalities and should not routinely be done.[4] Transcervical sampling may be more difficult after 12 weeks of menstrual age due to the increasing distance between the cervix and placental site as uterine growth continues.

Both transabdominal and transcervical techniques are equally safe and efficacious, and the majority of patients can be sampled by either techniques (Figs 21.2A and B).

Patient Evaluation

All the indicated cases are evaluated and called for procedure between 10 and 12 weeks of gestational age.

Genetic evaluation: Initial patient contact is with the genetic counselors, where the risks, benefits and alternatives of testing, versus no testing are discussed. Background and procedure related losses are reviewed. Benefits and risks of CVS versus amniocentesis are also discussed. Patient is told that more than one sampling may be neessary. Informed written consent taken before the procedure.

Clinical evaluation: Detailed obstetric history is of utmost importance. Patient with previous abortions, genital warts, Herpes simplex or recent beta *Streptococcus* infection have increased risk. Small or theoretical risk of introduction of infection into the fetal-placental tissues is discussed.

Small subchorionic bleeding manifested by sonolucent areas, usually accompanied by history of vaginal spotting. We attempt to individualize every case, delay the procedure and avoid the area in question, and have found in general CVS can be performed safely in these patients.

Ultrasound evaluation: Fetal viability has to be confirmed. In about 7% of patients a blighted ovum or an anembryonic/ fetal demise may be documented at this time.

Gestational age is evaluated, size-date discrepancies are noted. Of great concern is the smaller than expected fetus. These fetusus are at increased risk for aneuploidy.

Size of the pregnancy also has implication for special DNA studies. In sickle cell disease or cystic fibrosis, increased amount of tissues (20–40 mg) are necessary.

Multiple gestations are also encountered at the time of initial ultrasound.

Chorion frondosum evaluation is of utmost importance to minimize the risk of chorionic injury, detachment, hematoma and subsequent pregnancy loss and above all

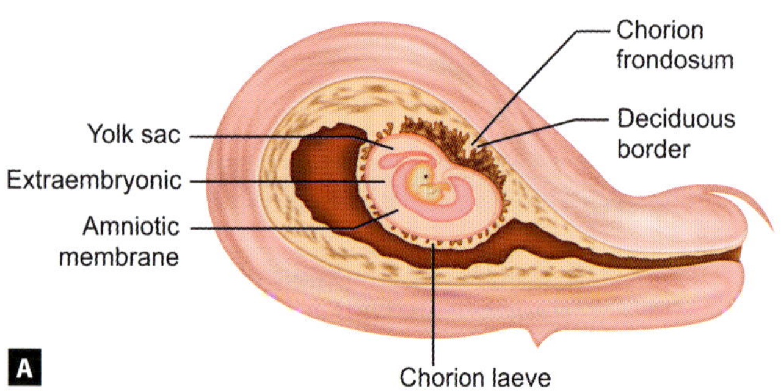

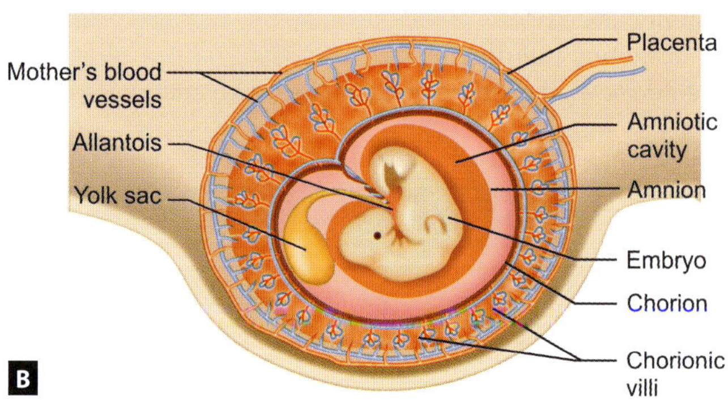

Figs 21.1A and B Procedure related anatomy

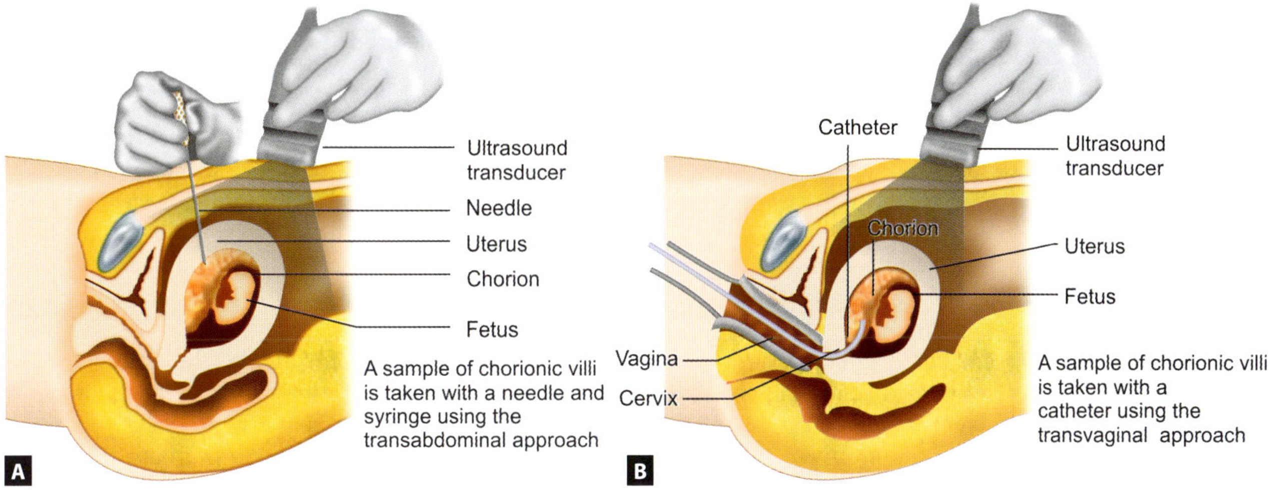

Figs 21.2A and B (A) Transabdominal CVS; (B) Transcervical CVS

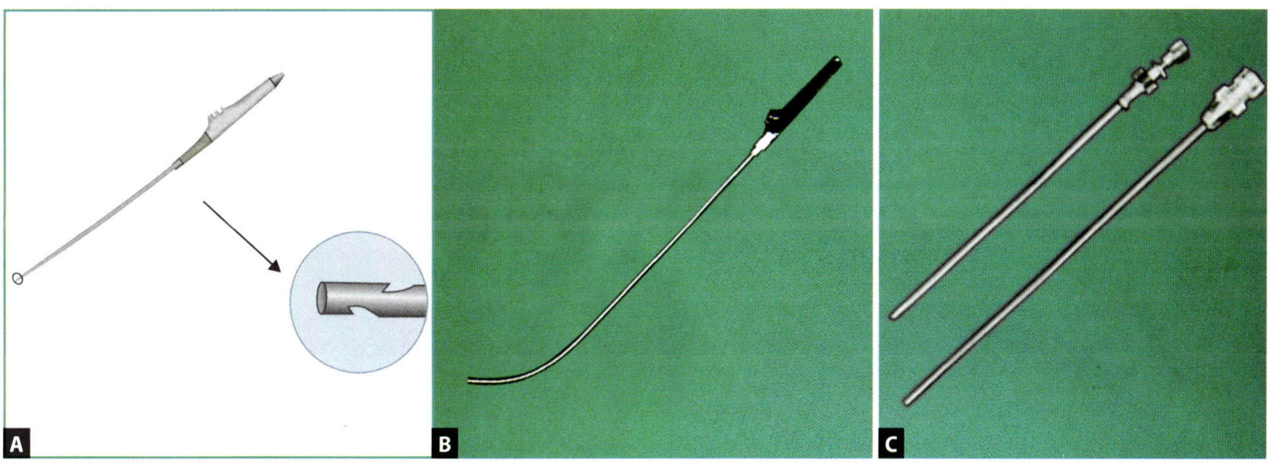

Figs 21.3A to C Types of cannulas

to determine whether the approach will be transcevical or transabdominal.

Last but not the least, intial ultrasound helps the obstetrician and the sonologist to orient the procedure of CVS.

Transcervical Sampling

Several techniques have been described for performing CVS, but only two methods are currently in widespread use.

1. These include the transcervical CVS by using a polyethylene catheter through which a stainlesssteel malleable stylet has been inserted. The stylet fits snugly through the catheter and provides sufficient rigidity for adequate passage through the cervix and into the frondosum. The stylet has a rounded, blunt end that protrudes slightly beyond the end of the catheter to prevent sharp edges that may potentially perforate the membranes. The catheter has a luerlock end to accommodate a syringe. However, this catheter has recently been removed from the market by the manufacturer, leaving the catheter manufactured by the Cook Company (Spencer, IN, USA) as the only commercially available TC sampling device. Also popular is the use of, economical, re-usable after autoclave, a stainless steel, mealeable, with olive tip cannula guage 16 mm.

   Modified PortexTC CVS Cannula/Cook TC CVS catheter/SS Malleable Cannula (Figs 21.3A to C).
2. Transabdominal, dispoable, spinal needle, guage 20/21, aspiration using mechanical suction.

Before performing the CVS procedure, ultrasound scanning confirms fetal viability and establishes the area of the chorionfrondosum. An approach is mentally mapped that allows catheter placement parallel to the chorionic membrane. Uterine contractions may be present and obstruct or alter the sampling path (Figs 21.4A and B). They may also alter the appearance and location of the placenta by pulling it.

The maternal bladder should be sufficiently full to provide an acoustic window through which the vagina, cervix, and uterus can be visualized. Overfilling makes retrieval more difficult by increasing patient discomfort.

The procedure is performed in the lithotomy position on a standard examination table with foot stirrups. A speculum is inserted, and the vagina and cervix are cleansed with antiseptic solution. The catheter is prepared by slightly curving its distal 3- to 5-cm part with the guidewire in place to allow easy insertion through the cervix. In most cases, only a minimal amount of curvature is required. The cervical canal is then reimaged by ultrasound, and the catheter is introduced through the cervix until loss of resistance at the internal os is felt. Once the sonographer clearly identifies the catheter tip, it is guided by real-time sector scanning to the placental site (Figs 21.5A and B). The catheter is directed by gently maneuvering the curved periphery of the gestational sac. Occasionally use of a single-tooth tenaculum on the cervix is needed to alter uterine position.

To ensure an adequate sample, the catheter should be advanced through the full length of the chorion. The guidewire is then removed, and a 20-cc syringe containing approximately 5 cc of a collection medium is attached.

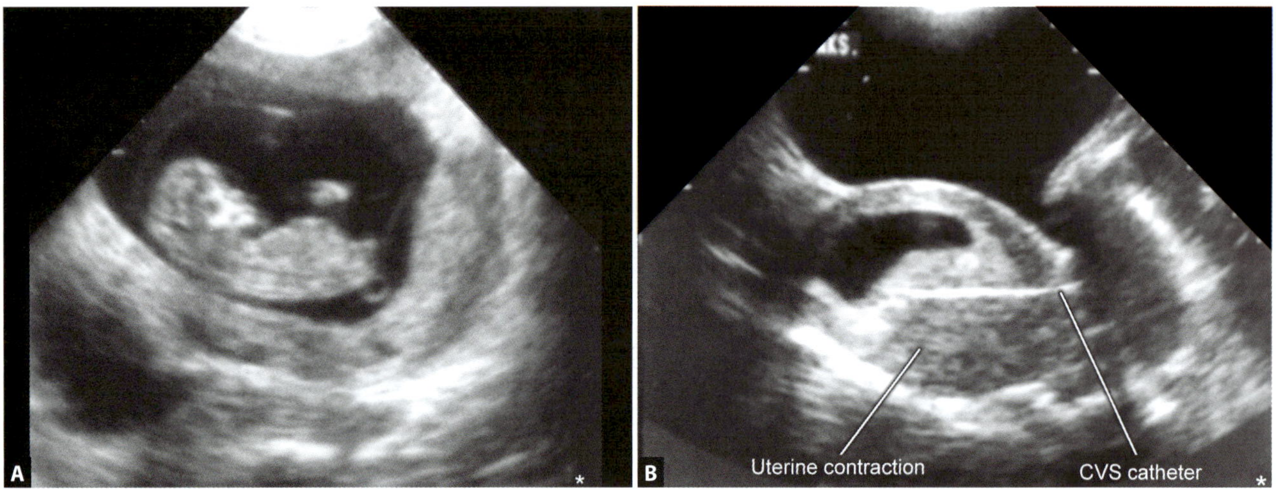

Figs 21.4A and B Uterine contraction affecting the procedure

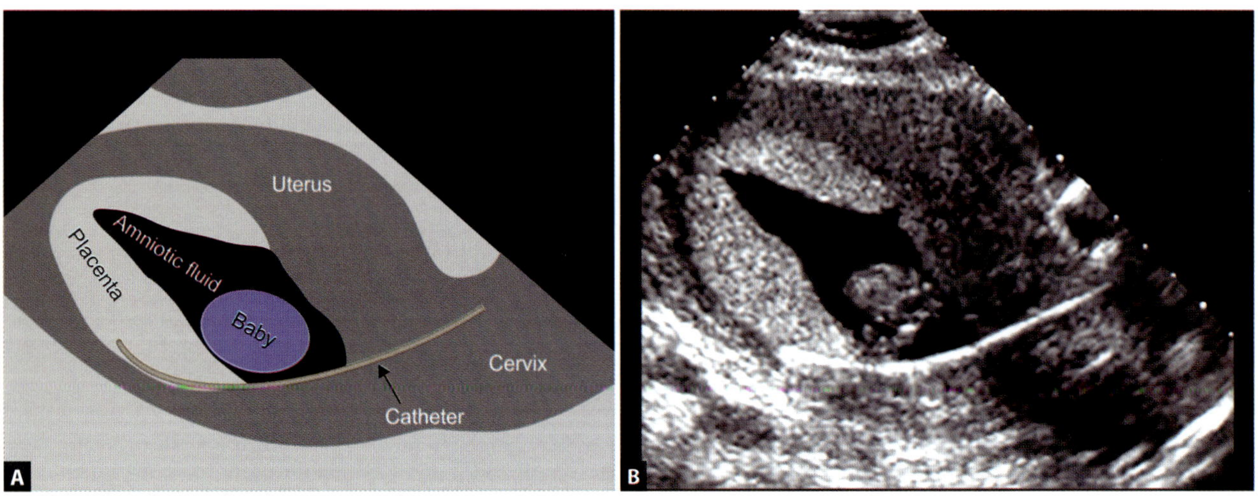

Figs 21.5A and B Showing diagrammatic and ultrasound placement of the catheters

The sample is collected by aspiration using negative pressure with to and fro movements and, as the catheter is slowly withdrawn.

DIFFICULTIES ENCOUNTERED: HOW TO OVERCOME?

Factors resulting to difficult procedure are, deviated uterus, retroverted fixed uterus, lateral location of chorion frondosum, previous cesarean with stenosed cervix, acute angulation of cervix with the uterus, cervical and uterine myoma, ultrasound artefacts, too little or too full urinary bladder.

Due to bladder: Urine in the bladder acts as an ascoutic window, it is very important that it should be adequately full. Too little may make procedure unclear and risky. Too full bladder may make procedure related manuarability difficult. Waiting for the bladder to adequately fill up or ultrasound guided empting of bladder may be required for safe procedure (Fig. 21.6).

Due to cervix and cervical canal: Long tubular and stenosed cervix may not only make entry of the olive tip cannula difficult, may also use up extra length of the cannula and also straighten the preformed curve of the malleable cannula desired for the procedure. A small myoma, just above the internal OS, may cause pain and initiation of a contraction may change the orientation for the procedure. Acutely anteverted and anteflexed cervicouterine angle makes negotiation of the cannula difficult. Cervical erosion with infection leads to bleeding on touch and may risk ascending infection. Adequate dilatation of cervix, adequate bladder, pre-treatment of any infection and relavent counseling makes procedure acceptable and safe (Fig. 21.7).

Due to uterus position and cervico uterine relation: Retroverted fixed uterus make procedure related mobility difficult and leads to in adequate sampling. Anticipating the difficulty one can preform the curve accordingly and orient, as an ink port approach, with in and out movement of the cannula sono guided in the chorion frondosum. Deviated uterus requires special expertise and obstetrician-sonologist coordination, all the way, from cervix upto the internal OS to lateral approch to the chorion frondosum. Intervening myoma along the path has to avoided by the sono-guided approach (Fig. 21.8).

Due to chorion frondosum location: For low lying chorion previa, it is best to delay the procedure until migration of the same upwards or opt for transabdominal approach. A sub-chorionic hematoma requires treatment and delay in the procedure. When chorion frondosum is not very obviously identified due to thin chorionic tissue all around, cord

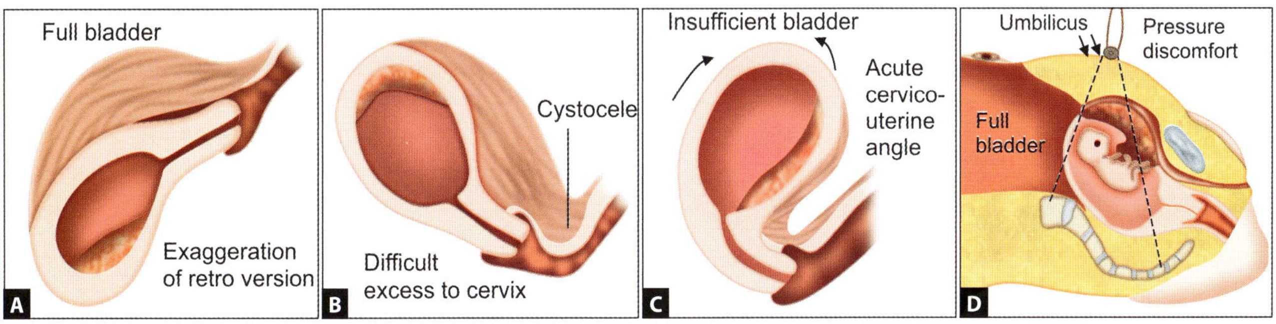

Figs 21.6A to D Difficulties encountered in the procedure due to urinary bladder

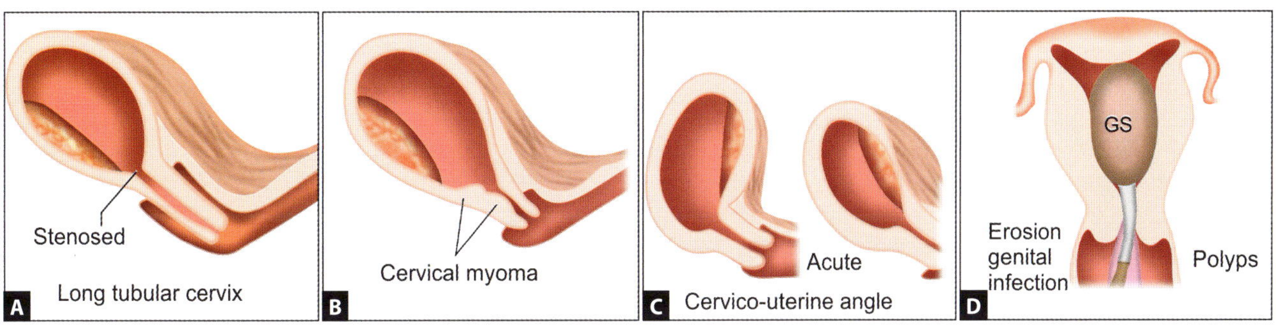

Figs 21.7A and B Difficulties encountered due to different types of cervices

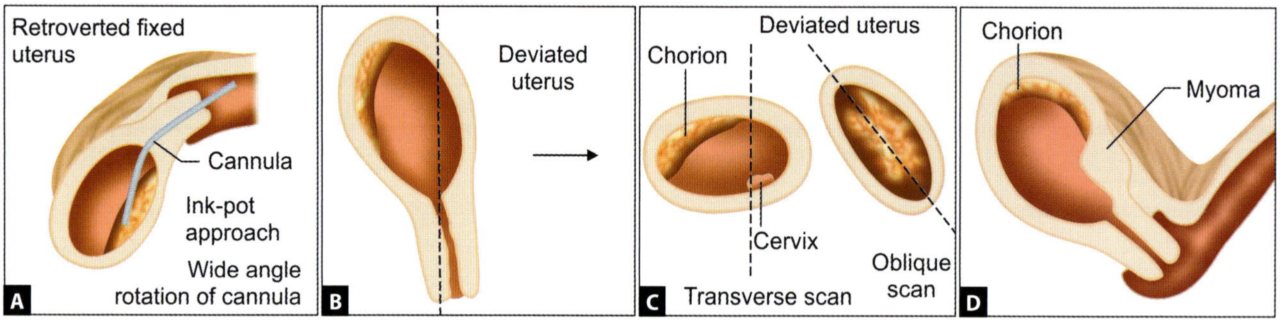

Figs 21.8A to D Difficulties encountered due to different types of uterine positions and myoma

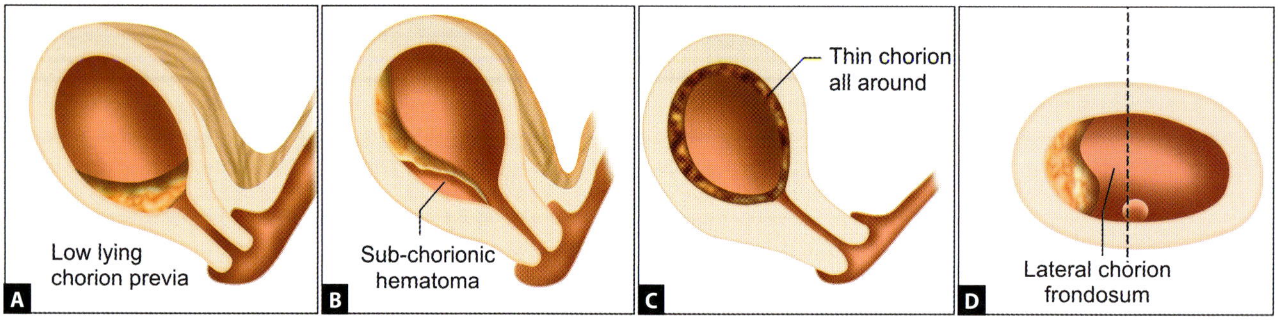

Figs 21.9A to D Difficulties encountered due to different kinds of chorion frondosum

insertion as a marker helps to identify the same. Counseling that a repeat procedure may be require if inadequate sample or unhealthy tissue is obtained. Lateral placement of chorion frondosum requires a well guided lateral path and approach for the procedure (Fig. 21.9).

Transcervical Contraindications

Cervical polyps, active cervical, or vaginal herpes.

Transabdominal Chorionic Villus Sampling

Two techniques for transabdominal (TA) sampling are presently used. In the single-needle approach a 20-gauge spinal needle is used.[5]Alternatively, some operators perform a double-needle technique that uses an outer guide needle (18-gauge thin wall standard spinal needle) and a smaller sampling needle (20 gauge).[6] In general, a 3.5-inch- long needle is sufficient for most patients, but a 5- or 6-inch-long needle should be available for very obese women.

With the single-needle technique, a sampling path is chosen so that the tip of the needle passes within the chorionfrondosum parallel to the chorionic membrane. Intervening bowel and bladder must be avoided. The needle tip is first inserted into the myometrium and then redirected parallel to the membrane. As with cervical sampling, the needle should be passed through as much villus tissue as possible and remain parallel to the chorionic membrane to avoid inadvertent puncture. Once appropriately placed within the chorion, the stylet is removed and a syringe containing 5 cc of media is attached. Under continuous suction, 4 or 5 to-and-fro passes within the frondosum are made. The needle is then removed from the abdomen while suction is continued. This “vacuuming” technique is required to ensure retrieval of sufficient villus tissue because the diameter of the 20-gauge needle is slightly smaller than that of a TC catheter.

The 2-needle technique uses a slightly larger-gauge spinal needle as a trocar, which is inserted into the myometrium. A thinner (19- to 20-gauge) and longer sampling needle is passed through the trocar into the chorion frondosum. The stylet of the sampling needle is then replaced with a syringe, and sampling is performed as with a single needle.

Sonogram illustrating transabdominal chorionic villus sampling. The needle is parallel to the chorionic plate (Figs 21.10A and B).

Transabdominal Contraindications

Patients undergoing transabdominal CVS were over all seen to be somewhat in less discomfort compared to transcervical CVS.

Operator difficulties were due to anterior wall uterine myoma and uterine contractions, posterior location of

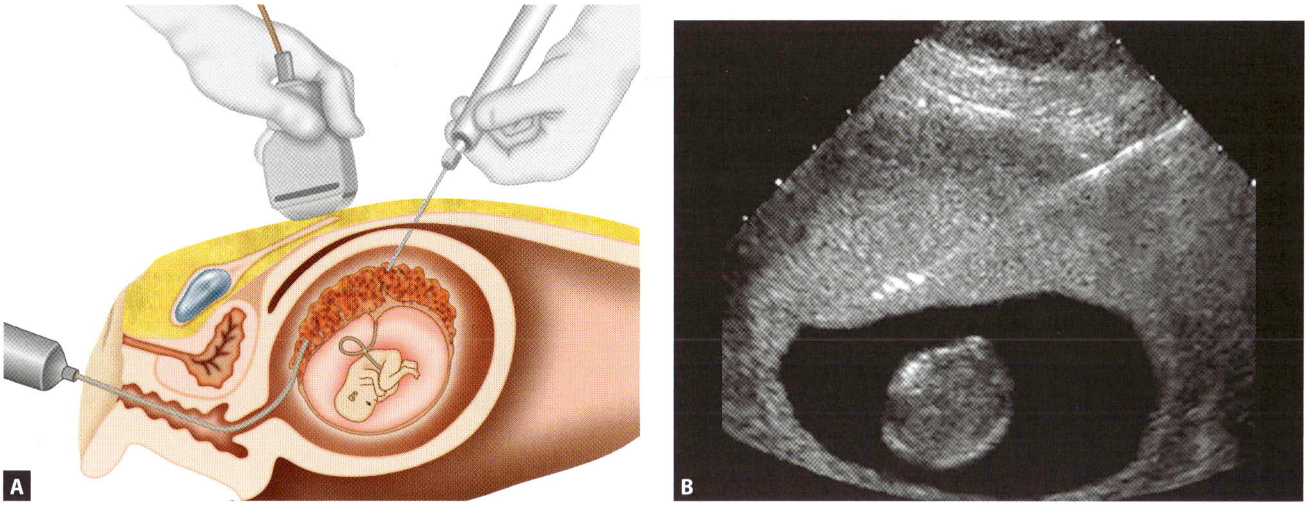

Figs 21.10A and B Diagrammatic and ultrasound images of a transabdominal CVS

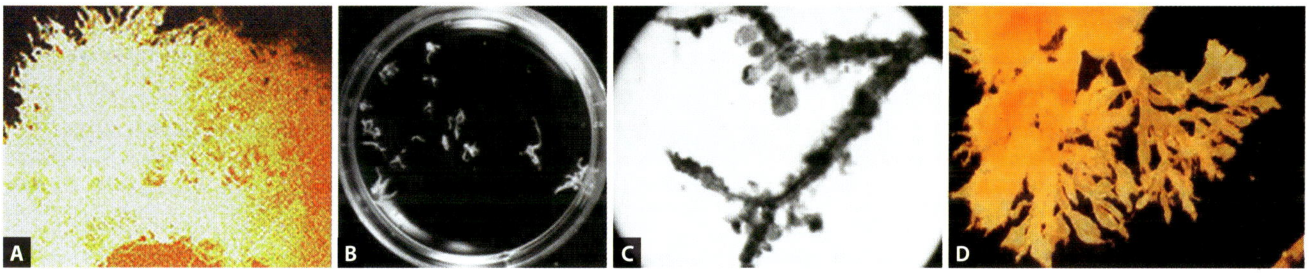

Figs 21.11A to D Vascular and mesencymal structures of the chorionic villi

chorion frondosum, interceding bowel, obesity, previous surgical scars and requirement of mechanical suction.

Confirmation of Adequate Tissue Retrieval

The presence of adequate villus tissue can usually be confirmed by visual inspection of the syringe contents or empting the same in a sterile petri dish placed on a vertical torch, but occasionally the sample may need to be evaluated under a dissecting microscope. Samples typically contain a mixture of predominantly villi with a small amount of maternally derived decidua. The chorionic villi appear as free-floating, white structures with fluffy, filiforme branches. Contaminating decidua tissue has a more amorphous appearance and lacks distinct branches. Although these 2 tissues can usually be grossly distinguished by virtue of their respective morphology, confirmation under a dissecting microscope is required if there is uncertainty that adequate villi have been retrieved.

Microscopically, the villi have a distinctive frond-like, branched appearance. Their surface is punctuated by small buds consisting of an outer syncytiotrophoblast covering and a core of mitotically active cytotrophoblast cells. Within the center of each villus is the mesenchymal core, through which capillaries carrying fetal blood cells course (Fig. 21.11).

A minimum of 10–15 mg of villus tissue when weighed wet is required for most genetic analyses. If insufficient villi are present with the initial attempt, a second aspiration may be performed without additional risk.[3] Pregnancy loss rates increase significantly when more than 2 insertions are required.

Patients may resume normal physical activity after CVS, although strenuous exercise should be avoided for 24 hours. Sexual abstinence is recommended for a week or two of time to minimize any risk of ascending infection. Patients may have some mild vaginal bleeding after CVS; therefore, they should be counseled about this possibility before sampling.

RISKS ASSOCIATED WITH CHORIONIC VILLUS SAMPLING

Bleeding

Vaginal bleeding is uncommon after TA CVS but is seen in 7–10% of patients sampled transcervically. Minimal spotting is a common occurrence and may occur in almost one-third of cases, the bleeding is self-limited and the pregnancy outcome is excellent.

Infection

Since the initial development of TC CVS, there has been concern that transvaginal passage of an instrument would introduce vaginal flora into the uterus.[7-9] However, in clinical practice, the incidence of post-CVS chorioamnionitis is low.[10] Infection after TA CVS also occurs and has been demonstrated, at least in some cases, to be secondary to bowel flora introduced by inadvertent puncture by the sampling needle.

Ruptured Membranes

Acute rupture of the membranes, documented by either obvious gross fluid leakage or a decrease in measurable amnionic fluid on ultrasound evaluation, is a very rare complication of CVS. Experimental attempts to rupture membranes intentionally with a TC catheter have confirmed that the chorion can withstand significant punishment without perforation.

Elevated MSAFP

An acute rise in MSAFP after CVS has been consistently reported, implying a detectable degree of fetal maternal bleeding.[11-13] The elevation is transient, occurs more frequently after TA CVS, and appears to be dependent on the quantity of tissue aspirated.

Rh Isoimmunization

In Rh-negative women, the otherwise negligible fetal maternal bleeding that follows CVS accrues special importance because Rh-positive cells in volumes as low as 0.1 mL have been shown to cause Rh sensitization.[13,14] Because all women with even a single pass of a catheter or needle show detectable rises in MSAFP, it seems prudent that all Rh-negative nonsensitized women undergoing CVS receive Rho (D) immunoglobulin subsequent to the procedure.

Pregnancy Loss

Multiple reports from individual centers have demonstrated the safety and low pregnancy loss rates after CVS.[3,15-22] In experienced centers, the rate of miscarriage from the time of CVS until 28 weeks of gestation is approximately 2–3%.[23] However, to determine the incidence of procedure-induced pregnancy loss, adjustments for the relatively high background loss at this gestational age must be made.

The consensus of the recent literature indicates that with experienced operators, the procedural complication rates with CVS and amniocentesis is comparable; however, CVS is more difficult to learn.[24]

RISK OF FETAL ABNORMALITIES AFTER CHORIONIC VILLUS SAMPLING

It has recently been suggested that CVS may be associated with the occurrence of specific fetal malformations. CVS and limb abnormality were observed when CVS was performed prior to 8.6 weeks gestation as reported, this could be due to vascular insult, resulting to incomplete morphogenesis and disrupted normal embryo. To ensure safety, CVS should be performed between 10 and 11 weeks of gestation.

PERINATAL RISKS AND IMPACT ON LONG-TERM DEVELOPMENT OF THE INFANT

No increases in preterm labor, mid-trimester oligohydramnios, premature rupture of the membranes, small-for-gestational-age infants, maternal morbidity, or other obstetric complications have occurred in sampled patients.

LABORATORY ASPECTS OF CHORIONIC VILLUS SAMPLING

CVS is now considered a reliable method of prenatal diagnosis, but early in its development incorrect results were reported.[25-27] The major sources of these errors included maternal cell contamination and misinterpretation of mosaicism confined to the placenta. Today, genetic evaluation of chorionic villi provides a high degree of success and accuracy, in particular with regard to the diagnosis of common trisomies.

Chorionic villi have 3 major components: (1) an outer layer of hormonally active and invasive syncytiotrophoblast, (2) a middle layer of cytotrophoblast from which syncytiotrophoblast is derived, and (3) an inner mesodermal core containing blood, capillaries for oxygen, and nutrient exchange (Figs 21.12A and B).

After collection, the villi are cleaned of any adherent decidua and then exposed to trypsin to digest and separate the cytotrophoblast from the underlying mesodermal core. The cytotrophoblast has a high mitotic index, with many spontaneous mitoses available for immediate chromosomal analysis. The liquid suspension containing the cytotrophblast

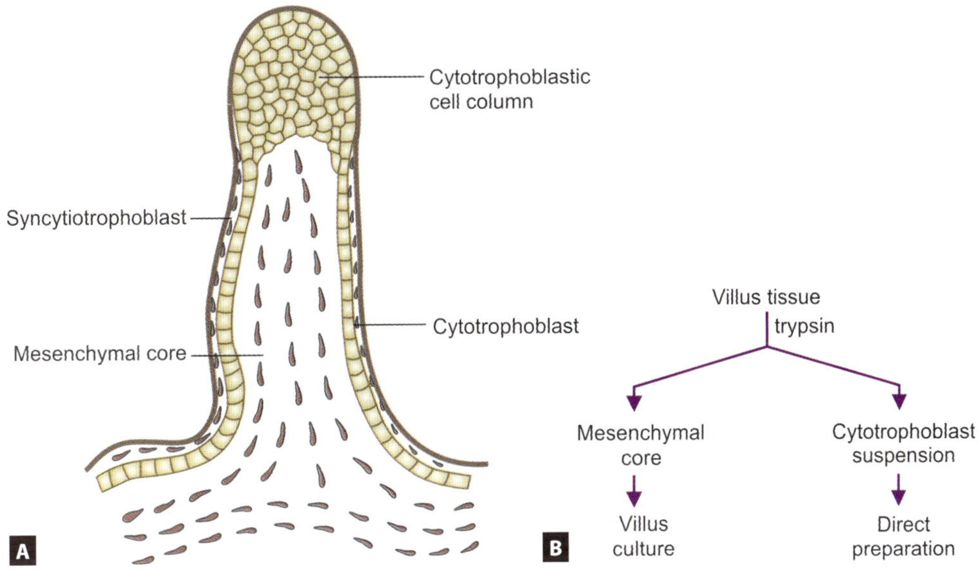

Figs 21.12A and B Anatomy of a villi

is either dropped immediately onto a slide for analysis or may undergo a short incubation.[28-31] This "direct" chromosomal preparation can provide preliminary results within 2–3 hours. However, most laboratories now use overnight incubation to improve karyotype quality and thus report results within 2–4 days. The remaining villus core is placed in tissue culture and is typically ready for harvest and chromosome analysis within 1 week. The direct method has the advantage of providing a rapid result and minimizing the decidual contamination, whereas tissue culture is better for interpreting discrepancies between the cytotrophoblast and the actual fetal state.

CONFINED PLACENTAL MOSAICISM

The CVS mosaic results require diligent follow-up by amniocentesis or fetal sampling to determine their clinical significance because, in most cases, if the mosaic results are confined to the placenta, fetal development will be normal. However, if the mosaic cell line also involves the fetus, there may be significant phenotypic consequences. Mosaicism occurs in about 1% of all CVS samples[32-35] but is confirmed in the fetus in only 10–40% of these cases.

BIOCHEMICAL AND DNA PROCEDURES

Most biochemical and molecular diagnoses that can be made from amnionic fluid or cultured amniocytes can also be made from chorionic villi. In many cases, the results will be available more rapidly and more efficiently by using villi, because sufficient enzyme or DNA is present in villus samples to allow direct analysis rather than wait for tissue culture.

CHORIONIC VILLUS SAMPLING IN MULTIPLE GESTATIONS (FIGS 21.13A TO C)

Chorionic villus sampling is a safe and effective approach to examining twins. Not only does it provide results early in pregnancy, but, if discordancy is discovered, the medical and psychological difficulties encountered with selective termination can be minimized. However, it can be technically more demanding because it requires an experienced operator and sonographer. The ideal time to perform a twin CVS is similar to that for singletons. Ultrasound initially identifies placental locations, determines chorionicity, and confirms fetal sizes and viability. Sampling of each sac is independently performed by either a TC or TA approach, with separate passes of a new sampling instrument for each attempt. Because no unique marker is available to ensure that the samples have been retrieved from distinct placentas, it is imperative that insertion of the instrument into each frondosum is certain. Longitudinal and transverse scanning planes should be used to ensure proper location. One has to limit the aspiration sites to ensure tissue from desired gestational sac. If any doubt exists, a repeat procedure is required, but with increased experience, the need for repeat procedure is rare.[36]

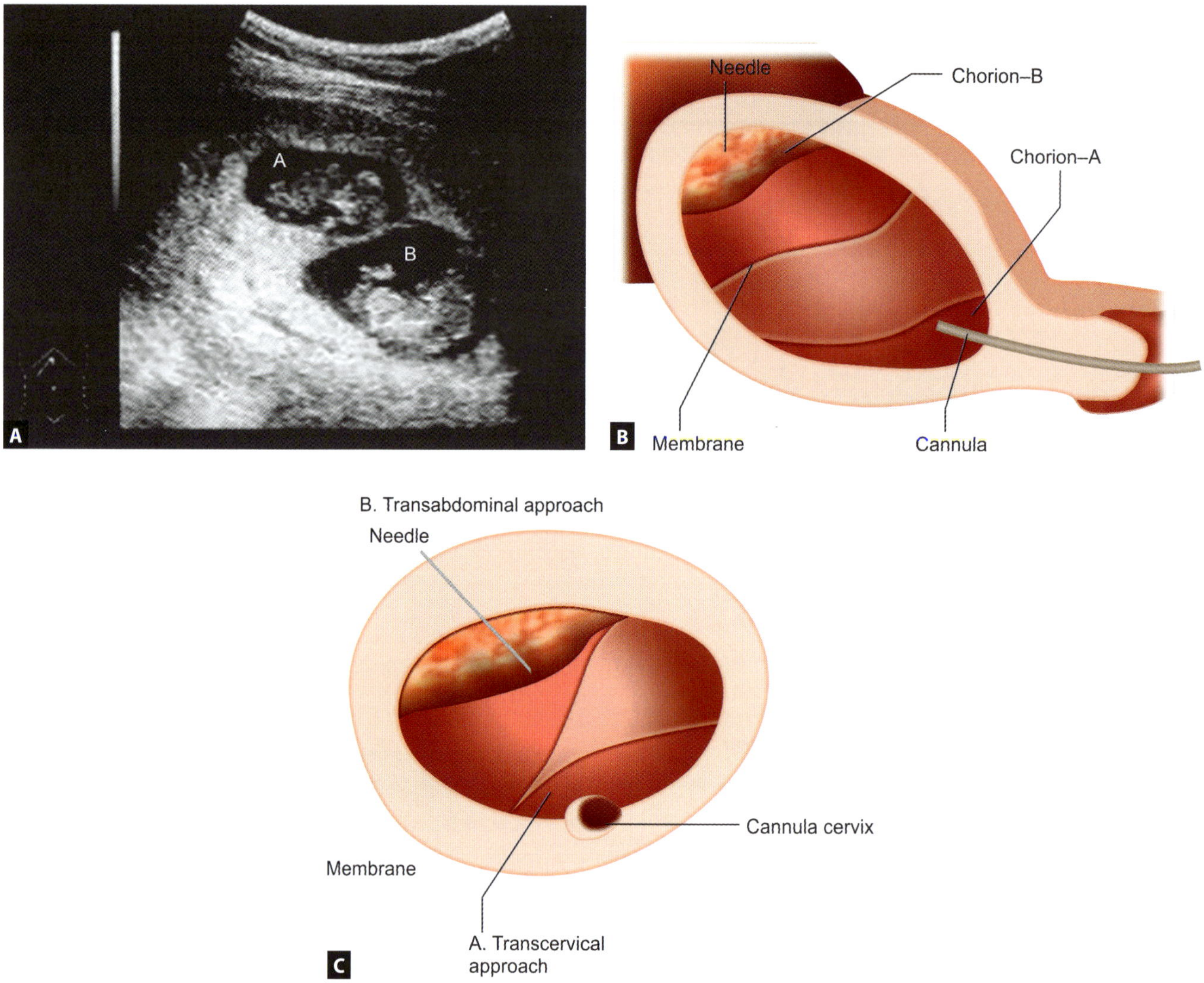

Figs 21.13A to C Procedure of CVS in multifetal pregnancy

CHORIONIC VILLUS SAMPLING AND MULTIFETAL PREGNANCY REDUCTION

Multifetal pregnancy reduction (MFPR) to improve perinatal outcome is an unfortunate but accepted part of reproductive medicine. As with selective termination, MFPR is most safely performed in the first-trimester.[37] Therefore, in high-order gestations at increased risk for a genetic abnormality, CVS before a reduction can avoid the potential need for a later selective termination. The CVS can be performed between 10 weeks and 11.5 weeks of gestation, and a rapid karyotype can be available within 24–48 hours, after which the MFPR is performed.

SUMMARY

Chorionic villus sampling is a safe technique for first-trimester prenatal diagnosis of genetic disorders. Real-time sonography and technologic advances of sampling instruments have been critical in establishing a safe technique for retrieving villus tissue for genetic analysis. Clinical trials suggest that CVS carries a low risk of pregnancy loss, which is comparable to that of second-trimester amniocentesis. An understanding of the laboratory techniques and human embryology is essential in avoiding diagnostic errors related to confined placental mosaicism.

To maximize outcome, CVS should be performed by an experienced team of physicians, ultrasonographers, and genetic laboratory technicians. Before initiating a CVS program, operators should have considerable experience in the placement of the catheter, which can be achieved either in a formal training program with observation of 50 procedures followed by close hands-on supervision of another 100 cases,[3] or by supervised practice on pregnancies undergoing subsequent abortion. In addition, it is advisable to limit the number of ultrasonographers assigned to assist in this procedure, because sampling success is equally dependent on skillful ultrasound guidance. Similar to the physician retrieving the villi, the guiding sonographer should be knowledgeable in the didactics of CVS sampling and should obtain adequate hands-on training before beginning work in this area. This can be achieved in a formal training program or by visiting centers performing this procedure.[3] In this setting, CVS will continue to be an important, reliable, and safe contributor to prenatal genetic diagnosis.

- Chorionic villus sampling has a low complication rate comparable to mid-trimester amniocentesis in experienced hands. The learning curve is more difficult with CVS.
- CVS is the preferable method of fetal aneuploidy testing in the first trimester.
- CVS is generally performed after 10 completed weeks of gestation. In this setting, there does not seem to be an increased risk of limb reduction defects.
- CVS may be performed either transabdominally or transcervically.
- Caution should be exercised in the interpretation of a mosaic of chromosomal findings from CVS.
- The complications of CVS include miscarriage, bleeding, rupture of membranes, and infection.

REFERENCES

1. American College of Obsetetricians and Gynecologists. Invasive prenatal testing for aneuploidy. ACOG Practice Bulletin 88, Washington, DC: 2007.
2. Hahnemann N, Mohr J. Genetic diagnosis in the embryo by means of biopsy from extraembryonic membranes. Bull EurSoc Hum Genet. 1968;2:23-9.
3. Boehm FH, Salyer SL, Dev VG, et al. Chorionic villus sampling: quality control-m-A continuous improvement model. Am J Obstet Gynecol. 1993;168:1766-77.
4. Jackson LG, Zachary JM, Fowler SE, Desnick RJ, Golbus MS, Ledbetter DH, et al. A randomized comparison ot transcervical and transabdominal chorionic-villus rampling. N Engl J Med. 1992;327(9):594-8.
5. Evans MI, Andriole S. Chorionic villus sampling and amniocentesis in 2008. Curr Opin Obstet Gynecol. 2008;20(1):164-8.
6. Smidt-Jensen S, Hahnemann N. Transabdominal chorionic villus sampling for fetal genetic diagnosis. Technical and obstetric evaluation of 100 cases. Prenat Diagn. 1988;8:7.
7. Brambati B, Matarrelli M, Varotto F. Septic complications after chorionic villus sampling. Lancet. 1987;i(8543):1212a.
8. Wass D, Bennett MJ. Infection and chorionic villus sampling. Lancet. 1985;ii:338.
9. Scialli AR, Neugebauer DL, Fabro SE. Microbiology of the endcervix in patients undergoing chorionic villus sampling. In: Fracearo M, Simoni G, Brambati B (Eds). First Trimester Fetal Diagnosis. Berlin: Springer-Verlag. 1985. pp. 69-73.
10. Rhoads GG, Jackson IG, Schlesselman SE, et al. The safety and efficacy of chorionic villus sampling for early prenatal diagnosis of cyto- genetic abnormalities. N Engl J Med. 1989;320:609-9.
11. Blakemore KJ, Baumgarten A, Schoenfeld-Dimaio M, et al. Rise in maternal serum alpha-fetoprotein concentration after chorionic villus sampling. Lancet. 1985;ii:339.
12. Bramabati B, Guercilena S, Bonacchi I, et al. Fetomaternal transfusion after chorionic villus sampling: clinical implications. Hum Reprod. 1986;1:37.
13. Shulman LP, Meyers CM, Simpson JL, et al. Fetomaternal transfusion depends on amount of chorionic villi aspirated but not on method of chorionic villus sampling. Am J Obstet Gynecol. 1990;162:1185.
14. Zipursky A, Israels LG. The pathogenesis and prevention of Rh immunization. Can Med Assoc J. 1967;97:1245-57.
15. Clark BA, Bissonnette J, Olson SB, et al. Pregnancy loss in a small chorionic villus sampling series. Am J Obstet Gynecol. 1989;161:301.
16. Green JE, Dorfman A, Jones SL, et al. Chorionic villus sampling: 66. Mastroiacovo P, Botto LD, Cavalcanti DP. Limb anomalies following chorionic villus sampling: a registry based case control study. Am J Med Genet. 1992;44:856-63.
17. Gustavii B, Claesson V, Kristoffersson U, et al. Risk of miscarriage after chorionic biopsy is probably not higher than after amniocentesis. Lakartidningen. 1989;86:4221.
18. Jahoda MGJ, Pijpers L, Reuss A, et al. Evaluation of transcervical chorionic villus sampling with a completed follow-up of 1550 con-secutive pregnancies. Prenat Diagn. 1989;9:621.
19. Young SR, Shipley CF, Wade RV, et al. Single-center comparison of results of 1000 prenatal diagnoses with chorionic villus sampling and 1000 diagnoses with amniocentesis. Am J Obstet Gynecol. 1991;165:255.
20. Hogge WA, Schonberg SA, Golbus MS. Chorionic villus sampling: experience of the first 1000 cases. Am J Obstet Gynecol. 1986;154(1):249-52.
21. Jackson LG. CVS Newslett. 1988;25-7.
22. Wade RV, Young SR. Analysis of fetal loss after transcervical chorionic villus sampling: A review of 719 patients. Am J Obstet Gynecol 1989;161:513-9.
23. Jackson LG, Zachary JM, Fowler SE, et al. Randomized comparison of transcervical and transabdominal chorionic villus sampling. N Engl J Med. 1992;327:594-8.

24. Evans MI, Andriole S. Chorionic villus sampling and amniocentesis in 2008. Curr Opin Obstet Gynecol. 2008; 20(1):164-8.
25. Martin AO, Simpson JL, Rosinksy BJ, et al. Chorionic villus sampling in continuing pregnancies II: cytogenetic reliability. Am J Obstet Gynecol. 1986;154:1653-62.
26. Simoni G, Gimelli G, Cuoco C, et al. Discordance between prenatal cytogenetic diagnosis after chorionic villi sampling and chromoso-mal constitution of the fetus. In: Fraccaro M, Simoni G, Brambati B, eds. First Trimester Fetal Diagnosis. Heidelberg: Springer-Verlag. 1985. pp. 137-43.
27. Cheung SW, Crane JP, Beaver HA, et al. Chromosome mosaicism and maternal cell contamination in chorionic villi. Prenat Diagn. 1987;7:535-42.
28. Simoni G, Brambati B, Danesino C, et al. Efficient direct chromo- some analyses and enzyme determinations from chorionic villi sam-ples in the first trimester of pregnancy. Hum Genet. 1983;63:349.
29. Ford JH, Jahnke AB. Handling of chorionic villus for direct chromo- some studies. Lancet. 1983;2:1491.
30. Gregson NM, Seabright N. Handling of chorionic villi for direct chromosome studies. Lancet. 1983;2:1491.
31. Chang HC, Jones OW, Masui H. Human amniotic fluid cells grown in a hormone-supplemented medium: suitability for prenatal diag- nosis. Proc Natl Acad Sci USA. 1982;79:4795.
32. Mikkelsen M, Ayme S. Chromosomal findings in chorionic villi. In: Vogel F, Sperling K, eds. Human Genetics. Heidelberg: Springer-Verlag. 1987;597.
33. Ledbetter DH, Zachary JL, Simpson MS, et al. Cytogenetic results from the US collaborative study on CVS. Prenat Diagn. 1992;12:317.
34. Vejerslev LO, Mikkelsen M. The European collaborative study on mosaicism in chorionic villus sampling: data from 1986-1987. PrenalDiagn. 1989;9:575.
35. Breed ASPM, Mantingh A, Vosters R, et al. Follow-up and pregnancy outcome after a diagnosis of mosaicism in CVS. Prenat Diagn. 1991;11:577.
36. Wapner RJ, Johnson A, Davis G, et al. Prenatal diagnosis in twin gesta- tions: a comparison between second trimester amniocentesis and first trimester chorionic villus sampling. Obstet Gynecol. 1993;82:49-56.
37. Evans MI, Wapner RJ, Carpenter R, et al. International collaboration on multifetal pregnancy reduction: dramatically improved outcomes with increased experience. Obstet Gynecol. 1999;180:S28.

CHAPTER

22 Amniocentesis

Ankesh R Sahetya, Divya A Sahetya

INTRODUCTION

Amniocentesis was introduced in clinical practice in the 19th century for the treatment of polyhydramnios. The technique was subsequently used in the 1930s for amniography and elective termination of the pregnancy, whereas the specific interest in obtaining amniotic fluid for prenatal diagnosis began in the 1950s with the management of pregnancies complicated by isoimmunization. The first prenatal diagnosis of a chromosomal anomaly, a balanced translocation, was reported by Jacobson and Barter in 1967.[1]

The relative simplicity of the method and widespread availability of ultrasonographic equipment and expertize made amniocentesis the most widely used invasive method for prenatal diagnosis.

INDICATIONS[1,2]

The most common indication is prenatal diagnosis, more specifically the diagnosis of chromosomal anomalies and neural tube defects in the early second trimester. In the third trimester, most of the procedures are performed to assess fetal lung maturity.

- Late first and second trimester diagnosis—cytogenetic diagnosis, diagnosis of neural tube defects, diagnosis of metabolic disorders.
- Late second and third trimester diagnosis—evaluation of the severity of isoimmunization, evaluation of fetal lung maturity, diagnosis of intra-amniotic infection, confirmation of ruptured membranes.
- Therapeutic—drainage of polyhydramnios, medical treatment of fetal disorders.

AMNIOCENTESIS FOR CYTOGENETIC DIAGNOSIS[3,4]

Cytogenetic diagnosis is routinely offered to women 35 years of age and older, to couples with chromosomal rearrangements, to women with a previous offspring affected by a chromosomal disorder, to women carrying an X-linked disease and to parents with a recessive gene for a metabolic disease or hemoglobinopathy. When amniocentesis is used for cytogenetic diagnosis it is usually performed after 15 weeks, most commonly between 16 and 18 weeks. Cytogenetic studies are usually completed in 1–2 weeks, allowing timely interruption of the pregnancy in case of a positive diagnosis.

Midtrimester Amniocentesis[3,4]

Technique (Figs 22.1 to 22.4)

Selecting a puncture site: Ultrasound is performed prior to amniocentesis to determine the number of fetuses, viability, placental location and the amount of amniotic fluid. The presence of uterine and fetal anomalies are specifically sought, since they may interfere with performance of the procedure. A site of puncture avoiding placental tissue or umbilical cord in the needle path is selected. In case a transplacental puncture is necessary, the place with the least amount of placental tissue should be selected.

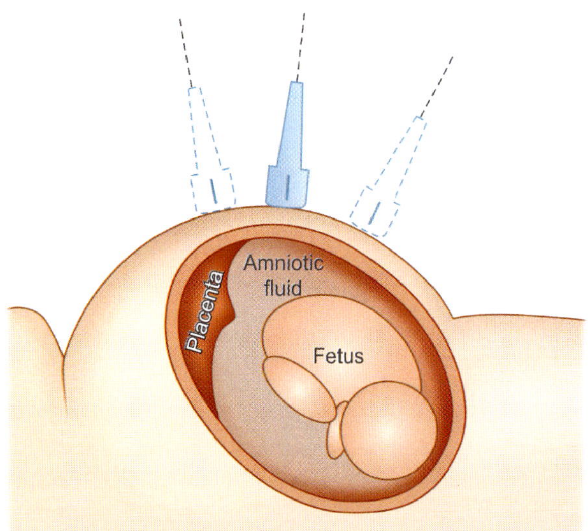

Fig. 22.1 Transverse sweep of the maternal abdomen with ultrasound probe

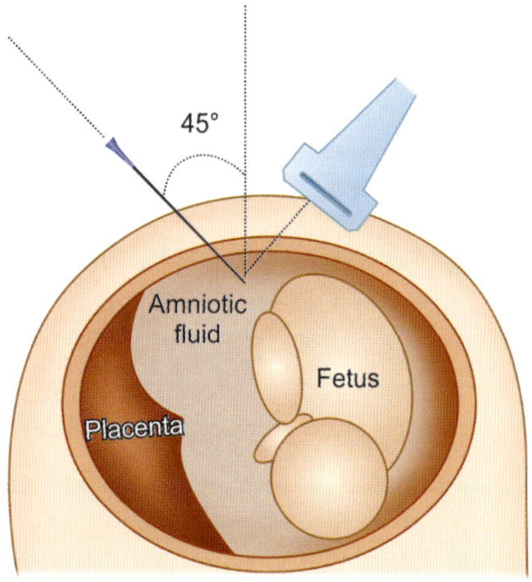

Fig. 22.2 Puncture of the maternal abdomen

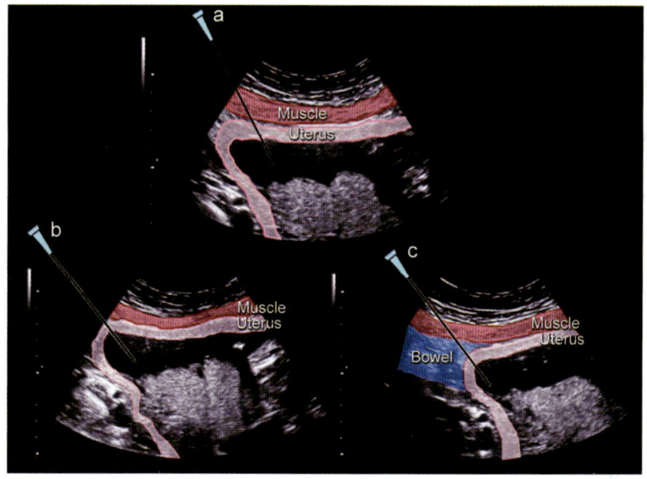

Fig. 22.3 The correct technique

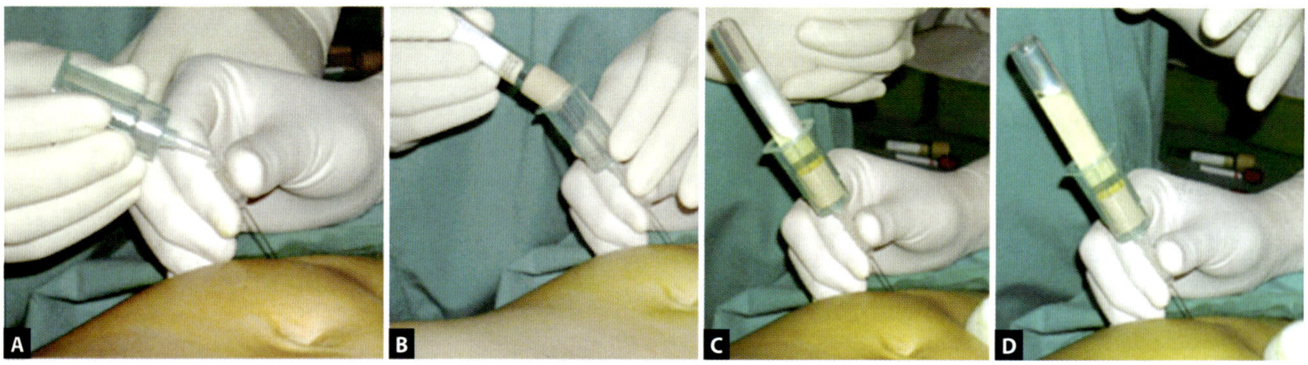

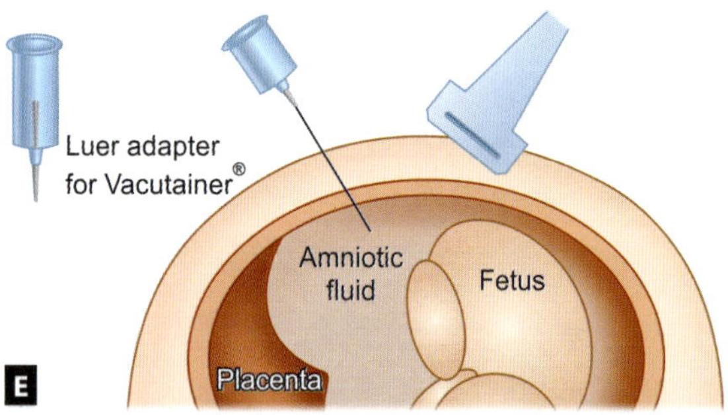

Figs 22.4A to E Amniotic fluid aspiration with the Vacutainer system

Selecting a needle: Needle selection is dependent upon the size of the patient and the amount of fluid to be retrieved. In the majority of cases a regular 20–22 gauge spinal needle with a standard length of 8.89 cm excluding the hub.

Needles with especially prepared tips designed to improve ultrasonographic visualization and side orifices to accelerate fluid withdrawal are commercially available.

Monitoring the needle insertion and placement: Once a puncture site is selected, asepsis of the skin is performed with wide boundaries and the field is draped. Two approaches may be used:

1. Ultrasonographic-guided amniocentesis
2. Ultrasonographic-monitored amniocentesis.

Ultrasonographic: Guided amniocentesis refers to the preselection of a puncture site with ultrasound before proceeding with blind insertion of the needle. Ultrasonographic-monitored amniocentesis refers to the continuous monitoring of needle insertion and fetal movements with real-time ultrasound. Monitoring the needle position with ultrasound reduces the frequency of bloody and dry taps and the risk of fetal injuries.

Convex, sector or linear: Array transducers may be used to monitor the procedure with slight modifications of the technique. Irrespective of transducer selection, a nonsterile coupling agent is applied to the transducer surface before placing it inside a sterile glove or plastic bag. A sterile coupling agent is then applied to the patient's skin and the puncture site is re-evaluated.

Amniotic fluid aspiration: Once the stylet is removed, an extension tube (which allows the needle to float free in the amniotic cavity, decreasing the likelihood of fetal injury) is attached to the hub of the needle and connected to the syringe. The first 0.5 mL of amniotic fluid is discarded in order to avoid maternal cell contamination. The recommended amount of fluid to be withdrawn is 1 mL/week of gestation. After obtaining the fluid, the stylet is relocated, the needle removed and fetal cardiac activity documented. The same technique is used for procedures performed during the late second and third trimesters.

EARLY AMNIOCENTESIS

Early amniocentesis refers to procedures performed before 15 weeks of gestation, allowing the diagnosis of anomalies at a time when suction termination is still possible and before fetal movements are perceived. Other potential advantages include the opportunity to screen for neural tube defects, by measurement of amniotic fluid alpha-fetoprotein and acetylcholinesterase after 13 weeks. However, the risk of spontaneous fetal loss rate for chromosomally normal fetuses within 2 weeks of the procedure and also before 28 weeks of gestation has been found to be greater than midtrimester amniocentesis. Early amniocentesis therefore is not really done these days as a better alternative, chorion villous sampling is available.

COMPLICATIONS[5,6]

Fetal Loss

Fetal loss can be idiopathic or a result of direct fetal injury with subsequent exsanguination or infection. Amniocentesis may lead to intra-amniotic infection by introducing microorganisms into the amniotic cavity. Alternatively, if amniocentesis results in rupture of the membranes, ascending infection may occur. Fetal loss rate for midtrimester amniocentesis range from 0.3% to 2.8%. Multiple needle insertions and intra-amniotic bleeding has also been implicated as causes for an increased pregnancy loss rate.

The use of continuous ultrasonographic monitoring and increased operator experience have been shown to reduce the number of attempts needed to obtain amniotic fluid as well as the number of bloodstained taps.

Fetal Injury[4,7,8]

A wide range of fetal injuries, from mild skin dimples to fetal death due to exsanguination, have been attributed to amniocentesis. Although fetal injuries are generally associated with bloody taps, they have also been reported after clear taps and even with the use of sonographically monitored technique.

Several ocular injuries have been attributed to amniocentesis. Typically these are unilateral lesions detected after birth. Thoracic lesions associated with amniocentesis include hemothorax, pneumothorax and fetal cardiac tamponade. In the abdomen, injuries have ranged from laceration of the liver, kidney and spleen to ileocutaneous fistula with ileal atresia. Limb lesions have included disruption of the patellar tendon, gangrene of one arm (perforation of the subclavian artery) and an arteriovenous fistula with ileal atresia.

Limb lesions have included disruption of the patellar tendon, gangrene of one arm and an AV fistula between the popliteal artery and vein. The most frequent lesion associated with amniocentesis is skin puncture. Although cause and effect is difficult to establish, needle injuries should be suspected of the shape of the lesion resembles a needle tract or a depressed punctiform scar.

Amniotic Fluid Leakage (Fig. 22.5)

Membrane rupture or amniotic fluid leakage are potential complications of amniocentesis. It has been suggested that the perinatal and maternal outcomes for membrane rupture and amniotic fluid leakage are better than the outcomes for patients who experience spontaneous rupture of the membrane in the second trimester of pregnancy.

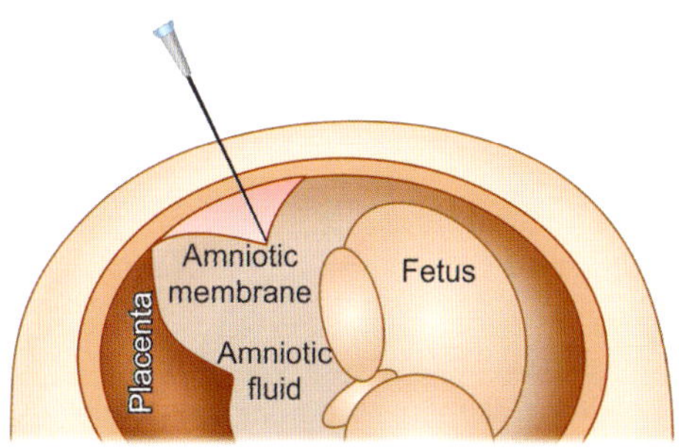

Fig. 22.5 Introduction of the needle into the uterine cavity and tenting of the membrane

Bloody Taps[7]

Bloody amniotic fluid can be a result of contamination with maternal or fetal blood. As mentioned earlier, the prevalence of this complication also decreased with the use of ultrasonographic monitoring.

The incidence of pregnancy loss when fetal blood contamination occurred was greater than when maternal blood contamination was documented.

Fetomaternal Transfusion

Fetomaternal transfusion is important because it may lead to isoimmunization and an increased risk of pregnancy loss.

Discolored Amniotic Fluid

Brown and green stained amniotic fluids are occasionally obtained during midtrimester amniocentesis. Although the possibility that some green-stained amniotic fluid could be due to meconium passage, compelling evidence suggests that green and brown stained amniotic fluids are a result of an intra-amniotic hemorrhage.

DIFFICULTIES

- A small or retroverted uterus
- The presence of overlying bladder or bowel
- A decreased amniotic fluid volume
- A history of recent bleeding or cramping
- The presence of severe contractions prior to the procedure and obesity may pose difficulties and are considered additional and are considered additional indications for rescheduling amniocentesis in some patients.

Amniotic Fluid Culture

Depending on laboratory experience, the interval between amniocentesis and culture ranges from 6 days to 21 days.

Amniocentesis and Isoimmunization

Fetal red blood cells contain the D antigen on their surface and are capable of immunizing the Rh-negative mother after fetomaternal transfusion in the midtrimester. This event can occur spontaneously during pregnancy or after an amniocentesis. The world health organization (WHO) and the American College of Obstetricians and Gynecologists (ACOG) have recommended the administration of anti-D IgG to women after midtrimester amniocentesis. There is no agreement on the dose; WHO recommends 50 µg, while the ACOG recommends 300 µg.

The basis for this recommendation is that midtrimester amniocentesis has been associated with an increased incidence of transplacental hemorrhage, a risk factor for isoimmunization.

Amniocentesis in Multiple Gestation

Before amniocentesis is carried out in a multiple gestation, the possible outcome, risks and management need to be discussed with the patient. The major problem to be considered is the possibility of discrepant results regarding cytogenetic diagnosis. If only one fetus is affected, the options available to the patient include abortion of both fetuses, continuation of pregnancy or selective feticide of the affected fetus. Feticide is associated with potential complications, such as infection, DIC and spontaneous abortion. Under these circumstances, pregnancy termination implies the abortion of an unaffected fetus. The technique for amniocentesis varies from that of a singleton pregnancy, depending on the location of the placentae and intra-amniotic membrane, and fetal biometry.

Several techniques have been proposed to ensure that fluid is retrieved from each amniotic cavity. In majority of centers, after amniotic fluid is obtained from the first sac and before removing the needle, an indicator dye is injected into the cavity. Indigo carmine is presently the dye of choice; alternatives are congo red and Evans blue. The use of solution of maternal hemoglobin as a dye has also been reported. The use of methylene blue is discouraged because of the risk of fetal hemolytic anemia due to methemoglobinemia and a possible association with gastrointestinal obstruction.

Clear amniotic fluid should be obtained when the second sac is punctured. The same procedure is applicable to amniocentesis for a multiple gestation with more than 2 fetuses. The technique consists of sequential injections of dye into different sacs before removal of needle. The number of clear amniotic fluid aspirations should be equal to the number of fetuses.

A difficult situation arises when an intra-amniotic membrane cannot be identified. This can occur in the setting of polyhydramnios and in monoamniotic twins. A practical approach consists of sampling two sites in close proximity to each fetus but distant from each other.

Before injection, the dye is diluted with 10 mL of amniotic fluid. The mixture is then injected into the amniotic cavity, producing a typical particulate image that identifies the boundaries of the sac. The operator must be ready to proceed with the second puncture because the image is short lived.

Amniocentesis for the Diagnosis of Microbial Invasion of the Amniotic Cavity[2,3,8]

The amniotic cavity is normally sterile and isolation of any microorganism from the amniotic fluid therefore constitutes evidence of microbial invasion.

The method of amniotic fluid collection for microbiological studies is critical. The 2 techniques that have been used are transabdominal amniocentesis and transcervical retrieval either by needle puncturing of the membranes or by aspiration through an intrauterine catheter. Transcervical amniotic fluid collection is associated with an unacceptable risk of contamination with vaginal flora and its contra-indicated in patients with preterm labor and patients with premature rupture of membranes (PROM) but not in labor. Successful retrieval of amniotic fluid by ultrasonographically monitored amniocentesis is possible in virtually all patients with preterm labor with intact membranes and over 90% of patients with preterm PROM, making it the method of choice to obtain fluid from these patients.

Post-procedure Recommendations[9,10]

Fetal viability must be assessed continuously and any bleeding at the point of insertion must be evaluated by ultrasound. Maternal blood group must be confirmed and entered in the woman's records and all maternal history and clinical data required by the laboratory for sample processing must be verified, as must the woman's name and patient number. The woman must be informed regarding the time required for sample processing and who will deliver to her the results of the rapid test (QF-PCR or FISH), karyotype, array comparative genomic hybridization (array-CGH) or infection studies.

Recommendations for the woman after the procedure are as follows:

- Anti-D immunoglobulin (300 μg) in RhD-negative women.
- Specific anti-HBV immunoglobulin (600 IU intramuscularly in the first 24 hours post-procedure) may be administered in women with positive HBsAg (hepatitis B surface antigen) in the case of HBeAg (hepatitis B 'e' antigen) or positive viral load (HBV-DNA), in cases in which transplacental insertion was unavoidable or when third-trimester amniocentesis was performed, although evidence for its prophylactic use in invasive procedures is lacking.

Pearls of Practice

- A 20–22 G needle must be used under continuous ultrasound guidance.
- An amniocentesis must be performed or supervised by an experienced operator, in order to diminish the risk of complications.
- The procedure must be performed from 16 weeks of gestation onwards, as confirmed by ultrasound.

REFERENCES

1. ACOG Practice Bulletin No. 88, December 2007. Invasive prenatal testing for aneuploidy. Obstet Gynecol. 2007;110:1459-67.
2. Mujezinovic F, Alfirevic Z. Technique modifications for reducing the risks from amniocentesis or chorionic villus sampling. Cochrane Database Syst Rev. 2012;8: CD008678.
3. Ghidini A. Diagnostic amniocentesis. In: Basow D (Ed). up to date: Waltham, MA, 2013.
4. Lopez M, Coll O. Chronic viral infections and invasive procedures: Risk of vertical transmission and current recommendations. Fetal Diagn Ther. 2010;28:1-8.
5. Davies G, Wilson RD, Desilets V, Reid GJ, Shaw D, Summers A, et al. Amniocentesis and women with hepatitis B, hepatitis C, or human immunodeficiency virus. J Obstet Gynaecol Can. 2003; 25:145-52.
6. Carlin AJ, Alfirevic Z. Techniques for chorionic villus sampling and amniocentesis: A survey of practice in specialist UK centres. Prenat Diagn. 2008;28:914-9.
7. Ville Y, Cooper M, Revel A, Frydman R, Nicolaides KH. Development of a training model for ultrasound-guided invasive procedures in fetal medicine. Ultrasound Obstet Gynecol. 1995;5:180-3.
8. Mann K, Ogilvie CM. QF-PCR: Application, overview and review of the literature. Prenat Diagn. 2012;32:309-14.
9. Royal College of Obstetricians and Gynaecologists. Amniocentesis and chorionic villus sampling. Green-top Guideline No. 8. RCOG: London, 2010.
10. Gramellini D, Fieni S, Casilla G, Raboni S, Nardelli GB. Mid-trimester amniocentesis and antibiotic prophylaxis. Prenat Diagn. 2007;27:956-9.

CHAPTER

23

Cordocentesis

Purnima Satoskar, Shilpa Agrawal

INTRODUCTION

Cordocentesis (i.e. fetal blood sampling, percutaneous umbilical blood sampling and funipuncture) is a procedure for sampling fetal blood from the umbilical cord by a needle that is inserted through the maternal abdominal wall under continuous ultrasonographic monitoring.

Prenatal diagnosis of 2–5% of all pregnancies with several congenital and genetic defects is now an important component of antenatal care. Direct access to the fetal vascular circulation allows improvement of prenatal diagnosis and therapy. Despite its advantages and high acceptance, fetal blood sampling is relatively invasive and limited to the skilled perinatologist.

Cordocentesis was first described in the early 1980.[1] It was first performed by Fernand Daffos in the 1980s.[2] In 1963, Liley[3] was the first to treat fetal anemia by intraperitoneal transfusion of blood. In 1979, Rodeck and Campbell[4] described the ability to perform fetal blood sampling (FBS) utilizing a fetoscopic approach, while 4 years later, Daffos et al.[2] introduced the technique of ultrasound guided FBS. The emergence of newer, less invasive testing modalities and development of molecular genetic techniques have greatly decreased the need for FBS. Nevertheless, it still has an important role in prenatal diagnosis and therapy.

INDICATIONS (TABLE 23.1)

Mainly divided into:

1. Diagnostic (Table 23.2)
2. Therapeutic

Tongsong et al. analyzed 1,320 cordocenteses performed between 1989 and 1999 at Maharaj Nakorn Chiang Mai Hospital, Thailand. The most common indication in that study was the fetal risk of thalassemia (61.1%) followed by rapid karyotyping (27.1%).[5]

Table 23.1 Indications of cordocentesis

Indications	Comment
Diagnose and treat fetal severe anemia	Most common indication for FBS
Diagnose and evaluate therapeutic response in NAIT	
Evaluate nonimmune fetal hydrops	Only in selected case specially if MCA –PSV is elevated
Historical and less common indications	
Fetal aneuploidy for karyotyping	Rarely used in current practice; largely replaced by CVS or amniocentesis with FISH, or by NIPT
Determine fetal blood type and platelet antigen status	Largely replaced by other tests, e.g., NIPT, CVS, or amniocentesis, and molecular testing Diagnose genetic disorders
Diagnose genetic disorders (e.g. hemophilia, thalassemia)	Largely replaced by CVS or amniocentesis for molecular genetic diagnosis
Measurement of biochemical or other serum markers for fetal disease (e.g. fetal infection, thyroid function)	Largely replaced by amniocentesis and PCR (e.g. infection); rarely needed (e.g. thyroid function)

Table 23.2 Indications for diagnostic cordocentesis

Indication	Percent
Rapid karyotype	50.7
Hemolytic disease	33.7
Severe growth retardation	21.7
Congenital infection	16.9
Miscellaneous indications	4.2

Diagnostic Indications

Fetal Anemia

Suspected severe fetal anemia is the most common current indication for FBS in the United States. Direct measurement of fetal hemoglobin, and therefore accurate diagnosis of fetal anemia, can only be made by FBS. Anemia may be suspected due to the presence of maternal alloantibodies, maternal parvovirus exposure or infection, other viral infections, or due to ultrasound findings such as fetal hydrops or elevated peak systolic velocity (PSV) of the fetal middle cerebral artery (MCA) by Doppler studies. Maternal anti-D alloimmunization remains the most common cause of fetal anemia.[6]

Current management of the pregnancy at risk for fetal anemia typically involves assessment with Doppler velocimetry of the fetal MCA. A MCA PSV of ≥1.5 multiples of the median is generally considered indicative of moderate or severe fetal anemia, and FBS is warranted to directly measure fetal hemoglobin (or hematocrit) levels and determine the need for intrauterine transfusion (IUT).[7]

Thrombocytopenia

The diagnosis of fetal thrombocytopenia caused by neonatal alloimmune thrombocytopenia (NAIT) in the current pregnancy can only be made with FBS.

Neonatal alloimmune thrombocytopenia (NAIT) is a disorder in which transplacental passage of maternal antiplatelet antibodies causes fetal (and neonatal) thrombocytopenia. Severe fetal thrombocytopenia as a result of alloimmune thrombocytopenia may lead to cerebral hemorrhage before, during, or after birth and may cause mental handicap or death. Currently, maternal intravenous immunoglobulin, sometimes in conjunction with corticosteroids, is administered to increase the fetal platelet count. FBS can be used to assess the response to maternal therapy provided benefits outweigh the risks of FBS and if vaginal delivery is considered.[8]

Fetal Hydrops

Fetal anemia is one of the most common causes of hydrops. The differential diagnosis of fetal hydrops is extensive[9] but fetal anemia, aneuploidy, and infection are relatively common causes. Initial work-up of hydrops involves maternal serum analyses, detailed ultrasound examination and fetal MCA-PSV. It is reasonable to offer FBS in the setting of nonimmune hydrops, especially if the rest of the work-up is negative and the fetal MCA-PSV is elevated.

Chromosomal Abnormalities

White blood cells divide at a rapid rate providing rapid (48–72 hrs.) and good banding. Because of the risks associated with FBS, it is rarely used in current practice and is largely replaced by CVS or amniocentesis with FISH, or by NIPT. If at all used, the indications are possible mosaicism, culture failure after either amniocentesis or placental biopsy, woman who seeks care late in pregnancy.

Single-Gene Defects

It includes mainly diagnosis of hemoglobinopathies, coagulopathies, severe combined immunodeficiency, chronic granulomatous disease, and some metabolic disorders.[6] Usually they are diagnosed earlier in gestation by applying various DNA techniques to amniocytes. FBS is important for at-risk patients who seek care late in pregnancy and when DNA analysis is not possible.

Inherited Anemias or Hemoglobinopathies: With the advent of modern molecular genetic techniques, fetal diagnosis can reliably be made using DNA obtained via CVS or amniocentesis.[10] In some parts of the world, sophisticated molecular techniques may be unavailable and hemoglobinopathies relatively common, so FBS continues to be routinely used in the diagnosis of alpha- and beta-thalassemia. In 1 recent study reported from Thailand, for example, more than 2000 cordocenteses were performed from 1989 through 2010; more than 75% of these were done due to a risk of fetal thalassemia.[11]

Hypoxia and Acidosis

Suspected fetal hypoxia or acidemia can be confirmed or refuted by fetal blood gas analysis. Fetal acidemia may be excluded by Doppler studies of the fetal vasculature. Increasing evidence shows that chronic fetal acidemia is associated with impaired long-term neurodevelopment. However, no convincing evidence shows that the benefits of fetal acid-base status outweigh the risks of FBS, and it is rarely indicated.

Fetal Infection

Appropriate fetal blood tests (e.g. infection-specific fetal immunoglobulin M or detection of specific genomic material by PCR) can determine whether maternal infection has led to fetal infection. However, the difference between being "infected" and "affected" (i.e., damaged) must not be forgotten. Amniotic fluid culture and/or PCR are currently the primary diagnostic modalities. In settings in which polymerase chain reaction (PCR) is not readily available, FBS has been used for diagnosis, for example in rare cases of fetal varicella with measurement of varicella-zoster virus-specific IgM and viral culture.[12]

Therapeutic Indications

Monitoring of Transplacental Therapy

Some fetal diseases are treated by drugs that are given to the mother, cross the placenta, and achieve therapeutic concentrations in the fetus. Examples include antiarrhythmic agents to correct fetal tachyarrhythmia and γ-globulin to improve low fetal platelet counts. An accurate assessment of placental transfer and monitoring of the success of therapy may require FBS.[13]

Fetal Therapy

Access to the fetal circulation offers the possibility of infusing biologic (e.g. blood transfusion) or pharmacologic agents for therapeutic purposes.

There are limited conditions for which a single dose of a medication is useful, and serial or chronic intravascular fetal therapy is impractical. Fetal hydrops due to supraventricular tachycardia, where trans placental therapy is less effective and a single injection may resolve the arrhythmia.[14] In general, FBS has rarely been used for medical therapies other than transfusions or refractory arrhythmias, and evidence for benefits from these other therapies is lacking.

Multiple Gestations

In multiple gestations, in which one of the fetuses is abnormal, cordocentesis is also applied for selective termination by potassium chloride injection, which causes cardiac arrest.[15]

COUNSELING

- Prenatal counseling concerning risks and benefits of screening versus invasive diagnostic testing
- Counseling regarding alternative invasive tests if can be used.
- Counseling of women with chronic hepatitis B or C virus infections, or human immunodeficiency virus infection.
- Nondirective counseling concerning pregnancy termination.

FETAL BLOOD SAMPLING

Technique

Fetal blood sampling was first performed under fetoscopic guidance, but fetoscopy carried a 2–5% risk of serious complications.[16] Ultrasound-guided needling is considered safer than fetoscopy and is the preferred technique.[17] It can be performed as early as 16 weeks of gestational, though it is technically more difficult prior to 18 weeks of gestation. In general, cordocentesis is commonly performed between 18 and 22 weeks of gestation for prenatal diagnosis.

Preprocedure

After reviewing the benefits, risks, and options, an informed written consent is obtained. Before the procedure, detailed ultrasound examination is performed using the convex transducer of 3.5–5 MHz to determine the number of fetuses, fetal viability, fetal biometry, fetal normality, placenta and umbilical cord locations.[18]

Technical Aspects (Table 23.3)

Operator Experience

Fetal blood sampling should be performed only by physicians who have extensive experience with other obstetric, ultrasound-guided needle procedures (e.g. amniocentesis, transabdominal CVS). Units that offer this service must perform enough cases to maintain expertise; 20 procedures per year is a reasonable minimum. This typically requires a center with many referrals.[19]

Location

Little information exists about the choice of physical location (e.g. operating room, ultrasound suite, office) for the

Table 23.3 Technical aspects of fetal blood sampling

Prophylactic antibiotics	Insufficient evidence to recommend
Maternal sedation	Used infrequently
Local anesthesia	Used by some centers
Skin preparation	Preprocedural antibacterial skin preparation and aseptic technique are recommended
Needle guidance	Both needle guide instrument and freehand techniques have been reported and are acceptable; direct needle into target (e.g. umbilical vein) under continuous ultrasound guidance; avoid umbilical arteries if feasible
Needle gauge and length	20- or 22-gauge; gauge and length depend on indication, suspicion of thrombocytopenia, gestational age, maternal body habitus, and distance from skin to target
Sampling site	Umbilical vein usually preferred, either at PCI or ACI, or into free loop, intrahepatic vein, fetal heart (cardiocentesis)

procedure. Once viability is reached, it is prudent to perform the procedure in close proximity to or within an available operating room should the need for emergency cesarean delivery arise. The decision to use prophylactic steroids for fetal lung maturity prior to FBS is also not well documented, but should be considered when FBS is performed around 23 0/7 to 33 6/7 weeks, given the increased risk of preterm birth. Cordocentesis is done on an outpatient basis in a location with close proximity to the delivery suite. A relaxed, informal setting helps to alleviate the mother's anxiety, which tends to improve her cooperation.

Prophylactic Antibiotics

There are no randomized trials on the efficacy of prophylactic antibiotic for FBS. In the American Congress of Obstetricians and Gynecologists Practice Bulletin on invasive testing for aneuploidy, there is no recommendation for the use of antibiotics to prevent intrauterine infection prior to invasive procedures.[20]

Maternal Position and Sedation

The mother should be positioned to avoid supine hypotension; hyperventilation and sedation should be avoided in a recumbent position with a lateral tilt.

Skin Preparation

The majority of studies endorse using an aseptic technique, including a preprocedural antibacterial skin preparation to reduce the risk of infection.[21] The abdomen is cleaned with an antiseptic solution and draped.

Local Anesthesia

Use of local anesthesia varies depending on the preference of the operator, as well as type of procedure (diagnostic sampling or IUT). While some centers use regional anesthesia after a viable gestational age and depending on the clinical circumstances, there are no data or clinical reports to support this practice.[22]

Needle Guidance

There are two standard methods for cordocentesis; free hand and the use of a fixed needle guide[23] with either method, the operator can control the transducer with one hand and the needle with the other, or an assistant can control the transducer and find the appropriate place for a needle insertion attempt. The majority of studies seemed to describe the freehand technique, which may allow for greater flexibility, although no trials exist comparing the two methods. Needle is guided into the umbilical vein without puncturing one of the arteries as these may constrict when punctured, leading to fetal bradycardia and a subsequent emergency delivery.

Needle Gauge and Length

Most centers use a 20- or 22-gauge spinal needle, depending on the indication for procedure (diagnostic vs therapeutic IUT), and suspicion for thrombocytopenia. Other important considerations when choosing the appropriate needle are gestational age, maternal body habitus, and distance from skin to target. For example, at an earlier gestational age (e.g. <24 weeks), it might be preferable to use a 22 gauge needle instead of 20 gauge given the smaller umbilical cord vessels. In women with a thick panniculus, a larger-bore 20-gauge needle may be useful to prevent bending of the needle and to improve visualization. The distance from skin to target is also important to measure to determine if the standard 9 cm spinal needle length is appropriate, or if a longer needle is needed. Finally, some operators prefer to run heparin through the needle prior to sampling to prevent the formation of a blood clot within the needle.[22]

Sampling Site

The target portions of umbilical cord location are classified in 3 subgroups, which are (1) placental origin of umbilical cord, (2) free loop of umbilical cord and (3) fetal origin of umbilical cord. There are currently no published randomized controlled trials comparing the efficacy and safety of these techniques. Advantages of sampling at the PCI are the relative stability of the cord for easier insertion and shorter procedure time.[21] A disadvantage is the possibility of contamination by maternal blood, and need to confirm that the sample obtained is indeed of fetal origin. FBS performed from a free loop of cord may result in more bleeding and longer bleeding time due to piercing of the wall of the vessel, although it has the advantage of avoiding placental penetration, and avoiding the need for confirmation of fetal origin.[24] The fetal origin of the umbilical cord is problematic because there is no length to buffer the effect of fetal movement after puncture. In addition, the proximal few centimeters of the umbilicus are sympathetically innervated, theoretically increasing the risk of bradycardia.

Cordocentesis is easiest when the placenta is anterior because access to the target portion of the cord with a posterior placenta may be hampered by the fetus.

The puncture site does not affect the difficulty if it is chosen on the basis of accessibility and quality of visualization. The major difficulties were apparently related to maternal obesity, resulting in poor sonographic images; the active fetal movement, and the presence of polyhydramnios, making the puncture site more difficult to access.[18]

Placental Penetration

A transplacental approach usually provides the easiest route to the placental cord origin, unless the placenta is entirely posterior. However, in women with red cell alloimmunization, transplacental puncture boosts the maternal antibody titer as a result of fetal-maternal hemorrhage.[25] Therefore, it is best to avoid the placenta unless transfusion is anticipated in an alloimmunized woman. Concerns for placental penetration during FBS involve the potential increased risk for fetomaternal hemorrhage, and potential for higher fetal death rates.[22]

Use of Paralytic Agents

Agents such as pancuronium, atracurium, or vecuronium are used as paralytic agents to reduce fetal movements during the procedure mainly intrauterine transfusion. Pancuronium is a long-acting agent, while atracurium and vecuronium are both short-acting. Atracurium may be beneficial in fetuses with hydrops because it is not eliminated by the liver, and has the added benefit that the breakdown products do not have significant cardiovascular and neuromuscular effects.[26] Paralytic agents may be particularly useful when large transfusion volumes (and therefore longer operating times) are anticipated, or when vigorous fetal movements make the procedure more challenging. They are not usually necessary when FBS is performed for indications other than potential IUT, or when an anterior placenta and cord insertion are present.

Procedure of Taking Fetal Blood

After the needle is in the umbilical vein, the needle tip is visualized within the lumen of the umbilical cord and the stylet is removed. If the needle is ideally sited, blood will fill the hub. The syringe may be primed upon the indications with a small amount of anticoagulant, such as heparin or citrate. A 1 mL syringe is applied tightly to the hub, and blood is withdrawn. After 20 weeks, 5 mL may be removed without concern (maximum of 6–7% of the fetoplacental blood volume for that gestational age). However, before 20 weeks, the volume removed should be the minimum necessary for the specific tests. Often, no blood is obtained initially and the operator must assess whether the needle tip has passed through the vessel lumen or perhaps is located in Wharton's jelly. The needle is sharply advanced or gently withdrawn, and the shaft is rotated 180° between the operator's finger and thumb while suction is maintained.

Needle Adjustments

Occasionally, amniotic fluid is obtained when the needle tip appears intraluminal. With the freehand technique, the needle is moved side-to-side in search of cord movement. With a needle guide, an up-and-down movement of the needle produces the same result. Cord movement indicates that the needle has passed through the cord. It is withdrawn until no more amniotic fluid is aspirated, the syringe is changed (because even a small amount of amniotic fluid is a very powerful coagulant), and the procedure is continued. If the needle has passed through the side of the cord without entering a vessel lumen, it is withdrawn slightly and its path adjusted. If the tip is lateral to the umbilical cord, it is withdrawn and the needle used to touch the vein before the puncture attempt is repeated.[27]

Identification of Vessel

If blood gas results are to be interpretable, it is essential to identify the vessel that has been entered. If the puncture is performed at either the placental or the fetal origin of the umbilical cord, the vessel can usually be identified by the direction of turbulence after rapid injection of up to 1 mL normal saline.[28]

Fetal Blood Specimen

Techniques such as measuring mean corpuscular volume (MCV) and the Kleihauer-Betke test have been successful in determining fetal origin. When the IHV, a free umbilical cord loop, or ACI are accessed, or if fetal cardiocentesis is performed, there is no need for verification of fetal blood since these sites assure a lack of maternal blood contamination[29] but done in cases where the sampling site is placental cord insertion. Before the procedure, the operator should determine which studies are desired and should rank them in importance. The samples are taken in rank order in case the needle slips out of the lumen or a complication occurs, causing the procedure to end prematurely. In the case of suspected fetal anemia, the blood is sent for immediate analysis of hemoglobin/ hematocrit to determine the amount of blood needed for IUT.

Umbilical venous pressure is measured by attachment of a pressure transducer to the needle. The value obtained should be corrected for amniotic fluid pressure. This measurement is very useful in evaluating nonimmune hydrops.[30]

Team Approach

Cordocentesis involves a team approach. Expert personnel are needed to support the mother through the procedure and to assist the operator. The laboratories must be familiar with the analysis of small volumes of blood and must recognize the need for efficient and rapid service. Should there be a complication, the team must be familiar with resuscitative procedures and be prepared to move rapidly to perform a cesarean delivery. Likewise, the delivery suite staff should be aware that a procedure is taking place and be ready to provide anesthesia and nursing personnel as necessary.

Postprocedure Monitoring

The puncture site is observed ultrasonically for bleeding after the needle is removed. Bleeding is common after transamniotic cordocentesis, but is usually brief and without clinical significance. After bleeding has stopped, the fetal heart rate is measured.

If the fetus is previable, the woman should wait in the hospital until she feels well, and then return home. There are no special precautions or restrictions. If a local anesthetic is used, she should be warned to expect a bruised sensation in a few hours. Acetaminophen (paracetamol) or another nonprescription analgesic can be used safely.

If the fetus is viable, the heart rate pattern is assessed by cardiotocography for at least 30 minutes before discharge. Pancuronium causes a nonreactive tracing, with mild fetal tachycardia. The mother should be warned that perceptible movement might not return for several hours.[28] Before being discharged, the mother is counseled to call if she has contractions, leakage of fluid, bleeding, fever, or uterine tenderness. If the patient is Rh-negative, the fetus should be typed and RhoGAM administered when appropriate.

Complications (Table 23.4)

Postprocedure Loss Rates

Fetal blood sampling does carry risk of procedure related pregnancy loss, usually defined as the risk of pregnancy loss/ fetal demise within 2 weeks of the procedure.[31] Loss and complication rates are clearly related to the indication for sampling and the final fetal diagnosis. The background risk of intrauterine death is high when there is a severe structural malformation or a major chromosomal abnormality.

Table 23.4 Risks of fetal blood sampling[22]

Risk	Comments
Bleeding from puncture site (e.g. umbilical cord)	20–30%; usually self-limited
Abnormal fetal heart rate	5–10% bradycardia; majority resolve within 5 minutes
Pregnancy loss	1.3% if no structural anomalies or hydrops and no placental penetration
Vertical transmission of maternal infection (e.g. hepatitis B, hepatitis C, or HIV)	Insufficient information to estimate risk

Gestational age at sampling is also an important determinant because a viable fetus can be delivered if a complication arises.

For example, fetuses with nonimmune hydrops have a higher procedure-related loss (25%) compared with fetuses with severe growth deficiency (13.8%), structural anomalies (6.6%), or those where the indication for cordocentesis was prenatal diagnosis (1.3%).[32] Fetuses with nonimmune hydrops, however, also have a high perinatal loss rate (70–90%) if nothing is done. Therefore, patients should be counseled regarding the background loss rate for the particular problem, as well as the additional procedural loss rate.

Fetal Bleeding

Bleeding from the umbilical cord puncture site is most common and has been reported to be 20–30% and is usually self-limiting, unless thrombocytopenia is present. Duration of bleeding from the artery is reported to be longer than that from the vein.[33] Differences among centers with respect to bleeding may relate to the size of the needle used (25-gauge, Bovicelli; 22-gauge, Weiner; 20-gauge, Daffos) and the technique employed (needle-guided, Bovicelli and Weiner; freehand, Daffos). The needle-guided technique likely reduces trauma to the cord because of the lack of lateral mobility of the needle.

Fetal Heart Rate Abnormality

An abnormal fetal heart rate can also occur after the procedure. Bradycardia is more common than tachycardia, with a reported incidence of 5–10%.[34] The majority of fetal bradycardias resolves within 5 minutes and usually requires no further intervention.

The incidence of bradycardia may be related to the size of the needle vessel, (umbilical artery or vein) punctured, severe growth restriction. Work from the University of Iowa reveals that the incidence of bradycardia is higher if the umbilical artery is punctured, rather than the vein (21% vs 3.4%, respectively). Bradycardia is also more common in severely growth-restricted fetuses. Fetuses experiencing a bradycardia have as a group lower blood pH levels, lower pO_2 levels, and higher pCO_2 levels before the onset of the bradycardia, as well as a higher umbilical artery systolic-to-diastolic ratio than fetuses that do not experience a bradycardia. These findings imply that the increased procedure-related loss rate for severely growth-restricted fetuses may be related to the increased incidence of bradycardia. It has been theorized that the umbilical arterial smooth muscle is more at risk for spasm than is muscle in the vein and that, in a hypoxic environment; it has an exaggerated response to catecholamines.[33]

Chorioamnionitis

It is usually caused by *Staphylococcus epidermidis*. It typically causes myalgia, arthralgia, and a low fever 4–10 days after the procedure. There is no evidence to support prophylactic antibiotic administration. The risk of amnionitis after cordocentesis should be equal to the risk of amnionitis after amniocentesis if an equal number of skin to amniotic sac punctures are made and the time and amount of manipulation required to obtain the sample is the same. The risk of amnionitis is approximately 1% when the freehand technique is used and less than 0.3% when the needle-guided technique is used.[33] Rarely, chorioamnionitis can lead to the development of maternal sepsis and adult respiratory distress syndrome.

Cordocentesis in Maternal Infections

Invasive prenatal diagnostic tests performed in women chronically infected with hepatitis B, hepatitis C, or human immunodeficiency virus (HIV) carry a theoretical risk of vertical transmission. Very limited information is available about the risk of vertical transmission during FBS. From small studies of amniocentesis, the procedure-related risks of vertical transmission of HIV, hepatitis B, and hepatitis C appear to be exceedingly low, and related to maternal viral load.[35] The risk of vertical HIV transmission is higher in women who are not taking antiretroviral therapy, compared with women who are being treated and have undetectable viral loads.[36] In patients for whom no alternative exists to FBS, e.g. severe fetal hemolytic disease requiring IUT, the potential risks of FBS related to vertical transmission should be discussed prior to the procedure. Treatment aimed at decreasing the viral load for both HIV and hepatitis B virus in patients with these infections should be considered. When performing FBS in a patient with one of these infections, efforts should be made to avoid traversing the placenta with the needle, if possible.

Maternal

The main maternal risk associated with FBS is red cell alloimmunization. The fetal blood type should be tested in at-risk women, and anti-D immunoglobulin should be given if the fetus is Rhesus-positive. Chorioamnionitis or emergency cesarean section can create secondary maternal risks. When FBS or transfusion is undertaken and the fetus is considered viable, maternal aspects of emergency delivery should be considered. Needle injury to the maternal intra-abdominal organs, such as intestines, or vessels may be more common than recognized, but significant morbidity has not been reported after FBS. Maternal intra-abdominal infection and bleeding would be expected to occur at the same rate as that for amniocentesis.

TAKE HOME MESSAGES

Preprocedure counseling is must and the patient should be made aware of the risks and benefits involved. Also if alternative less invasive test is available and applicable, option should be given to them.

- It should be attempted only if the operator has considerable experience with related procedures.
- A team approach is needed.
- FBS is indicated when the potential benefits outweigh the procedure-related risks.
- The risks and benefits to both the fetus and the mother should be considered.
- The most important determinant of the fetal loss rate is the indication for sampling.

When invasive testing is planned for suspected severe fetal anemia or thrombocytopenia, FBS is procedure of choice, with availability of immediate transfusion if confirmed.

COMPLICATIONS OF CORDOCENTESIS[30]

- Fetal death
- Bradycardia
- Amnionitis
- Cord hematoma
- Umbilical cord bleeding
- Fetal maternal hemorrhage
- Premature rupture of membranes
- Preterm labor
- Abruptio placentae
- Complications secondary to premature delivery
- Maternal sepsis, followed by adult respiratory distress syndrome
- Risk of emergency cesarean section
- Failure to obtain sample.

REFERENCES

1. Bang J, Bock JE, Trolle D. Ultrasound-guided fetal intravenous transfusion for severe rhesus hemolytic disease. Br Med J (Clin Res Ed). 1982;284:373-4.
2. Daffos F, Capella-Pavlovsky M, Forestier F. A new procedure for fetal blood sampling *in utero*: preliminary results of fifty-three cases. Am Obstet Gynecol. 1983;146:985-7.
3. Liley AW. Intrauterine transfusion of fetus in hemolytic disease. Br Med J. 1963;2:1107-9.
4. Rodeck CH, Campbell S. Umbilical-cord insertion as source of pure fetal blood for prenatal diagnosis. Lancet. 1979;1:1244-5.
5. Tongsong T, Wanapirak C, Kunavikatikul C, Sirirchotiyakul S, Piyamongkol W, Chanprapaph P. Cordocentesis at 16–24 weeks of gestation: experience of 1,320 cases. Prenat Diagn. 2000; 20:224-8.
6. Nicolaides KH. Cordocentesis. Clin Obstet Gynecol. 1988; 31:123-35.

7. Mari G, Deter RL, Carpenter RL, et al. Noninvasive diagnosis by Doppler ultrasonography of fetal anemia due to maternal red-cell alloimmunization; collaborative group for Doppler assessment of the blood velocity in anemic fetuses. N Engl J Med. 2000;342:9-14.
8. McQuilten ZK, Wood EM, Savoia H, Cole S. A review of pathophysiology and current treatment for neonatal alloimmune thrombocytopenia (NAIT) and introducing the Australian NAIT registry. Aust NZ J Obstet Gynaecol. 2011; 51:191-8.
9. Santo S, Mansour S, Thilaganathan B, et al. Prenatal diagnosis of non-immune hydrops fetalis: what do we tell the parents? Prenat Diagn. 2011;31:186-95.
10. Leung TY, Lao TT. Thalassemia in pregnancy. Best Pract Res Clin Obstet Gynaecol. 2012;26:37-51.
11. Boupaijit K, Wanapirak C, Piyamongkol W, Sirichotiyakul S, Tongsong T. Effect of placenta penetration during cordocentesis at midpregnancy on fetal outcomes. Prenat Diagn. 2012; 32:83-7.
12. Sanchez MA, Bello-Munoz JC, Cebrecos I, et al. The prevalence of congenital varicella syndrome after a maternal infection, but before 20 weeks of pregnancy: a prospective cohort study. J Matern Fetal Neonatal Med. 2011;24:341-7.
13. Nicolini U, Nicolaidis P, Fisk NM, et al. Fetal blood sampling from the intrahepatic vein: Analysis of safety and clinical experience with 214 procedures [comment]. Obstet Gynecol 1990;76:47-53.
14. Dangel JH, Roszkowski T, Bieganowska K, Kubicka K, Ganowicz J. Adenosine triphosphate for cardioversion of supraventricular tachycardia in two hydropic fetuses. Fetal Diagn Ther. 2000; 15:326-30.
15. Evans MI, Goldberg JD, Dommergues M, et al. Efficacy of second-trimester selective termination for fetal abnormalities: international collaborative experience among the world's largest centers. Am J Obstet Gynecol. 1994;171:90-4?
16. Soothill PW, Nicolaides KH, Rodeck CH. Invasive techniques for prenatal diagnosis and therapy. J Perinat Med. 1987; 15:117-27.
17. Nicolaides KH, Soothill PW, Rodeck CH, Campbell S. Ultrasound-guided sampling of umbilical cord and placental blood to assess fetal wellbeing. Lancet. 1986;1(8489):1065-7.
18. Chiang Mai. Review article Cordocentesis; Indications, Techniques, Complications and a Training Course Fuanglada Tongprasert, MD. Med J. 2007;46(3):119-27.
19. Whittle MJ. Cordocentesis. Br J Obstet Gynaecol. 1989; 96:262-4.
20. American College of Obstetricians and Gynecologists. ACOG practice bulletin no. 88, December 2007: invasive prenatal testing for aneuploidy. Obstet Gynecol. 2007;110:1459-67.
21. Tangshewinsirikul C, Wanapirak C, Piyamongkol W, Sirichotiyakul S, Tongsong T. Effect of cord puncture site in cordocentesis at mid-pregnancy on pregnancy outcomes. Prenat Diagn. 2011;31:861-4.
22. Society of Maternal and Fetal Medicine, Berry SM, Stone J, Norton ME, Johnson D, Berghella V. Fetal blood sampling. Am J Obstet Gynecol. 2013;209(3)170-80.
23. Weiner CP. Cordocentesis In: Evans MI, Johnson MP, Yaron Y, Drugan A (Eds). Prenatal Diagnosis. New York: McGraw-Hill; 2006. p. 443-7.
24. Sikovanyecz J, Horvath E, Sallay E, Gellen J, Pal A, Szabo J. Fetomaternal transfusion and pregnancy outcome after cordocentesis. Fetal Diagn Ther. 2001;16:83-9.Level II-2.
25. Weiner C, Grant S, Hudson J, et al. Effect of diagnostic and therapeutic cordocentesis on maternal serum alpha-fetoprotein concentration. Am J Obstet Gynecol. 1989; 161:706-8.
26. Mouw RJ, Klumper F, Hermans J, Brandenburg HC, Kanhai HH. Effect of atracurium or pancuronium on the anemic fetus during and directly after intravascular intrauterine transfusion: a double blind randomized study. Acta Obstet Gynecol Scand. 1999;78:763-7.
27. Aina-Mumuney AJ, Holcroft CJ, Blakemore KJ, et al. Intrahepatic vein for fetal blood sampling: one center's experience. Am J Obstet Gynecol. 2008;198:387.e1-6.
28. Hunter A, Soothild P. Invasive procedures for antenatal diagnosis. In: James DK, Steer PJ, Weiner CP, Gonik B (Eds). High Risk Pregnancy-Management Options, 4th edn. Elsevier Saunders, 2010.
29. Nicolaides KH, Soothill PW, Rodeck CH, Campbell S. Ultrasound-guided sampling of umbilical cord and placental blood to assess fetal wellbeing. Lancet. 1986;1(8489):1065-7.
30. Henderson J, Weiner C, Glob. libr. women's med. (ISSN: 1756-2228) 2008; DOI 10.3843/GLOWM.10212.
31. Sarno AP Jr, Wilson RD. Fetal cardiocentesis: a review of indications, risks, applications and technique. Fetal Diagn Ther 2008;23:237-44.
32. Maxwell DJ, Johnson P, Hurley P, et al. Fetal blood sampling and pregnancy loss in relation to indication. Br J Obstet Gynaecol. 1991;98:892.
33. Weiner CP, Wenstrom KD, Sipes SL, Williamson RA. Risk factors for cordocentesis and fetal intravascular transfusion. Am J Obstet Gynecol. 1991;165:1020.
34. Han JY, Nava-Ocampo AA. Fetal heart rate response to cordocentesis and pregnancy outcome: a prospective cohort. J Matern Fetal Neonatal Med. 2005;17:207-11.
35. Towers CV, Asrat T, Rumney P. The presence of hepatitis B surface antigen and deoxyribonucleic acid in amniotic fluid and cord blood. Am J Obstet Gynecol. 2001;184: 1514-20.
36. Panel on Antiretroviral Guidelines for Adults and Adolescents. Guidelines for the use of antiretroviral agents in HIV-1-infected adults and adolescents. Department of Health and Human Services. HIV infected women. Available at: *http://aidsinfo.nih.gov/contentfiles/lvguidelines/AdultandAdolescentGL.pdf. Accessed Aug. 7, 2013.*

CHAPTER

24

Fetoscopy

S Suresh, Uma Ram

Fetoscopy is a technique by which a small endoscope is introduced percutaneously into the pregnant uterus to visualize the fetus, umbilical cord and the placental surface with the vessels. It is especially useful to identify the placental vascular anastomoses in a monochorionic twin.

HISTORICAL PERSPECTIVE

The first fetoscopy was performed in the year 1954 by Westin,[1] when a 10 mm hysteroscope was introduced through the cervix between 14–18 weeks of gestation. This was done as a purely experimental technique on women who were undergoing abortion. Subsequently, Madelbaum[2] in the year 1957 used a transabdominal approach and attempted to perform endoscopic guided intrauterine transfusion for Rh disease. In 1972, Valenti coined the term 'endo amnioscope'. This instrument was 5 mm in diameter and was modified from a pediatric cystoscope. He demonstrated that this technique could be used for obtaining samples from the fetal skin for diagnosing genodermatoses. In 1973, Valenti demonstrated for the first time[3] the use of a 1.7 mm scope for performing fetal blood sampling under local anesthesia for diagnosis of hemoglobinopathies. At about the same time, Scrimgeour coined the term 'fetoscope'.[4] He used a 2.2 mm needle scope and introduced it though the uterus after a laparotomy in 6 women who were at high risk for neural tube defect. In this group there were three healthy babies and one spina bifida was detected. Mitchell Golbus et al.[5] from the USA used fetoscopic skin biopsy for diagnosis of epidermolysis bullosa and Rodeck[6] did a fetal liver biopsy to diagnose ornithine carbamyl transferase deficiency. For over a decade after this, as ultrasound skills improved, the use of fetoscopy for fetal anomalies reduced but was still used for fetal blood sampling and skin biopsy. However, in 1983, Daffos et al.[7] initiated ultrasound guided fetal blood sampling, which subsequently has become the standard of care. In 1988 De Lia pioneered fetoscopic laser occlusion of the 'chorioangiopagus' vessels (FLOC) and by 1991, this was introduced by Nicolaides in UK and Yves Ville in France.

APPLICATIONS OF FETOSCOPY

The most common application of fetoscopy is for laser photocoagulation of the anastomotic vessels in twin-to-twin transfusion syndrome (TTTS) or sometimes in selective intrauterine growth restriction (IUGR). Today there are several centers across the world performing fetoscopy which has helped reduce mortality in complicated monochorionic twins. Fetoscopy is also used during bipolar cord occlusion, dividing amniotic bands and for complete transection of the cord in momo twins. The technique has now been extended to perform endoscopic balloon occlusion of the trachea for diaphragmatic hernia, fetal cystoscopic fulguration of the posterior urethral valves. A few centers have now embarked on minimally invasive *in utero* surgery for repair of meningomyelocele.

Instrumentation

The European Commission initiated a EUROFETUS project as part of its biomed 2 program. In this program, a manufacturer of medical equipment was partnered with and with leading medical experts in the field, set out to design special instruments to make fetoscopic procedures safer with reduced size of the instruments. From 25 mm scopes in the 1950's, the size has been reduced to 1–2 mm.

Fetoscopic instrumentation typically consists of a sheath with a working channel for introducing the laser fiber, a telescope for viewing, typically 1.3 mm or 2.0 mm. The sheath can be introduced directly using a sharp introducer along with the sheath. Alternatively a Seldinger technique may be used with a guidewire and a 10 Fr introducer set (Fig. 24.1).

Anesthesia for fetoscopy: Fetoscopic procedures can be done under local anesthesia with maternal sedation. In some centers it has been performed under epidural or rarely general anesthesia.

Procedures: Fetoscopy for laser photocoagulation of anastomotic vessels in TTTS.

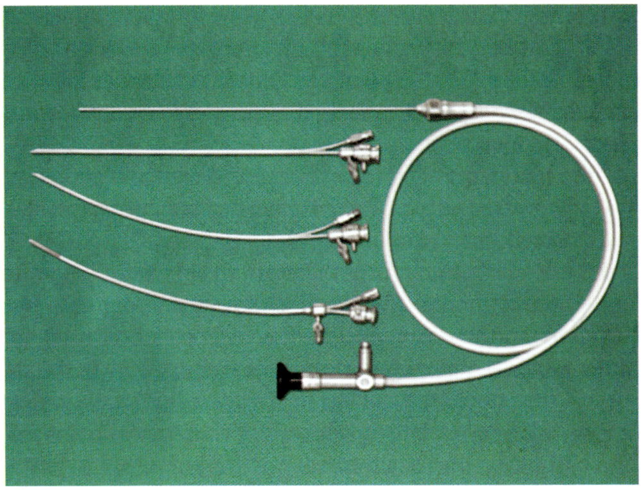

Fig. 24.1 A 2 mm fetoscope with sheaths

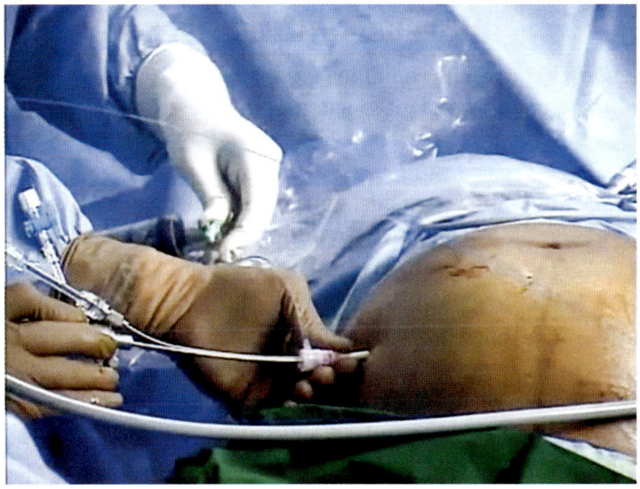

Fig. 24.2 External marking of site of entry

The diagnosis of TTTS is based on quintero staging as explained in the chapter for TTTS.

There are two types of systems that can be used. In one system the telescope, and sheath are separate and depending on anterior or posterior placenta, the telescope can be used using a curved or straight sheath. This can be introduced either by a Seldinger technique or directly by using a sharp introducer that goes into the sheath.

In the second system, there is a straight and curved telescope at 30° angle integrated with working channels. This can be used only through a flexible trocar introduced by the Seldinger technique.

In addition to the above, a light source and camera is required as for laparoscopic procedures.

Laser fibers of 400 nm or 600 nm can be used. The laser equipment can be a 60 w Diode Laser or an Nd:YAG Laser 60–100 Watts. The laser fibers come as disposable fibers or reusable fibers and the usage policy is as per the institution's policy. The reusable fibers are autoclavable and the tip can be cut after each procedure to expose a fresh tip.

Step 1: Preprocedural ultrasound confirming chorionicity and the diagnosis and marking the placenta, cord insertion sites and the position of the babies.

Step 2: Planning the site of entry (Fig. 24.2)—This is determined based on the sites of cord insertion and the position of the intertwin membrane. The intention is to enter the recipient sac perpendicular to the intertwin membrane. Care is to be taken to ensure that we do not go through the placenta or through the donor sac as the membrane can sometimes be flat against the uterine wall.

Step 3: Entry—Entry can be direct (if using a scope with a sharp introducer) or by using a Seldinger technique using a flexible trocar. Entry is always into the recipient sac, under ultrasound guidance. Once the entry is made, amnioinfusion is done if necessary and the fetosocpe is introduced (Fig. 24.3).

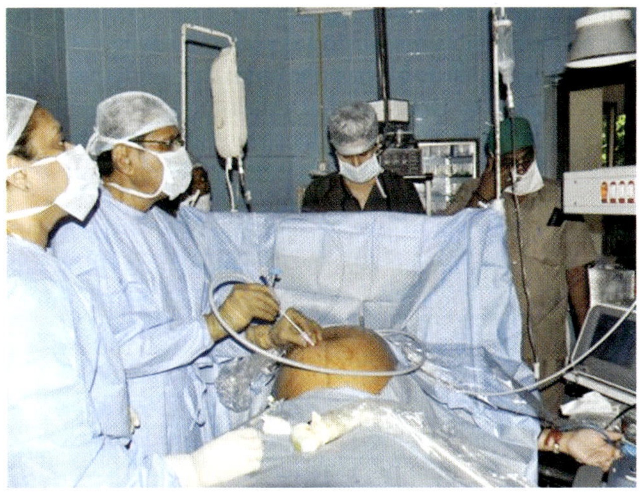

Fig. 24.3 Set up with fetoscope introduced

Step 4: Identifying the membrane, cord insertion sites and anastamoses sites.

Once the fetoscope is in, it is important to get a good orientation to the placental circulation. This is achieved by identifying the dividing membrane and both cord insertions. All vessels that cross the membrane along this full length are followed to identify the anastamoses.

Step 5: *Coagulation of anastomotic vessels*—Laser energy (20–40 Watts from a diode or YAG laser) is delivered to the vessels through a 400–600 micron quartz fiber that is introduced through an operating channel in the fetoscope. A second channel allows irrigation to promote visualization.

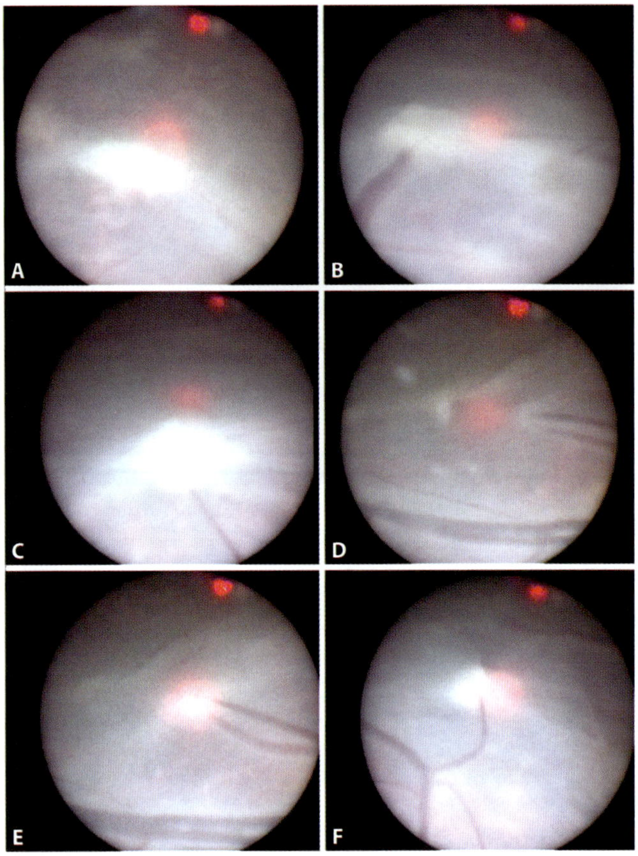

Figs 24.4A to F Laser coagulation done of anastomotic sites

It is important to ensure that all anastomotic sites are coagulated and sometimes it may be necessary to release some of them to ensure complete coagulation (Figs 24.4A to F).

Step 6: *Amnioreduction*—At the end of the procedure, after we pull out the scope, amnioreduction is done in a controlled fashion.

Bipolar Cord Occlusion

Bipolar cord occlusion is a procedure done for selective fetal reduction of a monochorionic twin. Severe selective IUGR and monochorionic diamniotic (MCDA) twins discordant for anomaly and twin reversed arterial perfusion (TRAP) sequence are the most common indications.

This is essentially done under ultrasound guidance through a 10 french trocar that is introduced using Seldinger technique. The cord is held under ultrasound guidance and cessation of flow on the cord is the point of completion of the procedure.

A take-Apart bipolar forceps of diameter 3 mm is used since the trocar is in place, we can use a fetoscope to check the site of the coagulation and ensure that we have indeed got the full thickness of the cord. More recently an optical bipolar forceps has been introduced to provide visibility on the scope as the forceps is being introduced. In a series of 118 pregnancies, Fanna et al. reported an overall survival of 71% with 9% neonatal deaths.[8]

In monoamniotic twins requiring selective fetal reduction, it is important to transect the cord after a bipolar occlusion to prevent cord entanglement. Transection of the cord is done under fetoscopic vision using a laser.

Amniotic Bands

Amniotic bands can occur spontaneously or after a fetoscopic laser for TTTS. The procedure is not done for bands, which have caused multiple severe anomalies. It is done in cases where the bands are causing constriction around the limbs and potentially can cause neurological and ischemic damage of the distal portion. The procedure is done fetoscopically using a special scissors or using a low wattage laser. Extreme care is to be taken when using laser as potential damage to the underlying limb is possible.

Fetal Endoscopic Tracheal Occlusion

Fetal endoscopic tracheal occlusion (FETO) is a procedure done for antenatal management of congenital diaphragmatic hernia. In diaphragmatic hernia, compression of the fetal lungs causes egress of lung liquid which over a period of time results in pulmonary dysfunction. The FETO procedure helps to expand the lungs and preserve the lung liquid which can potentially improve outcomes. In this procedure under local anesthesia, through a fetoscope, a small balloon is placed in the trachea of the fetus. A specially designed 3 mm fetoscope with a working channel is used.

In a series of 210 cases, Jani et al reported a high rate of preterm premature rupture of membranes (PPROM) (47.1%) and preterm labor (16.7%).[9] The procedures were done at a median gestational age of 27 weeks with a range of 23–33 weeks. Prior to delivery the balloon has to be decompressed either through a repeat fetoscopic procedure at 35 weeks or by puncture of the balloon under ultrasound guidance or an exit procedure. All this entails a team of fetal medicine specialists, pediatric surgeon, neonatologist and the obstetrician work very closely together and can be available at short notice when required and delivery should take place at a tertiary center with neonatal care facilities.

Fetal Cystoscopy

In 1995, Quintero et al.[10] described the technique of fetal cystoscopy for bladder outlet obstruction using a flexible fiberoptic cystoscope. In a series of 11 cases, either a urethral shunt was placed or vesicoamniotic shunting was done. They also noted that this technique helped to identify the cause of obstruction which could not be done with ultrasound. They concluded that fetal cystoscopy was feasible and could potentially be used to define management in lower urinary tract obstruction.

Martinez et al. in 2015[11] reported a series of 20 cases of fetal cystoscopic fulguration of posterior urethral valves. Technically they were able to access the urethra in 95% of the cases and normalization of bladder size and amniotic fluid volume could be achieved in 80% of the cases. Even though all cases had severe oligohydramnios prior to the procedure, there were no cases of pulmonary hypoplasia at birth and all were alive at 15–110 months. 72.7% of them had normal renal function and 27.3% have renal failure awaiting transplantation. This study shows that fetal cystoscopic fulguration of posterior urethral valves could potentially be a prenatal therapeutic option. Sananes N et al.[12] reported that urological fistulas as a potential complication in 10% of the cases. These occurred with less operator expertize, later gestational age at surgery and usage of higher laser power. They reported a survival rate of 85.7% in a series of 23 fulgurations.

Even though fetal cystoscopic procedure has distinct advantages over vesicoamniotic shunting, better instrumentation and larger studies are required to recommend it as a procedure of choice.

Fetoscopy is a procedure that needs training. There are few centers in the world that have the skill to perform the more complicated type of fetoscopic procedures. There is a mismatch between the availability of these procedures across the world. Given that the complexities of training, different models of training are being looked at. Telementoring and simulater based training are some of the models that seem to work well.

As with any complex surgical procedure, it is best that fetoscopy is done by trained personnel in units that have a good volume to ensure that skill sets and standards are being maintained. In a country such as India, it is vital to ensure that the growth and availability of fetoscopic surgery is structured. Resources and expertize should be pooled to ensure regional centers are developed that work within accepted protocols of management.

REFERENCES

1. Westin B. Hysteroscopy in early pregnancy. Lancet. 1954;11:872.
2. Mandelbaum B. Pontarelli D, Brushenko A. Amnioscopy for prenatal transfusion. Am J Obstet Gynecol. 1967;98:1140.
3. Valenti C. Antenatal detection of hemoglobinopathies. Am J Obst Gynecol. 1973;115:851.
4. Scrimgeour JB. Other techniques for antenatal diagnosis. In: Emery AEH (Ed). Antenatal Diagnosis of Genetic Disease. Edinburgh: Churchill Livingstone; 1973. p. 49.
5. Golbus MS, Sagebiel RW, Filly RA, et al. Prenatal diagnosis of congenital bullous ichthyosiform erythroderma (epidemolytic hyperkeratosis by fetal skin biopsy. New Eng J Med. 1979; 302:93.
6. Rodeck CH, Patrick AD, Pembrey ME y cols. Fetal liver biopsy for prenatal diagnosis of ornithine carbamyltransferace deficiency. Lancet. 1982(1):189-94.
7. Daffos F, Cappella-Pavlovsky M, Forestier F. Fetal blood sampling via the umbilical cord using a needle guided by ultrasound. Report of 66 cases. Prenat Diagn. 1983;3:271-7.
8. Lanna MM, Rustico MA, Dell'avanzo M, Schena VS, Faiola D, Consonni A. Ferrazzi bipolar cord coagulation for selective feticide in complicated monochorionic twin pregnancies: 118 consecutive cases at a single center. Ultrasound Obstet Gynecol. 2012;39:407-13.
9. Jani JC, Nicolaides KH, Gratacós E, Valencia CM, Done E, Martinez JM, et al. Severe diaphragmatic hernia treated by fetal endoscopic tracheal occlusion. Ultrasound Obstet Gynecol. 2009;34:304-10.
10. Quintero RA, Johnson MP, Romero R, Smith C, Arias F, Guevara-Zuloaga F, et al. In-utero percutaneous cystoscopy in the management of fetal lower obstructive uropathy. Lancet. 1995;346(8974):537-40.
11. Martínez JM, Masoller N, Devlieger R, Passchyn E, Gómez O, Rodo J, et al. Laser ablation of posterior urethral valves by fetal cystoscopy. Fetal Diagn Ther. 2015;37(4):267-73. doi: 10.1159/000367805. Epub 2015 Jan 21.
12. Sananes N, Favre R, Koh CJ, et al. Urological fistulas after fetal cystoscopic laser ablation of posterior urethral valves: surgical technical aspects. Ultrasound Obstet Gynecol. 2015;45(2):183-9. doi: 10.1002/uog.13405.

SECTION

5

Laboratory Techniques

CHAPTER

25

Genetic Testing: Indications, Types and Principles

Nandini Vaz Fernandes, Hema Purandarey, Vishalakshi Kamat

INTRODUCTION

Genetic testing involves identification of changes in the chromosomes, genes or proteins produced by the genes. Genetic testing is essential to either confirm or rule out suspected genetic conditions or determine the risk associated with inheritance pattern. Today, more than 1000 genetic tests are in use and there is ongoing research to still develop more and more tests mostly at molecular level.

Genetic testing is slowly gaining importance in the Indian society because of increasing awareness about the availability of the tests. It is now more important for obstetricians and gynecologists as clinical cytogenetics has direct effects on diagnosis, prognosis, management and prevention of many genetic disorders. Since medicolegal responsibilities are associated with counseling, screening and diagnosis of chromosomal disorders, thus medical fraternity need to have sound knowledge about the important concepts, developments in cytogenetics and their applications in the practice.

In fact, general awareness is now encouraging people to resort to voluntary genetic testing for risk assessment. Genetic testing has multiple benefits in terms of managing the disease and assessing the future risk and understanding the mode of transmittance. Though these tests have some limitations and risks, it has multiple benefits too. A medical practitioner/physician can recommend individuals to a geneticist or a genetic counselor to provide information about the pros and cons of the test and discussing the social and emotional aspects of testing.

IMPORTANCE

Genetic diagnosis has tremendous benefits. However appropriate pre test genetic counseling is essential to select a test, time, tissue and turn around time for the results. Many diseases and medical conditions have genetic basis. As most genetic disorders cannot be cured, early detection and informed choices of management is the only option. There are over nine hundred genetic tests available today and newer tests are being added periodically. Most of the genetic tests are carried out on blood, bone marrow or fetal samples prenatally or postnatally. An appropriately qualified geneticist can explain in detail the benefits, risks, and limitations of a particular test as well as interpreting the reports. The importance of genetic diagnosis to the practice of obstetrics and gynecology has dramatically increased, during the past three decades because clinical cytogenetics had direct affects on diagnosis, management and prevention of many genetic disorders. Since medicolegal responsibilities are associated with counseling, screening and diagnosis of chromosomal disorders, obstetricians and gynecologists need to have sound knowledge about the important concepts, developments in cytogenetics and their applications in the practice of obstetrics and gynecology.

Genetic testing can be done at different levels. The major levels are given in Figure 25.1.

Diagnostic testing: It is offered when an individual has a clinical suspicion of a genetic disorder, diagnostic genetic test is ordered to confirm the diagnosis. Chromosomal aberrations numerical or structural can be identified by karyotyping or advanced tests of chromosome microarray, e.g. Philadelphia chromosome in chronic myeloid leukemia, Down's syndrome, Turners syndrome, Klinefelter syndrome etc., which may involve numerical or structural abnormalities of the chromosome. While metabolic tests are used by biochemical methods for suspected inborn errors of metabolism.

Predictive testing: Also known as presymptomatic testing. Usually in this category there is a family history of a certain disorder, the members of family can be screened for a specified genetic mutation study by molecular testing. Such a study can be useful in early intervention and management. Some commonly known disorders are: Familial breast cancer (BRCA-1 and BRCA-2) or colon cancer. The risk to other family members of Huntington disease, an adult neurological genetic disorder inherited as an autosomal dominant condition expressing in midlife, can also be detected by predictive testing.

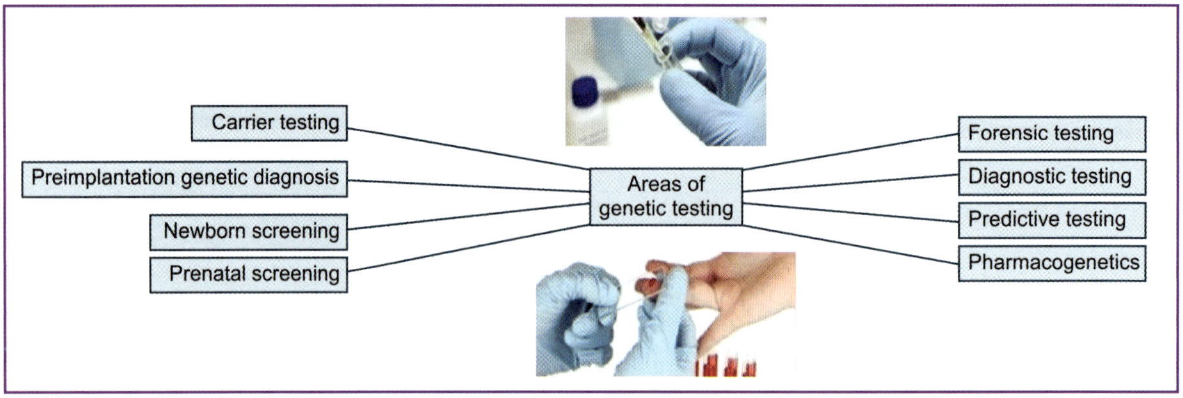

Fig. 25.1 Areas of genetic testing

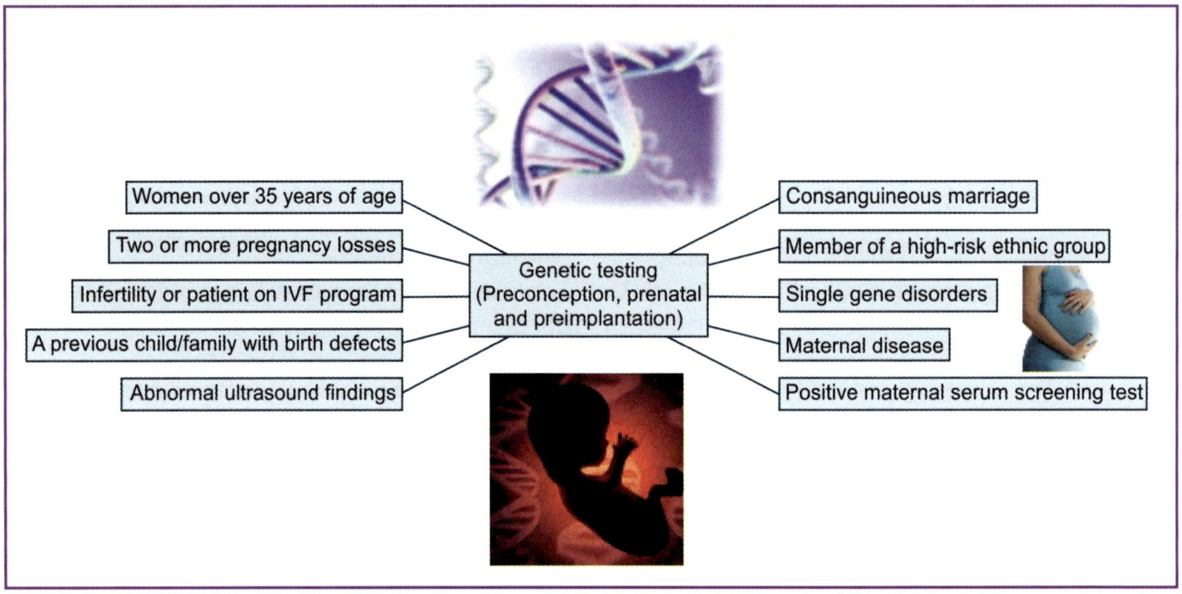

Fig. 25.2 Genetic testing for fetal anomalies

Carrier testing: It is offered to check if one is a carrier or evaluate the risk of transmission of a disease carrying gene in the offspring after an affected child is born for recurrence risk and prenatal diagnosis. Carrier testing is also used in population screening, e.g. thalassemia is known to be prevalent in mediterranean region and population screening can pick up high-risk cases and be offered prenantal diagnosis in the first trimester.

Prenatal screening: Maternal Serum screening and has become a standard care in obstetric practice today. It is offered as Dual marker test (11–14 weeks), Triple marker test and Quadruple marker test (15–17 weeks) based on maternal serum analysis (Fig. 25.2). It is used in risk prediction for commonly known chromosome aneuploidies like Down's syndrome (Trisomy 21), Edwards syndrome (Trisomy 18), Patau syndrome (Trisomy 13) and neural tube defects. The predictivity is 84–92%. Patients screened positive are offered confirmatory tests by fetal karyotype by amniocentesis or chorionic villus sampling. A high end screening test known as noninvasive prenatal testing has been newly developed. In here, cell free fetal DNA is extracted from maternal blood after 10 weeks; though reliability for chromosome aneuploidies is 99% all positive cases need confirmatory test.

Pharmacogenetics: It is the study of inherited genetic differences in drug metabolic pathways which can affect individual's responses to drugs both in therapeutic or adverse effects. The drug and dosage can be adjusted accordingly to yield the best results.

Newborn screening: This screening is recommended to identify genetic metabolic disorders which can be treated if detected on newborn screening and confirmed by advanced test. The time period for testing is within first few days of life, ideally within 24–48 hours of birth. Basic screening is available for hypothyroidism, congenital adrenal hyperplasia, galactosemia, biotinidase deficiency, maple syrup urine disease, cystic fibrosis, phenylketonuria (PKU), G6pd, thyroid and more. It is done on a drop of blood from heel puncture.

Preimplantation genetic diagnosis (PGD): It is a very specialized technique on a single cell biopsy—blastomere biopsy performed on embryos of IVF pregnancies at 8-celled stage, to reduce the risk of having a child with a particular genetic or chromosomal disorder. The selected healthy embryos are then implanted.

Forensic testing: It is a highly reliable test on DNA isolated from biological evidence samples whether freshly collected, dry or frozen, regardless of age. The extracted DNA's quantity is evaluated and then specific regions are amplified by polymerase chain reaction. PCR produces millions of copies for the DNA segment of interest and helps in examination of even very minute DNA amount. Multiple STR regions can be examined simultaneously to increase the informativeness of the DNA test. The test is also called identity testing and is used to identify missing individual from forensic material from crime site, blood, hair, semen or any body tissue. Types of DNA evidence analysis: Polymerase chain reaction, short tandem repeats, Y-chromosome, mitochondrial DNA

In conclusion, above genetic tests are beneficial whether the results are positive or negative for a tested gene mutation. Negative results can provide a reassurance. On the other hand, if the test is positive, the doctors can direct a person toward available prevention, monitoring, and possible treatment options.

Predictive testing helps risk assessments, may help people to change their lifestyle to postpone the onset of the disease like in hypercholesteremia and therefore increase their life span, or help plan a sedentary profession in Huntington's disease.

Carrier testing can also help prospective parents to make important decisions about child bearing and reproductive options.

Prenatal testing enables diagnosis of genetic disorders and helps in voluntary decision making in abnormal results.

The newborn screening tests identify some metabolic disorders early in life, so treatment can be started early and mental retardation can be prevented in relevant cases.

INDICATIONS AND COUNSELING

Genetic tests are suggested to individuals for the indications discussed further.

Preconception, prenantal and preimplantation:

- Consanguineous marriage
- Member of a high risk ethnic group
- Maternal disease
- Single gene disorders
- Infertility or patients on IVF program
- Two or more pregnancy losses
- A previous child/family with birth defects
- Positive maternal serum screening test (Double/Triple/Quadruple)
- Abnormal ultrasound findings
- Women over 35 years of age.

Infants, children, adolescents and adults:

- Developmental delay
- Ambiguous genitalia; puberty disorders
- Dysmorphic features; mental retardation
- Growth retardation
- Suspected metabolic disorders
- Blindness or deafness
- Primary and secondary amenorrhoea
- DNA parentage studies
- Cancer, diabetes and schizophrenia.

METHODS

Today, there are several different genetic tests performed in the genetic laboratories. The choice of the test will depend on type of abnormality that is being measured or depends on the reason for the genetic test. The genetic tests can be discussed at three different levels viz. cytogenetic, biochemical, and molecular testing.

Cytogenetic testing: This test involves the examination of chromosomes and their abnormalities. Chromosomes are obtained from the cultured white blood cells, specifically T lymphocytes, and analysed for numerical and structural abnormalities. Cells from other tissues such as bone marrow, amniotic fluid, and other tissue biopsies can also be cultured for cytogenetic analysis. Chromosomes obtained are fixed, spread on microscope slides and then stained and analysed using karyotyping software. The arranged chromosomes are called as karyotype.

Karyotyping is the most reliable cytogenetic test. Here the chromosomes are analyzed for detecting chromosomal aberrations on account of change in chromosome number or chromosome structure. Numerical chromosomal abnormalities include extrachromosomes (e.g. Down's syndrome) or missing chromosomes (Turner's syndrome). Structural abnormalities would include deletions, translocations, inversions, substitutions, etc. It can be performed on almost all the body tissues.

Chromosomal testing can be recommended for diagnostic testing, prenatal screening, preimplantation genetic diagnosis and newborn screening.

Molecular cytogenetics: Fluorescent *in situ* hybridization (FISH) is a molecular cytogenetic test which involves hybridization of the probes for specific abnormality/disease detection. The probe is tagged with specific color fluorescence. FISH allows chromosomal and nuclear localization of specific DNA sequences to be seen through the microscope. FISH technology permits the detection of specific nucleic acid sequences in morphologically preserved chromosomes, cells and tissues. This procedure can be used to detect the abnormality/disease using chromosome plates or even the cells. Probe used here is a portions of chromosomes tagged with fluorescent molecules to identify chromosomal abnormalities (e.g. insertions, deletions, translocations and amplifications). FISH is commonly used to identify specific chromosomal deletions associated with pediatric syndromes such as DiGeorge syndrome (del22) and cancers such as chronic myelogenous leukemia (BCR-ABL 9;22) (Fig. 25.3) and B cell Lymphoma (IgH-BCL2 14;18).

Another molecular cytogenetic technique used includes *'spectral karyotyping'(SKY)*, which involves whole chromosome paint. Each chromosome is colored with a specific color (Fig. 25.4). This enables detection of minute structural abnormalities and for assigning the origin of the marker chromosomes detected through karyotyping. Thus SKY or M-FISH allows all the 24 human chromosomes to be painted in different colors. By making use of various combinations and concentrations of fluorescent dyes, it is even possible to give every single chromosome a different color (SKY) which can be of particular use when dealing with complex aberrations often associated with various types of solid tumors. SKY or M-FISH enables production of chromosome-specific 'paints': combines fluorochromes to produce 24 color combinations, one for each chromosome (Reid et al. 1992) and hence multicolor analyses.

Certain specific disorders that can be detected by chromosomal and/or molecular cytogenetic testing include: a group of disorders called microdeletion syndromes, Angelmen syndrome, DiGeorge syndrome, Miller-Dieker syndrome, Prader-Willi syndrome, Smith-Magenis syndrome, Velocardiofacial syndrome, Williams syndrome, Cri du Chat syndrome, Wolf-Hirschhorn syndrome, Fanconi anemia, trisomy 21, trisomy 13 syndrome, trisomy 18 syndrome, trisomy 21 syndrome, sex chromosome aneuploidy (Klinefelter syndrome, Turner syndrome, etc.) all have probes that can help in quick identification of aneuploidy.

Molecular genetic tests: These tests can also be referred to as gene tests. This is the next level at which genetic disorders can be detected. It involves the study of single gene or short lengths of DNA to identify variations or mutations that lead to genetic disorders. *Gene mutation test* is not available for all disorders. DNA analysis is possible for only those disorders whose gene sequence is known. DNA test generally can be performed on small quantity of any tissue sample.

Polymerase chain reaction-based assays: Molecular technologies used for gene mutation detection include direct sequencing, polymerase chain reaction-based assays (PCR), and hybridization. PCR involves amplification of targeted segments of DNA through repeated cycles of denaturation, annealing and elongation. The amplified product is then digested with a restriction enzyme and subjected to gel electrophoresis to detect the presence of a mutation/polymorphism.

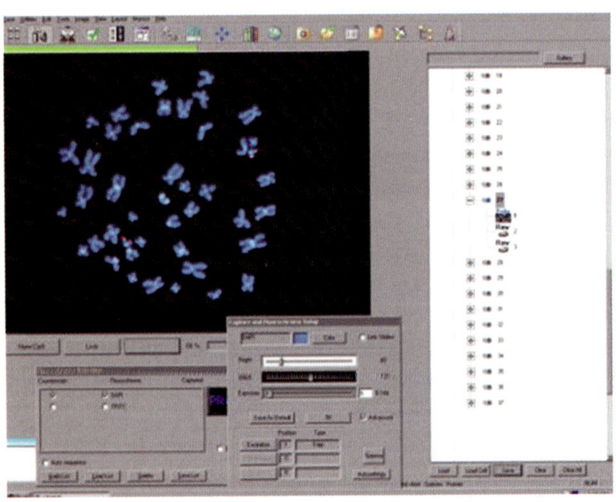

Fig. 25.3 FISH metaphase

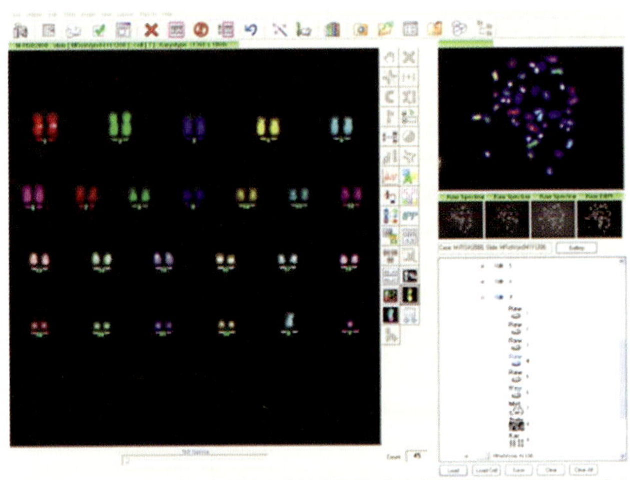

Fig. 25.4 Spectral karyotype

Microarrays test: Another important molecular genetic test includes DNA "chips" or microarrays test. Microarrays have been used as a possible testing for multiple mutations. In this technology, single DNA strands including sequences of different targets are fixed to a solid support in an array format. Interpretation of this test requires special lab expertise.

Multiplex ligation-dependent probe amplification (MLPA): MLPA is commonly applied to screen deletions and duplications of up to 50 different genomic DNA or RNA sequences.

For some genetic diseases, many mutations can occur in the same gene and result in the same disease, making molecular testing challenging. For example, more than 800 mutations in the cystic fibrosis transmembrane conductance regulator (CFTR) can cause cystic fibrosis (CF). It would be impractical to sequence the entire CFTR gene to identify the causative mutation since the gene is quite large. Today around 200 syndromes can be identified by microarray analysis.

Biochemical genetic tests: Some genetic disorders include change in the metabolic regulations. These disorders can be detected by performing biochemical tests. These tests study the amount or activity level of proteins involved. This is a technique that examines the protein instead of the gene. Many biochemical genetic diseases are known as 'inborn errors of metabolism' since they are present at birth and disrupt a key metabolic pathway. The types of biochemical test to be recommended depend on the type of disease suspected or considered for evaluation. These tests require a tissue sample such as blood, urine, amniotic fluid, or cerebrospinal fluid. Because proteins are more unstable the sample must be collected and stored properly and shipped promptly according to the laboratory's specifications.

A variety of technologies enable both qualitative detection and quantitative determination of metabolites such as high performance liquid chromatography (HPLC), gas chromatography/mass spectrometry (GC/MS), and MS/MS. In addition, bioassays may employ fluorometric (e.g. beta-galactosidase), radioisotopic (e.g. galactosemia), or thin layer chromatography (e.g. mucopolysaccharidosis) methods.

PROCEDURES (FLOW CHARTS 25.1 AND 25. 2)

Sample Handling and Transport for Genetic Testing

Sample for genetic testing may be received in the laboratory or may be collected in the laboratory. The received sample or collected sample needs to be labeled accurately and logged

Flow chart 25.1 Basic steps in cytogenetic testing

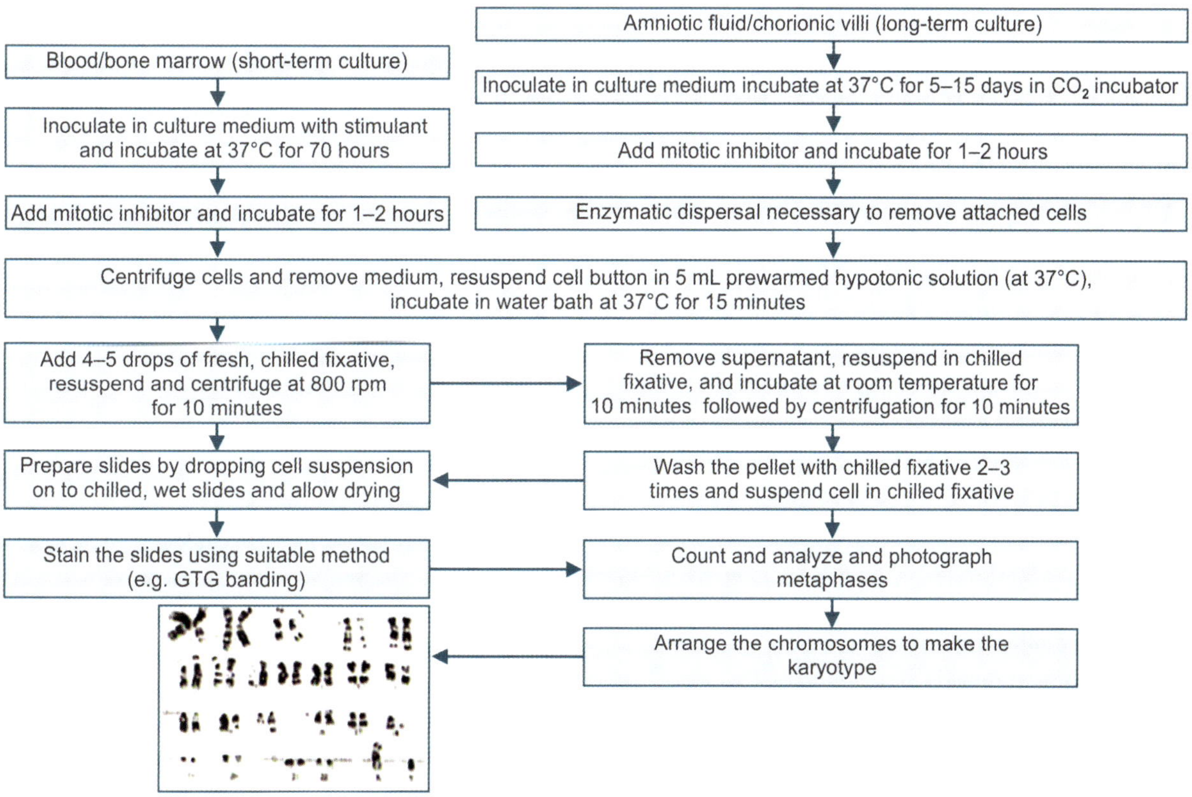

Flow chart 25.2 Basic steps in FISH

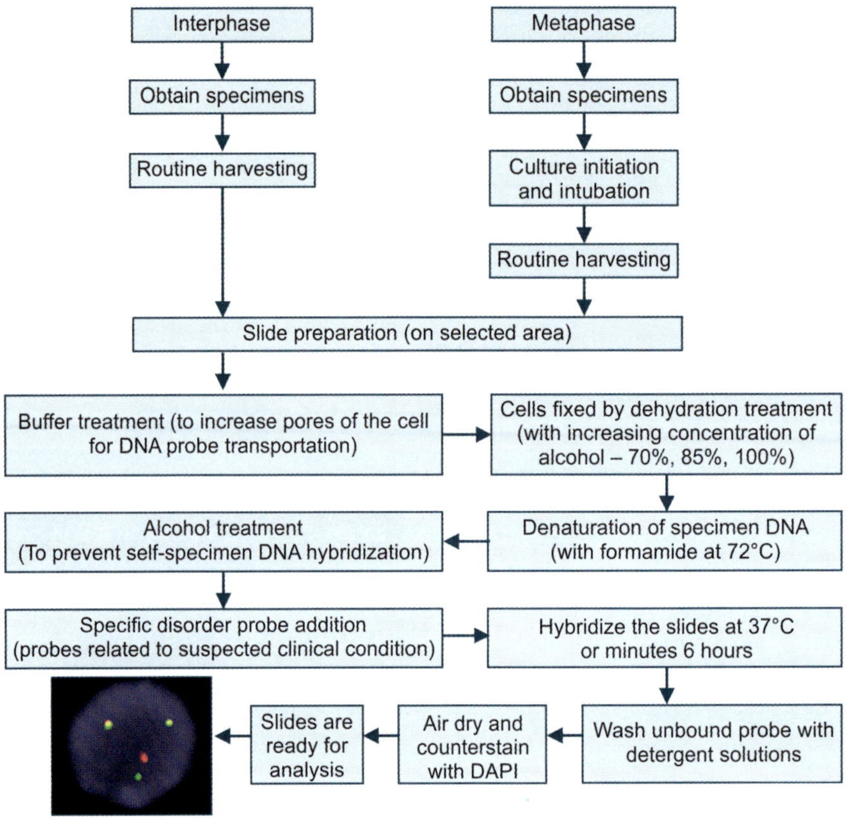

in the database of the laboratory. Specimens must be labelled with the patient's full name (or unique code number in the case of anonymous testing) and one other unique identifier such as the admission/identification or accession number.

Method of Sample Collection

- *Peripheral blood (chromosome and/or FISH analysis):* Usually, 2–5 mL blood sample should be collected in Sodium heparin tubes (green top vacutainer), labeled and transported.
- *Peripheral blood chromosomal microarray (CMA):* Around 3 mL whole blood per tube needs to be collected into one purple-top (EDTA) and one green-top sodium heparin vacutainer.
- *Amniotic fluid:* 10–25 mL of amniotic fluid needs to be collected at 14 weeks of gestation or greater in a sterile syringe. The fluid can then be transferred to sterile centrifuge tubes in 3–4 sterile aliquots and transported to the laboratory within 24 hours.
- *Chorionic villi specimens (CVS)*: Approximately 20–30 mg of chorionic villi are collected either transabdominally or transcervically. These villi are placed in CVS transport media and transported at room temperature to the laboratory within 24 hours.
- *Bone marrow specimens (chromosome and/or FISH analysis)*: Two mL of bone marrow aspirate are collected into a heparinized syringe using the first draw or a repositioned needle and placed in containers of medium supplied by the laboratory. Alternatively sodium heparinized vacutainer can also be used.
- *Product of conception:* 3–10 mm^3 of tissue from spontaneous abortions, stillborns, terminations or autopsy specimens is collected aseptically and placed in tissue transport media in a sterile container. Villi are preferred, although fetal cartilage, membrane or tendon is also acceptable. Since living cells are required, the specimen should not be dropped into fixative or formalin.

It is important that following criteria needs to be observed while choosing a centre for sending the samples, namely the centre should have experienced medical geneticist to interpret the reports, accreditations, reliable reporting and interaction with the physician.

SUGGESTED READING

1. Archana Sharma, Geeta Talukdar. Laboratory procedures in human genetics. Volume 1 Chromosome methodology. The Nucleus, 1974.
2. Barch M, Knutsen T, Spurbeck J. AGT Manual, 3rd edn. New York, Lippincott-Raven Publishers, 1997.
3. Gardner RJM, Sutherland GR. Chromosome Abnormalities and Genetic Counseling, 3rd edn. New York, NY: Oxford University Press; 2004:117-8.
4. Lisa Shaffer, Jean McGowan-Jordan, Michael Schmid: ISCN 2013. An International System for Human Cytogenetic Nomenclature. Karger Publishers, 2013.
5. Online Mendelian Inheritance in man, OMIM. McKusick-Nathans Institute of Genetic Medicine, Johns Hopkins University (Baltimore, MD) and National Center for Biotechnology Information, national Library of Medicine (Bethesda MD), URL: *http://www.ncbi.nlm.nih.gov/omim/*.
6. Purandare H, Chakravarty A. Human Cytogenetic Techniques and Clinical Applications. Mumbai, Bhalani Publishing House, 2000.
7. Schinzel A. Catalogue of Unbalanced Chromosomal Aberrations in Man, 2nd edn. New York, NY: Walter De Grutter GmbH & Co.; 2001:954-5.

CHAPTER

26 Preimplantation Genetic Diagnosis

Prochi F Madon, Arundhati S Athalye, Firuza R Parikh

INTRODUCTION

Preimplantation genetic diagnosis (PGD) was introduced for couples at high risk of having children with genetic disorders, to avoid pregnancy termination after prenatal diagnosis. It has become an alternative to traditional prenatal diagnosis and also an integral part of assisted reproduction. PGD is an efficient tool for improving the success of *in vitro* fertilization (IVF) by avoiding transfer of genetically affected embryos. It thus eliminates the risk of passing on genetic disorders to a child before the woman gets pregnant. PGD is the earliest form of genetic diagnosis of chromosomal and inherited single gene disorders as it is carried out on embryos which are only three to five days old. Single blastomeres biopsied from cleavage stage embryos or a few trophectoderm cells obtained by blastocyst biopsy are used for genetic analysis. Embryos which are normal, or not affected (heterozygous carriers) by the familial genetic disorder being tested, are selected for transfer to the uterus. PGD thus helps to eliminate the need for repeated abortions of affected natural pregnancies, when an abnormality is detected by prenatal diagnosis on a chorionic villus sample (CVS), amniotic fluid or cord blood. The genetic abnormalities can be as small as a single-base mutation in just one gene, or they can involve structural and numerical chromosome abnormalities. Intracytoplasmic sperm injection (ICSI) is necessary for PGD, to prevent misdiagnosis due to DNA contamination from residual sperm. Every year, an estimated 8 million infants (6% of total births worldwide) are born with serious birth defects of genetic or partially genetic origin, according to the March of Dimes global report on birth defects. PGD is carried out to help prevent such birth defects.

Advances in IVF such as blastocyst biopsy, vitrification of biopsied embryos and transfer of unaffected embryos in subsequent cycles, together with recent genetic techniques like chromosome microarray (CMA) and next generation sequencing (NGS) have led to the increasing use of PGD.[1-10] The easy availability of these genetic techniques now to diagnose mutations and the carrier status in a large number of single gene disorders, has increased the scope and demand for PGD.

WHO NEEDS PREIMPLANTATION GENETIC DIAGNOSIS/PREIMPLANTATION GENETIC SCREENING?

Preimplantation genetic diagnosis can be carried out on fertile couples who are carriers of genetic mutations of single gene disorders. These are usually detected after the birth of an affected child in the family. It is also used if one of the partners is a carrier of a structural chromosome rearrangement. The term preimplantation genetic screening (PGS) was introduced later, to differentiate chromosome aneuploidy screening from diagnosis of inherited disorders. Thus PGS covers 24-chromosome aneuploidy screening or comprehensive chromosome screening (CCS), which can be carried out even in the absence of a familial genetic disorder. PGS helps to increase the chances of live births in IVF cycles, as it detects aneuploid embryos which have a trisomy or monosomy of any of the 23 pairs of chromosomes and even duplications, deletions and multiple chromosome aneuploidies. Such embryos are not transferred as they generally lead to failed implantation, early miscarriage or a child with developmental delay and congenital malformations.

PGS is particularly useful in cases of advanced maternal age.[11] It is also useful in couples with aneuploidy in a previous child, or a miscarriage. After PGD for single gene disorders, unaffected embryos can further undergo PGS from the left over DNA to eliminate the chromosomally abnormal ones too. As couples undergoing PGD combined with PGS are generally fertile, if genetic problems of both the single gene disorder and aneuploidy are eliminated, the chances of a successful IVF with the best embryos selected are good. The chances of success with single embryo transfer to reduce multiple offspring are also higher after PGD combined with PGS.

GENETIC COUNSELING

Genetic counseling plays an important role even in PGD. The counselor talks to the couple regarding the genetic disorder in the family. Pedigree charting helps to identify the pattern of inheritance in cases of single gene disorders, and determine the risk of recurrence. When a child is affected with autosomal recessive disorders such as thalassemia, cystic fibrosis, sickle cell anemia, spinal muscular atrophy (SMA), oculocutaneous albinism, Gaucher disease, Wilson disease and many others, both parents are likely to be carriers of the same mutation or different mutations in the same gene. They have a 25% risk of recurrence in every pregnancy and cases of consecutive abnormal pregnancies are known to occur. As carriers are asymptomatic, a couple may not be aware that both have the trait for a particular disorder till they have an affected child. It is necessary to know the mutations of the affected child and parents in advance, in order to carry out PGD when the couple plans to have another child. Hence DNA analysis of an affected child and even of POC of recurrent miscarriages is very important. Once the mutations in the affected child are known, the couple needs to be tested to confirm the carrier status.

Awareness is spread that blood of a very sick child should be collected in EDTA (purple top tube) at least for DNA extraction and storage before the child passes away. The blood sample could also be stored in the refrigerator for a few days till it is sent to a laboratory for DNA extraction. Mutation analysis could be carried out later, followed by confirmation of the couple's carrier status. If DNA of a deceased child affected by a genetic disorder is not available, the mother could initially undergo detailed genetic testing such as NGS or single nucleotide polymorphism (SNP) microarray to identify a heterozygous mutation. X-linked mutations can simultaneously be detected if the female partner is tested first, to cut costs. If an autosomal recessive mutation is detected, the male partner could then be checked for mutations only in that particular gene. As the chance of both partners being carriers of the same mutation in a particular gene is higher in consanguineous marriages, targeted mutation analysis of the other partner is likely to pick up the same mutation. In cases of male infertility due to congenital absence of the vas deferens (CAVD), the husband is likely to be a carrier of a mutation in the *CFTR* gene for cystic fibrosis. Hence in this case too, the wife could be sequenced first to check for a pathogenic mutation. If it is absent, PGD is not required. If a mutation is detected, the husband is also checked.

In autosomal dominant conditions such as Huntington disease, achondroplasia and neurofibromatosis, PGD is carried out when either partner is a carrier of the mutation. The risk of recurrence in these cases is 50% for both males and females. In X-linked disorders like hemophilia, Duchenne muscular dystrophy, G6PD deficiency and Norrie disease, PGD is done when the wife is a carrier of the mutation. In the case of Fragile X, a triplet repeat disorder, she is a carrier of a premutation, with CGG repeats between 55–200. The number of repeats in the *FMR1* gene expands in every generation and its expression is seen only when an affected child with >200 repeats is born. This phenomenon is known as genetic anticipation. Fragile X carriers are known to have premature ovarian failure or primary ovarian insufficiency. In X-linked recessive conditions, there is a 50% chance in each pregnancy for the son to be affected or the daughter to be a carrier. On the other hand, in X-linked dominant conditions such as Rett syndrome and certain types of ornithine transcarbamylase deficiency (OTC), the disorder is lethal in males, while females are affected. There is a 50% chance of stillbirths or early neonatal deaths of male children and a 50% chance of affected female children.

Genetic counselors determine the pattern of inheritance, decide on the genetic tests to be carried out, coordinate and facilitate the testing at specialized laboratories in different cities by sending out samples, following up the test results and explaining the reports to the couple. The various procedures by which the birth of an affected child can be prevented are put forth, so the couple can make an informed choice. Other close family members at risk of being carriers and who need testing are identified. If PGD is an option, a pre-PGD workup of the couple is coordinated with the laboratory where the biopsied cells of the embryos are to be tested. The entire procedure of PGD is explained to the couple, together with the risks, benefits and limitations. They are made aware that in very rare cases, all the embryos may turn out to be abnormal after PGD and PGS, in which case the cycle would have to be repeated. Informed consent is taken and smooth transport of biopsied cells from the embryology to the genetics laboratory for PGD is coordinated.

HISTORY

Gardner and Edwards (1968) in UK first demonstrated the PGD technique by biopsy of rabbit blastocysts to check for the presence of Barr bodies and replaced them into recipient female rabbits.[12] PGD was first clinically applied in 1989 when an English couple who were at high risk of having sons with a form of severe X-linked mental retardation, opted to have only a daughter. The Y-specific DNA amplification technique was used at that time.[13] In cases of X-linked disorders such as Duchenne muscular dystrophy (DMD) and hemophilia, where only males were at 50% risk of being affected, PGD helped in selection of female embryos for transfer, prior to the refinement of molecular methods of genetic diagnosis from DNA of a single cell.[14] The development of fluorescence *in situ* hybridization (FISH) and the commercial availability of prelabeled probes aided in rapid identification of common aneuploidies such as trisomy 21, trisomy 18, trisomy 13 and sex chromosome aneuploidies such as Turner and Klinefelter syndromes in prenatal and preimplantation samples.[15]

PGD/PGS for chromosome aneuploidies and translocations became widely available from the nineties by the FISH technique.[16-20] It was shown that PGD helped to improve success rates of IVF, especially in women of the older age group who were at a higher risk of chromosome aneuploidies.[21-28] Simultaneously, the development of single cell PCR analysis facilitated the detection of Mendelian disorders. By 2001, Verlinsky's team from Chicago reported the first successful PGD with HLA matching a sib with Fanconi anemia by haplotype analysis.[29] The advent of whole genome amplification (WGA) and chromosome microarray (CMA) technology or array-CGH, led to the development of comprehensive chromosome screening (CCS) for aneuploidy of all the 24 chromosomes.[30-39] Now NGS is also being used for CCS.[1, 4, 6, 7] Targeted NGS based PGD of monogenic disorders is an emerging technology which has shown a high level of consistency with established methodologies.[40]

REQUIREMENTS OF A PREIMPLANTATION GENETIC DIAGNOSIS CENTER

Patients Need

- Genetic and specific PGD counseling
- Pre-PGD work-up on blood of affected child and couple
- A highly successful IVF unit
- Biopsy performed by trained embryologists
- Fixation of single cells and FISH performed by trained cytogeneticists
- Extraction of deoxyribonucleic acid (DNA) from a single cell, polymerase chain reaction (PCR), array-comparative genomic hybridization (CGH), sequencing, diagnosis and interpretation by an experienced molecular biologist
- Excellent communication between IVF center and genetic laboratories.

PGD Cycle

The female partner is treated with hormonal stimulation in order to obtain a fairly large number of oocytes, which are then picked up under anesthesia. Intracytoplasmic sperm injection (ICSI) is performed, whereby a single sperm is injected into the cytoplasm of each mature egg manually in the embryology laboratory under a special microscope fitted with a micromanipulator and a laser. This is followed by incubation to allow fertilization and formation of the embryo.

For FISH analysis, a single cell is biopsied on the third day and processed in the genetics laboratory, while the embryo continues growing in the IVF laboratory. The FISH result is available by the fifth day and three fresh unaffected embryos are selected for transfer to the uterus. Additional normal embryos are frozen for future use.

Embryo Biopsy

A blastocyst biopsy is the current method of choice for PGD. At the blastocyst stage (Day 5–6), the embryo has differentiated into the inner cell mass of fetal cells and the trophectoderm which will form the placenta.

An opening is created in the zona of the embryo (hatching) using a noncontact diode LASER system attached to the micromanipulator. The blastocyst stage embryo is further incubated till the trophectoderm cells come out from the opening (herniation). Around 4–8 trophectoderm cells are separated from the embryo. All the above steps are carried out in the embryology laboratory. The trophectoderm cells are either put in separate tubes (tubing) to carry out molecular analysis, or fixed on slides to check for chromosomal aneuploidies or translocations by FISH. As trophectoderm cells herniate out from the blastocyst to form the placenta, removal of 4–8 trophectoderm cells will not affect the development of the fetus.

The biopsied embryos are cryopreserved by vitrification till the genetic results are available. The analysis of 4–8 trophectoderm cells helps to overcome the problem of misdiagnosis due to allele drop-out. In addition, cryopreservation of embryos allows more time for genetic analysis.

A cleavage stage biopsy is done on day-3 when a single cell (blastomere) is biopsied mainly for chromosome testing of aneuploidies and translocations. Cleavage stage biopsy gives us the advantage of embryo transfer in the same cycle. However, only 2 days are available for analysis. A polar body biopsy can also be carried out, though this will reveal only the maternal component. Polar body biopsies were generally used in countries where embryo biopsy was banned.

Embryo biopsies are technically challenging and are limited to centers experienced in micromanipulation and vitrification. The procedure of actual PGD is very delicate as a very small amount of genetic material is available for analysis. Also, there is a high risk of extraneous DNA contamination, hence extreme care needs to be taken to avoid this.

Tubing of Biopsied Cells for Molecular Techniques

For PGD of single gene disorders or PGS by CMA/NGS, the biopsied cells are 'tubed', i.e. put in small tubes containing buffer, and transported to a molecular laboratory experienced in single cell analysis. Whole genome amplification is carried out to increase the quantity of DNA. Then the amplified product is subjected to further testing for the single gene disorder or chromosomal aneuploidy screening. The parental genetic markers are also matched with the embryonic markers in cases of single gene disorder testing.

Genetic Analysis of Biopsied Cells

PGS of all chromosomes is now possible by CMA or NGS techniques. Prior to this, aneuploidy screening of about 12 chromosomes was carried out by FISH.[27]

PGS by the FISH Technique

For PGS by FISH, single blastomeres are biopsied from cleavage stage embryos on day-3, treated with hypotonic solution and fixed on slides with a 3:1 mixture of methanol and acetic acid in a very delicate procedure where the intact nucleus is exposed after removing the cytoplasm. The success of FISH and accurate interpretation of results after relocating the single cells under the microscope depends mainly on a good fixation, which is a crucial step. Rapid hybridization for a few hours is carried out with multicolor probes, where 5 chromosomes can be checked together. The slide is washed using a buffered detergent solution at specified temperatures and mounted in antifade. Colored images are captured under the oil immersion lens of a fluorescence photomicroscope with the help of software. The signals are washed off after analysis and another round of FISH with different probes is set up on the same cells. This procedure can be repeated for 3–4 rounds, depending on the quality of the fixed nuclei. In case of a doubtful interpretation of a particular signal, FISH can be repeated on the same cell with another probe of that particular chromosome. This procedure is known as 'no result rescue'. Though CCS or 24 chromosome aneuploidy screening is superior, FISH is also offered as a cheaper alternative for testing limited aneuploidies, familial microdeletions and translocations.

PGS by Microarray

Tubed biopsied cells are subjected to whole genome amplification (WGA). The test sample (WGA product) is further processed for comparison with reference male and female DNA. The slides are placed in the microarray reader for analysis. The data is interpreted using software to check gain or loss in any particular chromosome. The technique can also be adapted for detection of unbalanced translocations.

PGS by NGS

For NGS, a library of test DNA is prepared by fragmenting the sample into different sizes. These fragments are processed further and finally sequencing is carried out. The end results are obtained by subjecting the raw data to bioinformatics tools.

RISKS AND LIMITATIONS

Even though the benefits of PGD/PGS are considerable, there are some associated risks and limitations. One cannot guarantee a healthy baby or eliminate the risk for miscarriage, stillbirth or a child with a genetic abnormality. After stimulation, some female individuals may show the presence of multiple follicles on a scan due to ovarian hyperstimulation. Also, very few oocytes may be available after retrieval. All oocytes may not be mature. Fertilization failure, embryonic arrest and bad quality embryos are some of the setbacks which could occur in a PGD cycle. The quality of genetic material present in the biopsied cell/cells may be poor or degenerating which may lead to a "No DNA and hence no result" situation. In such cases a repeat biopsy may help. Assay failure is another possibility which may lead to an uninformative situation.

PGD may not always result in a pregnancy after transferring unaffected embryos. The possibility of spontaneous abortion, abnormal USG findings, intrauterine growth retardation (IUGR) or intrauterine fetal death (IUFD) cannot be ruled out. Hence standard ultrasound evaluation and follow-up by dual/triple/quadruple marker testing during pregnancy is important. PGD is done to avoid medical termination of pregnancy (MTP) due to a known familial genetic mutation, and not as a replacement for prenatal and postnatal testing. The couple is advised to undergo prenatal diagnosis for confirmation. They should be aware of the possibility of a misdiagnosis due to chromosome mosaicism.[41] There is also a possibility that none of the embryos tested are normal and the cycle would have to be repeated. All these factors should be explained to the couple and an informed consent taken.

A pictorial summary of steps involved in PGD is shown in Figures 26.1 and 26.2.

INDIAN SCENARIO

The state-of-the-art technique of PGD was introduced in India in 1999 and was progressing slowly at a few centers, while awareness was being spread.[42-53] Our department of Assisted Reproduction and Genetics at Jaslok Hospital and Research Center was consistently at the forefront, being the first center in India offering PGD by the FISH technique for inherited chromosome translocations and inversions (ivfclinicindia.com). The first livebirths in India after PGD for Robertsonian and reciprocal translocations, and inversions were reported by our team.[54-56] Our center is also experienced in vitrification of biopsied blastocysts followed by frozen embryo transfer (FET) resulting in livebirths, especially in cases of PGD for single gene disorders.[57] With the recent availability in India of PGS for 24 chromosomes by microarray technology (igenomix.co.in) or NGS (supratechlabs.com),

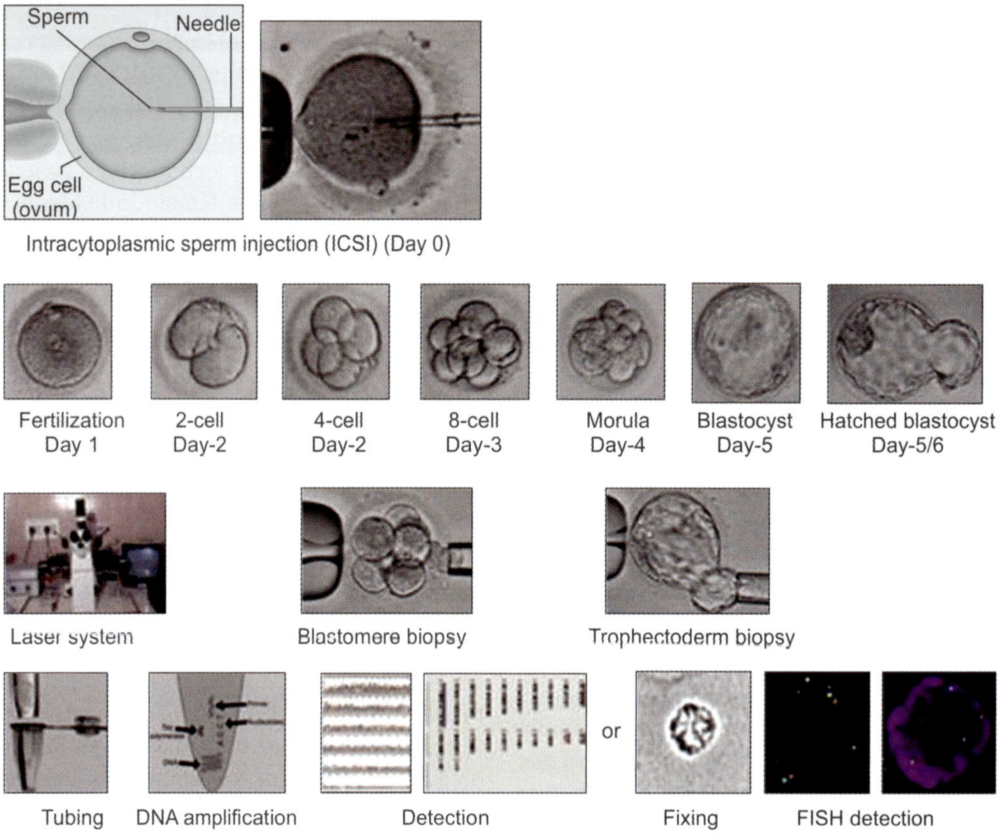

Fig. 26.1 Intracytoplasmic sperm injection, early development of the embryo, biopsy and tubing of cells for genetic analysis

and the possibility of testing single gene disorders from tubed blastocyst biopsies, the field has now opened up in India and will benefit many more couples. We have a series of couples with beta-thalassemia trait undergoing PGD for eliminating the risk of thalassemia major in their offspring.

Awareness of the availability and uses of PGD/PGS needs to be spread by genetic counselors, fetal medicine specialists, pediatricians, general practitioners and others, so that affording couples can avail of the benefits of PGD. Misuse of PGD for preconception sex selection is prohibited in India as per the amendment of the Pre-conception and Pre-natal Diagnostic Techniques Act in 2003. All the centers offering PGD/PGS need to be registered for the various procedures they carry out, and maintain the required documentation.

SAVIOR SIBLING

Hematological disorders such as thalassemia or Fanconi anemia are now curable in small children if bone marrow transplantation with human leukocyte antigen (HLA) matching donors is carried out to avoid graft rejection. It is difficult to get a perfect HLA matched sibling through a natural conception. However, this is possible though PGD for both-the familial disorder and for the selection of a HLA matched prospective donor sibling. A large number of embryos are required and multiple cycles may be necessary for success.[58-61] There are ethical issues too as some feel that such tailor made children may not feel wanted once the objective of the parents in curing the elder child is achieved. However, others feel that these are savior siblings and the family will be ever grateful to them and shower their love on them.[62]

PREIMPLANTATION GENETIC DIAGNOSIS FOR CANCER PREDISPOSITION

In hereditary cancer predisposition syndromes such as colon, breast and ovarian cancers, neurofibromatosis and retinoblastoma, once the mutation in the genes such as *APC*, *NF1*, *BRCA1* and *TP53* is identified, patients and unaffected relatives who carry the same mutation have the option of PGD in order to select embryos without the familial cancer-predisposing mutations.[63-65] Despite ethical objections and arguments, PGD for adult-onset cancer and other disorders such as Huntington disease is a reality today. Prenatal diagnosis and selective pregnancy termination for adult-onset

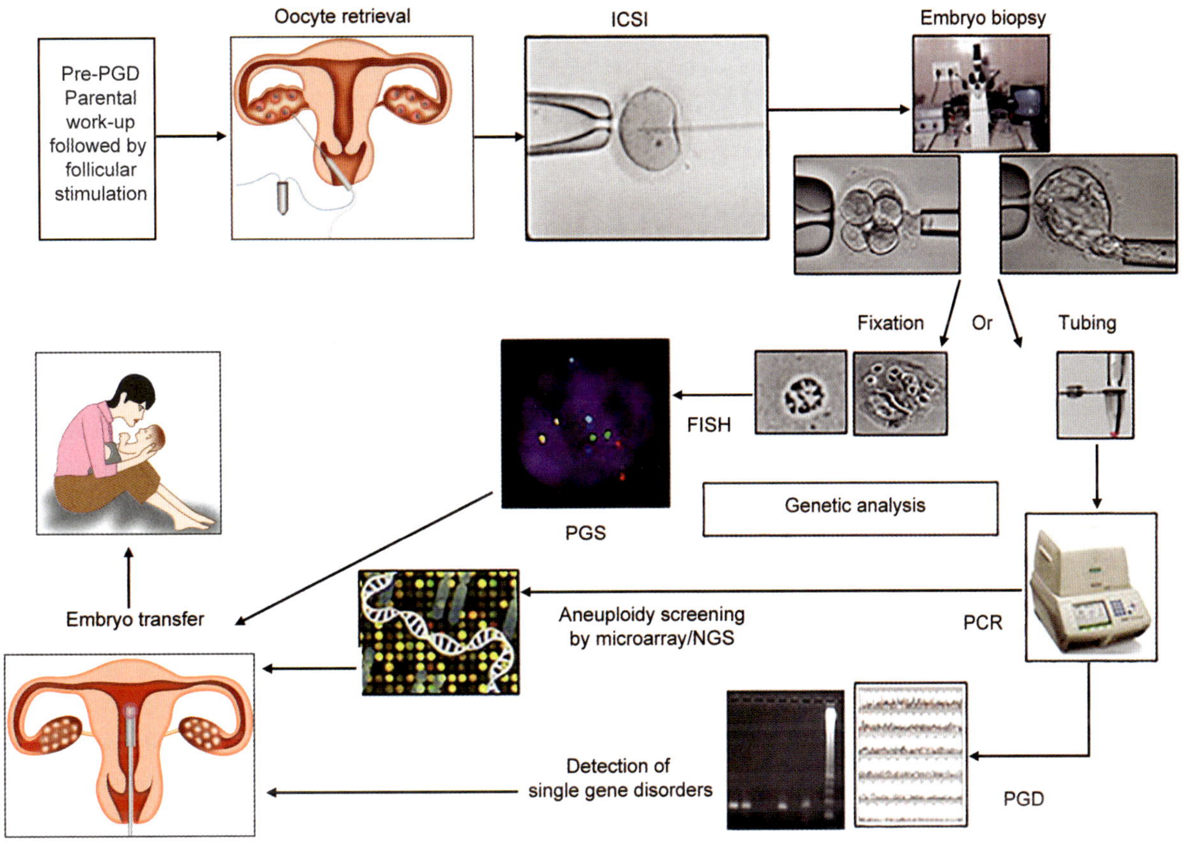

Fig. 26.2 Steps involved in PGD

disorders is emotionally difficult and, in some cases, socially not well accepted.[66] Preimplantation genetic diagnosis (PGD) appears as an attractive alternative to prenatal diagnosis (PND), as it ensures the establishment of a pregnancy free of the mutation from the onset, circumventing the potentially difficult decision of termination of pregnancy.

MITOCHONDRIAL DNA

PGD for mitochondrial DNA (mtDNA) disorders is still in the research phase. Interpretation of the test results may be difficult. In such cases, PGD then may contribute to a reduction of reproductive risk by selecting the embryos with the highest probability of leading to a healthy child. Specific ethical questions are generated by the characteristics of mtDNA genetics, such as heteroplasmy, which is a mixture of normal and mutant mtDNA, the level of which can differ among tissues. The current opinion is to allow PGD for mtDNA mutations as there is no high risk of serious harm to the future child, though this is still in the research phase. At present, the consensus is for a cutoff point of 80%. If the mutant mitochondrial DNA is more than 80%, the child has a high probability of being affected.[67,68]

TAKE HOME MESSAGE

PGD and PGS have a wide scope today for preselection of genetically normal embryos for transfer, using assisted reproduction techniques. Both chromosomal and single gene disorders can be tested. Though it is expensive, the trauma of recurrent abortions of affected pregnancies can be avoided. PGS helps to improve the success rate of IVF especially in cases of advanced maternal age. Awareness needs to be spread that PGD is now available for all genetic disorders in India.

REFERENCES

1. Zheng H, Jin H, Liu L, Liu J, Wang W. Application of next-generation sequencing for 24-chromosome aneuploidy screening of human preimplantation embryos. Molecular Cytogenetics. 2015;8:38.
2. Yang Z, Lin J, Zhang J, et al. Randomized comparison of next-generation sequencing and array comparative genomic hybridization for preimplantation genetic screening: a pilot study. BMC Med Genomics. 2015;8:30.
3. Thornhill A, Ottolini C, Harton G, Griffin D. Aneuploidy testing by array-CGH. In: Markus Montag (Ed). A Practical Guide to Selecting Gametes and Embryos. CRC Press. 2014;255-68.

4. Fiorentino F, Bono S, Biricik A, et al. Application of next-generation sequencing technology for comprehensive aneuploidy screening of blastocysts in clinical preimplantation genetic screening cycles. Hum Reprod. 2014;29:2802-13.
5. Halam S, Nelson H, Greger V, et al. Validation for clinical use of, and initial clinical experience with, a novel approach to population-based carrier screening using high-throughput, Next-Generation DNA Sequencing. J Mol Diagn. 2014;16:180-9.
6. Wells D. Next-generation sequencing: the dawn of a new era for preimplantation genetic diagnostics. Fertil Steril. 2014;101:1250-1.
7. Rubio C. Next-generation sequencing: challenges in reproductive genetics. FertilSteril. 2014;101:1252-3.
8. Wells D, Alfarwati S, Fragouli E. Use of comprehensive chromosomal screening for embryo assessment: microarrays and CGH. Mol Hum Reprod. 2008;14:703-10.
9. Harper JC, Sengupta SB. Preimplantation genetic diagnosis: state of the art 2011. Hum Genet. 2012;131:175-86.
10. Taylor A. A guide to preimplantation genetic diagnosis. Galton Institute occasional papers, 2008; Third series, No.1.
11. Harton GL, Munne S, Surrey M, et al. Diminished effect of maternal age on implantation after preimplantation genetic diagnosis with array comparative genomic hybridization. Fertil Steril. 2013;100:1695-1703.
12. Gardner RL and Edwards RG. Control of the sex ratio at full term in the rabbit by transferring sexed blastocysts. Nature. 1968;218:346-8.
13. Handyside AH, Kontogianni EH, Hardy K, Winston RM. Pregnancies from biopsied preimplantation human embryos sexed by Y-specific DNA amplification. Nature. 1990;344: 768-70.
14. Griffin DK, Handyside AH, Penketh RJ, Winston RM, Delhanty JD. Fluorescent *in situ* hybridization to interphase nuclei of human preimplantation embryos with X and Y chromosome specific probes. Hum Reprod. 1991;6:101-5.
15. Grifo JA, Boyle A, Tang YX, Ward DC. Preimplantation genetic diagnosis. *In situ* hybridization as a tool for analysis. Arch Pathol Lab Med. 1992;116:393-7.
16. Munne S, Lee A, Rosenwaks Z, Grifo J, Cohen J. Diagnosis of major chromosome aneuploidies in human preimplantation embryos. Hum Reprod. 1993;8:2185-91.
17. Verlinsky Y, Cieslak J, Frieidine M, et al. Pregnancies following pre-conception diagnosis of common aneuploidies by fluorescence in-situ hybridization. Human Reprod. 1995;10:1923-7.
18. Munné S, Magli C, Bahçe M, et al. Preimplantation diagnosis of the aneuploidies most commonly found in spontaneous abortions and livebirths, XY, 13, 14, 15, 16, 18, 21, 22. Prenatal Diagn. 1998;18:1459-66.
19. Gianaroli L, Magli C, Ferraretti A P, Munné S. Preimplantation diagnosis for aneuploidies in patients undergoing in-vitro fertilization with a poor prognosis-identification of the categories for which it should be proposed. Fertil Steril. 1999;72:837-44.
20. Munné S, Sandalinas M, Escudero T, et al. Outcome of preimplantation genetic diagnosis of translocations. Fertil Steril. 2000;73:1209-18.
21. Munné S, Sandalinas M, Escudero T, et al. Improved implantation after preimplantation genetic diagnosis of aneuploidy. Reprod Biomed Online. 2003;7:91-7.
22. Verlinsky Y, Cohen J, Munne S, et al. Over a decade of experience with preimplantation genetic diagnosis: A multicenter report. Fertil Steril. 2004;82:292-4.
23. Verlinsky Y, Tur-Kaspa I, Cieslak J, et al. Preimplantation testing for chromosomal disorders improves reproductive outcome of poor prognosis patients. Reprod Biomed Online. 2005;11:219–25.
24. Munné S, Chen S, Fischer J, et al.Preimplantation genetic diagnosis reduces pregnancy loss in women 35 and older with a history of recurrent miscarriages. Fertil Steril. 2005;84:331-5.
25. Munné S, Fischer J, Warner A, Chen S, Zouves C, Cohen J. Referring centers PGD group. Preimplantation genetic diagnosis significantly reduces pregnancy loss in infertile couples, a multi-center study. Fertil Steril. 2006;85:326-32.
26. Rubio C, Buendía P, Rodrigo L, et al. Prognostic factors for preimplantation genetic screening in repeated pregnancy loss. Reprod Biomed Online. 2009;18:687-93.
27. Colls P, Goodall N, Zheng X, Munné S. Increased efficiency of preimplantation genetic diagnosis for aneuploidy by testing 12 chromosomes. Reprod Biomed Online. 2009;19:532-8.
28. Munné S, Fragouli E, Colls P, Katz-Jaffe M, Schoolcraft W, Wells D. Improved detection of aneuploid blastocysts using a new 12-chromosome FISH test. Reprod Biomed Online. 2010;20:92-7.
29. Verlinsky Y, Rechitsky S, Schoolcraft W, Strom C, Kuliev A. Preimplantation diagnosis for Fanconi anemia combined with HLA matching. JAMA. 2001;285:3130-3.
30. Wells D, Delhanty JD. Comprehensive chromosomal analysis of human preimplantation embryos using whole genome amplification and single cell comparative genomic hybridization. Mol Hum Reprod. 2000;6:1055-62.
31. Le Caignec C, Spits C, Sermon K, et al. Single-cell chromosomal imbalances detection by array CGH. Nucleic Acids Res. 2006;34:e68.
32. Hellani A, Abu-Amero K, Azouri J, El-Akoum S. Successful pregnancies after application of array-comparative genomic hybridization in PGS-aneuploidy screening. Reprod Biomed Online. 2008;17:841-7.
33. Wells D, Alfarawati S, Fragouli E. Use of comprehensive chromosomal screening for embryo assessment: Microarrays and CGH. Mol Hum Reprod. 2008;14:703-10.
34. Schlenker T, Stevens J, Rawlins M, McCormick S, Katz-Jaffe MG, Schoolcraft WB. Clinical success with vitrification following trophectoderm biopsy for comprehensive chromosomal screening. Fertil Steril. 2009;92:Suppl, S-71.
35. Schoolcraft WB, Fragouli E, Stevens J, Munné S, Katz-Jaffe MG, Wells D. Clinical application of comprehensive chromosomal screening at the blastocyst stage. Fertil Steril. 2010;94:1700-6.
36. Fragouli E, Alfarawati S, Katz-Jaffe M, et al. Comprehensive chromosome screening of polar bodies and blastocysts from couples experiencing repeated implantation failure. Fertil Steril. 2010;94:875-87.
37. Fragouli E, Alfarawati S, Daphnis DD, et al. Cyto-genetic analysis of human blastocysts with the use of FISH, CGH

and aCGH-scientific data and technical evaluation. Human Reprod. 2011;26:480-90.
38. Scott RT Jr, Ferry K, Su J, Tao X, Scott K, Treff NR. Comprehensive chromosome screening is highly predictive of the reproductive potential of human embryos: A prospective, blinded, nonselection study. Fertil Steril. 2012;97:870-5.
39. Handyside AH. 24-chromosome copy number analysis: A comparison of available technologies. Fertil Steril 2013;100:595-602.
40. Treff NR, Fedick A, Tao X, Devkota B, Taylor D, Scott RT Jr. Evaluation of targeted next-generation sequencing-based preimplantation genetic diagnosis of monogenic disease. Fertil Steril 2013;99:1377-84.
41. Munné S, Sandalinas M, Escudero T, Marquez C, Cohen J. Chromosome mosaicism in cleavage stage human embryos: evidence of a maternal age effect. Reprod Biomed Online. 2002;4:223-32.
42. Parikh FR, Naik NJ. Uttamchandani SA, et al. Preimplantation Genetic Diagnosis using the Diode Laser in a couple with a family history of Haemophilia. In: The Indo-European Seminar cum Workshop on Advances in Human Cytogenetics, SGPGI Lucknow, 1999; poster.
43. Parikh FR, Madon PF, Athalye AS, et al. Preimplantation genetic diagnosis of chromosome abnormalities by multicolour fluorescence *in situ* hybridization. J Indian Med Assoc. 2001;99:441-4.
44. Parikh FR, Madon PF. Preimplantation genetic diagnosis: PGD. Modern Medicare. 2004;1:24-6.
45. Athalye AS, Parikh FR, Naik NJ, Madon PF. Preimplantation genetic diagnosis. Health Screen. 2006;2:19,34-6.
46. Madon PF, Athalye AS, Naik NJ, Parikh FR. Preimplantation genetic diagnosis. In: Telang M (Ed). Atlas of Human Assisted Reproductive Technologies, India. Jaypee, 2007;167-74.
47. Madon PF. Conventional and molecular cytogenetics in India. In: Kumar D (Ed). Genomics and Health in the Developing World. UK. Oxford Monographs on Medical Genetics, 2012;1096-111.
48. Malhotra N, Shah D, Pai R, Pai H, Bankar M. Assisted reproductive technology in India: A 3 year retrospective data analysis. J Hum Reprod Sci. 2013;6:235-40.
49. Sharma S, Sharma R. Preimplantation genetic diagnosis. In: Talwar P (Ed). Manual of Assisted Reproductive Technologies and Clinical Embryology. Jaypee, 2012;327-33.
50. Gopinathan KK. Preimplantation genetic diagnosis for single gene disorders. In: Arora S, Merchant R, Allahbadia GN (Eds). Reproductive Medicine: Challenges, solutions and breakthroughs. India. Jaypee, 2014;393-400.
51. Govindarajan M. Preimplantation genetic diagnosis: Clinical applications. In: Arora S, Merchant R, Allahbadia GN (Eds). Reproductive Medicine: Challenges, solutions and breakthroughs. India. Jaypee, 2014;410-14.
52. Gunasheela S. Preimplantation genetic diagnosis: The current state of the art. In: Arora S, Merchant R, Allahbadia GN (Eds). Reproductive Medicine: Challenges, solutions and breakthroughs. India. Jaypee, 2014;415-22.
53. Gada SS, Sarnath D. Preimplantation genetic diagnosis using fragment analysis for β-thalassemia in an Indian couple with β-globin gene mutations: a case report. J Hum Reprod Sci. 2012;5:289-92.
54. Madon PF, Athalye AS, Naik NJ, Naik DJ, Parikh, FR. PGD for a Robertsonian translocation by FISH: First successful pregnancy from India. J Prenat Diagn Ther. 2010;1:20-2.
55. Naik DJ, Madon PF, Naik NJ, Athalye AS, Parikh FR. PGD by FISH for a reciprocal translocation: First baby from India. J Fetal Med. 2014;1:41-3.
56. Madon P, Athalye A, Sanap R, Naik D, Naik N, Parikh F. Preimplantation genetic diagnosis by FISH in India: The Jaslok Hospital experience. Cytogenet Genome Res. 2014;142:226.
57. Athalye AS, Madon PF, Parikh FR. Preimplantation genetic diagnosis for single gene disorders. In: Agarwal MB, (Ed). Hematology Today—A case-based approach. 2015;125-8.
58. Van de Velde H, De Rycke M, De Man C, et al. The experience of two European preimplantation genetic diagnosis centres on human leukocyte antigen typing. Hum Reprod. 2009;1:1-9.
59. Fiorentino F, Kahraman S, Karadyani H, et al. Short tandem repeats haplotyping of the HLA region in preimplantation matching. Eur J Hum Genet. 2005;13:953-8.
60. Kahraman S, Beyazyürek C. PGD for selecting HLA compatible embryos. In: Arora S, Merchant R, Allahbadia GN (Eds). Reproductive Medicine: Challenges, solutions and breakthroughs. India. Jaypee, 2014;401-9.
61. Kahraman S, Beyazyürek C, Tac H, Pirkevi C, Cetinkaya M, Gülüm N. Recent advances in preimplantation genetic diagnosis. Advances in Genomics and Genetics. 2015;5: 189-203.
62. Zierhut H, MacMillan ML, Wagner JE, Bartels DM. More than 10 years after the first 'savior siblings': parental experiences surrounding preimplantation genetic diagnosis. J Genet Couns. 2013;22:594-602.
63. Konstantopoulou I, Pertesi M, Fostira F, Grivas A, Yannoukakos D. Hereditary cancer predisposition syndromes and preimplantation genetic diagnosis: where are we now? J BUON. 2009;14(Suppl 1):S187-92.
64. Spits C, De Rycke M, Van Ranst N, et al. Preimplantation genetic diagnosis for cancer predisposition syndromes. Prenat Diagn. 2007;27:447-56.
65. Verlinsky Y, Rechitsky S, Verlinsky O, et al. Preimplantation diagnosis for neurofibromatosis. Reprod Biomed Online. 2002;4:218-22.
66. Winkelman WD, Missmer SA, Myers D, Ginsburg ES. Public perspectives on the use of preimplantation genetic diagnosis. J Assist Reprod Genet. 2015;32:665-75.
67. Bredenoord A, Dondorp W, Pennings G, Die-Smulders C, Smeets B, De Wert G. Preimplantation genetic diagnosis for mitochondrial DNA disorders: ethical guidance for clinical practice. Eur J Hum Genet. 2009;17:1550-9.
68. Hellebrekers DM, Wolfe R, Hendrickx AT, et al. PGD and heteroplasmic mitochondrial DNA point mutations: a systematic review estimating the chance of healthy offspring. Hum Reprod Update. 2012;18:341-9.

CHAPTER

27 Intrauterine Infections Leading to Increased Fetal Morbidity and Mortality

Maya Lulla

INTRODUCTION

Infection is important cause of neonatal mortality and morbidity. Prevention of infection should be primary goal, early recognition followed by prompt and aggressive treatment are keys to improve the perinatal outcome.[1]

Common causes are:

Antenatal period	Toxoplasmosis, rubella cytomegalo virus (CMV), syphilis, malaria, human immunodeficiency virus (HIV)
Intrapartum	Group B *Streptococcus*, herpes simplex virus (HSV), cytomegalovirus (CMV), *Gonococcus*
Postnatal	Acquired bacterial vaginosis, Candidiasis.

Clinical Manifestations[2]

Skin lesions	Umbilical stump infection, skin rash, eruptions
Gastrointestinal lesions	Necrotizing enterocolitis, diarrhea, vomiting
Eyes	Ophthalmia neonatorum
Respiratory system	Bronchiolitis, pneumonia
Others	Urinary tract infections, meningitis encephalitis septicemia, telangiectasias.

Congenital Anomalies and Fetal Damage

Which could be attributed to TORCH, which includes toxoplasmosis, syphilis varicella-zoster virus, parvovirus, hepatitis B virus, rubella, CMV, HSV.[3]

Most infections are asymptomatic and cause minimal maternal morbidity but have serious fetal consequences. The infection may be severe enough to cause more damage to fetus than his/her mother, degree of damage depends on gestational age at which disease is contracted.

TORCH continues to be popular essay with perinatologists and pediatricians, in spite of the known limitations in clinical practice. The rational of doing TORCH panel is being questioned by obstetricians as it has low diagnostic yield. However, knowledge of these diseases will help clinicians to counsel mothers on preventive measures to avoid these infections and potential for adverse fetal outcome when these infections are contacted during pregnancy.

Indications for screening: Routine screening not indicated, however screening must be carried out for certain cases as listed in Table 27.1.

Placenta forms a big barrier between mother and fetus during first trimester of pregnancy that protects fetus by humoral and cell mediated immunological response. Fetus may get immunity from virus in first trimester but fetus may get seriously infected by virus from second trimester onwards due to lack of immunity. The damage to fetus depends on factors like gestational age at which infection occurs and whether it is primary infection, reactivation of latent infection (Secondary infection) immunological status and other associated infections like HIV transplant patients on immune suppressive therapy. Primary infection causes more damage than secondary infection.[5]

Table 27.1 Obstetric indications for screening[5,6]

- Signs of infection in mother
  - Fever with or without skin rash
  - Lymph adenopathy
- Exposure or contact with infected person
- Pregnant woman at high-risk of TORCH infection in pregnancy
  - Immunocompromised
  - Handling pets (Toxoplasma)
- Preconception or routine screening in pregnancy
- Presence of ultrasound markers of infection
  - Hydrocephalus
  - Microcephaly
  - Nonimmune hydrops
  - Cardiac anomaly
  - Calcification
  - Polyhydramnios
  - Oligohydramnios
  - Intrauterine growth restriction (IUGR)[3,4]

Serology plays an important role to determine syphilis and CMV, cultures although expensive, not easily available and reports take long to come, may not be of much use in clinical practice.

Polymerase chain reaction (PCR) is diagnostic for rubella, HSV and Toxo. Material needed for testing are mother's blood, cord blood obtained by cordocentesis, amniotic fluid, placenta, cord blood after birth for interpretation of results.

Interpretation of results is as follows:

- *No infection*: IgG, IgM negative. This is ideal time to advice vaccination, if a vaccine is available, e.g. rubella vaccination.
- *Recent infection*: IgM positive initially followed by appearance of IgG antibodies and declining IgM antibodies.
- *Past infection*: IgM negative, IgG positive.
- *Reactivation of old infection*: Low titers of IgM antibodies with 2–4 fold rise in IgG antibodies.

TOXOPLASMOSIS (TABLES 27.2 TO 27.4)

- *Causative organism*: *Toxoplasma gondii* is an obligate intracellular protozoan
- Incubation period is 5–18 days
- Clinical symptoms are low grade fever with lymphadenopathy
- *Mode of infection*: Fecal matter of cat, eating raw meat, unwashed vegetables, contaminated water, soil, unpasteurized goat milk.

If a woman is pregnant with active toxoplasmosis infection there is possibility that parasites can cross placenta and infect fetus, although damage is not apparent at birth. 70–90% infants will develop clinical illness in adulthood. There are three types of strains of which type I and type II are found in humans and type III is found in animals.[5]

Symptoms

Risk of transmission is 6% in 1st trimester, and increases to 60–81% in 3rd trimester. Disease severity highest in 1st trimester and gradually declines in 3rd trimester. Only 10–15% of infants will show clear symptoms like skull anomalies, encephalitis, neurological deficit, and eye anomalies and stillbirth.[8,9] Only 5% will demonstrate severe complications like thrombocytopenia, anemia, jaundice, hepatomegalia, maculopapular rash, CNS sequelae. Classic triad of hydrocephalus, chorioretinitis and intracranial calcifications is rarely seen.[4] If a woman contacts Toxoplasma infection in 3rd trimester, infant is usually asymptomatic at birth.[3,9]

Table 27.2 Infective organisms

Viruses	Rubella, CMV, human parvovirus B-19, varicella zoster, HSV, HIV
Bacteria	Syphilis
Protozoa	Toxoplasmosis, *Plasmodium, vivax, P. falciparum*

Table 27.3 Specific technique of detection of TORCH disease[5]

TORCH disease	Serology	Culture	Histo-pathology	Polymerase chain reaction (PCR)
Toxoplasmosis	–	++++	+	+
Rubella	–	++++	+++	+++
CMV	++++	+	–	+
HSV	+/-	+++	–	+
Syphilis	+++	+	–	+

Table 27.4 Clinical manifestations in fetus are dependent on organism involved[4,7]

Symptoms	Organisms
Intracranial calcification	CMV, toxoplasmosis
Cataract	Rubella, HSV
Chorioretinitis	Toxoplasmosis, CMV
Bone lesions	Syphilis, rubella
Microcephaly	CMV
Hydrocephalus	Toxoplasmosis
Vesicles	HSV, syphilis, varicella zoster virus (VSV)
Blueberry muffin lesions	Rubella

Diagnosis

IgM antibodies persist for 3 months, while IgG will remain detectable for lifetime producing immunity or reducing severity of reinfection in mother. Presence of IgM antibodies during pregnancy indicates recent active infection. Causative organism can be isolated from placenta, serum and cerebrospinal fluid.

Diagnostic test for the fetus can be done at 18 weeks of pregnancy by amniotic fluid study using DNA PCR, cordocentesis IgM antibodies, calcification can be diagnosed by computed tomography (CT) scan of the head.

Diagnostic test for neonate: Evaluation of placenta, elevation of proteins in CSF after delivery, rising levels of IgM and IgG antibodies in cord blood or serum of neonate.

Treatment for Mother

Spiramycin 1500 mg, 12 hourly, as fetal prophylaxis to prevent placentitis and thus prevent spread of infection from mother to fetus.

If fetus is found to be infected then treatment is combined with pyrimethamine 50 mg/day + sulfadiazine 3 g/day along with supplements of folic acid to prevent bone marrow depression caused by pyrimethamine and sulfdiazine.

Three weeks of course with spiramycin alternating with 3 sulfadiazine + pyrimethamine throughout the pregnancy.

These drugs are not to be used in first trimester as they are teratogenic.

Health Education

Spread public awareness for maintaining proper hygienic conditions. Women planning a pregnancy should be tested for Toxoplasma IgG and IgM antibodies.

Women who plan pregnancy should be counseled about eating properly cooked meals, fruits and vegetables to be thoroughly washed and skin to be peeled before eating. Avoid eating raw meat, wearing gloves, washing hands with warm water and soap after handling soil, vegetables and raw meat, and avoid handling cats or new kittens, or their litters. If she is toxoplasmosis positive, advised to avoid pregnancy for 6 months.[3]

SYPHILIS (TABLES 27.2 TO 27.4)

Causative organism: Gram-negative spirochetes *Treponema pallidum*.[3] It has 100% vertical transmission rating.

Mode of infection: Direct contact with spirochete containing lesion sexually or transplacentally.[3] Incubation period is 10 days to 3 months

Spirochete organism affects an individual in 3 stages clinically:

1. *Primary infection*: Appearance of syphilitic chancre with lymphadenitis.
2. *Secondary infection*: Rash on hands and feet after 2–10 weeks of chancre.
3. *Tertiary stage*: Neurological, cardiovascular manifestations, gummatous lesions (granulomas) of skin and musculoskeletal system.

Primary and secondary stages are contagious and can lead to fetal and neonatal infection. Tertiary stage is not contagious. Risk of transmission is rare before 16 weeks however fetal affectation is 75%, if mother is in active stage of disease.[10]

Congenital syphilis has 2 stages:

1. *Early disease*: Clinical manifestations within 2 years.
2. *Late disease*: Clinical manifestations after 2 years.

Symptoms of early disease are hemorrhagic nasal discharge (sniffles) hepatosplenomegaly, jaundice, raised liver enzymes, lymphadenopathy, hemolytic anemia, thrombocytopenia, osteochondritis, periostitis, rash, chorioretinitis, nephritis, nephrotic syndrome, CNS abnormalities, failure to thrive Parrot's pseudoparalysis.[7]

Symptoms of late disease are Hutchinson's teeth (small teeth with an central groove) mulberry molars (bulbous protrusion of molar teeth resembling mulberries) hard palate perforation. Eighth nerve deafness, interstitial keratitis, bony lesions, saber shins due to chronic periostitis.[3]

Diagnosis

- Direct tests on lesions, placenta and cord
  - Dark field microscopy
  - Direct immunofluorescent assays of samples
- Indirect tests done on blood
  - Blood venereal disease research laboratory (VDRL), pallidum hemagglutination assays (TPHA)
  - Rapid plasma reagin (RPR) test
  - Enzyme linked immune assay ELIA
  - PCR.

Treatment

Ten days course of aqueous penicillin treatment of mother can eliminate risk of infection in neonates. Follow-up of infant is important till tests are negative.[4]

Patient can be treated with long-acting benzathine penicillin 2.4 m units weekly for 3 weeks to prevent fetal infection in 98% cases. Treatment failure is usually due to associated other infection, e.g. namely HIV. Effectiveness of successful treatment can be ascertained by serological testing at 3–6 weeks which should demonstrate 4-fold drop in titers.

As a preventive measure every pregnant woman should be advised to undergo VDRL test at first antenatal visit.

VARICELLA ZOSTER (CHICKEN POX) (TABLES 27.2 TO 27.4)

Organism is HZV virus, a member of herpes virus family.

Mode of infection: Direct physical contact, air borne contact with droplets of respiratory infection. Newly infected candidates are infective from 1 day to 2 days before onset of rash. Incubation period is 14–16 days.

Clinical symptoms are vesicular rash, high grade fever, respiratory symptoms, pneumonia.

After resolution of primary infection virus enters latent phase and remains dormant in sensory thoracic ganglia.

Reactivation may occur along the sensory dermatomes leading to "shingles".[11]

Risk of transmission is 0.5% in 1st trimester, 1.4–2% in 2nd trimester, 0% in 3rd trimester.

Clinical Manifestations

Chicken pox shingles, hemorrhagic rash, viral pneumonia, meningitis, encephalitis hepatitis and possibility of vertical transmission to fetus.

Fetal Manifestations

Limb hypoplasia, paresis, microcephaly hydrocephalus, microphthalmia, duodenal stenosis, jejunal dilatation, microcolon, atresia of sigmoid colon, cicatricial lesions of skin/hypoplasia of tissues in dermatomal distribution, cataract, chorioretinitis, seizures, hypotonia, hyporeflexia, encephalomyelitis, dorsal radiculitis, Homer's syndrome, bulbar dysphagia. Nystagmus corneal opacities, anophthalmia, atrophy of optic disc optic atrophy, squint, gastrointestinal reflux, sphincter malfunction, neurogenic bladder and micrognathia.

Diagnosis by VZV PCR of tissues or amniotic fluid 1 month after viremia, cord blood can be subjected to IgG and IgM assays.

Treatment

In case of severe maternal infection acyclovir can be given to mother and combination of acyclovir with immunoglobulins to the fetus or neonate.

Counseling

It involves history taking to confirm if she has suffered from chicken pox in childhood or taken vaccine.

Vaccine is available to give lifelong immunity to sero-negative women. In a sero-negative woman vaccine can be given in immediate postpartum period and breastfeeding is not contraindicated.

Preconceptional stage patient should do serological test and if it is negative she should take vaccine and avoid pregnancy for one month. However, if she becomes pregnant there is no need to recommend termination.

If a woman comes in contact with infected patient 2 days before or 5 days after appearance of rash, her immune status should be ascertained and if she is sero-positive (lifelong immunity due to vaccination or exposure to infection in the past) there is no need for any treatment, however, if she is sero-negative, she should be given immunoglobulins VZIG. The immunoglobulins must be given within 10 days of exposure to be effect. If a pregnant woman is given VZIG, she should be managed as potentially infectious from 8 days to 28 days after VZIG, and 8 days to 21 days if no VZIG has been given.

Management of a pregnant woman who develops chicken pox during pregnancy calls for acyclovir 800 mg 5 times a day for 7 days to prevent associated morbidity like pneumonia, hepatitis and encephalitis and vertical transmission to the fetus. Acyclovir can only be prescribed after 20 weeks of gestation and that too if they consult obstetrician within 24 hour of onset of rash. There is no place for VZIG once rash has appeared. Elective delivery should be avoided for 5–7 days after onset of rash, to allow passive transfer of antibodies from mother to fetus. If birth occurs within 7 days of rash or mother develops rash within 7 days of delivery, neonate should be given VZIG and infant should be monitored for 28 days for sign and symptoms of chicken pox. Neonatal infection should be treated with acyclovir.[12]

PAROVIRUS B19 VIRUS (TABLE 21.2)

- It is a DNA virus
- Incubation period 3–7 days
- Mode of infection is transmission through air and contaminated blood. Mothers get this infection by coming in contact with children suffering from erythema infectiosum infection.

Clinical features in mother: It may lead to miscarriage or nonimmune hydrops fetalis development. Asymptomatic in 50% of cases, Classic "slapped face" appearance with maculopapular rash of face and or trunk and peripheral, poly arthropathy of hands feet and knees.

Diagnosis by serology IgM antibodies persist for 3–4 months and IgG life long.

Fetal transmission risk 30%. Risk of hydrops fetalis is 0–12.5%

Clinical features of infection in fetus and neonate are polyhydramnios. Nonimmune hydrops, raised middle cerebellar artery (MCA), pulsatile systolic velocity (PSV) suggesting fetal anemia. Virus interrupts production of RBCs thus leading to anemia which causes cardiac arrest.[2]

Diagnosis of fetal affection by PCR of HPV B19 viral DNA or RNA in amniotic fluid, fetal blood or tissues of the infant using enzyme-linked immunosorbent assay (ELISA) and RIA methods, or cord blood.

After diagnosis of infection in pregnancy weekly follow-up by sonography till 10 weeks of pregnancy.

Risk of fetal complications is more if infection occurs before 22 weeks. Fetal monitoring of middle cerebral artery to detect fetal anemia which appears before onset of hydrops, if fetal anemia is detected there is place for *in utero* transfusion.

Only one transfusion will be enough as condition is transient and hematopoiesis returns to normal once fetal infection subside.[13] Fetal hydrops may also occur due to associated myocarditis. Long-term follow-up has shown there may be developmental delay in some infants (11%) cases.

Treatment

There is no specific treatment for B19 virus infection, intravenous immunoglobulin may be beneficial to some extent.[2]

HEPATITIS B

- Organism involved is DNA containing virus belonging to hepadnavirus family.
- Mode of infection contaminated blood or body fluids during process of delivery.

Incubation period is 2–5 months.

Symptoms are fatigue, malaise, fever, anorexia, nausea, and icterus.

Diagnosis by deranged liver function tests and HbsAg positivity.

Risk of transmission during childbirth varies from 30% to 85%.

Symptoms or morbidity is inversely proportional to gestational age. If gestational age increases at time of infection, risk of chronic infection decreases. Chronic stage can lead to cirrhosis or hepatocellular carcinoma.

Diagnosis routine HbsAg testing in pregnancy and in sero-positive woman rapid immunization of infant with vaccine and immunoglobulins, within 12 hours of birth is recommended.

No specific treatment for disease except lamivudine recommended for chronic HBV in children more than 2 years of age.

RUBELLA (GERMAN MEASLES) (TABLES 27.2 TO 27.4)

- Rubella virus is RNA virus.
- Incubation period is 2–3 weeks.
- Mode of infection direct contact or air borne droplets from respiratory system.

Symptoms are fever, malaise urinary tract infection URTI, lymphadenopathy (sub-occipital), and conjunctivitis, rash, arthralgia, arthritis, encephalitis thrombocytopenia, neuritis, orchitis.

Rubella is contagious disease and in pregnancy virus may spread through placenta and infect fetus.

Fetal occurrence is
- 90% in 1–11 weeks
- 50% in 11–20 weeks
- 37% in 20–35 weeks
- 100% in last month of pregnancy.

Clinical management depends on period of gestation, e.g. MTP is recommended in first trimester. However, if patient declines MTP immunoglobulins may be given as supportive therapy.[14]

In 2nd trimester advise sonography to rule out any cardiac anomalies.

Congenital rubella syndrome (CRS) rate is low less than 1% between 16 and 20 weeks of pregnancy and may manifest as neurologic deafness in newborn. Sonography plays important role to detect fetal cardiac anomalies.

After 20 weeks, there is no evidence of CRS so patient needs to be reassured allowed to continue with pregnancy.

Clinical manifestation are fever with rash, rash is minute discrete macular, nonconfluent appears initially on face and then spreads to trunk and extremities.

Diagnosis by Serology IgM and IgG Titers

Risk of fetal transmission 85% up to 12 weeks of gestation and rare beyond 20 weeks.

Fetal manifestations are IUGR, rash, petechiae, hepato-splenomegaly, chorioretinitis cataract, deafness, and cardiac abnormalities.[7]

Diagnosis of maternal infection is isolate the virus from nasopharyngeal swab, and detecting IgM antibodies, this estimation is important at 23 weeks of gestation.

Diagnosis of fetal affectation by amniotic fluid rubella virus RNA PCR or chorionic villi.[4]

Counseling: When patient visits for premarital counseling rubella IgG should be done and if it is positive she is immunized. However, if it is negative she should be advised to take vaccine and avoid pregnancy for 3 months post-vaccination. The rubella vaccine gives protection for 18 years. However, if she becomes pregnant within 3 months of vaccination, it does not call for termination of pregnancy.[15]

CYTOMEGALOVIRUS (TABLES 27.2 TO 27.4)

This virus is a member of HS family. It is the most common infection in USA.

Mode of infection: Transmitted to infant by ingestion of infected human milk, direct contact with urine or saliva, spread from "day care centers", crèches and nurseries and families having many young children.[3]

Incubation Period is 4–8 Weeks

It may cause severe illness in immunocompromised individuals and transplant patients.[3]

Clinical manifestations fever, fatigue, muscle aches, lymphadenopathy, especialy in neck region.

Diagnosis by serology IgM and IgG: Risk of vertical transmission is 30–40% in primary infection and 2% in recurrent infection.

Clinical manifestations in fetus and newborn are IUGR, rash, petechiae, jaundice hepatosplenomegaly hydrocephaly, intracranial calcification, optic atrophy impaired hearing. Fetal morbidity is high if mother suffers from primary infection in pregnancy.[7]

Diagnosis of fetal infection by amniotic fluid CMV DNA by PCR (applicable after 21 weeks of gestation). Virus is shed from functioning fetal kidney and urinary tract into amniotic fluid and urine contributes significantly to amniotic fluid volume only after 20 weeks.[7]

Sonography plays an important role to assess fetal infection in the form of hydrocephaly and intracranial calcification.

There is no vaccination available as yet and no effective treatment. CMV HIG hyperimmunoglobulin may be given to mother to prevent fetal transmission. Postdelivery neonate may be treated with ganciclovir. Some studies have demonstrated some improvement or less deterioration in hearing in infants.[16,17]

Additional investigations on neonate include testing body fluids, urine, pharyngeal secretions in first 3 weeks of birth by PCR to rule out congenital infection. After 3 weeks, it will be very difficult to differentiate congenital infection from postnatal acquired infection.

Counseling involves practicing good personal hygiene such as avoiding intimate contact with salivary secretions of infected individuals. All women working in nurseries or crèches and handling small babies should observe good hand hygiene and wash hands frequently.

HERPES (TABLES 27.2 TO 27.4)

Causative organism herpes simplex virus (HSV).

There are 2 variants:

1. *Type 1* associated with extra genital lesions
2. *Type 2* associated with genital lesions.

Incubation period is 2–10 days.

Mode of infection: Direct contact with infected lesions.

- Neonatal infection occurs due to vaginal secretions.
- Postnatal infection may occur due to kissing touching the infant.

Clinical manifestations: 50% are asymptomatic 20% develop vulvo-vaginitis and less than 30% develop vesicular and ulcerative lesions on genitalia, blister like vesicular lesions which rupture leading to many shallow ulcers which heal by scab formation. New lesions may continue to develop in crops for a week.

Herpes virus can besides skin lesions give CNS manifestations like calcification, encephalomalacia, ventriculomegaly, microcephaly, hemorrhage, seizures, meningoencephalitis and hypertonia/spasticity. Eyes may be involved in the form of keratoconjuctivitis, chorioretinitis, cataracts, renal detachment.[7]

Diagnosis

- Diagnosis by presence of lesions.
- Diagnosis confirmed by serology IgM and IgG antibodies.

Urine, saliva, nasopharyngeal secretions from infected people can be sent for cultures. PCR can be done on CSF.

Treatment: Once diagnosis is confirmed, treat with acyclovir for 14–21 days 20 mg/kg body weight. CBC to be monitored and adequate hydration to avoid kidney damage.[18]

Management at Term

Avoid procedures like fetal scalp monitoring, avoid rupture of membranes to prevent ascending infection of the fetus.

If active lesions present by pass the route and do LSCS, elective or within 4 hours of spontaneous rupture of membranes. To avoid LSCS one may put the patient on acyclovir 400 mg thrice a day or 200 mg 4 times a day from 36 weeks onwards and plan a vaginal delivery.[18]

Recent studies have recommended valacyclovir to suppress genital lesions rapidly in dose of 500 mg orally twice a day.

Woman can breastfeed the newborn provided there are no active lesions on breast.

If patient presents with preterm premature rupture of membranes (PPROM) there is a role for IV acyclovir in conservative management of pregnancy.

Risk of fetal affection during delivery process is 30–50% for primary infection compared to less than 1% in recurrent infection. Clinical features of fetal or neonatal infection are petechiae, rash, hepatosplenomegaly, meningoencephalitis, chorioretinitis, cataract and deafness.

Investigations include serology of blood and CSF, PCR on urine saliva and nasopharyngeal secretions. HSV cultures of the lesions.

Treatment of infected neonate with acyclovir for 14–21 days, CBC to be monitored with adequate hydration to prevent renal damage.

HUMAN IMMUNODEFICIENCY VIRUS (TABLES 27.2 TO 27.4)

- Incubation period is few months to 6 years
- Usually patients asymptomatic susceptible to become symptomatic due to immune suppression
- Diagnosis by western blot test
- Risk of *in utero* transmission *in utero* 10%, during delivery 20% and breastfeeding 15–29%
- There are no clinical features of infection in mother, fetus or neonate.

Diagnosis of fetal infection by HIV, DNA, PCR within 48 hours of birth, at 2 weeks, 1–2 months and 3–6 months after birth. Two separate samples should test positive to consider infant as infected.

Counseling: Preconception counseling in HIV positive patient calls for avoiding pregnancy till HIV, RNA levels are undetectable and CD 4 cell count more than 200 for 6 months. It indicates that there is no likelihood of any opportunistic infection. She should be recommended a folate supplement.

Women with CD 4 cell count more than 350 does not need antiretroviral drugs ARV however once she becomes pregnant she has to be put on antiretroviral drugs ARV to prevent vertical transmission.

Three prophylactic drugs are recommended as shown in Table 27.5.

Nevirapine to be avoided in 1st trimester as it is teratogenic. Zidovudine is recommended in all regimens. Nevirapine if CD 4 cell count falls below 200/cu mm. If patient misses taking drugs in 1st trimester and comes for consultation in 2nd trimester antiretrovirals should be started immediately and may be only zidovudine.

Important investigations are CD 4 cell count, HIV RNA levels, CBC and liver function tests (LFT).

Opportunistic infection prophylaxis if CD 4 cell count falls below 200.

Table 27.5 Prophylactic drugs

Zidovudine	100 mg 5 times a day
Nevirapine	200 mg once daily for 14 days thereafter twice a day
Lamivudine	150 mg twice a day or 300 mg once daily

Lower segment cesarean section (LSCS) is recommended if more than 1000 copies of HIV RNA are present at 34 weeks. LSCS to be timed at 38 weeks. Vaginal delivery is recommended if patient has been on anti-retrovirals drugs with undetectable HIV RNA copies from 28 weeks. Patient is put on IV zidovudine 3 hours prior to LSCS or when in labor. Avoid fetal scalp blood sampling, ARM, operative vaginal delivery to be avoided and augmentation of labor with syntocinon is recommended.

Nevirapine is highly potent remains in circulation for 21 days after injection. Neonate to be put on zidovudine to prevent MTCHT of virus. Post-delivery lamivudine for 7 days will reduce drug resistance. Fetus may develop neutropenia as a result of drugs.

Neonate to be treated with zidovudine till 6 weeks. Women should be counseled against breastfeeding if not on retroviral drugs. If a woman is on retroviral drugs breastfeeding may be allowed but there is no place for "mixed" feeding.

MALARIA

Clinical symptoms are fever and chills, headache, anemia, pulmonary edema, jaundice, seizures. Incubation period is 12–17 days.

Diagnosis by peripheral smear examination, *P. falciparum* antigen detection by ELIZA and PCR technique, rapid blood test using dipstick.

Transmission rate is 0–33%.

Clinical implication of infection in pregnancy is IUGR, majority of them asymptomatic at birth. Some may exhibit pallor, hypothermia, lethargy, inability to feed, respiratory distress, splenomegaly and neonatal sepsis.

Ideally a pregnant woman should not travel to endemic areas, or she should be put on chloroquine prophylactic treatment 2 weeks prior to travel to endemic areas, and continue up to 4 weeks post-travel in dose of 500 mg/week and once a week. In areas with chloroquine resistant *P. falciparum* mefloquine 250 mg weekly may be recommended in the same schedule.

During pregnancy, it is important to assess period of gestation when malaria occurs. Chloroquine safest drug 80% of falciparum are resistant to the drug. Quinine in therapeutic doses is safe in 1st trimester. Antifolate drugs like sulfadoxine tyrimethamine or sulfamethoxazole trimethoprim work synergistically with 2 enzymes of *P. falciparum* organism, but they are teratogenic in 1st trimester. Sulfa drugs can cause kernicterus in newborn so they can be given only in 2nd or early 3rd trimester. Artinisan new drug found to be effective but it is teratogenic so cannot be given in 1st trimester but safely given in 2nd and early 3rd trimester.

CONCLUSION

If obstetrician decides to screen a woman for TORCH infections, it should done either in nonpregnant stage or in early pregnancy as intrauterine infections can cause congenital anomalies which may warrant termination. It can also lead to increased morbidity for which timely intervention and management is essential and it also helps neonatologist to implement corrective treatment to the neonate to prevent adverse outcome or improve neonatal outcome.[1]

REFERENCES

1. Yadav RK, Maity S, Saha S. A review of TORCH group of congenital infections during pregnancy. J of Scientific Innovations and Research 2014;3(2): 258-64.
2. Boyers SG, Boyers KM. Update on TORCH infection in new born infants. Newborn and Infant Nurs Rev. 2004;4:70-80.
3. Pizzo JD. Focus on diagnostics, Congenital infections. Pediatric Review. 2011;32:537-42.
4. Wilson-Davis ESW, Aitken C. When should the TORCH study be requested. Pediatric and Child Health. 2013;23:226-8.
5. Chiodo F, Veruchi G, Mori F, et al. Infective diseases during pregnancy and their teratogenic effects. Ann 1st Super Sanita. 1993;29:57-67.
6. Sadik MS, Fatima K, Jamil C Patil. Study of TORCH profile in patients with bad obstetric history. Biology and Medicine. 2012;4:95-101.
7. Sher A. Congenital and perinatal infections; throwing new light with an old TORCH. Indian J Pediatrics. 2011;78(1):88-95.
8. Brown ED, Chau JK, Atashband S, et al. A systemic review of neonatal toxoplamosis exposure and sensorineural hearing loss. Int J Pediatr Otorhinolaryngol. 2009;73(5):707-11.
9. Di Carlo P, Romano A, Schimmenti MG, et al Maternofetal Toxoplasma gondii infection; critical review of available diagnostic methods. Infez Med. 2008;16(1):28-32.
10. William JL, Mehmet G. Syphilis in pregnancy. Sex Transm Infect. 2000;76:73-9.
11. Gardella C, Brown ZA. Managing, varicella zoster infection in pregnancy. Cleveland Clinical J Medicine. 2007;74:290-6.
12. Miller E, Cradock-Watson JE, Ridehalgh MK. Outcome in newborn babies given anti varicella zoster immunoglobulins after perinatal maternal infection with varicella zoster virus Lancet. 1989;2:371-3.
13. Nagel HT, de Haan TR, Vandenbussche FP, et al. Long term outcome after fetal transfusion for hydrops associated with parovirus B-19 Infection. Obstet Gynecol. 2007;109(1):42-7.
14. Rubella and Pregnancy ACOG technical bulletin number 171-August 1992. Int J Gynecol Obstet. 1993;42:60-6.
15. Reef SE, Plotkin S, Cordero JF, et al. Preparing for congenital rubella syndrome elimination in United States Cli. Infect Dis. 2000;31:85-95.
16. Nigro G, Adler SP, La Torre R, et al. Passive immunization during pregnancy for congenital cytomegalovirus infection. N NGL J Med. 2005;353:1350-2.
17. Adler SP, Nigro G, Pereira L. Recent advances in prevention and treatment of congenital cytomegalovirus infection. Semin Perinatol. 2007;31:10-8.
18. Sheffield JS, Hollier LM, Hill JB, et al. Acyclovir prophylaxis to prevent herpes simplex virus recurrence at delivery; a systematic review. Obstet Gynecol. 2003;102:1396-403.

SECTION

6

Antenatal Use of Fetal Therapy

CHAPTER

28 Principles of Fetal Therapy and Multifetal Pregnancy Reduction

Vandana Bansal

INTRODUCTION

Fetal therapy is defined as any fetal intervention, whether medical or surgical, that attempts to treat a disorder *in utero* with an aim to improve perinatal outcome.

In the past, once a disorder was diagnosed prenatally options available were either termination of pregnancy or continuation till term and have the appropriate pediatric specialist and neonatal care team ready to manage the neonate with the birth defect. However, many such abnormalities are progressive *in utero* and by the time the neonate is delivered, the disorder is either uncorrectable or correctable with residual disease which may compromise quality of life or the fetus may deteriorate to death *in utero*.

With technological advancement in ultrasound, we have not only been able to diagnose disorders *in utero* but also understand fetal development process and the natural history of disease detected prenatally. Fetal therapeutic interventions were aimed at correcting *in utero* progression of disorder so as to reduce damage to the fetus and subsequently improve long-term outcome.

Fetal therapy was first attempted by Liley et al. by performing intraperitoneal transfusion for fetal anemia under X-ray control in 1963.[1] In past two to three decades, advances in ultrasound technology, magnetic resonance imaging and improvement in minimal invasive techniques have allowed more successful and less invasive fetal interventions. Diseases which are amenable to *in utero* intervention maybe structural abnormality, cardiac defects or rhythm disorder, fetal metabolic, hematological and hormonal disorders or abnormalities of placental vessels.

Most fetal therapies whether medical or surgical are interim procedures intended to allow the fetus to remain *in utero* until it is mature enough to survive delivery, neonatal period and postnatal surgical procedure.

Fetal therapy may be categorized into:

- Fetal medical therapy
- Fetal surgery.

Routes of fetal interventions may be:

- Noninvasive transplacental route
- Ultrasound-guided interventions
- Fetoscopic surgery
- Open fetal surgery.

MEDICAL THERAPY

Transplacental Route

Route where maternal administration crosses placenta and treats the fetus. It is a noninvasive intervention.

- *Steroids for lung maturity* in fetuses at risk for preterm delivery is the best known pharmacological intervention for preventing hyaline membrane disease and reduce the incidence of intraventricular hemorrhage.[2]
- *Transplacental transport of folic acid supplementation* has a protective effect on neural tube defect.
- *Maternal administration of intravenous immunoglobulin G (IVIg G)* to mothers who are alloimmunized against fetal platelets antigen inherited from father to the fetus.
- *Maternal administration of magnesium sulfate (Magsulf)* in pre-eclampsia and extreme preterm for neuroprotection and reducing risk of cerebral palsy.[3]
- *Congenital adrenal hyperplasia:* Differentiation of external genitalia starts at 7–8 weeks, hence all mothers of fetuses at risk of congenital adrenal hyperplasia (parents carrier, previous affected fetus) are initiated on 0.25 mg dexamethasone orally as early as 7–9 weeks which transfers to the developing fetus transplacentally. Steroids are continued through pregnancy only in female fetuses found to be affected at chorionic villus sampling.
- *Maternal HIV:* Maternal administration of zidovudine started at 14 weeks of gestation and continued throughout pregnancy, intrapartum period and to the neonate reduces rate of vertical transmission.
- *Thyroid disorders:*
  - *Hyperthyroidism* in the fetus may occur due to transplacental transfer of thyroid stimulating antibodies

from a mother with Graves' disease to the fetus. This may be diagnosed on ultrasound by the presence of fetal tachycardia, fetal growth restriction and hydrops and confirmed on cordocentesis for TSH values. The hyperthyroid fetus is then treated by maternal administration of higher doses of propylthiouracil or methimazole. If the mother becomes hypothyroid, supplementation with thyroxine may be needed.

- *Hypothyroid fetus:* Fetus *in utero* becomes hypothyroid in mothers who are thyrotoxic on antithyroid drugs, mothers who have received radioactive radioiodine in pregnancy, euthyroid mother with fetal dysgenesis/agenesis of thyroid gland. Presence of goiter in the fetus with or without polyhydramnios on ultrasound would initiate an amniocentesis/cordocentesis to evaluate the fetal thyroid status. Increased levels of TSH in the amniotic fluid or fetal cord blood is diagnostic. Intra-amniotic instillation of L Thyroxine (500 μg) every 2 weeks or 200 μg weekly may help in regression of goiter, polyhydramnios and normalization of hormonal levels (Figs 28.1A to C).

- *Fetal arrhythmias*
  - *Supraventricular tachycardia:* Most fetal arrhythmias are intermittent and benign in nature. 90% are due to atrial extrasystole and require only observation. Persistent supraventricular tachycardia may evolve into fetal hydrops and hence must be treated *in utero* or delivered, if pregnancy is close to term.

    Transplacental treatment of fetus is done by administering digoxin to the mother under supervision of an adult cardiologist. Mother should be admitted and investigated with ECG, renal function and electrolyte prior to the loading dose as the impact of the drug on the mother should be monitored. Digoxin is widely accepted as the first line antiarrhythmic drug for fetal therapy. Recently sotalol, flecainide and amidarone are being used as second-line treatment when either

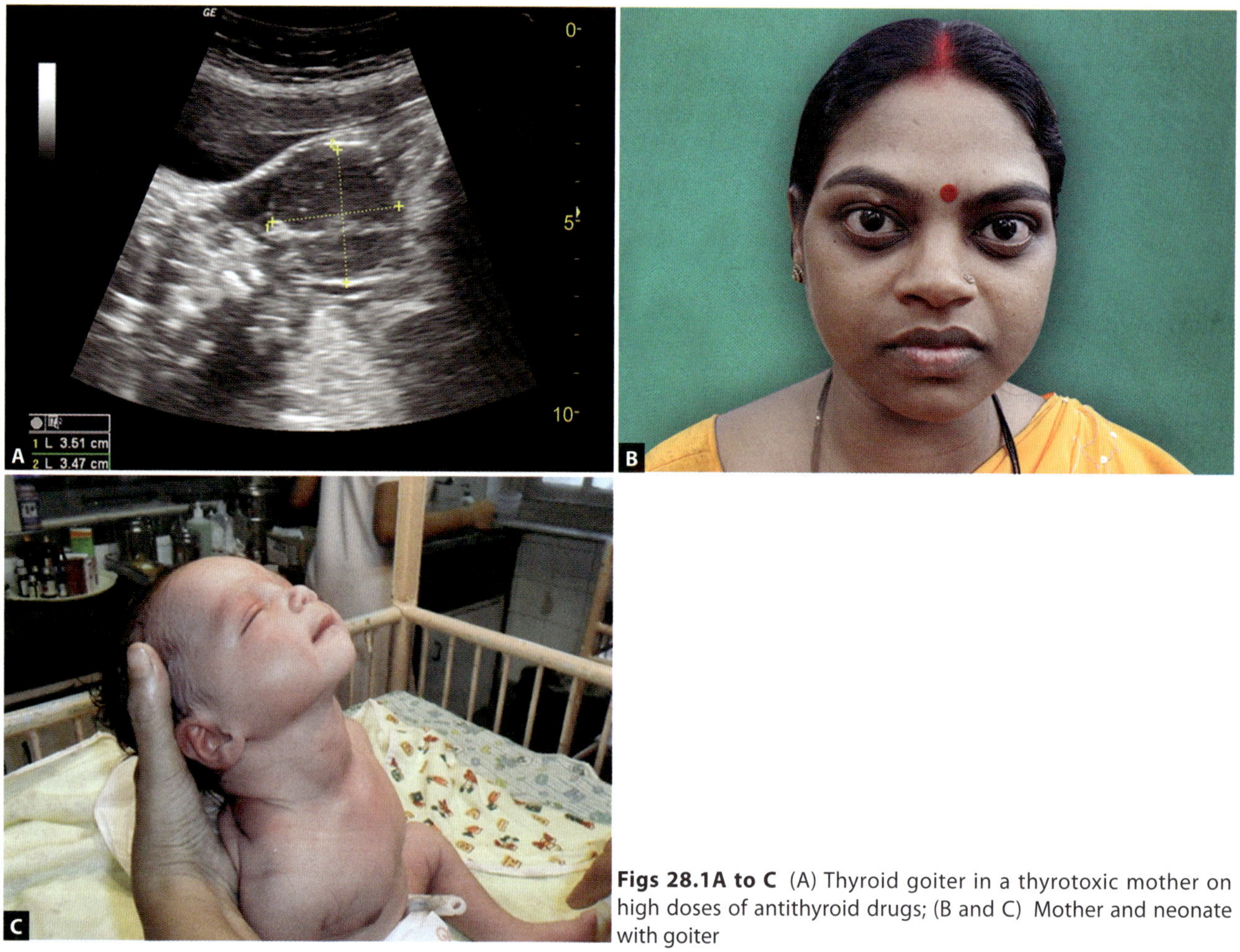

Figs 28.1A to C (A) Thyroid goiter in a thyrotoxic mother on high doses of antithyroid drugs; (B and C) Mother and neonate with goiter

digoxin is ineffective or when correction is attempted after hydrops develops.

- *Complete heart block* in the fetus is seen in association with maternal autoimmune disease (Systemic lupus erythematosus, Sjögren syndrome) with maternal serum positive for Anti-Ro and/or Anti-La antibodies. These antibodies cause fetal myocarditis and damage the conduction fibers leading to dissociation of atrial and ventricular rhythm. Prior to any prenatal intervention in a complete heart block, structural cardiac anomalies associated in about 50% of cases like atrioventricular canal defect, ventricular septal defects, transposition of great vessels must be ruled out. Maternal administration of steroids (Dexamethasone 4 mg) or β_2-stimulants transplacentally to the fetus have been reported as effective with variable results.[4]

ULTRASOUND-GUIDED MEDICAL INTERVENTION

Intrauterine Transfusion

Hemolytic disease of the fetus and newborn is due to maternal alloantibodies directed against paternal antigen on fetal cells resulting in hemolysis of fetal RBC causing anemia. Intrauterine transfusion of blood to these anemic fetuses is one of the best fetal therapy available with extremely good results.

Rh-negative isoimmunized mother with previously affected fetus or those with Rh-antibodies titers above critical levels are monitored noninvasively by Doppler of middle cerebral artery-peak systolic velocity (MCA-PSV) to identify moderate-to-severe anemia prior to development of hydrops. MCA-PSV correlates well with the degree of fetal anemia. A cut-off value of MCA-PSV of 1.5 MoM for the period of gestation or evidence of hydrops on ultrasound indicates severe anemia (Hematocrit <30%) requiring intrauterine transfusion (Fig. 28.2A).

If untreated the anemic fetus would develop hepatosplenomegaly, cardiomegaly, placentomegaly, polyhydramnios and end-stage hydropic fetus which may die *in utero* or postnatally of cardiac failure or develop kernicterus with its sequelae.

Under ultrasound guidance, intrauterine transfusion is done of double packed (Hematocrit of 75–80%) fresh-O-negative blood, leukodepleted, cytomegalovirus (CMV) negative cross-matched with mother's blood into the intravascular (cord insertion site or hepatic portal vein) or intraperitoneal compartment. Volume of blood to be transfused is calculated depending on the initial fetal hematocrit, donor hematocrit and fetoplacental blood volume. In experienced hands, intrauterine transfusion is considered relatively safe with survival rates of about 90% for red cell alloimmunization (Fig. 28.2B).[5]

Intrauterine transfusion may also be used in anemic fetuses secondary to parvovirus infection, large fetomaternal hemorrhage, Twin anemia polycythemia syndrome, intrauterine fetal demise of single fetus in monochorionic twins, placental and fetal tumors such as chorioangioma and sacrococcygeal teratoma.

Multifetal Pregnancy Reduction and Selective Fetal Reduction

With increasing use of assisted reproduction and advanced maternal age, there is a boom of higher order multiple

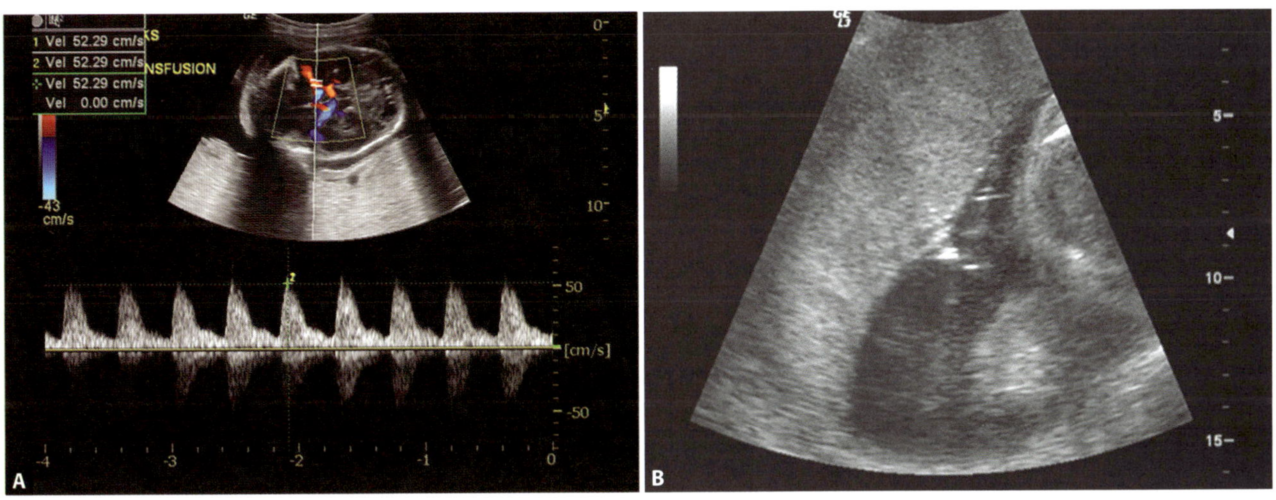

Figs 28.2A and B (A) Middle cerebral artery peak systolic velocity for determining fetal anemia; (B) Intravascular transfusion in the placental cord insertion site

gestation in the past two decades. From 1980 to 2009, twin rates increased by 76% (18.9 to 33.3/1000 livebirths). Triplets or higher order births have increased 400% from 1980 to 1998, followed by a slight decrease by 29% due to restrictions on number of embryos transferred at IVF and the use of multifetal pregnancy reduction (MFPR).[6]

The risk of preterm delivery (<37 weeks) for singleton is about 10% and it increases to 50% for twins and 80% for triplets.[7] Average gestational age at delivery decreases from 35 weeks for twins to 32 weeks for triplets and 29 weeks for quadruplets. Average birth weight in triplets, quadruplets and higher order fetuses is 1666, 1371 and 1253 respectively. Risk of spontaneous loss of entire pregnancy is 25% for quadruplets, 15% for triplets and 8% for twins. Rate of fetal growth restriction reported is 14–25% for twins and increases to 50–60% for triplets and quadruplets. Higher preterm and growth restriction in higher order multiple births are major contributors to neonatal major handicap, cerebral palsy, learning disability and death before one year of age.[8]

Maternal morbidity and mortality increases with presence of each additional fetus and is related to higher rates of gestational diabetes, pregnancy induced hypertension, admission for preterm and premature rupture of membrane, higher operative delivery, postpartum hemorrhage and higher postpartum depression.

Multifetal pregnancy reduction (MFPR) is defined as first or early second trimester procedure for reduction of one or more normal fetuses so as to increase the likelihood of survival and reduce morbidity of remaining fetuses. In addition, it reduces maternal morbidity.

Multifetal pregnancy reduction to twins increases gestational age at delivery by 4 weeks and significantly improves maternal and fetal outcome. A comparative study between reduced and non-reduced triplets showed a total pregnancy loss rate of 20.7% in non-reduced group compared to 8.7% in reduced group. A mean gestational age at delivery was 33.5 weeks in the conservative group versus 36.7 weeks in the reduced group. The benefit of fetal reduction of triplets and higher order fetuses exceeds the risk involved in the procedure.[9]

The inherent risk of pregnancy loss in MFPR is directly proportional to the higher starting number of fetuses, number of fetuses reduced and finishing fetal numbers. The risk reduces with the experience and expertise of the operator. The average risk of pregnancy loss due to the procedure at <26 weeks is about 4–5%.[10]

International Federation of Gynecology and Obstetrics Committee states that it is ethical to reduce the number of fetuses if they are three or more.

Preprocedure Assessment and Counseling

A detailed ultrasound is performed before MFPR to confirm gestational age, determine number of fetuses, labeling them, assessing growth of each fetus, chorionicity determination, early evaluation for structural defects and screening for aneuploidy by Nuchal translucency. Nuchal translucency has a detection rate of 70% with a false positive rate of 5% for trisomy 21. Additional soft markers will increase specificity and it would be beneficial to assess nasal bone, ductus venosus flow and tricuspid regurgitation in the higher order fetuses planning a reduction as maternal serum screening is not useful for theses higher order pregnancies. Some centers routinely perform chorionic villus sampling for karyotype for all the fetuses prior to the procedure. This may further increase the risk of pregnancy loss (Fig. 28.3A).

Determining chorionicity is most important before fetal reduction as MFPR with intracardiac KCl can only be done in dichorionic fetuses. Presence of the twin peak sign in the initial evaluation would confirm dichorionicity.

Detailed nondirective counseling is extremely necessary prior to the procedure and the benefits, risks and alternatives should be explained. Finally, the autonomy of the mother must be respected. An informed consent is to be documented.

Choosing the Fetus to be Reduced

Fetal reduction is done on the fetus that, on initial evaluation, is relatively smaller in size (early fetal growth restricted) or structurally abnormal or fetus with increased nuchal translucency. However, if all fetuses are similar in above assessment, then the fetus that is easily approachable, fundal and away from the cervix is targeted for reduction.

Technique

Place

MFPR is an outpatient procedure and is done in the ultrasound department.

Timing

Although the procedure can be done from 8 weeks to 20 weeks, the ideal timing for the procedure is between 11 weeks and 13 weeks. The advantage of pregnancy reduction after 11 weeks (crown rump length >45 mm) include:

- Most spontaneous fetal loss would have already occurred
- Procedure is technically easier
- Identification of many structural anomalies and aneuploidy screening can be done
- Risk of procedure loss rate is least.

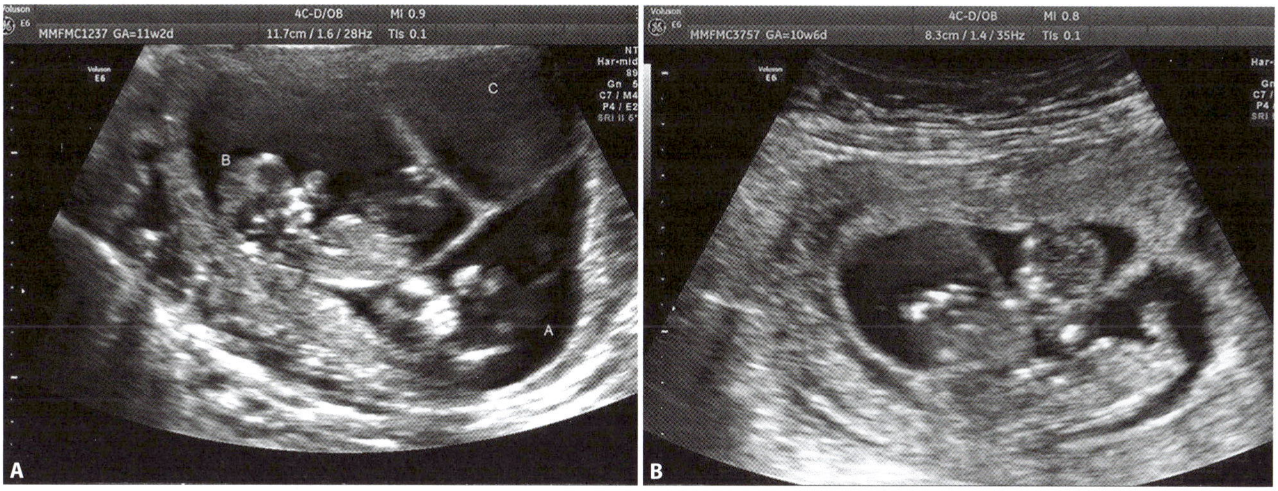

Figs 28.3A and B (A) Assessment of triplets for size, position, labeling, chorionicity and aneuploidy screen prior to multifetal pregnancy reduction; (B) Fetal instillation of KCl into the heart of the triplet near the fundus. Note the needle traversing the skin, amniotic fluid and thorax of the fetus

Route

Multifetal pregnancy reduction can be done transabdominal or transvaginal depending on the expertise of the operator. However, pregnancy loss rates are higher in transvaginal route than transabdominal (13.3 vs 3.5%).[11] Hence, transvaginal route is rarely used unless there is severe maternal obesity or approach to the fetus to be reduced requires it.

Procedure

Under ultrasound guidance and under aseptic precautions, a 20–22 Gauze spinal needle is inserted into the heart or thorax of the fetus and 0.2–0.5 mL potassium choride (KCl) is injected. Needle is not withdrawn till asystole is achieved. Patient is rescreened on ultrasound after 1/2 to 1 hour to ensure asystole in the reduced fetus and normal cardiac activity in the remaining fetuses. Procedure may have to be repeated, if the cardiac activity reverts (Fig. 28.3B).

Risks

- Amniotic fluid leak
- Chorioamnionitis
- Damage of the fetus without death
- Death of rest of the fetuses, if chorionicity determination was inappropriate
- Threatened miscarriage and bleeding
- Loss of entire pregnancy.

Postprocedure

In view of risk for chorioamnionitis a broad-spectrum antibiotic is given prior to the procedure and continued for 5 days. Giving progestrone/tocolysis are individual decisions. Patient is advised on restricted activity for few days and to report if fever/bleeding/leaking/or pain abdomen.

Patient should be informed that leaking of amniotic fluid is not uncommon over the first 24 hours and it spontaneously resolves.

Follow-up ultrasound is done after 2 weeks. Reduced fetus continues to be seen on ultrasound for few weeks to months. Malformation along with cervical length assessment is to be done at 18 weeks followed by routine monitoring for growth and Doppler as in any twin pregnancy.

Reduction in Monochorionic Fetuses

In monochorionic twins, intracardiac KCl will cross over to the other fetus through vascular communications and cause fetal demise of the co-twin also. In these cases, if indicated, selective cord occlusion is the treatment of choice but carries a higher risk of pregnancy loss.

Selective Feticide

This is a term used distinctly for reduction done in a twin fetus for discordant fetal anomaly. Selective feticide is indicated in fetuses whose anomaly is nonlethal but with morbidity or if the defect has a potential for affecting the other fetus and course of pregnancy.

FETAL SURGERY

Before deciding on a therapeutic intervention the questions that need to be answered are:

- Will the therapy benefit the fetal short or long-term outcome?

- Does the benefit to the fetus outweigh the harm to the mother?
- Can the treatment wait till delivery?

If the answer to first two questions is in affirmative and third answer is no, then therapy can be considered.

Distinct advantages of fetal surgery are:

- Intervene before progressive damage
- Surgical healing is better with no scars
- Fetus has the ideal postoperative environment in the mothers womb.

Three approaches are used for fetal surgical intervention.

1. Open fetal surgery
2. Fetoscopic surgery
3. Percutaneous ultrasound-guided surgery using shunts.

Principles of Fetal Surgery

Prenatal intervention is justified, only if:

- Accurate diagnosis is made
- Disease is severe enough to warrant risk of intervention
- The malformation interferes with organ development
- If alleviated will allow normal development
- Fetus cannot be safely delivered at that point of time.

Prerequisite for Fetal Surgery

- *Nondirective counseling*: Although the final goal of fetal intervention is to improve the health of the fetus, any fetal intervention *in utero* has implications on the mothers health. Hence, the women and the family should be informed in detail about the risks and benefits. The informed consent should involve thorough discussion of the options available including fetal intervention, postnatal therapy, palliative nature of the therapy, residual disease and its long-term implications and also options of pregnancy termination.
- *Coexisting anomalies and chromosomal abnormalities* are ruled out.
- Prenatal diagnostic procedure is done to *determine the functional status* of the organ system, which needs treatment.
- *Tertiary level obstetric, anesthetic and neonatal care* available.

Conditions Amenable to Surgery with Proven Results

- Pleuroamniotic shunt in primary hydrothorax
- Twin-to-twin transfusion syndrome
- Twin reversed arterial perfusion sequence
- Ovarian cyst aspiration.

Conditions Amenable to Surgery with Mixed Results

- Vesicoamniotic shunt for obstructive uropathy
- Thoracoamniotic shunt for congenital pulmonary airways malformation (CPAM, initially called CCAM)
- Fetal tracheal occlusion for congenital diaphragmatic hernia
- Surgery for meningomyelocele
- Surgery for sacrococcygeal teratoma.

Conditions Amenable to Surgery with Disappointing Results

- *Ventriculomegaly:* Aqueductal stenosis
- *Structural cardiac defects:* Balloon valvuloplasty/ septoplasty.

OPEN FETAL SURGERY

Open fetal surgery was first attempted in 1960. It involves an initial hysterotomy under general anesthesia where the fetus is extracted partially without disconnecting from the placenta and undergoes fetal surgery intrapartum for the disorder. Fetus is then returned back to the amniotic cavity and the uterus with membranes is resutured. Mother has to be under high doses of intravenous tocolysis for the procedure as well as subsequently to tide over the extremely high-risk of preterm labor. Subsequently, the mother will need a second surgery lower segment cesarean section (LSCS) for delivery of the baby.

Conditions correctable with open fetal surgery are:

- Meningomyelocele
- Repair of congenital diaphragmatic hernia
- Ligation of sacrococcygeal teratoma.

Fetal Surgery for Meningomyelocele

Meningomyelocele can cause hydrocephalus as well as motor impairment and loss of bowel and bladder control. These have been postulated to aggravate due to exposure of spinal cord to the trauma of amniotic fluid *in utero*. Covering of meningomyelocele (initially in sheep and later in human fetus) has been shown to reduce the need for ventriculoperitoneal shunts, slow the progress of ventriculomegaly, resolution of hindbrain hernia and improved motor outcome in short-term follow-up of 30 months. There has been a return of open fetal surgery for meningomyelocele after a randomized multicentric trial by Bebbington et al. in 2010 which showed reduced neonatal and childhood morbidity.[12]

Surgery for Sacrococcygeal Teratoma

Sacrococcygeal teratoma causes large arteriovenous shunting of blood leading to high output cardiac failure, hydrops and death. Traditionally, the tumor was resected by open technique followed by fetoscopic route. Attempts have been made towards percutaneous minimal invasive coagulation of tumor vessels.

Risk involved with open surgery include:

- High chances of preterm labor
- Premature rupture of membrane
- Bleeding per vaginum
- Chorioamnionitis
- Pulmonary edema and complications of anesthesia
- Need for LSCS for present as well as all subsequent pregnancies.

FETOSCOPIC FETAL SURGERY

Open fetal surgery gave way to fetoscopic surgeries as they were relatively less invasive than open fetal surgery. Fetoscopic surgery was a spin off of general endoscopic procedure. Hobbins was the first person to insert an endoscope inside the uterus and subsequently fetoscopic surgeries reached heights in 1970–80s. However, with better ultrasound imaging and guided needle procedures, fetoscopy quickly became redundant. Fetoscopy was revisited by Delia in 1990 for treatment of twin-to-twin transfusion syndrome.

Fetoscopic surgery is done under epidural/local anesthesia. It requires specialized fetoscopic instruments, atraumatic ports and working fluid media (saline/ringer). There is no mandatory need for LSCS later as compared to open surgery.

Indications

- *Fetoscopic tracheal occlusion for treatment of congenital diaphragmatic hernia (Fetendo technique):* The aim is to temporarily plug the trachea using clips or balloon so as to cause obstruction to lung secretion and subsequently cause expansion of lungs pushing the herniated abdominal viscera back into the abdomen.
  An *ex utero* intrapartum procedure (EXIT) to remove the clips and intubate the trachea is performed at term during LSCS, while the partially delivered fetus is still receiving placental supply
- *Fetoscopic balloon valvuloplasty of critical aortic stenosis* in the fetus has been attempted to prevent progression to hypoplastic left heart syndrome with mixed results.
- About 10–15% of all monozygous twins have twin-to-twin transfusion syndrome (TTTS) where there are unbalanced vascular anastamosis between both the fetuses. Without treatment, perinatal mortality reaches 63–80%. Fetoscopic surgery has re-emerged as the treatment of choice for twin-to-twin transfusion syndrome where *selective laser photocoagulation of communicating vessels* are done. The Eurofetus randomized control study published in 2004 showed significant survival benefits as well as lesser neurological damage in fetoscopic laser ablation of communicating vessels group over other surgical techniques in TTTS.[13] Today fetoscopic laser for TTTS is the most common fetal surgical procedure being carried out.
- *Fetoscopic cord occlusion/ligation of acardiac twin* is also a successful surgical modality. Twin reversed arterial perfusion sequence is seen in 1% of monozygous twins and is associated with cardiac failure in the pump twin with perinatal mortality as high as 55%. Recently, intrafetal interstitial laser in the acardiac fetus under ultrasound guidance using laser fibers inserted via 18-gauze needle has become the treatment of choice as it is simple, safer and more effective.
- Fetoscopic fulguration of posterior urethral valves.

Limitations of Fetoscopic Surgery

- Invasive
- Limited depth and field of vision
- Intra-amniotic bleed may obscure vision
- Risk of preterm labor and premature rupture of membranes slightly more than USG-guided procedures but less than open fetal surgery
- Maternal and fetal injury with the trocar
- Potential teratogenic effect of light and heat.

PERCUTANEOUS ULTRASOUND-GUIDED FETAL SHUNTS

Ultrasound-guided interventional procedures are done under local anesthesia.

Complication low as compared to above procedures and include:

- Preterm, premature rupture of membranes
- Fetal injury
- Shunt block or displacement
- Chorioamnionitis.

Indications

- *Primary pleural effusion (Chylothorax):* Extrinsic compression on the developing lungs may lead to pulmonary hypoplasia and hydrops. Pleuroamniotic shunt is a double pigtail catheter which is placed under ultrasound guidance with one end of the shunt in the

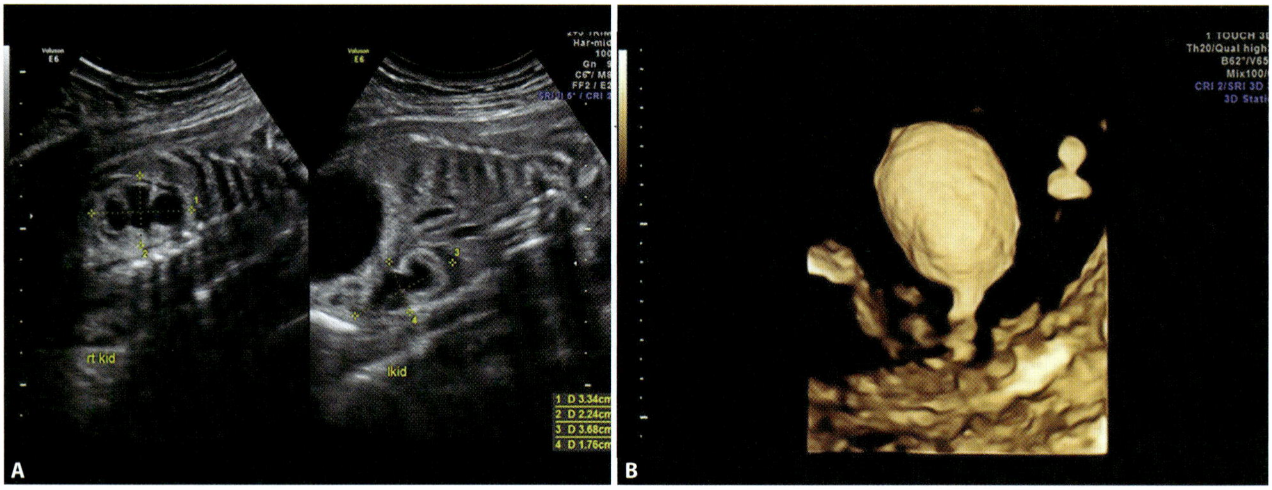

Figs 28.4A and B Severe obstructive uropathy in a case of posterior urethral valve at 25 weeks requiring vesicoamniotic shunt

pleural cavity and other end in the amniotic cavity. About 60% survival rates have been achieved in carefully selected cases of primary pleural effusion.[14] Another approach in fetal chylothorax is performing pleurodesis by administering OK-432 in the pleural cavity.

- *Obstructive uropathy*: Severe bilateral obstruction to outflow of urine may cause backpressure changes leading to nonfunctional dysplastic kidneys *in utero* and pulmonary hypoplasia due to oligohydramnios (Potter's syndrome). Vesicoamniotic shunts aim to release back pressure effect in the urinary tract, restore urinary outflow and improve liquor and pulmonary development (Figs 28.4A to C).

Intervention justified only, if the obstruction is severe, bilateral, causing progressive oligohydramnios and deteriorating renal function on serial ultrasound remote from term. Some amount of residual renal function must be preserved before intervention. Fetal karyotype must be done and any other disorders ruled out.

Prenatal shunts for obstructive urinary system are not indicated in unilateral obstruction or bilateral partial obstruction with normal liquor or in nonfunctioning fetal kidneys.

Renal function is assessed by fetal vesicocentesis where initially urine in the distended fetal bladder is completely aspirated. Subsequent urine sample is analyzed for sodium, chloride and β_2-microglobulin. Nonfunctional kidneys are salt wasters and β_2-microglobulin of >2 mg/L is the best predictor of poor renal function.

Ultrasound-guided vesicoamniotic shunt is done under local anesthesia using double pigtail shunt where one end is in the fetal bladder and other in the amniotic fluid. The percutaneous shunting in lower urinary tract obstruction (PLUTO) trial compared conservative treatment with vesicoamniotic shunts in singleton fetuses less than 28 weeks. Survival seemed to be better in the intervention group at 28 days of life. However, the authors concluded that there were substantial short- and long-term morbidity in both groups due to poor renal residual function.

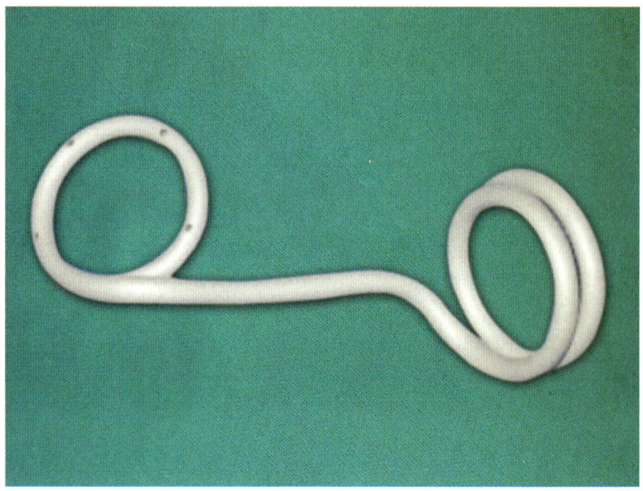

Fig. 28.4C Harrison shunt for vesicoamniotic shunt

Relieving obstruction temporarily may prolong gestational age at delivery, improve pulmonary maturity but renal damage already done and its sequel may remain. The child may subsequently develop chronic renal failure requiring dialysis.

Other options are open or fetoscopic fulguration of posterior urethral valves.

- *Ventriculoamniotic shunts* have been evaluated for decompression in obstructive hydrocephalus but have poor results and has been abandoned.
- *Congenital pulmonary airway obstruction (CPAM/ CCAM):* The natural history of this lung lesion may be progression/regression or remains stable antenatally. Large cysts involving a large part of the lung may cause lung compression, mediastinal shift, hydrops and fetal mortality. These progressive, macrocystic, large lung cysts maybe drained via a cystoamniotic shunt under ultrasound guidance and thus help in regression and improve lung growth.

CONCLUSION

Prenatal medical therapy has good post-intervention results with minimal risk to the mother. Intrauterine transfusion in Rh-isoimmunized anemic fetus has a survival rate as high as 70–80%. Fetal reduction procedures are extremely important for risk reduction in patients with higher order pregnancies.

However, fetal surgeries have a potential risk to mother and fetus and need an extensive presurgical counseling of parents and family. It necessitates careful case selection, well-coordinated team, extensive expertise in the field and hence is limited to few specialized centres in India and worldwide.

Fetoscopy has re-evolved with its use in treating complications of monochorionic twins. Fetoscopic laser ablation of unbalanced communicating vessels in TTTS is today the most common fetal surgical procedure carried out.

REFERENCES

1. Liley AW. Intrauterine transfusion of fetus with in hemolytic disease. Br Med J. 1963;2:1107-9.
2. Report on the Consensus Development Conference on the Effect of Corticosteroids for Fetal Maturation on Perinatal Outcomes. US Department of Health and Human Services, Public Health Service, NIH Pub No. 95-3784, November 1994.
3. The Antenatal Magnesium Sulphate for Neuroprotection Guideline Development Panel. Antenatal magnesium sulphate prior to preterm birth for neuroprotection of the fetus, infant and child: National Clinical Practice Guidelines. The Australian Research Centre for Health of Women and Babies, The University of Adelaide; 2010.
4. Breur JM1, Visser GH, Kruize AA, et al. Treatment of fetal heart block with maternal steroid therapy: case report and review of the literature. Ultrasound Obstet Gynecol. 2004;24(4):467-72.
5. Oepkes D, Adama van Scheltema P. Intrauterine fetal transfusions in the management of fetal anemia and fetal thrombocytopenia. Semin Fetal Neonatal Med. 2007;12:432-8.
6. Luke B. The changing pattern of multiple births in the United States: maternal and infant characteristics, 1973 and 1990. Obstet Gynecol. 1994;84:101-6.
7. Births: Final data for 2010. Natl Vital Stat Rep. 2012;61:1.
8. ACOG Committee on Practice Bulletin. Obstetrics ACOG Practice Bulleitin No 56. Multiple gestation: complicated twins, triplets and higher order multifetal pregnancy. Clinical Management Guidelines for Obstetrician-Gynecologists. Obstet Gynecol. 2004;104(4):869-93.
9. Lipitz S, Reichmann B, Uval J, et al. A prospective comparison of the outcome of triplet pregnancies managed expectantly or by multifetal reduction to twins. Am J Obstet Gynecol. 1994;170:874-9.
10. Evans ML, Berkowitz RL, Wapner RJ, et al. Improvement in outcome of multifetal pregnancy reduction with increased experience. Am J Obstet Gynecol. 2001;184:97-103.
11. Timor Tritsch IE, Bashiri A, Monteagudo A, et al. Two hundred and ninety consecutive cases of multifetal pregnancy reduction: Comparison of transabdominal versus the transvaginal approach. Am J Obstet Gynecol. 2004;194:2085-9.
12. Adzick NS, Thomas EA, Spong CY. A Randomized trial of prenatal versus postnatal repair of myelomeningocele. New England Journal of Medicine. 2011;364:11.
13. Ville Y, for the Eurofoetus Group. Treatment of twin-to-twin-transfusion syndrome. The end of a long-standing misunderstanding. Ultrasound Obstet Gynecol. 2003;22(Suppl 1): 64(OC241).
14. Smith RP, Illanes S, Denbow ML, et al. Outcome of fetal pleural effusions treated by thoracoamniotic shunting. Ultrasound in Obstetrics and Gynecology. 2005;26:63-6.

CHAPTER

29

Intrauterine Transfusion

Purnima Satoskar, Shilpa Agrawal

Present-day guidelines for the administration of Rhesus (Rh) immune globulin (RhIG) to every Rho(D)-negative women at 28 weeks' gestation and postpartum have greatly reduced the incidence of red blood cell alloimmunization.[1]

Intrauterine transfusion (IUT) is a highly specialized area of medical practice requiring close collaboration between experts in fetal medicine, hematology and blood transfusion, and rapid access to blood counting. Even in the most expert hands IUT carries a risk of fetal death of 1–3% per procedure and fetomaternal hemorrhage may cause further sensitization and worsening of hemolytic disease the fetus and newborn (HDFN). IUT was the first effort at *in utero* treatment of the human fetus. During the last 30 years, it has become the treatment of choice for patients alloimmunized to red blood cell antigens in whom severe fetal anemia develops remote from term.[2]

HISTORY

In the early 1960s, intrauterine treatment of fetal anemia due to red cell immunization by percutaneous intraperitoneal transfusion was introduced by Liley. Initially, Liley[3] devised bilirubin extinction in amniotic fluid as a diagnostic tool for fetal alloimmune anemia.[4] At one occasion, erroneously he collected ascites instead of amniotic fluid and this event brought him the idea that intraperitoneal blood transfusion could be an effective method to correct fetal anemia. Fetal position was determined by X-ray to visualize the persistence of swallowed water-soluble contrast medium 'urografin' in the fetal gut, which was combined with fat-soluble contrast medium to visualize the outline of the skin. Under local anesthesia, a needle was inserted into the fetal peritoneum. Although survival rates improved, outcome, especially of hydropic and very young anemic fetuses, remained poor. The currently used technique, intravascular intrauterine transfusion (IUT) into the umbilical cord, was first described by Rodeck et al.[5] in 1981 using guidance of the needle by fetoscopy. Advances in the resolution of ultrasound enabled pioneers such as Ferdinand Daffos in Paris and Jens Bang in Copenhagen to perform ultrasound-guided cordocentesis and blood transfusion directly into the umbilical vein.[6] IUT into the intrahepatic portion of the umbilical vein was first described by Nicolini et al.[7] in 1990, and it can be a safe alternative for umbilical cord transfusion in particular in case of a posterior placenta.[8] In the Netherlands, IUT was introduced in 1965 by Bennebroek Gravenhorst et al.[9] From 1987 onwards the intravascular technique became the method of choice.[10] Consequently IUT continues to be the cornerstone of treatment for fetal anemia for a variety of causes.

INDICATIONS

Fetal anemia is a serious complication in pregnancy and associated with perinatal mortality and morbidity. During 25 years of worldwide experience with intravascular intrauterine blood transfusion, a variety of indications have been described. Intrauterine transfusion (IUT) treatment is considered most successful for fetal anemia due to red cell alloimmunization.

Treatment of Fetal Anemia due to Hemolytic Disease of the Fetus and Newborn

The most common indication for intrauterine blood transfusion, hemolytic disease of the fetus and newborn (HDFN) results from maternal alloimmunization to red cell antigens, for which mother and fetus are incompatible. Maternal red cell IgG antibodies pass the placenta into the fetal circulation and may cause hemolysis. More than 50 red cell antigens have been associated with HDFN. The most prevalent red cell antibodies are RhD, Kell and Rhc. Other antibodies associated with severe HDFN are anti-Rh-e/E (Rhesus), Fy(a)/Fy(b) (Duffy blood group), Kidd(Jka) and anti-M (MNS system).[11]

Recently, a larger follow-up study (LOTUS study) analyzed outcome after a total of 1,284 IUTs performed in 451 fetuses in a 20-year period.[12] Alloimmunization was due to RhD in 80%, Kell in 12% and Rhc in 5% of the cases. Twenty-six percent of the fetuses were hydropic at the first transfusion and the mean gestational age at first transfusion was 26 weeks; the mean number of transfusion was 3. The vast majority (>95%) of children had a normal neurodevelopmental outcome. The major preoperative risk factor for neurodevelopmental impairment was the presence of hydrops. Prevention of fetal hydrops by timely detection and treatment may improve long-term outcome. The high rate of intact survival confirms the success of IUT for alloimmune anemia.

Parvovirus Infection

Human parvovirus B19 causes erythema infectiosum (fifth disease) in children. One-third of infected pregnant women will remain asymptomatic and will not manifest the exanthem typical of this disease. Parvovirus suppresses the fetal bone marrow and inhibits fetal erythropoiesis with the subsequent development of aplastic anemia, nonimmune hydrops, and fetal death.

Maternal parvovirus infection is often confirmed by detection of a specific IgM antibody that appears 3–4 days after the onset of clinical disease and persists for 3–4 months. Fetal infection usually occurs 4–6 weeks after maternal infection, although hydrops fetalis has been reported as late as 12 weeks after the maternal illness. If maternal infection has been confirmed, the fetus should undergo weekly ultrasound examinations for the presence of hydrops fetalis for a total of 12 weeks. If hydrops is noted, donor red blood cells and platelets should be prepared, and cordocentesis performed. Studies of fetal blood usually show a negative direct Coombs' test, severe anemia, occasional thrombocytopenia, an inappropriately low reticulocyte count, normal serum bilirubin, elevated total IgM, and elevated liver enzymes.[13] Under the electron microscope, viral particles may be observed in fetal ascitic fluid or blood.[14] Using probes specific for human parvovirus B19, viral DNA also can be identified in some fetal body fluids. Spontaneous resolution of hydrops fetalis secondary to fetal parvovirus infection has been reported by several authors.[15] Thus, if the fetal reticulocyte count is elevated before the first IUT, a second procedure is not necessary because recovery of the fetal bone marrow is ongoing. Nonimmune hydrops due to *in utero* parvovirus infection may require several weeks to resolve after the fetal hematocrit has returned to normal.

Fetomaternal Hemorrhage

Fetomaternal hemorrhage (FMH) is defined as the passage of fetal blood into the maternal circulation and is a serious rare complication in pregnancy. Massive fetomaternal hemorrhage is the cause of fetal death in 1 per 1000 births and results in significant fetal morbidity in at least 1 per 800 deliveries.[16] A Kleihauer test to estimate the volume of hemorrhage and Doppler evaluation of fetal flow velocities (MCA PSV) to detect fetal anemia may aid in disease management.[17] IUT corrects fetal anemia and can prolong gestation until a more mature gestational age is reached. Perinatal death varies between 31% and 50%.[18] The outcome of long-term survivors after severe anemia due to FMH is not well known but includes neurological sequelae[18]

Twin-twin Transfusion Syndrome

Fetofetal transfusion due to communicating vascular anastomoses in MC twin pregnancies may result in fetal anemia of the donor twin and polycythemia in the recipient: twin anemia polycythemia sequence (TAPS). Treatment with IUT may help to correct the donor twin's anemia, but may potentially deteriorate the plethoric twin's condition.[19] Therefore, a combination of IUT to the donor with an exchange transfusion in the recipient twin can be considered.[20] Follow-up data on the long-term neurodevelopmental outcome in TAPS are lacking. More studies are necessary to determine whether IUT is a successful option in the management of TAPS.

Placental and Fetal Tumors

Large chorioangiomas are clinically significant and may cause serious complications, such as fetal anemia, hydrops and fetal death. Fetal anemia may be a result of FMH (shunting of large volumes of blood to the tumor) and/or hemolysis because of the entrapment and destruction of fetal erythrocytes in the vascular network of the chorioangioma. Treatment with IUT may improve fetal condition and may prevent preterm delivery.

Fetal sacrococcygeal teratoma may lead to anemia due either to hemorrhage or hemolysis within the tumor and is associated with poor survival.

Rare Causes of Fetal Anemia

Rarely, IUT has also been used to treat severe fetal anemia due to α thalassemia.[21]

Platelets for Neonatal Alloimmune Thrombocytopenia

Neonatal alloimmune thrombocytopenia (NAIT), a disease process analogous to red blood cell alloimmunization, complicates 1 per 1000–2000 livebirths.[22] In this situation, transplacental passage of maternal antibodies to fetal platelet antigens of paternal origin results in severe fetal and neonatal thrombocytopenia. Unlike Rh alloimmunization, the first fetus may already be severely affected; maternal antibody titers are not predictive of the degree of fetal thrombocytopenia.[23] Currently, fetal platelet count and antigen status of any subsequent pregnancy are determined most commonly by cordocentesis at 20 weeks' gestation. Unfortunately, this approach is not without risk. Maternal platelets for immediate transfusion should be available at the time of cordocentesis should excessive streaming of blood occur from the umbilical vessel puncture site. Alternatively, if the fetal platelet count can be assessed rapidly while the cordocentesis needle is still in place, platelet transfusion should be performed for counts less than 50,000/mm^3. This threshold is based on neonatal courses complicated by bleeding in infants born to women with autoimmune thrombocytopenia.[24]

Rh-Negative Sensitized Women

Noninvasive Evaluation

The prediction of fetal risk by combining the maternal obstetric history and serologic examination is an imprecise art. The magnitude of fetal and neonatal disease typically progresses from one pregnancy to another.

Maternal Titer

The maternal titer is the first step in the evaluation of the Rh D-sensitized patient. The human antiglobulin titer (Indirect Coombs') is used to determine the degree of alloimmunization. The critical titer for a laboratory is the titer below which no fetal death has been observed. When this is present, further testing with more invasive techniques is required. A critical value for anti-D between 1:8 and 1:32 is usually used.

Middle Cerebral Artery Doppler

Hydrops fetalis can be detected easily by ultrasonography, but unfortunately this is a late sign of fetal anemia when hemoglobin values have declined to more than 7 g/dL below the norm for gestational age. Mari et al. were the first to propose that Doppler assessment of the peak velocity in the fetal middle cerebral artery (MCA) could determine accurately whether the human fetus was anemic. A value more than 1.5 multiples of the median (MoM) for gestational age detected all cases of moderate to severe anemia with a false-positive rate of only 12%. Technically, the determination of the MCA peak systolic velocity (MCA PSV) is relatively straightforward.

Measurements can be initiated as early as 15 weeks of gestation and should be repeated at 1-week–2-week intervals. Because the normal peak MCA Doppler velocity increases with advancing gestational age, data should be adjusted for the time in pregnancy when the study is undertaken. This can be achieved by plotting the value on a standardized graph. After 35 weeks of gestation, there appears to be a higher false-positive rate in the detection of fetal anemia. Therefore, late in gestation, a normal MCA velocity can be followed with repeat measurements. If an elevated value is noted, amniocentesis for ΔOD450 and fetal lung maturity testing should be undertaken to determine whether delivery is indicated.

Invasive Evaluation

Two invasive methods are used to search for fetal anemia secondary to hemolytic disease:

1. *Indirect*: Spectrophotometry (the ΔOD450) using a specimen of amniotic fluid obtained by ultrasound-guided amniocentesis.
2. *Direct*: Fetal blood studies using a sample obtained by cordocentesis.

When to Transfuse?

Fetal transfusion therapy should not be undertaken in the absence of hydrops without first confirming that the fetus has significant anemia. A hematocrit below 30% is usually used because it is below the 2.5 percentile for all gestational ages greater than 20 weeks. These procedures should be performed whenever possible only by individuals with considerable and regular experience, namely 8–10 transfusions per year as a minimum.[25]

How to Transfuse?

Techniques[26]

- Intraperitoneal
- Intravascular by cordocentesis
  - Exchange transfusion
  - Simple direct transfusion
- Intravascular by intrahepatic venous puncture
  - Simple direct transfusion
- Intracardiac by fetal cardiocentesis
  - Simple direct transfusion
  - Combined approaches
  - Exchange intravascular transfusion followed by intraperitoneal transfusion
  - Simple direct intravascular transfusion followed by intraperitoneal transfusion
- Exchange transfusions are associated with a high risk of serious complications so it is not the recommended form of therapy.

How Much to Transfuse?

The volume infused is a compromise between the amount necessary to correct the estimated hemoglobin deficit and the amount that will safely fit into the intra-abdominal cavity. A final fetal hematocrit of 50–60% is usually the goal when intravascular transfusion (IVT) alone is performed. A rise in fetal whole-blood viscosity during transfusion can be minimized by restricting the post-transfusion fetal hematocrit to approximately 50–55%. The final target hematocrit in the combined IVT/IPT approach is usually approximately 40%. This is more physiologic because the fetal hematocrit normally ranges from 33% at 17 weeks' to 47% at 40 weeks' gestation.[27]

The formula of Bowman is quite practical and recommended:

$$\text{Volume} = (\text{weeks gestation} - 20) \times 10 \text{ mL}$$

The required amount of donor blood (Vdonor) is determined by the formula proposed by Rodeck et al.[5]

$$\text{Vdonor} = \text{FPVinitial} \times (\text{desired Ht} - \text{initial Ht})/\text{Ht donor blood}$$

The initial fetoplacental blood volume (FPVinitial) is based on estimated fetal weight and normal values for fetoplacental blood volume as proposed by Nicolaides et al.[28]

Usually, Rodeck's formula underestimates the required donor volume, to reach desired hematocrit, since the formula does not take an increase in blood volume during transfusion into account.

Initial Fetal Investigations[25]

Cordocentesis is performed with complete preparation for intrauterine transfusion depending on the reports. Intrauterine treatment should be implemented only in cases where the fetus is not mature enough for extrauterine life.

First Specimen

- ABO and Rh type
- Direct Coombs test
- Complete blood count (CBC)
- Manual reticulocyte counts (%RBCs)
- Total bilirubin.

Subsequent Specimens

- Complete blood count (CBC)
- Manual reticulocyte counts (%RBCs)
- Total bilirubin.

Preprocedure Requirements

- Thorough counseling of the parents regarding the procedure, risks and complications involved, follow-up, need of repeat procedure and outcome is mandatory.
- Written, informed valid consent is taken.

Donor Blood

- Confirm fetal hematocrit <30%
- Preparation of donor blood O Rh negative, as fresh as possible and compatible with both mother and fetus
- Buffy coat poor, washed in saline × 3, irradiated. Final hematocrit 70–80%
- Preparation two sets of tubing for transfusion and measurement of umbilical venous pressure (UVP). Filters are mandatory.

Preparation

- The procedure should be performed in a sterile room under strict aseptic precautions. Diazepam, 5–10 mg slow IV for maternal comfort if needed, though used rarely
- Lateral displacement of the uterus, support lower back
- Acetone wipes to remove ultrasound contact gel from the skin
- Povidone or alcohol surgical preparation of the skin
- Drape as desired and prepare surgical tray
- 20 gauge Tuohy needle 25 cm long
- 20 mL syringe
- 3 Way connector and extension tubing
- 5 mL normal saline
- 20 gauge spinal needle
- Pancuronium, 0.3 mg/kg estimated fetal weight
- Sterile prepare ultrasound transducer.

TRANSFUSION[25]

Intraperitoneal

Intraperitoneal transfusion is used when approach to cord is difficult as in cases of obesity, posterior placenta and early gestation.

Target fetal abdomen between umbilicus and bladder; avoid liver. Administer pancuronium intramuscularly targeting the fetal buttock. Insert Tuohy needle into selected site. Confirm intra-abdominal, extravascular location by injecting saline. Infuse donor blood in 1 mL aliquots over 10 min checking the fetal heart rate after each aliquot.

Continue transfusion until planned volume infused calculated by: volume = (wk. gestation - 20) × 10 mL.

Follow-up

Document complete absorption of donor blood by serial ultrasonography. Examinations every 2–3 days. Second transfusion after complete absorption; thereafter, repeat at 4-week intervals.

Intravascular

Though most fetuses tolerate a hematocrit of 25% or lower without clinically significant sequelae, cut-off point of <30% has proved a pragmatic threshold.

Procedure

Flush three syringes with heparin (100 U/mL); fill one with lidocaine (1%) and fill one with desired dose of pancuronium (0.3 mg/kg sonographically estimated fetal weight) for IM use or vecuronium 0.1 mg/kg for IV use.

Puncture umbilical vein at most accessible site, usually placental end of cord. Immediately administer vecuronium—paralysis will be rapid.

Aspirate 1 mL for complete blood count, Keilhauer stain and reticulocyte count; check hematocrit immediately. Aspirate 1 mL for venous blood gases. Begin infusion of packed red blood cells after double checking there is no air in the system. Infuse half the estimated requirement and repeat blood sampling. Measurement of umbilical venous pressure is useful in severely anemic fetus and can be repeated at midtransfusion. Halt transfusion if the rise in the umbilical venous pressure (UVP) has exceeded 10 mm Hg; check heart rate to rule out bradycardia as an explanation.

If UVP acceptable calculate remaining volume necessary to achieve a hematocrit of 50%; infuse that volume. Repeat blood sampling and pressure measurement; remove needle if UVP at acceptable level. Monitor fetus frequently until spontaneous movement resumes.

Repeat Transfusion

Middle cerebral artery (MCA) Doppler is not as useful as in untreated patients due to changes in circulatory hemodynamics due to earlier transfusion. The decline in hematocrit after transfusion is more rapid and variable between the first and second transfusions compared to subsequent procedures. This variability results from the differing rates of destruction of disparate amounts of fetal antigen positive and banked antigen negative red blood cells. Except for the hydropic fetus, the second transfusion is performed 2 weeks after the first. Subsequently, the decline in hematocrit per week is predictable for any given fetus. The factor useful for determining the subsequent transfusion is the hemoglobin level directly and the fact that the concentration of fetal hemoglobin in blood decreases at the rate of 0.3 gm% per day.

When to Deliver?

The timing of delivery in fetuses undergoing serial IUTs has undergone considerable change. During the era of IPT, fetuses affected by hemolytic disease were delivered routinely at 32 weeks' gestation. Hyaline membrane disease and hyperbilirubinemia necessitating neonatal exchange transfusion were frequent complications. The widespread use of IVT during the past decade has led many centers to perform the final procedure at approximately 35 weeks' gestation with delivery planned approximately 3 weeks later. This change in management has virtually eliminated hyaline membrane disease and the need for neonatal exchange transfusions for elevated bilirubin. The addition of at least 10 days of maternal phenobarbital (30 mg three times daily) has resulted in a 75% reduction in the need for neonatal exchange tranfusions.[29] Once fetal viability is reached, IUTs should be undertaken close to the labor and delivery suite so that an immediate cesarean section can be performed in cases of fetal distress.

Hydrops

Because most hydropic fetuses have myocardial dysfunction that prevents them from tolerating the required infusion volume,[30] the target hematocrit after their first transfusion is only 25%. Twenty-four hours later, the hematocrit can be safely brought to 50% during a second transfusion.

Delivery

The obstetric philosophy need not be altered for the nonanemic, transfused fetus. Antenatal transfusion is not a reason to deny a vaginal birth after cesarean section. If the final hematocrit at the end of the last transfusion was 50%, it will be in the mid-30s in the umbilical cord at delivery. Typically, the neonatal hematocrit increases approximately 15% within 8 hours of delivery, reflecting a massive shift of extracellular and intravascular fluid. The hematocrit then declines to or below the delivery level over the next few days to weeks.[25]

Need for Neonatal Top-up Transfusion

Weekly hematocrit and reticulocyte determinations should be performed for the first 2 months of life in infants with a history of IUT.[31] Infants with hemoglobin of less than 5–6 g/dL clearly should be transfused, even if they are symptom-free. Infants showing signs related to severe anemia, such as failure to thrive and lethargy, also are candidates for transfusion. Scaradavou and colleagues[32] reported the use of erythropoietin to treat late anemia caused by suppression of erythropoiesis due to IUT for Rh alloimmunization. Subcutaneous injection of 200 U erythropoietin per kilogram of body weight three times per week, combined with ferrous sulfate and folic acid supplementation was effective in markedly decreasing the need for postnatal transfusion.

COMPLICATIONS

Acute

Fetal distress during or after the procedure is the most serious complication and may result in fetal death or emergency delivery with the risk of prematurity, neonatal asphyxia or death. Fetal distress can occur after local cord accidents (rupture, spasm, tamponade from a hematoma or excessive bleeding), volume overload, chorioamnionitis, preterm rupture of membranes or preterm labor.[33] Fetal demise after intrauterine treatment may be the result of an already compromised fetal state or due to the invasive procedure itself.

Long-term Complications

Neonates treated with IUT require more top-up red blood cell transfusions during the first 6 months of life, which may be explained by the suppression of fetal erythropoiesis.[34] Red blood cell donor transfusions have a minimal but theoretical risk for anaphylactic reactions and transmission of viral diseases. IUT, transplacental puncture in particular, is also associated with the formation of new red cell antibodies.[35] Additional antibodies are formed by small FMH after IUT. The prevalence of additional maternal red cell antibodies is 19–26% and may complicate present and subsequent pregnancies and future transfusions.[36] The presence of additional antibodies causes problems in selecting compatible red blood cells for fetal and maternal transfusions, and the antibodies are capable of inducing delayed hemolytic transfusion reactions.

TAKE HOME MESSAGES

1. Intrauterine transfusion is an invasive procedure which should only be performed for well-defined indications by a skilled and experienced fetal medicine specialist.
2. Intravascular transfusion is the procedure of choice.
3. The risks of transfusion should be balanced with morbidity and mortality of preterm delivery after 32 weeks and detailed counseling done.
4. Careful monitoring by laboratory tests and ultrasonography are important both before and after the procedure.
5. Site of transfusion should be chosen after careful consideration in individual patients.
6. In case of unexpected technical difficulties an intraperitoneal transfusion may be done or the procedure rescheduled to reduce procedural complications.
7. Successful transfusion eliminates the antenatal and, largely, the postnatal complications of fetal hemolytic disease.
8. By maintaining the hematocrit at the high end, fetal erythropoiesis is minimized, reducing the risk of postnatal hyperbilirubinemia.
9. The neonate should be checked for anemia fortnightly till 3 months of age and given packed cell transfusions if needed.

REFERENCES

1. American College of Obstetricians and Gynecologists. Prevention of D Isoimmunization. Technical Bulletin No. 147, ACOG, Washington, DC, October, 1990.
2. Moise K Jr. Changing trends in the management of red blood cell alloimmunization in pregnancy. Arch Pathol Lab Med. 1994;118-421-8.
3. Liley AW. Intrauterine transfusion of foetus in haemolytic disease. Br Med J. 1963;2(5365):1107-9.
4. Liley AW. Liquor amnii analysis in the management of the pregnancy complicated by rhesus sensitization. Am J Obstet Gynecol. 1961;82:1359-70.
5. Rodeck CH, Nicolaides KH, Warsof SL, Fysh WJ, Gamsu HR, Kemp JR. The management of severe rhesus isoimmunisation by fetoscopic intravascular transfusion. Am J Obstet Gynecol. 1984;150:769-74.
6. Bang J, Bock JE, Trolle D. Ultrasound-guided fetal intravenous transfusion for severe rhesus haemolytic disease. Br Med J. 1982;284:373-4.
7. Nicolini U, Nicolaidis P, Fisk NM, Tannirandorn Y, Rodeck CH. Fetal blood sampling from the intrahepatic vein: analysis of safety and clinical experience with 214 procedures. Obstet Gynecol. 1990;76:47-53.
8. Van Kamp IL, Klumper FJ, Oepkes D, Meerman RH, Scherjon SA, Vandenbussche FP, Kanhai HH. Complications of intrauterine intravascular transfusion for fetal anemia due to maternal red-cell alloimmunization. Am J Obstet Gynecol. 2005;192:171-7.
9. Bennebroek Gravenhorst J, Kanhai HH, Meerman RH, Ruys JH, Eernisse JG, Stroes TJ, van Nieuwaal K. Twenty-two years of intra-uterine intraperitoneal transfusions. Eur J Obstet Gynecol Reprod Biol. 1989;33:71-7.
10. Van Kamp IL, Klumper FJ, Meerman RH, Oepkes D, Scherjon SA, Kanhai HH. Treatment of fetal anemia due to red-cell alloimmunization with intrauterine transfusions in the Netherlands 1988–1999. Acta Obstet Gynecol Scand. 2004;83: 731-7.
11. Koelewijn JM, Vrijkotte TG, van der Schoot CE, Bonsel GJ, de Haas M. Effect of screening for red cell antibodies, other than anti D, to detect hemolytic disease of the fetus and newborn: a population study in the Netherlands. Transfusion. 2008;48: 941-52.
12. Lindenburg IT, Smits-Wintjens VE, van Klink JM, Verduin E, van Kamp IL, et al. LOTUS study group: Long-term neurodevelopmental outcome after intrauterine transfusion for hemolytic disease of the fetus/newborn: the LOTUS study. Am J Obstet Gynecol. 2012;206:141.e1-141.e8.
13. Peters MT, Nicolaides KH. Cordocentesis for the diagnosis and treatment of human fetal parvovirus infection. Obstet Gynecol. 1990;75:501.
14. Naides SJ, Weiner CP. Antenatal diagnosis and palliative treatment of non-immune hydrops fetalis secondary to fetal parvovirus B19 infection. Prenat Diagn. 1989;9:105.
15. Humphrey W, Magoon M, O'Shaugnessy R. Severe non-immune hydrops secondary to parvovirus B-19 infection:

Spontaneous reversal *in utero* and survival of a term infant. Obstet Gynecol. 1991;78:900.
16. Renaer M, Van de Putte I, Vermylen C. Massive fetomaternal hemorrhage as a cause of perinatal mortality and morbidity. Eur J Obstet Gynecol Reprod Biol. 1976;6:125.
17. Sueters M, Arabin B, Oepkes D. Doppler sonography for predicting fetal anemia caused by massive fetomaternal hemorrhage. Ultrasound Obstet Gynecol. 2003;22:186-9.
18. Kecskes Z. Large fetomaternal hemorrhage: clinical presentation and outcome. J Matern Fetal Neonatal Med. 2003; 13:128-32.
19. Nakata M, Sumie M, Murata S, Miwa I, Kusaka E, Sugino N. A case of monochorionic twin pregnancy complicated with intrauterine single fetal death with successful treatment of intrauterine blood transfusion in the surviving fetus. Fetal Diagn Ther. 2007;22:7-9.
20. Genova L, Slaghekke F, Klumper FJ, Middeldorp JM, Steggerda SJ, Oepkes D, Lopriore E. Management of twin anemia-polycythemia sequence using intrauterine blood transfusion for the donor and partial exchange transfusion for the recipient. Fetal Diagn Ther. 2013;34:121-6.
21. Wang C, Ryan G. Transfusion medicine illustrated: intrauterine transfusion for homozygous alpha thalassemia reverses hydrops fetalis. Transfusion. 2009;49:1043.
22. Blanchette VS, Chen L, de Friedberg ZS, et al. Alloimmunization to the PLA1 platelet antigen: Results of a prospective study. Br J Haematol. 1990;74:209.
23. Deaver JE, Leppert PC, Zaroulis CG. Neonatal alloimmune thrombocytopenia purpura. Am J Perinatol. 1986;3:127.
24. Scott JR, Cruikshank DP, Kochenour NK, et al. Fetal platelet counts in the obstetric management of immunologic thrombocytopenic purpura. Am J Obstet Gynecol. 1980;136:495.
25. Weiner CP. Fetal hemolytic disease. In: James DK, Steer PJ, Weiner CP, Gonik B (Eds). High Risk Pregnancy: Management Options, 4th edition. Elsevier, 2009.
26. Moise K Jr, Glob. libr. Women's med. (ISSN: 1756-2228) 2011; DOI 10.3843/GLOWM.10213.
27. Nicolaides KH, Thilaganathan B, Mibashan RS. Cordocentesis in the investigation of fetal erythropoiesis. Am J Obstet Gynecol. 1989;161:1197.
28. Nicolaides KH, Clewell WH, Rodeck CH. Measurement of human fetoplacental blood volume in erythroblastosis fetalis. Am J Obstet Gynecol. 1987;157(1):50-3.
29. Trevett TN Jr, Dorman K, Lamvu G, et al. Antenatal maternal administration of phenobarbital for the prevention of exchange transfusion in neonates with hemolytic disease of the fetus and newborn. Am J Obstet Gynecol. 2005;192(2):478-82.
30. Weiner CP, Pelzer GD, Heilskov J, et al. The effect of intravascular transfusion on umbilical venous pressure in anemic fetuses with and without hydrops. Am J Obstet Gynecol. 1989; 161:149E.
31. Millard DD, Gidding SS, Socol ML, et al. Effects of intravascular, intrauterine transfusion on prenatal and postnatal hemolysis and erythropoiesis in severe fetal isoimmunization. J Pediatr. 1990;117:447.
32. Scaradavou A, Inglis S, Peterson P, et al. Suppression of erythroblastosis by intrauterine transfusions in hemolytic disease of the newborn: Use of erythropoietin to treat the late anemia. J Pediatr. 1993;123:279.
33. Lindenburg I, van Kamp I, van Zwet E, Middeldorp J, Klumper F, Oepkes D. Increased perinatal loss after intrauterine transfusion for alloimmune anaemia before 20 weeks of gestation. BJOG. 2013;120:847-52.
34. Rath ME, Smits-Wintjens VE, Lindenburg I, Brand A, Oepkes D, Walther FJ, Lopriore E. Top-up transfusions in neonates with Rh hemolytic disease in relation to exchange transfusions. Vox Sang. 2010;99:65-70.
35. Schonewille H, Klumper FJCM, van de Watering LMG, Kanhai HHH, Brand A. High additional maternal red cell alloimmunization after Rhesus- and K-matched intrauterine intravascular transfusions for hemolytic disease of the fetus. Am J Obstet Gynecol. 2007;196:143.e1–143.e6.
36. Watson WJ, Wax JR, Miller RC, Brost BC. Prevalence of new maternal alloantibodies after intrauterine transfusion for severe Rhesus disease. Am J Perinatol. 2006;23:189-92.

CHAPTER

30

Management of Multifetal Pregnancies

Shantala Vadeyar

Multifetal pregnancies are on the rise due to assisted reproductive techniques in combination with advanced maternal age. Such pregnancies are high risk as there is an increased risk of adverse outcomes as compared to singleton pregnancies. Good antenatal and intrapartum management of these high risk pregnancies along with good neonatal care is vital in optimizing outcomes.

INCIDENCE

The incidence of multifetal pregnancies varies worldwide, the average frequency quoted in 1:80 pregnancies. In Japan, it is the lowest at 6.7 per 1000 deliveries and it is the highest in Nigeria at 40 per 1000 deliveries. The rate is on the rise due to assisted reproductive techniques (ART) being used, especially in cases of advanced maternal age, polycystic ovaries, etc. The rate of monozygous twinning is constant and is 3.5 per 1000 births. The dizygous twinning rates vary depending on race, parity, maternal age and use of ART. Early ultrasound scans often show "vanishing twin" embryos, thus, the rates of twin conceptions is probably much higher than the above mentioned figures.

RISKS/COMPLICATIONS

Multifetal pregnancies are at higher risk of maternal and fetal complications/adverse outcomes as detailed in Table 30.1.

Thus, multifetal pregnancies are very high risk pregnancies that need to be managed in a multidisciplinary setting, preferably by a Maternal and Fetal Specialist with good neonatal intensive care (NICU) facilities.

CLASSIFICATION

Zygosity: Twins could be monozygous (identical, uniovular) or dizygous (fraternal, binovular). Monozygous twins would have the same genotype and hence, of the same gender whilst dizygous twins could be of the same of different genders. Occasionally, monozygous twins could have differences in their genotype due to postzygotic nondysjunction. Blood group studies and genetic DNA fingerprinting can identify zygosity.

Chorionicity and amnionicity: Twins can be classified according to number of placentae (chorionicity) and number of amniotic sacs (amnionicity).

Pregnancies with dizygous twins will have two placentae and two sacs (dichorionic diamniotic twins). Monozygous twins, on the other hand, may have varying types of presentations depending on when the zygotic mass splits to form the twins. If the splitting happens within 3 days of fertilization, this results in two placentae and two sacs (dichorionic diamniotic twins). If the splitting happens from days 4 to 7 after fertilization, the resulting twins are monochorionic diamniotic. If the splitting occurs between

Table 30.1: Risks/complications associated with multifetal gestation

Maternal	Fetal
Increased symptoms of pregnancy	Abortion/early fetal loss
Hyperemesis gravidarum	Vanishing twin
Hypertensive disorders of pregnancy	Chromosomal abnormality
Anemia	Congenital anomalies
Gestational diabetes	Growth discordance
Polyhydramnios	Growth restriction
Antepartum hemorrhage	Intrauterine demise, single or both
Placenta previa	Preterm birth
Abruptio placentae	Malpresentations, malpositions
Prelabor preterm rupture of membranes	Twin-twin transfusion syndrome (TTTS)
Increased cesarean section rates	Twin reverse arterial perfusion (TRAP)
Postpartum hemorrhage	Twin anemia polycythemia sequence (TAPS)
Postnatal depression	Selective growth restriction (sIUGR)
Maternal mortality	Cerebral palsy

days 8 and 11 postfertilization, this results in a monochorionic monoamniotic twin pregnancy. Finally, if the splitting happens after day 12, this results in incomplete division, leading to various types of conjoint twins.

DETERMINATION OF CHORIONICITY

Since zygosity cannot be ascertained *in utero*, chorionicity determination is vital as this directly impacts the risks and potential complication rate in the multifetal pregnancy.

Chorionicity determination is done by ultrasound examination, preferably in the first trimester. Dichorionic twins are identified with the demonstration of the "lambda" or "twin peak" sign. This corresponds to a triangular wedge of chorionic tissue that is seen between the two membranes at their point of insertion into the placenta. Monochorionic twins would have a thin membrane inserting directly onto the placenta, without the chorionic tissue, thus simulating a "T" sign (Figs 30.1 and 30.2). The accuracy of ultrasound chorionicity determination is best before 14 weeks, can be done up to 19 weeks, but is significantly less accurate after 20 weeks. Accuracy rates are as high as 96–100% in determining chorionicity in first trimester using ultrasound.

Other means of identifying chorionicity is as follows:

- *Determination of gender*: If different genders are seen, it would clearly confirm a dizygous, and hence a dichorionic twin pregnancy.
- Two separate placentae, with no connection at all, would also identify dichorionic gestation.
- Thickness of the membranes has also been proposed, as dichorionic (DC) twins would have a thicker dividing intertwin memebrane as compared to monochorionic (MC) twins. Counting of the membrane layers has been done, but this is not very easy nor is it accurate.

The importance of determining chorionicity is tremendous—it guides the obstetrician in the management of multifetal pregnancy as the risks/complications differ greatly between DC and MC twins. Thus, depending on the chorionicity, parents can be counseled regarding potential complication rates, place and timing of delivery and also the frequency of maternal and fetal surveillance required during the pregnancy.

ANTENATAL MANAGEMENT

General Principles, Frequency of Visits

Regular antenatal care with an increased frequency of visits is accepted good practice for multifetal pregnancy management. Specialized "Multiple Pregnancy" clinics have been set up in High Risk Centers with Maternal-Fetal Medicine specialists managing these pregnancies. Chorionicity determination by ultrasound before 14 weeks sets the stage for the subsequent plans for antenatal management.

Dichorionic twins should be seen 4 weekly and can be delivered at 37–38 weeks if maternal and fetal monitoring remains normal. Monochorionic diamniotic (MCDA) twins need to be seen at least 2 weekly and monitored very carefully for specific complications. Delivery in MC twins is aimed at 36–37 weeks if no other complications are detected. Monoamniotic twins (MCMA) have to be followed up extremely carefully, especially in the late second and third trimester as there is a high risk of sudden demise. Delivery of MCMA twins is advised at 35–36 weeks. Antenatal steroid administration is accepted, though no definite data exists for their use in twin pregnancies. If delivery is required between 28 and 32 weeks, antenatal magnesium sulfate could be used for fetal neuroprotection.

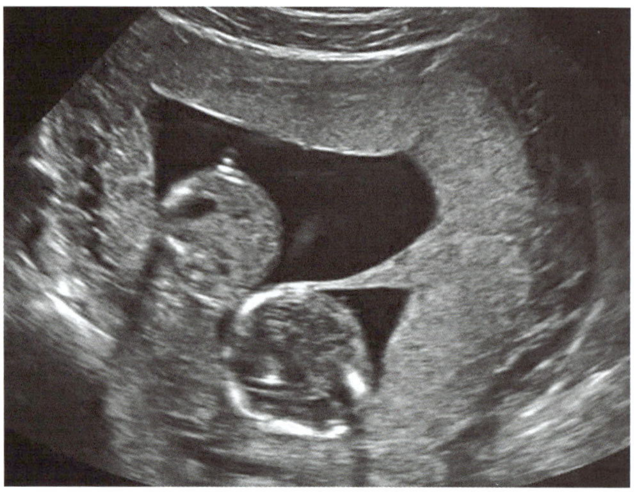

Fig. 30.1 "Lambda" or "twin peak" sign indicating dichorionic twin pregnancy

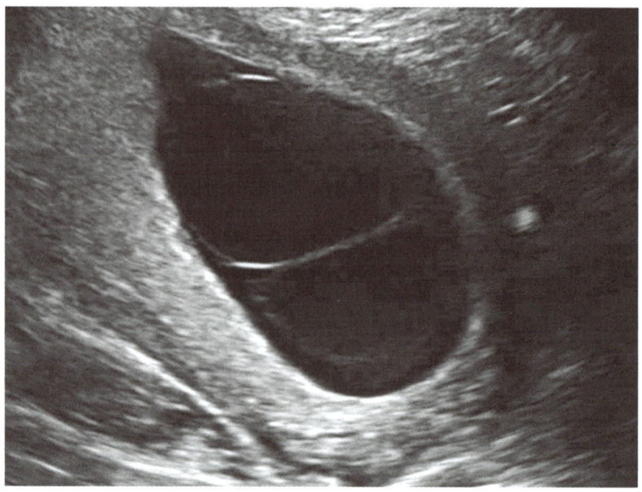

Fig. 30.2 "T sign" indicating monochorionic twin pregnancy

Role of Embryo Reduction

Higher order multifetal pregnancies pose significantly high perinatal and maternal mortality and morbidity risks. Hence, embryo reduction (ER) or multifetal pregnancy reduction has been proposed to reduce these risks, yet giving an optimal outcome for the resulting twin pregnancy. The main risk of these procedures is the risk of losing the entire pregnancy. The overall procedure related loss is 5–10% and the incidence of early preterm delivery between 25 and 28 weeks is 4–5%. Another concern is the risk of fetal growth restriction (FGR) in the remaining fetuses. A study by Depp et al showed that the risk of FGR was 36% in twins reduced from triplets, 42% in twins reduced from quadruplets and only 19% in nonreduced twins.

An ultrasound guided injection of intracardiac KCl is used to cause fetal cardiac asystole. The procedure is performed between 9 and 12 weeks, though it has been recommended to perform this procedure after the nuchal translucency (NT) scan, so as to select the fetuses with the highest NT. If any fetus has a smaller CRL, that one is chosen for ER. Otherwise, the fetuses that are most superior and accessible for the procedure are chosen. One fetus from a pair of MC twins cannot be selected for the ER.

Screening for Chromosomal Abnormalities

As there is more than one fetus in a multifetal pregnancy, the total risk of chromosomal abnormalities is higher in multiple pregnancies than that in a singleton pregnancy. Also, the association of multiple pregnancies with advanced maternal age, there is a higher risk of chromosomal abnormality.

Nuchal translucency scanning can be used in multiple pregnancies for screening for chromosomal abnormality. Using a combination of nuchal translucency (NT) and biochemical analytes [free beta human chorionic gonadotropin (hCG) and pregnancy-associated plasma protein-A (PAPPA) in the first trimester] the sensitivity of screening can be increased. The specific risks for each twin in a dichorionic pregnancy can be calculated by using the NT for each twin. For monochorionic twins, there is an overall risk for the entire pregnancy and the NT can be a predictor of twin-to-twin transfusion syndrome (TTTS).

High risk screening results can be followed up with diagnostic testing by chorionic villous sampling (CVS) or amniocentesis. Care must be taken whilst performing invasive procedures in multiple pregnancies and the fetuses should be mapped accurately. The fetal medicine expert performing the invasive procedures should be the one who will perform the selective reduction, if needed. The loss rate for invasive procedures in multiple pregnancies is slightly higher than that for singleton pregnancies.

Anomaly Scan

Congenital anomalies are commoner in twins than singleton pregnancies. The most frequent abnormalities noted are neural tube defects, congenital heart defects, genitourinary, abdominal wall, VATER and isolated limb abnormalities. The abnormalities in MC twins are higher and more lethal than in DC twins. Diagnosis of a lethal abnormality in DC twins can be managed by selective reduction of the affected fetus with an intracardiac injection of KCl. A lethal abnormality in MC twins can be selectively reduced only by cord banding.

TRAP/Acardiac Twin

Acardia or twin reverse arterial perfusion (TRAP) is a rare complication seen in 1:35000 pregnancies and 1% of MC twins. One of the twins has a normal structure whilst the other one has no cardiac structures. This twin therefore survives on the blood supply from the normal twin via the umbilical artery and iliac vessels. This results in deoxygenated blood supply to the acardiac twin with especially poor supply to the upper half of the body. The pump twin's heart may suffer from circulatory overload in perfusing two bodies and may result in hydrops in the normal twin. Mortality in the normal twin in up to 50% cases may be seen.

Management may be expectant, as spontaneous resolution may occur with complete cessation of blood flow to the acardiac twin. Polyhydramnios may be treated with serial amniodrainage and maternal indomethacin administration. Minimally invasive procedures aimed at complete circulatory cut-off between the two fetuses are increasingly being used to manage TRAP. Fetoscopic cord laser or ligation is the most effective of these, but carries a high risk of preterm premature rupture of membranes (PPROM). Ultrasound guided needle based cord coagulation (monopolar) is effective and poses a lesser risk of PPROM. Radiofrequency ablation of the cord has also been used successfully. Ultrasound guided bipolar cord coagulation with a small 2.4–3 mm bipolar forceps is another way, especially if the cord is thick. These procedures should be performed in specialized units with expertise and equipment, which can be tailored to suit the needs of each case.

Conjoint Twins

This rare disorder occurs 1 in 200 monozygotic twin pregnancies, 1 in 900 twin pregnancies and 1 in 25000 to 100,000 births. It is seen more in females (3:1) than males. Conjoint twins are of various types depending on the site of union – thoracopagus (joined at the chest), omphalopagus (joined at the anterior abdominal wall), ischiopagus (joined at ischium), craniopagus (joined at the head), pyopagus (joined at the buttocks) or rachipagus (joined at the spine). Termination of pregnancy is an option, especially if a heart is shared. In general, the outcome for conjoint twins is poor with high stillbirth (40%) and neonatal death (35%) rates.

Twin-to-Twin Transfusion Syndrome

This may occur in 10–15% of MC twins and is due to chronic imbalance in the net flow across the placental anastomoses in MC twins. It usually occurs between 15 and 26 weeks and is diagnosed by the following criteria:

- Hydramnios in the recipient sac (SDP > 8 cm prior to week 20 and >10 cm after week 20) due to polyuria
- Oligoamnios in the donor sac (SDP < 2 cm) due to oliguria
- Growth discordancy (donor twin smaller than recipient)
- Doppler abnormalities may be seen.

Quintero (1999) described a staging system to classify and prognosticate the severity of the condition.

Stage I: Oligopoly sequence, but donor bladder still visible.
Stage II: Donor bladder is absent, usually "stuck" twin.
Stage III: Severely abnormal Doppler studies-Absent/Reverse EDF in Umbilical artery of donor twin or abnormal venous Doppler–reverse flow in Ductus venosus or pulsatile venous flows in recipient twin.
Stage IV: Fetal hydrops.
Stage V: Death of one or both twins.

Generally, there is a very high perinatal mortality in untreated cases of twin-to-twin transfusion syndrome (TTTS). Early identification of TTTS is the key and timely treatment can improve outcomes (Qunitero et al. 2003). An increased NT (>95th centile) in the first trimester, discrepant crown-rump length (CRL) measurements, velamentous cord insertion and discordant amniotic fluid in the first trimester have all been used a predictors for development of TTTS.

Laser coagulation of the anastomotic vessels has been proven to be the most effective treatment for TTTS. Laser coagulation is performed percutaneously under local or regional anesthesia. Amniodrainage is also performed at the end of the procedure. The Eurofetus trial showed that both primary outcomes measures (fetal survival of at least one twin to 6 months of age) and secondary outcome measures (intact neurologic survival) were improved for the laser coagulation group as compared to the amniodrainage group (76.4% vs 51.4% and 52% vs 31% respectively), (Senat et al. 2004). Complications of laser coagulation include PPROM (28%), preterm birth (20%), twin anemia-polycythemia sequence (TAPS) (10%) and neurological sequelae. Careful monitoring of the pregnancy postlaser is vital.

Twin Anemia Polycythemia Sequence

This is a sequence occurring in MC twins which has chronic and severe hemoglobin (Hb) discordancy in the absence of amniotic fluid discordancy. This results from few small unidirectional arteriovenous (AV) anastomoses without compensating arterio-arterial (AA) anastomoses, resulting in a slow net transfusion of blood from one twin (donor) to the other (recipient). Typically, the Hb of the donor twin is low (<11 g/dL) and that of the recipient is high (>20 g/dL). Twin anemia polycythemia sequence (TAPS) can occur spontaneously or postlaser therapy for TTTS, when the small AV anastomoses have been missed. Severe case may lead to hydrops and fetal demise. Most cases can be managed conservatively, severe cases may be managed with an *in utero* transfusion. Redo laser therapy to coagulate the small anastomosing vessels is an option, but usually, not needed in practice.

Discordant Growth

This may occur both in MC or DC twins. In DC and MC twins, discordant growth could be due to unequal placental mass or genetic syndromes. In MC twins it is either selective FGR or TTTS. In DC twins, discordant growth could have one twin that grows appropriately, whilst the other is growth restricted or both are growth restricted but of a varying degree. Growth discordancy of more than 25% results in increased risk for adverse perinatal outcomes. Discordant growth may be of early-onset or the late-onset type, with the early onset growth discordancy having worse prognosis. The well being of the smaller twin should be monitored carefully and delivery is advised if signs of fetal distress arise. Elective delivery should be considered when the pregnancy reaches 34–36 weeks. If the cause is due to genetic syndromes, the delivery is planned depending on the wellbeing of the normal twin, as iatrogenic preterm delivery may harm the normal twin with no advantage to the abnormal one.

Single Intrauterine Device

This is a dreaded complication in a high risk multifetal pregnancy. It may occur due to maternal hypertension, abruption placentae, cord accidents, selective IUGR, etc. In DC twins it is possible to continue the pregnancy to 36 weeks provided no other reasons to effect delivery are present. Regular maternal monitoring for possible development of DIC should be instituted. In MC twins, however, single intrauterine device (IUD) can be disastrous for the survivor. This is because, death of one twin will cause sudden hypotension and this can lead to bleeding from the survivor into the dead twin by the anastomotic vessels. This, in turn, causes sudden hypotension leading to neurologic damage to the surviving twin. Hence, urgent delivery may help in sudden single IUD in a MC twin pair. However, if the hypotensive episode has occurred already, the neurologic damage may be seen, even if early delivery is performed. Delivery timing and mode is determined by the etiology and gestational age at which the sIUD is diagnosed.

Selective Fetal Growth Restriction/Selective Intrauterine Growth Restriction

A specific type of fetal growth restriction (FGR) in MC twins due to discordant placenatal sharing is selective IUGR (sIUGR). Gratocos (2004) has classified the types of sIUGR into three types:

Type I: Discordant growth with normal Dopplers.
Type II: Discordant growth with abnormal Dopplers.
Type III: Intermittent normal and abnormal Dopplers.

The Type III sIUGR are most unpredictable in terms of sudden IUD. They occur due to large AA anastomoses, which allow for some growth in the smaller twin, but also, may result in sudden unpredictable blood flows across them, which may cause sudden *in utero* demise. This will also result in sudden hypotension in the survivor causing neurologic damage, which can be diagnosed on ultrasound or MRI after 4–6 weeks of the IUD event.

Hence, laser coagulation of the large AA anastomoses may not be the best treatment strategy as it could lead to intrauterine demise of the smaller twin postlaser, due to cut-off of the "feeding" vessels.

Hypertensive Disorders of Pregnancy

The incidence of hypertension in multifetal pregnancies is twice that in singleton pregnancies, 13% versus 6% respectively (Sibai et al. 2000). Gestational hypertension is more common than proteinuric hypertension. If pre-eclampsia sets in, it happens earlier in onset and severity with higher risk of HELLP syndrome. The risk of hypertension, both proeinuric and non-proteinuric types, is higher in pregnancies resulting from ART (Ecchevery CJ, 2008). The management, as with singletons, consists of maternal surveillance by means of regular clinical and biochemical monitoring, therapy with antihypertensives, and fetal surveillance with growth assessments, amniotic fluid and Doppler assessments. The ultimate "cure" is delivery. The timing of delivery is determined by any signs of fetal or maternal compromise, or when the gestational age reaches 35–36 weeks, when the *ex utero* survival is optimal. Magnesium sulfate should be used in severe pre-eclampsia and HELLP syndrome as in singleton pregnancies. It is useful for maternal prevention of seizures and helps recovery, as well as fetal benefits of neuroprotection (prevention of intra-ventricular hemorrhage and cerebral palsy).

Preterm Labor Screening/Preterm Birth

Many multifetal pregnancies are delivered preterm (<37 weeks), some are spontaneous (due to preterm labor) whilst others could be iatrogenic (decision to deliver earlier for maternal or fetal reasons). Either way, nearly 57–60% of twins get delivered before 37 weeks. Hence, low birth weight complicates most multifetal gestations and this is a combination of prematurity with growth restriction. The gestational age at the time of birth decreases as the number of fetuses goes higher (Donovan et al. 1998). The most common neonatal complications of preterm birth are respiratory distress, hypothermia, necrotizing enterocolitis, intracranial hemorrhage, sepsis, persistent ductus arteriosus and retinopathy of prematurity.

Prophylactic cervical cerclage in twins has not been shown to reduce preterm delivery rates or improve outcomes. Screening for preterm birth can be performed by serial ultrasound scans from 14 weeks onwards. Transvaginal scans should be performed on an empty bladder, with minimal pressure, measuring the endocervical length over 2 minutes of scanning. Funneling of the internal os and/or shortening of the cervical length before 20–22 weeks are an indication for considering cervical cerclage. Beyond 22–24 weeks or if the cervical length is too short with prolapsing of the membranes into the vagina would make cervical cerclage very risky. The risks of cerclage include PPROM and infection, which in turn may lead to preterm labor and delivery.

Prophylactic progesterone therapy for prevention of preterm labor has not been proven to be of equal benefit as compared to singleton pregnancies. However, it is being widely used in many centers, as benefits may outweigh the risks.

Anemia

Maternal anemia is extremely common in multiple pregnancy. The iron demands of more than one fetus and placenta on the maternal system are huge and the intravascular expansion leading to hemodilution is larger. A combination of both these factors leads to anemia. This can be countered by iron and protein supplementation throughout the pregnancy. Incases of severe iron deficiency, if necessary, intravenous iron therapy could be administered in cases of intolerance to oral iron.

Postpartum Hemorrhage

Uterine hyperdistension leads to uterine atony, which is the prime cause of postpartum hemorrhage following the delivery of twins/triplets. Hence, twin deliveries at term, when there is maximum distension of the uterus, pose the maximum risk of postpartum hemorrhage (PPH). Prophylactic use of prostaglandins and oxytocin is recommended to reduce PPH in multiple pregnancy.

MANAGEMENT OF LABOR AND DELIVERY

Timing and Place of Delivery

Triplet pregnancies are usually delivered by cesarean section.

The risk of stillbirth in twins beyond 38 weeks is greater than the risk of neonatal death (Sairam et al. 2002). In general, therefore, if there are no maternal or fetal complications, delivery in DC twins could be planned at 37–38 weeks, MCDA twins at 36 weeks and MCMA twins at 34–35 weeks. However, usually, maternal complications like hypertension/pre-eclampsia, GDM, placenta previa, abruption placentae, etc. may necessitate early delivery. Fetal complications that will necessitate early delivery are growth restriction, discordant growth, oligoamnios, single IUD, etc.

Antenatal steroids for pulmonary maturity could be used, though there is less evidence of their efficacy in multiple gestation. However, since, the potential benefits outweigh the risks, most practioners use antenatal steroids prior to preterm birth of multiple pregnancies also. Magnesium sulfate can be used for fetal neuroprotection when preterm delivery is planned between 26 and 32 weeks.

Good maternal IV access is necessary for all twin deliveries. An anesthetist should be in attendance and epidural analgesia is recommended for vaginal birth, so as to be in preparation for operative delivery for second twin. Both fetuses should be monitored carefully and separate FHR should be documented. Preferably an ultrasound scan machine should be available in the labor room, so as to determine the presentation and position of the second twin after delivery of the first. Delivery should take place in a tertiary center well equipped with NICU facilities and with neonatologists in attendance.

Mode of Delivery

There is a high incidence of malpresentation in twin pregnancies hence overall, the incidence of cesarean births is higher.

When both twins are relatively mature and are presenting cephalic-cephalic, with no other contraindications, a vaginal birth is considered safe. If the first twin is presenting as cephalic, the second is noncephalic, vaginal birth can be allowed. This may result in an external cephalic version or an internal podalic version for the second twin. However, if unsuccessful, cesarean section may have to be done in an emergency situation, sometimes, with considerable risk to the second twin. Also, for a vaginal breech delivery, the estimated weight should be between 2000 g and 3000 g, have a flexed head, should be of a size smaller than the first twin. The main risk in the second twin's delivery is that of cord prolapse, which also needs immediate delivery. Hence, an anesthetist should always be in attendance of all twin births.

Appropriate counseling of parents is vital part of antenatal care. The various possibilities and complications in twin deliveries should be discussed early on, so as to prepare parents for the various emergencies that may arise.

TAKE HOME MESSAGES

1. Twin pregnancies are on the rise, these are high risk pregnancies and need expert management in a multi-disciplinary set up with fetomaternal specialists.
2. Chorionicity determination is vital and should be done and documented in the first trimester.
3. Monochorionic twins are at especially high risk due to complications of TTTS, TAPS, sIUGR, etc. and need expert fetomaternal advice.
4. Preterm delivery is the major cause of perinatal mortality and morbidity in multiple pregnancy.
5. Antenatal steroids and magnesium sulphate should be used in preterm gestation for improved neonatal outcomes.
6. The timing of delivery should take into consideration gestational age, maternal, fetal complications and neonatal facilities. If needed, *in utero* transfer to a tertiary care center is advised.
7. An anesthesiologist and neonatologist should be in attendance of multiple pregnancy deliveries.
8. Appropriate counseling of parents regarding the various possibilities and complications in twin deliveries should be discussed early on, so as to prepare parents for the various emergencies that may arise.

BIBLIOGRAPHY

1. Donovan EF, Ehrenkranz RA, Shankaran S, et al. Outcomes of very low birth weight twins cared for in the National Institute of Child Health and Human Development Neonatal Research Network's intensive care units. Am J Obstet Gynecol. 1998; 179:742-9.
2. Ecchevery CJ. In: Arias F, Daftary S, Bhide A (Eds). Multifetal Gestation in Practical Guide to High-Risk Pregnancy and Delivery, 2008.
3. GratocosE, Carreras E, Becker J, et al. Prevalence of neurological damage in monochorionic twins with selective intrauterine growth restriction and intermittent absent or reversed end-diastolic umbilical artery flow. Ultrasound Obstet Gynecol. 2004;24:159-63.
4. Quintero RA, Morales WJ, Allen MH, et al. Staging of twin-twin transfusion syndrome. J Perinatol. 1999;19:550.
5. Qunitero RA, Dickinson JE, Morales WJ, et al. Stage-based treatment of twin-twin transfusion syndrome. Am J Obstet Gynecol. 2003;188(5):1333-40.
6. Sairam S, Costeloe K, Thilaganathan B. Prospective risk of stillbirth in multiple-gestation pregnancies: a population based analysis. Obstet Gynecol. 2002;100(4):638-41.
7. Senat MV, Deprest J, Boulvain M, et al. Endoscopic laser surgery versus serial amnioreduction for severe twin-to-twin transfusion syndrome. N Engl J Med. 2004;351:136-44.
8. Sibai BM, Hauth J, Caritis S, et al. Hypertensive disorders in twins versus singleton gestations. Am J Obstet Gynecol. 2000; 182:938.

CHAPTER

31 Twin to Twin Transfusion Syndrome

Uma Ram, S Suresh, Roopa R Shinde

INTRODUCTION

Twin-twin transfusion syndrome (TTTS) is one of the most serious complications of monochorionic multiple gestations. It is associated with a very high-risk of fetal and neonatal problems. Monochorionic pregnancies are at a higher risk of complications essentially because of vascular connections that exist virtually in all monochorionic placentae. The other problems that arise from these vascular communications include, twin anemia polycythemia sequence (TAPS), twin reversed arterial perfusion sequence (TRAP) and selective intrauterine growth retardation (sIUGR). Also these vascular connections expose the co-twin to greater risk in cases of spontaneous single fetal demise.[1]

It is therefore absolutely vital to determine chorionicity in multiple pregnancies since it defines and dictates management. Chorionicity can be identified accurately in the first trimester and is best done at the 11-13 week scan. The "lambda" sign is indicative of dichorionicity and "T" sign is indicative of monochorionicity (Figs 31.1 and 31.2). After 20 weeks, there can be a loss of the "lambda" sign in 14% of pregnancies, making it essential to document chorionicity in the first trimester.

The first description of TTTS was as early as the era of the twin brothers Esau and Jacob. The first scientific paper was published in the 19th century by Friedrich Schatz; a German gynecologist who was the first to study the relationship of vascular anastomosis in TTTS.

TTTS complicates 10-15% of monochorionic twin pregnancies and 6% of monoamniotic pregnancies.[2] It is characterized by a gradual shift of blood volume from the donor twin to the recipient twin through inter-twin vascular anastomoses. If untreated, there is an extremely high fetal mortality from miscarriage, previable preterm delivery and fetal demise. Both the donor and recipient are at risk. Even those born alive have a significant risk of cardiac and

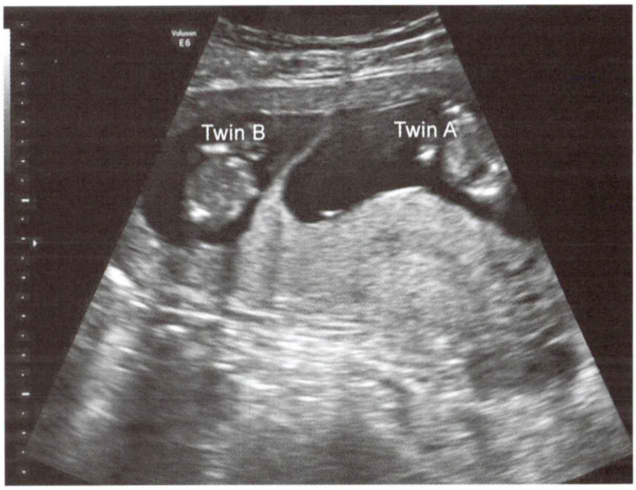

Fig. 31.1 Dichorionic diamniotic (DCDA) lambda sign

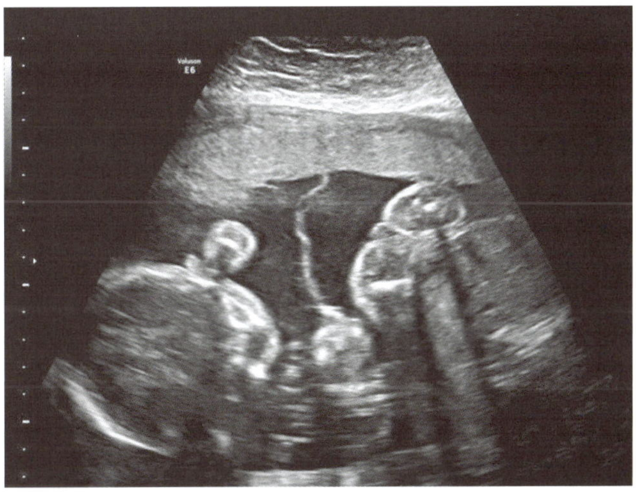

Fig. 31.2 Monochorionic diamniotic T sign

neurological morbidity. TTTS accounts for 17% of perinatal mortality, nearly 12% of neonatal deaths and 8.4% of infant deaths in twins.[3,4]

CLINICAL FEATURES AND DIAGNOSIS

The diagnosis of TTTS is made entirely on ultrasound examination of monochorionic pregnancies. It requires two important criteria—a monochorionic placentation and discordancy in liquor. The presence of oligohydramnios [maximum vertical pocket (MVP) < 2 cm] in one sac and polyhydramnios (MVP > 8 cm) in the other sac is diagnostic of TTTS. Maximal vertical pocket of 2 cm and 8 cm represent the 5th and 9th percentiles for amniotic fluid measurements, respectively (Fig. 31.3). In severe cases, this results in a "stuck" donor twin with the amniotic membrane lying against the body of the donor twin no or minimal liquor (Fig. 31.4).

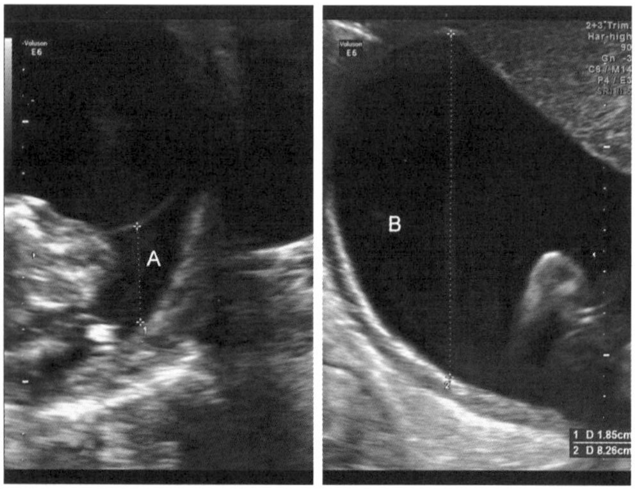

Fig. 31.3 Tops maximum vertical pocket

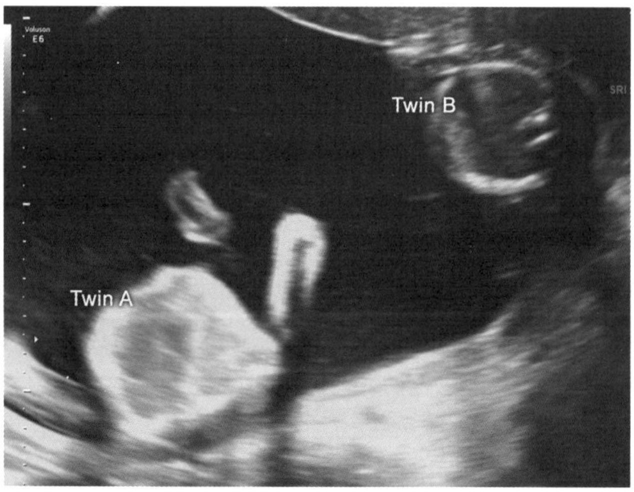

Fig. 31.4 Twin-twin transfusion syndrome stuck twin

The discordancy in bladder sizes and Doppler changes are used to help stage TTTS. Staging of TTTS is described in detail later in the chapter.

In the era prior to ultrasound, TTTS was diagnosed at birth as 20% discordance in weight and at least a 5 g/dL difference in hemoglobin concentrations between two twins of the same sex at birth. This obviously did not take into consideration, the more severe forms where there was fetal loss of both twins and took into consideration only the surviving twins. This criterion has now been abandoned.

PATHOPHYSIOLOGY

Placental intertwin vascular anastomoses play a key role in the pathophysiology of TTTS. The architecture of intertwin vascular connections has been the subject of many studies pertaining to complications associated with monochorionic twin pregnancies.[5,6]

Placental anastomoses are of three type's: (1) Arterioarterial, (2) Arteriovenous, and (3) Venovenous. Arterioarterial and venovenous anastomoses are superficial and bidirectional anastomoses. The term "superficial" means that they are visible on the surface of the chorionic plate, forming direct communications between the arteries and veins. They are "bidirectional" because they allow flow in both directions depending upon the vascular pressure gradients on both the sides.

An arterioarterial anastomosis is a flexible connection and therefore compensates for any imbalance that occurs over the unidirectional arteriovenous anastomoses. Venovenous anastomoses are rarer and its function is less established. A study done by Denbow ML et al. has stated that venovenous anastomoses may be associated with decreased perinatal survival and cause demise because of sudden changes in venous return. However, this association has not been confirmed by other studies.[7]

Arteriovenous anastomoses are referred to as deep and unidirectional anastomoses due to the fact that the anastomoses occur at the capillary level within a shared placental lobule and they allow flow in one direction only. It receives arterial supply from one twin and gives its well-oxygenated venous supply to the other twin. The supplying artery and draining vein can be visualized on the chorionic surface as an unpaired artery and vein that pierce the chorionic plate at close proximity of one other to supply the underlying shared placental lobule. By virtue of this anastomosis a monochorionic placenta actually has three parts, one each of the twin fetuses and one that is shared and supported by arteriovenous anastomoses. Because of their unidirectional nature, arteriovenous anastomoses can create a transfusion imbalance and this phenomenon if opposed by a bidirectional flow, adequate compensation

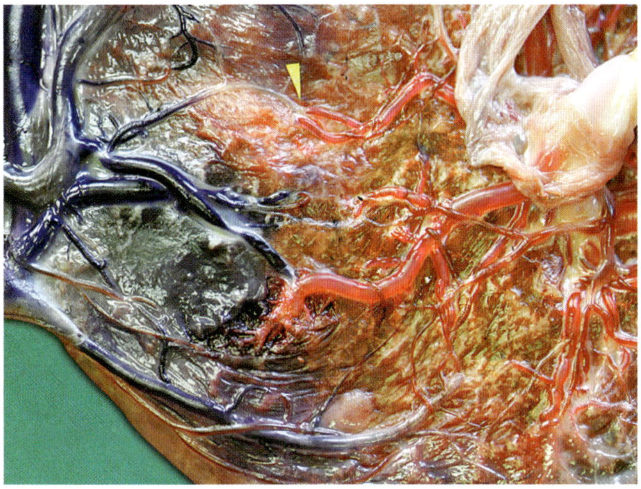

Fig. 31.5 Arteriovenous anastomoses twin-twin transfusion syndrome

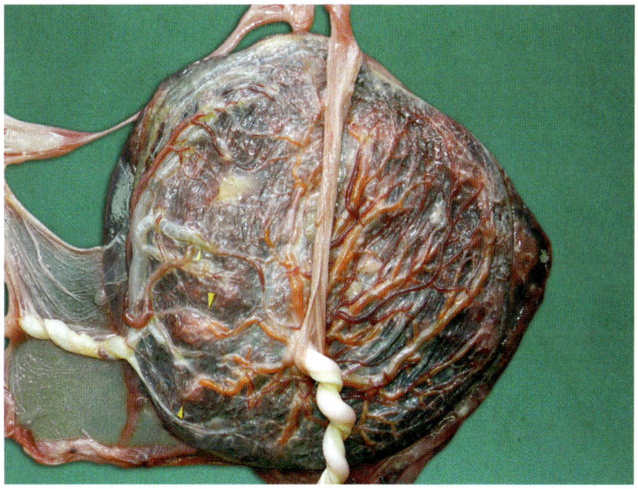

Fig. 31.6 Cord insertion sites twin-twin transfusion syndrome

takes place. About 90% of monochorionic placentas have several arteriovenous and venoarterial anastomoses in combination with an arterioarterial and/or venovenous anastomosis. In about 5% of monochorionic placentas, there are only arteriovenous anastomoses and in another 5% there are no anastomoses (Fig. 31.5).[7,8]

Apart from understanding these vascular connections, it is also important to know the characteristics of the vascular distribution patterns. Chorionic vascular patterns have been described as disperse, magistral or mixed. The disperse pattern is wherein a fine network of vessels branch out from the cord insertion to the various placental cotyledons and the magistral pattern has arteries of relatively uniform size that course across the placental surface nearly to the edge without diminishing in diameter. Mixed is when these two patterns coexist.

Studies have demonstrated that the prevalence of magistral/mixed vascular types was significantly higher in placentas of twins with TTTS compared with those without TTTS. Furthermore, in twin pairs with TTTS, donor twins were significantly more likely to have magistral/mixed vascular patterns than recipients (87% versus 33%). These observations suggest that the presence of a magistral/mixed vascular distribution pattern in one or both monochorionic diamniotic twins may be implicated in the development of TTTS.[9]

Though the vascular anastomoses are an anatomical prerequisite, the pathogenesis of TTTS is more complex than a simple net transfer of red blood cells, because both the twins usually have similar hemoglobin values. As mentioned earlier TTTS is a problem of discordant amniotic fluid overloaded recipient and a fluid depleted donor. Therefore, endocrine factors related to fluid and pressure homeostasis has been postulated to be involved in the pathogenesis of TTTS.

Because the fetal urine is hypo-osmotic, a vicious cycle of hypervolemia-polyuria-hyperosmolality is established leading to polyhydramnios and high output cardiac failure in the recipient. Cardiac overload and atrial dilatation in the recipient promotes secretion of atrial natriuretic peptide, which in turn inhibits the antidiuretic hormone thus worsening polyhydramnios. In addition, Mahieu Caputo et al.[10] speculated that the hypovolemia in the donor triggers the rennin angiotensin system, which in turn negatively, affects both the fetuses. In the donor, it worsens the hypoperfusion. It has been said that fetal hypertension and worsened the cardiac after load seen in the recipient can be partly due to the transfer of circulatory rennin from the donor to recipient.

The other metabolic changes noted were in that of erythropoietin and leptin levels. It was noted that the fetal erythropoietin concentrations were higher in the TTTS group and the leptin levels were higher in the recipients. It is unclear whether these findings are a consequence of TTTS or a trigger.[11]

The role of velamentous cord insertion in the genesis of TTTS has been highlighted by Fries et al.[12] Velamentous cord insertions are more common in twin-twin transfusion syndrome pregnancies and may contribute to the development of profound disparity in fluid volume because the membranously inserted cord can be easily compressed, reducing blood flow to one twin (Fig. 31.6).

In short, most authors believe that the pathophysiology of TTTS is believed to be due to unbalanced vascular anastomoses and specific placental vascular patterns that form the main basis for the condition. The renin angiotensin system is imbalanced with over function in the donor and down regulation in the recipient. The increase in atrial natriuretic peptide worsens polyhydramnios. Hypovolemia in the donor increases the antidiuretic hormone causing local vasoconstriction—oliguria, oligoamnios and renal tubular dysgenesis. The other anatomical placental characteristic that has been linked to the pathogenesis of TTTS are velamentous or marginal cord insertion and unequal sharing of the single-disc placenta.

MONITORING FOR TWIN-TWIN TRANSFUSION SYNDROME AND SURVEILLANCE OF MONOCHORIONIC TWINS

Establishing chorionicity is the fundamental first step in the management of twins. Once monochorionic twins have been identified increased monitoring and surveillance is put in place in order to pick up TTTS and other complications unique to monochorionic (MC) pregnancies.

At the 11–13 week scan, Crown-Rump Length (CRL), nuchal translucencies (NT) are noted. Anticipating hemodynamic imbalance as early as the first trimester of pregnancy, several screening models have been proposed to predict TTTS in the first trimester like inter twin discrepancies in NT or CRL. NT discordance alone as a marker for developing TTTS has low sensitivity (Table 31.1). CRL discordance is a marker for developing sIUGR and not of TTTS.

Considering the fact that TTTS is the consequence of a circulatory imbalance, the DV, as the main regulatory shunt of oxygenated blood, can add valuable information to fetal hemodynamic evaluation early in pregnancy. A study done by Matias and co-workers confirmed that the evaluation of ductus venosus (DV) flow was significant at 11–14 weeks in defining a group of monochorionic twins at risk of developing TTTS.[13] Abnormal DV blood flow in at least one fetus as the only marker, the relative risk of developing TTTS was found to be 15 times higher. Subsequently larger series have also analysed the same correlation.[14] The relative risk is 21 times for a combination of discordant DV and NT.

Table 31.2 shows the summary of few studies done on the screening parameters for TTTS in the first trimester.

After the first trimester scan, all monochorionic pregnancies should be followed up with a scan at 16 weeks and then every two-week thereafter. At 16 weeks, cord insertions are noted bladder and liquor volumes in both sacs documented. At 18 weeks, a detailed anatomical survey with fetal echo is also done. From this visit on, every 2 weeks, liquor, bladder and Doppler (Umbilical, MCA and DV) have to be done and documented. Biometry for growth is performed once in 4 weeks (Flow chart 31.1).

Table 31.1 Sonographic predictors of twin to twin transfusion syndrome in first trimester

Study done by	Predictors	Sensitivity	Specificity	Odds ratio
Sebire et al.[15,16]	Nuchal translucency thickness >95th percentile	28%	90%	3.4
Matias et al. 2000 and 2005[17,18]	Abnormal ductus venosus A-wave	100%	96–100%	—
Sebire et al.[19]	Folding of the intertwin membrane	91%	78%	38.3

Flow chart 31.1 Monochorionic diamniotic pregnancy follow-up

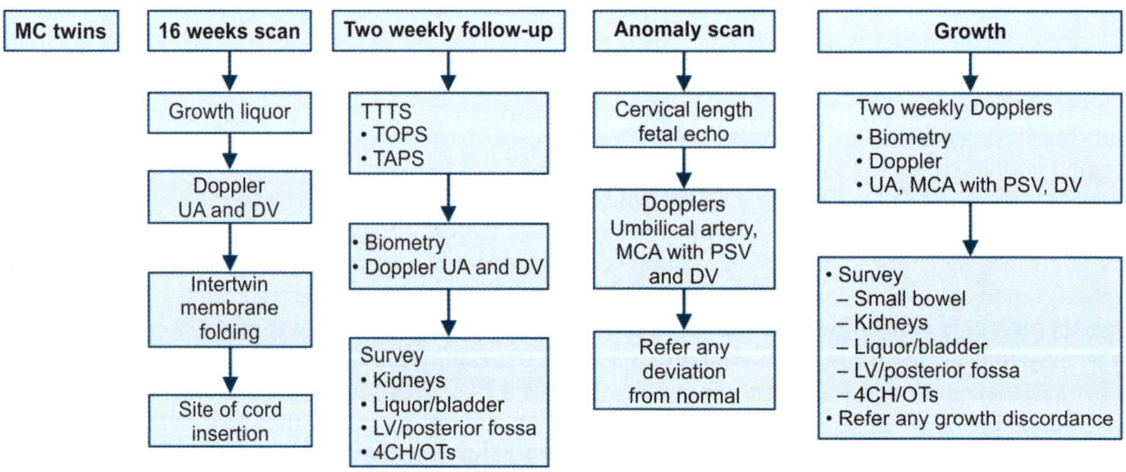

Abbreviations: MC: monochorionic; UA: umbilical artery; DV: ductus venosus; TTTS: twin-twin transfusion syndrome; TOPS: twin oligo-polyhydramnios sequence; TAPS: twin anemia-polycythemia sequence; LV: left ventricle; MCA: middle cerebral arterial; PSV: peak systolic velocity

In the second trimester, 50% of cases which had membrane folding, developed TTTS. Velamentous insertion of cord is also associated with TTTS in different studies. Evaluation of these predictors may potentially improve the detection rate.

Assessment

The ultrasound assessment of TTTS can be particularly challenging. The oligoamnios in the donor makes difficult imaging of the anatomy and Doppler analysis of this fetus. Polyhydramnios in the recipient with increase movement of the fetuses associated with polyhydramnios and maternal discomfort hinders detailed evaluation. Despite these limitations, it is mandatory to do a detailed assessment to come to a correct diagnosis and plan management. A careful assessment of sonographic details is necessary to avoid pitfalls. Quintero has enumerated the ultrasound of TTTS in different steps or levels, which includes diagnosis, staging, cervical length and preoperative mapping.[20]

It is important that the cervical length is documented only by transvaginal ultrasound unless and until there are specific contraindications for the same.

Identifying and noting cord insertions is important in all monochorionic pregnancies. The location of the cords, helps predict the location of dividing membranes and thus the vascular equator and the direction of anastomoses. This step is particularly important when an intervention is planned.

Staging

The most widely used staging for TTTS was developed by Quintero et al. in 1999, and is based on sonographic findings (Table 31.2).[21] The Quintero staging system includes 5 stages, ranging from mild disease with isolated discordant amniotic fluid volume to severe disease with demise of one or both twins. Though Quintero staging is the most commonly used, it has its limitations. A given case need not progress through the stages in a stepwise fashion. It has been stated that around three fourth of stage one TTTS resolve to normal or do not progress.[22,23] An advanced stage of TTTS especially if presented prior to 26 weeks is associated with high perinatal losses. Sometimes, atypical stages are seen such as the presence of Doppler abnormality without bladder discordance.

A cardiovascular scoring system has been reported from Children's Hospital of Philadelphia (CHOP score), based on echocardiographic and peripheral Doppler findings.[24] The Cincinnati modification of the Quintero staging system is another cardiovascular scoring system.[25]

MANAGEMENT OPTIONS OF TWIN-TWIN TRANSFUSION SYNDROME

Since the untreated mortality and morbidity for the fetuses is extremely poor in untreated TTTS, different therapeutic options have evolved.

Today fetoscopy and laser photocoagulation (LPC) of anastomotic vessels is the first line treatment for the management of TTTS. In the past, amnioreduction and septostomy have been used as management options. Total survival rates are better and neurological morbidity is lower with LPC than amnioreduction.

Expectant management may be offered for mild Stage 1 TTTS where there is no progression of the disease. The percentage of such cases vary and in some series, up to 70% of stage do not progress or regress and these cases could do well with expectant management.[26] Some case series though have shown that even in stable Stage 1, outcomes are better with intervention.[27]

Amnioreduction

Amnioreduction is basically removing the excess amniotic fluid from the recipient sac. In 1986, Feingold et al.[28] described two cases where 3500 and 4750 mL were removed and pregnancy was prolonged for 14 and 11 days respectively. Although two of the four fetuses died, these investigators concluded that decompression amniocentesis "can offer some hope in an otherwise hopeless situation".

Table 31.2 Staging of twin-twin transfusion syndrome by Quintero et al.[20]

Stage	Ultrasound parameter	Categorical criteria
I	MVP of amniotic fluid	MVP < 2 cm in donor sac; MVP > 8 cm in recipient sac
II	Fetal bladder	Nonvisualization of fetal bladder in donor twin over 6 minutes of observation
III	Umbilical artery, ductus venosus, and umbilical vein Doppler waveforms	Absent or reversed umbilical artery diastolic flow, reversed ductus venosus a-wave flow, pulsatile umbilical vein flow
IV	Fetal hydrops	Hydrops in one or both twins
V	Absent fetal cardiac activity	Fetal demise in one or both twins

Abbreviation: MVP, maximal vertical pocket

By reducing maternal over distension, amnioreduction reduces the risk of preterm labor. Also by reducing the pressure inside the amniotic cavity it improves placental perfusion. The outcomes from amnioreduction, while being superior to expectant management, are not as good as laser photocoagulation. Therefore, it is no longer the treatment of choice in TTTS. For gestations above 26 weeks, especially in the US, since FDA approval for fetoscopy is not there beyond 26 weeks, amnioreduction may be offered.

In earlier gestation and milder TTTS, it is prudent to avoid amnioreduction as complications from the procedure may preclude definitive treatment with fetoscopy and laser subsequently.

Technique: Under ultrasound guidance and local anesthesia, an 18 gauge needle is inserted into the recipient sac. Care is taken to avoid the placenta and to be away from the inter twin membrane. A sterile tubing is connected to a vacuum suction to ensure a closed sterile system and fluid is drained. Care is taken to ensure that there is not a rapid reduction in volume and the fetal heart rates are monitored for any bradycardia (Fig. 31.7).

Complications: The complications of amnioreduction include unintentional perforation of the intervening membrane, amnion-chorion separation, intra-amniotic bleeding, and preterm premature rupture of membranes (PPROM).

Septostomy

This technique was a result of an inadvertent puncture of the dividing membrane was made in error during amnioreduction. Subsequently this was used in some cases of TTTS.[29,30] There is equalization of pressure by removal of the dividing membrane, in effect creating a monoamniotic pregnancy.

Moise et al. explored the possibility of amnioseptostomy as a treatment option for TTTS. The study was stopped after 71 cases and it concluded that there was no difference with outcomes with regard to fetal death in the septostomy v/s amnioreduction group (13% v/s 12.5%) and also a higher need for combination therapies in the septostomy group 40% v/s 8% in the amnioreduction group. Septostomy is not currently recommended as a treatment option for TTTS.

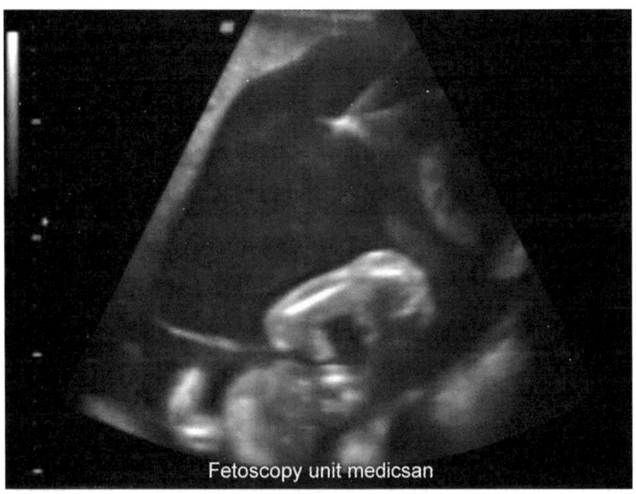

Fig. 31.7 Amnioreduction

Laser Photocoagulation of Anastomosis Vessels

Laser ablation of placental anastomoses, was first introduced by De Lia in 1990 and has gained widespread acceptance as the definitive treatment for severe TTTS between 16 weeks and 26 weeks of gestation.[31]

Procedure

Given the complexity of the condition a detailed counseling session is extremely important. In this session, it is important to explain the condition to the couple in a manner that they will understand. The outcome, if nothing is done and the risks and benefits of laser photocoagulation have to be discussed and informed consent obtained. The need for post-procedure follow-up also needs to be emphasized at this point itself. The couple must plan and have access to delivery in a center with good neonatal facilities as the possibility of preterm delivery is high.

Equipment Needed for the Procedure

- A 10/12 french torcar
- Fetoscopes (2 mm with straight or curved sheaths)
- High end camera, light source and laparoscope monitor as used in regular laparoscopy procedures
- 60 watt diode laser/ND YAG laser with 400–600 nm laser fibers.

Technique

The placental position and cord insertion sites are mapped on the maternal abdomen. This determines the entry point (Figs 31.8 and 31.9).

The procedure is usually done under local anesthesia, antibiotic prophylaxis and tocolysis. Epidural and sometimes sedation and general anesthetic have also been described. Some people use a direct entry but others use the seldinger technique under ultrasound guidance and a flexible trocar, ensuring that the entry of the trocar is perpendicular to the inter-twin membrane. Once the entry is made, amnioinfusion is done if necessary and the fetoscope is introduced.

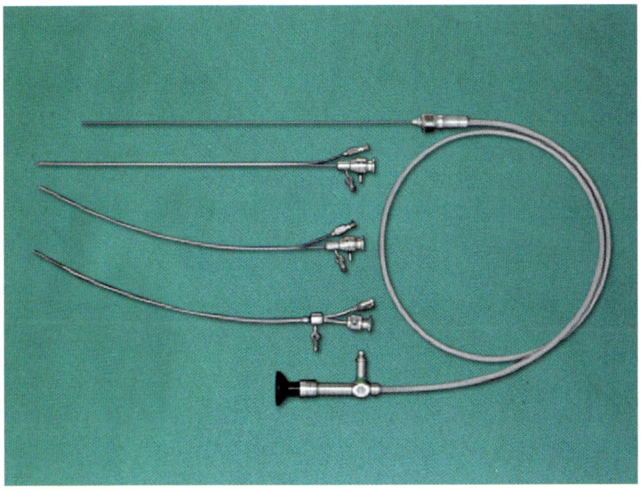

Fig. 31.8 Fetoscopy instruments

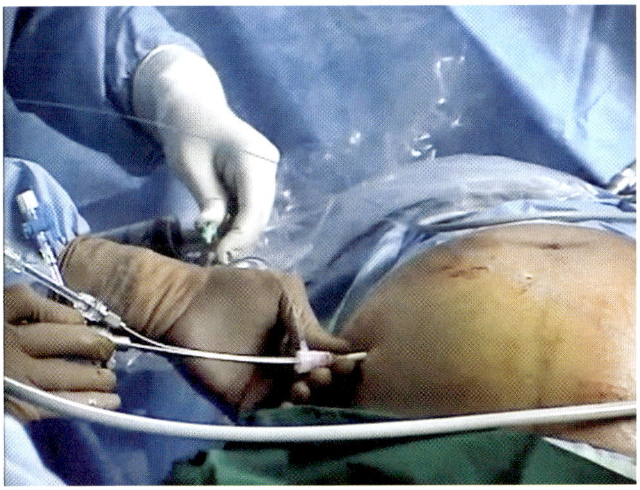

Fig. 31.9 Fetoscope entry

The choice of sheath is dependent on the position of the placenta with a curved sheath for anterior placentae.

Once the fetoscope is inserted, the dividing membrane is seen and both cord insertions identified (Fig. 31.10). The length of the membrane is visualized and all vessels that cross the membrane are followed to identify the ones that have anastamoses. These anastomoses are identified based on whether they are arteriovenous or arterioarterial. They are also classified based on the direction of flow as Donor to Recipient (DR) or vice-versa.

Laser energy is delivered to the anastamostic sites. A second channel allows irrigation to promote visualization.

Originally nonselective ablation of all vessels that crossed the dividing membrane was performed. Subsequently,

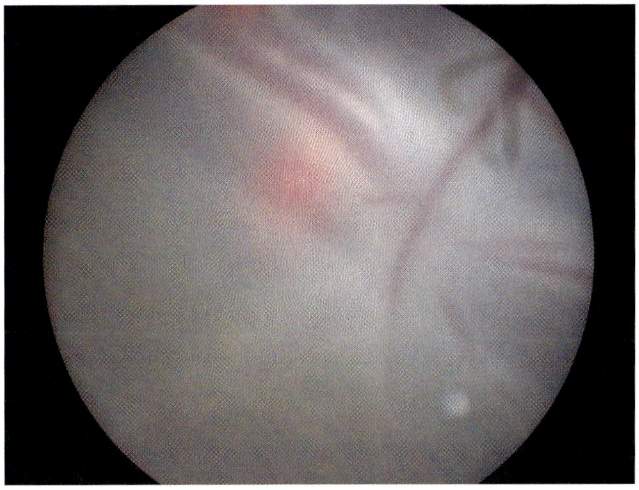

Fig. 31.10 Fetoscopy membrane

selective ablation of only the anastamoses was shown to have better outcomes. Today sequential selective ablation is performed as a further refined procedure.[32] This means, arteriovenous (AV), venoarterial (VA), and finally, arterioarterial (AA) anastomoses are coagulated in sequential order. It is recommended that the larger vessels are done first.

Equatorial dichorionization, or Solomon technique, is another approach. Here a line is drawn across the entire placental vascular equator on the surface of the chorionic plate between the main anastomotic channels after ablation of all visible intertwin anastomoses and vessels with uncertain course. This technique appears to decrease TTTS recurrence rates by targeting the placental territories left untreated by selective laser ablation.[33] On completion, it is normal to double check that all anastamoses are coagulated.

At the end of the procedure, after the scope is removed, amnioreduction is done in a controlled fashion. Both heart rates are documented.

Complications

Chorioamnionitis, preterm labor and PPROM are complications that are documented post-laser. TAPS is a complication seen post-laser and these need to have been discussed pre-procedure itself.

Follow-up: These babies are followed up closely in the fetal medicine unit initially a week following the procedure and after 2 weeks, will move back to every 2 weeks. The need for good quality neonatal care for these babies cannot be over emphasized.

Selective feticide: This is an option if one of the babies has an anomaly in addition to the TTTS. Sometimes, if there is significant cardiac dysfunction or severe selective IUGR as well, selective feticide could be performed by cord occlusion or interstitial laser.

Outcomes: Untreated severe TTTS has 95–100% mortality and hence treatment of TTTS will help in reducing mortality due to this condition.

The outcomes for amnioreduction are reported from the largest series of TTTS patients undergoing amnioreduction by the International Amnioreduction Registry[34] from 223 pregnancies from 20 centers. The fetuses were live born in 55% of pregnancies, one twin was live born in 31%, and both twins were stillborn in the remaining 14%. During the first four weeks of neonatal life, an additional 30% of live born twins succumbed. Intracranial abnormalities were seen in 25% of donors and 24% recipients at 4 weeks of life.

In 2004, Senat and co-workers, showed that compared with amnioreduction, laser photocoagulation has a higher chance of at least one live baby at 4 weeks of age and significantly less neurological problems at 6 months of age.[35]

A cochrane review in 2008 analysed the data from the Eurofetus and NIH trials, 182 pregnancies, 364 fetuses; and compared the outcomes between the Amnioreduction group and the Laser photocoagulation group. The overall results favored Laser coagulation as a treatment of choice in TTTS. Babies were twice as likely to survive after laser photocoagulation. Perinatal (26% v/s 44%) and neonatal deaths (7.6% v/s 26%) were less in the laser group when compared to the amnioreduction group. The laser group had an 80% less chance of neurological damage than those undergoing amnioreduction.[36]

A systematic review in 2011 states that the incidence of neurologic morbidity at birth was 6.1% with no significant differences between donors and recipients. The incidence of any degree of neurologic impairment at follow-up at 6 to 48 months of age was 11.1%, with no significant differences between donors and recipients or pregnancies with one versus two survivors. A subsequent follow-up publications showed that long-term neurological impairment was better, at age 5 years, in the infants treated by laser besides a nearly 40% reduction in fetal death.[37]

A more recent study published by Murakoshi et al. have demonstrated that by using a trocar assisted technique, careful mapping of vessels and drawing a virtual line with the laser along the hemodynamic equator helps improve outcomes. In a series of 171 cases, the overall survival rate was 78% and 5% neonatal morbidity. Both twins survived in 64% and one twin survival rate was 93%.[38]

Twin-twin transfusion syndrome is a challenging problem. Awareness and effective triaging help identify the problem early. Identification or indeed suspicion of the condition should result in a referral to a fetal medicine center with the expertise to manage the condition.

Detailed counseling, expertise to offer fetoscopy and laser as treatment and diligent follow-up can result in good outcomes. These mothers need to be taken care of for other maternal complications inherent to twin pregnancies. Good neonatal care is vital and these babies will need to be followed up for further neurodevelopmental assessment as well.

KEY MESSAGES

- Twin to twin transfusion syndrome (TTTS) is one of the most serious complications of monochorionic multiple gestations. It is associated with a very high-risk of fetal and neonatal problems.
- The presence of oligohydramnios (MVP < 2 cm) in one sac and polyhydramnios (MVP > 8 cm) in the other sac is diagnostic of TTTS. Maximal vertical pocket of 2 cm and 8 cm represent the 5th and 95th percentiles for amniotic fluid measurements, respectively.
- The pathophysiology of TTTS is believed to be due to **unbalanced vascular anastomoses** and specific placental vascular patterns that form the main basis for the condition. The renin angiotensin system is imbalanced.
- Two weekly assessments of MC pregnancies is recommended from 16 weeks onwards. Identifying and noting cord insertions is important in all monochorionic pregnancies. From 18 weeks, it is important to document Umbilical artery, MCA and DV Doppler's besides noting liquor and bladder in both babies.
- Quintero staging is most commonly used for TTTS.
- For stage II–IV TTTS before 26 weeks laser photocoagulation is the recommended treatment. Laser ablation results in greater prolongation of gestational age, higher neonatal survival, and improved long-term neurologic outcome. Sequential selective technique followed by the "Solomon" method assures complete dichorionization of the placenta.
- Postlaser regular and meticulous monitoring of babies is needed to identify the hemodynamic changes and other complications that may arise.
- Twin anemia polycythemia sequence may be seen post-laser and is identified by MCA Doppler at every follow-up visit.
- Maternal monitoring is needed especially for pre-eclampsia and preterm labor.
- Timing delivery, access to good neonatal care and subsequent neonatal follow-up are vital for overall good outcome.

REFERENCES

1. Chalouhi GE, Stirnemann JJ, Salomon LJ, et al. Specific complications of monochorionic twin pregnancies: twin-twin transfusion syndrome and twin reversed arterial perfusion sequence. Fetal Neonatal Med. 2010;15(6):349-56.
2. Lewi L, Lewi P, Diemert A, et al. The role of ultrasound examination in the first trimester and at 16 weeks' gestation to predict fetal complications in monochorionic diamniotic twin pregnancies. Am J Obstet Gynecol; 2008.
3. Baxi LV, Walsh CA. Monoamniotic twins in contemporary practice: a single-center study of perinatal outcomes. J Matern Fetal Neonatal Med. 2010;23(6):506-10.
4. Sebire NJ, Snijders RJ, Hughes K, et al. The hidden mortality of monochorionic twin pregnancies. BJOG. 1997;104:1203-7.
5. Ville Y. Monochorionic twin pregnancies: 'les liaisons dangereuses'. Ultrasound Obstet Gynecol. 1997;10:82-5.
6. Liesbeth Lewi, Jan Deprest, Kurt Hecher. The vascular anastomoses in monochorionic twin pregnancies and their clinical consequence, AJOG. 2013;208(1):19-30.
7. Denbow ML, Cox P, Taylor M, et al. Placental angioarchitecture in monochorionic twin pregnancies: relationship to fetal growth, fetofetal transfusion syndrome, and pregnancy outcome. Am J Obstet Gynecol. 2000;182(2):417-26.
8. Lewi L, Cannie M, Blickstein I, et al. Placental sharing, birth weight discordance and vascular anastomoses in monochorionic diamniotic twin placentas. Am J Obstet Gynecol. 2007;197:587.e1-8.
9. De Paepe ME, DeKoninck P, Friedman RM. Placenta vascular distribution patterns in monochorionic twin placentas. 2005;26:471e475 doi:10.1016/j.placenta.2004.06.014
10. Mahieu-Caputo D, Dommergues M, Delezoide AL, et al. Twin-to-twin transfusion syndrome role of the fetal renin-angiotensin system. American Journal of Pathology. 2000;156(2):629-36.
11. Bajoria R, Ward S, Sooranna SR. Erythropoietic in monochorionic pregnancy in relation to twin-twin transfusion syndrome. Human reproduction. 1995;16(3):574-80.
12. Fries MH, Goldstein RB, Kilpatrick SJ, Golbus MS, Callen PW, Filly RA. The role of velamentous cord insertion in the etiology of twin-twin transfusion syndrome. Obstet Gynecol. 1993;81(4):569-74.
13. Matias A, Montenegro N, Loureiro T, Cunha M, Duarte S, Freitas D, et al. Screening for twin-twin transfusion syndrome at 11–14 weeks of pregnancy: the key role of ductus venosus blood flow assessment. Ultrasound Obstet Gynecol. 2010;35:142-8.
14. Maiz N, Staboulidou I, Leal AM, et al. Ductus venosus Doppler at 11 to 13 weeks of gestation in the prediction of outcome in twin pregnancies. Obstet Gynecol. 2009;113:860-5.
15. Sebire NJ, Souka A, Skentou H, et al. Early prediction of severe twin-to-twin transfusion syndrome. Hum Reprod. 2000;15:2008-10.
16. Sebire NJ, D'Ercole C, Hughes K, et al. Increased nuchal translucency thickness at 10-14 weeks of gestation as a predictor of severe twin-to-twin transfusion syndrome. Ultrasound Obstet Gynecol. 1997;10:86-9. Level II-1.
17. Matias A, Ramalho C, Montenegro N. Search for hemodynamic compromise at 11-14 weeks in monochorionic twin pregnancy: is abnormal flow in the ductus venosus predictive of twin-twin transfusion syndrome? J Matern Fetal Neonatal Med.; 2005.
18. Matias A 1, Montenegro N, Areias JC. Anticipating twin-twin transfusion syndrome in monochorionic twin pregnancy. Is there a role for nuchal translucency and ductus venosus blood flow evaluation at 11-14 weeks. Twin Res. 2000;3(2):65-70.
19. Sebire NJ, D'Ercole C, Carvelho M, et al. Inter-twin membrane folding in monochorionic pregnancies. Ultrasound Obstet Gynecol. 1998;11:324-7.
20. Ruben A Quintero. Twin-Twin Transfusion Syndrome (TTTS), Publisher Taylor and Francis; 2007.
21. Quintero RA, Morales WJ, Allen MH, Bornick PW, Johnson PK, Kruger M. Staging of twin-twin transfusion syndrome. J Perinatol. 1999.
22. Bebbington MW, Tiblad E, Huesler-Charles M, Wilson RD, Mann SE, Johnson MP. Outcomes in a cohort of patients with stage I twin-to-twin transfusion syndrome. Ultrasound Obstet Gynecol. 2010;36:48-51. Level II-2.
23. Rossi C, D'Addario V. Survival outcomes of twin-twin transfusion syndrome in stage I: a systematic review of the literature. Am J Perinatol; 2012, July 26 [epub ahead of print]. Level II-1.
24. Rychik J, Tian Z, Bebbington M, Xu F, McCann M, Mann S, et al. The twin-twin transfusion syndrome: spectrum of cardiovascular abnormality and development of a cardiovascular score to assess severity of disease. Am J Obstet Gynecol. 2007;197(4):392.
25. Crombleholme TM, Lim FY, Habli M, Polzin W, Jaekle R, Michelfelder E, et al. Improved recipient survival with maternal nifedipine in twin-twin transfusion syndrome complicated by TTTS cardiomyopathy undergoing selective fetoscopic laser photocoagulation. Am J Obstet Gynecol. 2010;203(4):397.
26. O'Donoghue K, Cartwright E, Galea P, et al. Stage I twin-twin transfusion syndrome: rates of progression and regression in relation to outcome. Ultrasound Obstet Gynecol. 2007; 30(7):958.
27. Wagner MM, Lopriore E, Klumper FJ, Oepkes D, Vandenbussche FP, Middeldorp JM. Short- and long-term outcome in stage 1 twin-to-twin transfusion syndrome treated with laser surgery compared with conservative management. Am J Obstet Gynecol. 2009;201(3):286.
28. Feingold M, Cetrulo CL, Newton ER, Weiss J, Shakr C, Shmoys S. Serial amniocenteses in the treatment of twin-twin transfusion complicated with acute polyhydramnios. Axta Gen Med Gemellol. 1986;35:107-13.
29. Saade GR, Olson G, Belfort MA, et al. Amniotomy: a new approach to the 'stuck twin' syndrome. Am J Obstet Gynecol. 1995;172:429-31.
30. Saade GR, Belfort MA, Berry DL, et al. Amniotic septostomy for the treatment of twin oligohydramnios-polyhydramnios sequence. Fetal Diagn Ther. 1998;13(2):86-93.
31. De Lia JE, Cruikshank DP, Keye WR Jr. Fetoscopic neodymium: YAG laser occlusion of placental vessels in severe twin-twin transfusion syndrome. Obstet Gynecol. 1990;75(6):1046.

32. Quintero RA, Ishii K, Chmait RH, Bornick PW, Allen MH, Kontopoulos EV. Sequential selective laser photocoagulation of communicating vessels in twin-twin transfusion syndrome. J Matern Fetal Neonatal Med. 2007;20(10):763.
33. Baschat AA, Barber J, Pedersen N, et al. Outcome after fetoscopic selective laser ablation of placental anastomoses vs equatorial laser dichorionization for the treatment of twin-to-twin transfusion syndrome. Am J Obstet Gynecol. 2013;209(3): 234.e1.
34. Mari G, Roberts A, Detti L, Kovanci E, Stefos T, Bahado-Singh RO, et al. Perinatal morbidity and mortality rates in severe twin-twin transfusion syndrome: results of the International Amnioreduction Registry. Am J Obstet Gynecol. 2001;185(3):708.
35. Senat MV, Deprest J, Boulvain M, Paupe A, Winer N, Ville Y. Endoscopic laser surgery versus serial amnioreduction for severe twin-to-twin transfusion syndrome. N Engl J Med. 2004;351(2):136.
36. Roberts, Devender, Gates, Simon, Kilby, Mark, Neilson, et al. Interventions for twin-twin transfusion syndrome: a Cochrane review. Ultrasound in Obstetrics and Gynecology. 2008;31(6):701-11.
37. Salomon LJ, Örtqvist L, Aegerter P, et al. Long-term developmental follow-up of infants who participated in a randomized clinical trial of amniocentesis vs laser photocoagulation for the treatment of twin-to-twin transfusion syndrome. Am J Obstet Gynecol. 2010;203: 444.e1-7.
38. Takeshi Murakoshi, Hiroo Naruse, Satoru Nakayama, et al. The treatments of twin-twin transfusion syndrome in monochorionic twin pregnancies by the fetoscopic laser photocoagulation. J Health Med Informat; 2013.

CHAPTER

32 Pregnancy and Antiepileptic Drug Treatment

Ankesh R Sahetya

INTRODUCTION

Epilepsy is one of the most common chronic diseases accompanying humankind for centuries. For epileptic women, it is important to obtain appropriate information about possibility to have children and about risks connected with their pregnancy. Various population-based cohort studies have suggested decreased birth rate among patients with epilepsy. As both, disease and treatment, may induce inborn defect, it is essential to diminish their negative effects. Every chronic treatment during pregnancy increases estimation of the risk to offspring.

In various patients the risk perception during pregnancy with epilepsy, have made the couples afraid about transfer epilepsy onto the offspring or disability to care for a child. Thus, making it an important factor in the family planning and deciding to have fewer children. They were afraid another factor having effect on their decision is teratogenicity of drugs used for treatment. Women with epilepsy may benefit from discussion with their healthcare provider about the impact their epilepsy may have on children. Every physician should be informed about risk to the fetus that is associated with seizures and drugs used for treatment during pregnancy. Drug used in girls and young women should be chosen with the respect to the future reproduction, because the use of antiepileptic drugs (AEDs) in women with epilepsy is in fact a balance between seizure control and adverse effects of drugs.

HISTORY

Hydantoins has been used since 1938. Many new drugs were discovered subsequently. Apart from the fact, that anticonvulsant drugs have been used for many years, their embryotoxicity was not be described before 60th, when first case reports were published.[1,2] Fetal hydantoin syndrome was described in 1975 by Hanson and Smith. Similar inborn defects were described for all older anticonvulsant drugs (primidone, valproate, phenobarbital, phenytoin, carbamazepine, trimethadion). The frequency and severity of defects associated with use trimethadione were so high to warrant consideration of early elective termination of pregnancy. The teratogenic mechanism of AEDs is only partially understood.

FETAL ANTICONVULSANT SYNDROME[1-3]

Fetal anticonvulsant syndrome is associated with exposure to dilantin, diphenylhydantoin, phenytoin, hydantoin, and valproic acid during 1st trimester of pregnancy, in lower degree also with other (carbamazepine). The abnormalities include:

- *An increase of major congenital anomalies:* Congenital heart defects (septal defects, tetralogy of Fallot, aortic coarctation, etc.), cleft lip and palate, limb defects with hypoplasia of nails and distal phalanges, finger-like thumbs, abnormal palmar creases, dislocation of hip, malformation of brain, especially neural tube defects.
- Specific syndrome including facial dysmorphy with wide anterior fontanel, ocular hypertelorism, broad, depressed nasal bridge, short nose with bowed upper lip, midface hypoplasia, epicanthus, often also malformation of external genitalia and neural tube.
- Intrauterine growth retardation.
- Developmental disorders mainly affecting cognitive functions and behavior.

Small variations were noted according to the drug used. A significant association was seen between maternal use of valproic acid and spina bifida, and a weaker, non-significant one between carbamazepine and spina bifida. Facial clefts were associated with both diphenylhydantoin and phenobarbitone use and also with polytherapy.[4,5] As AEDs have effect also on cognitive development, children exposed to valproate have increased risk of delayed early development in comparison to the control group. It seems, that a distinctive pattern of abnormalities in infants is associated with the use of anticonvulsant drugs during pregnancy rather than with epilepsy itself.

EMBRYOTOXICITY AND ITS EVALUATION

Genetic Background as a Factor for Inborn Defect

Drug metabolizing enzymes and the genetic variants they carry are one of the factors that might be responsible for the efficacy and side effect of AED treatment in individual patients. They also modulate development and induce embryotoxicity. The speed and differences in metabolic inactivation may increase plasma level of AEDs up to embryotoxic threshold. Polymorphy in genes for enzymes involved in metabolic pathways for detoxification is suspected cause for development of birth defect in certain cases.

Phenytoin toxicity is dependent on epoxide hydrolase activity,[6,7] i.e. arena oxidase or on CYP2C19 specific cytochrome P-450 isoenzyme deficiency. Valproate toxicity is increased in ornithine trans-carbamylase deficiency. Drug competition or the induction of microsomal enzymes may change AED plasma level and increase the risk. High-risk for neural-tube defects such spina bifida and anencephaly after valproate or carbamazepine exposure has been assigned to the deficiency in folate dependent homocysteine metabolism. Polymorphism of MTHFR (methylenetetrahydrofolate reductase) is associated with high-risk for anticonvulsant syndrome. Mothers who are homozygous for MTHFR genotype 677T were found to have three to four high-risk compared with those that were homozygous for allele 677C. Other genes, for example *MTR 2756*, are involved in susceptibility to embryotoxic impairment. In present, we may conclude those woman having a child with valproate fetal syndrome is in high-risk of malformed child for the next pregnancy. In future, the genetic profile will be a goal for the optimal treatment of epileptic patients.

Ischemia and Re-perfusion Injury

The role of ischemia and re-perfusion producing tissue damage linked for example to neural tube defect has to become more evident in the past years. During an ischemic event, intracellular xanthin dehydrogenase is converted to xantin oxidase. When the ischemia resolves, xanthin oxidase metabolized purines in uric acid. By-products of this reaction are super-oxide radicals. They produce tissue damage directly or indirectly. As convulsions results in anoxia, higher rate of malformation was demonstrated in epileptic women without treatment and without seizure control in comparison with healthy population. Combination anoxia with teratogenic potential of drug even increases risk.[8]

FIRST GENERATION OF ANTIEPILEPTIC DRUGS CAUSING EMBRYOTOXICITY

Phenytoin[9-16]

Phenytoin is the most widely used hydantoin derivate with antiepileptic effect. The teratogenic potential of hydantoin and its derivatives is known since 1968.[1] The anomalies observed were described as "fetal hydantoin syndrome". In the case of phenytoin, it appears that fetal susceptibility correlates with the fetal level of the microsomal detoxifying enzyme epoxide hydrolase. Developmental toxicity is probably caused by concentration-dependent bradycardia and hypoxia related damage of embryonic tissue resulting in alteration of gene expression minimally, if not everywhere, in craniofacial region. In comparison with other AEDs, phenytoin produced higher incidence of fetal defects (20.9%) in animal study however risk occurring in epidemiological studies was lower.

The risk of phenytoin exposure during pregnancy has been well documented. It has been estimated to be two to three folds higher than that of mothers without treatment as has been confirmed in several studies. The prospective observation study made by 25 epilepsy centers in USA and UK from 1999 to 2004 determine risk of adverse outcomes for phenytoin on 10.7% (including fetal death), and major malformation on 7.1%. Phenytoin monotherapy increases the risk for cleft palate, but it has not been associated with microcephaly.

Barbiturates[17,18]

Barbiturates used for epilepsy treatment are phenobarbital, methylphenobarbital, and primidone, the pro-drug of phenobarbital to which is largely metabolized. In higher doses (50 mg/kg/day and more) primidone was teratogenic in mice increasing the incidence of cleft palate, other defects as exencephaly, fused ribs, and undescended testes were observed less frequently. The incidence of major malformation was dose dependent in primidone as well as phenobarbital. After exposure to primidone, the malformation typical for AEDs has been described in many case reports and studies. Increased risk for major malformations associated with primidone exposure was demonstrated in large prospective study North American Registry demonstrated a 6.5% risk after phenobarbital monotherapy in comparison with 1.6% for control population.

Ethosuximide[19]

Ethosuximide is recommended drug for petit mal treatment, only. In animal studies, the risk of major malformation was approximately as high as in primidone. There are only a few report of the ethosuximide therapy during pregnancy.

Study reporting on pregnancy outcome in ten women described two major malformation cleft lip in mothers treated ethosuximide in combination with primidone or phenobarbital.

SECOND GENERATION OF ANTIEPILEPTIC DRUGS

Valproic Acid[17,19]

Valproic acid (VPA) is widely used for treatment of a broad spectrum of epilepsy types, migraine as well as bipolar disorder. *In utero* exposure results in higher incidence of major and minor malformations. Malformations occurred not only after valproic acid but also after valproate conjugates with anticonvulsant activity in animal model with different intensity.

Fetal valproate syndrome was described in 1968. The most frequent malformations were hernia, ear/neck/face malformations, cleft lip, and spina bifida. Nowadays, the studies have been focused on the correlation between dose and teratogenic effect. Higher doses than 1400 mg/day have been proved to be more teratogenic.

Carbamazepine[14,16]

Carbamazepine (CBZ) is efficacious in treatment of a variety of CNS disorders, as well as epileptic seizures. CBZ is usually well tolerated and therefore is also used in pregnant women. Carbamazepine in dose that is corresponding to the therapeutic range in humans was not associated with negative pregnancy outcome in mice. It had no effect on fertility. Higher number of resorptions or higher risk of malformation was not detected. Similar findings were found in study after the exposure to higher doses (1.000, 1.500 and 2.000 mg/kg). In those doses, no specific pattern of malformation and no correlation between detected anomalies and dose were found.

A few studies described typical carbamazepine syndrome characterized by facial dysmorphic features and mild mental retardation that did not seem to be related to presence of maternal convulsions but more to the hereditary factors. Some studies reported a risk for spina bifida in women used carbamazepine that is ten times higher than in unexposed population. Many case reports describing occurrence of spina bifida or eye malformation may support the opinion.

Oxcarbazepine[14]

Oxcarbazepine (OCZ) is similar to carbamazepine in chemical structure, but it is metabolized in different metabolic pathway. A monohydroxy-derivative (MHD) is responsible for its clinical efficacy. Premarketing studies showed an increase in congenital malformations in the offspring of rats treated with oxcarbazepine at doses similar to those used in humans on a surface area basis. The abnormalities in the offspring included craniofacial, cardiovascular, and skeletal abnormalities. In rabbits, an increase in fetal mortality was noted at similar doses. Higher frequency of malformation was found also in mice.

Benzodiazepines[14,16]

Benzodiazepines are widely used as tranquilizers, hypnotics as well as AEDs. For epilepsy treatment are used currently diazepam, clonazepam, clobazam, and sulthiame. Diazepam cross easily placenta and it is present in blood in three time higher level than in mother. Case control studies indicate higher risk of major malformation, especially oral cleft, however meta-analysis demonstrated no association between benzodiazepine exposure and major malformations. No relevant information was published about clobazam and sulthiame.

THIRD GENERATION OF ANTIEPILEPTIC DRUGS

Lamotrigine

Resorption and reduction of fetal weight were seen both being dose dependent. Skeletal malformation found in these studies were assigned to the maternal toxicity, however neural tube defects (anencephaly), malformation related to the cranial crest cells, and caudal dysgenesis were probably induced by lamotrigine. Prenatal exposure to LTG induced altered brain structure in a dose-dependent manner at maternal plasma concentrations within the clinically occurring range.

Levetiracetam[10,12]

Some studies described a higher incidence of resorptions in rats at dose 500 mg/kg/day and dose-related decrease in fetal weight. They demonstrated malformations as supernumerable ribs, absent tail, anal atresia, cardiovascular defects, and impairment of ossification at dose 250 mg/kg /day and higher, that was six-fold higher than therapeutic dose for human and that was toxic for mother. Study in a mouse model did not reveal higher incidence of major malformations after levetiracetam treatment up to dose 2000 mg/kg/day. There was higher frequency of resorptions at high doses.

Topiramate[9,11]

As reported by the manufacturer (Janssen-Cilag), topiramate is teratogenic in mice, rats and rabbits. Similar findings revealed a study describing an adverse effect of topiramate (100 mg/kg/day) on developing embryos in rats increasing number of resorptions.

OTHER NEW ANTIEPILEPTIC DRUGS

Risk assessment for following new antiepileptic drugs is not possible due to lack of experience.

Vigabatrin

The animal experiments demonstrated significant teratogenic effect when drug was administered to mice during organogenesis. Lower doses were associated with disturbance of motor-cognitive behavior and lower weight of pups, however higher caused abortions. Since vigabatrin (VGB) exposure has been associated with retina damage, two small studies examined children exposed *in utero* to drug demonstrated no clear ophthalmic abnormalities. However, sample was to small to be able to confirm safety for fetus. According to the FDA recommendation, the treatment may be only short-term.

CONCLUSION

The management of the pregnant women suffering from epilepsy requires close cooperation between the neurologist and obstetrician. Women with epilepsy have a low complication rate except of that related to AEDs exposure. All of them in childbearing age should be informed about the rates of teratogenicity of AEDs, possibility of increased seizure frequency during pregnancy, and the risks of the pregnancy and labor. If almost half of pregnancies are not planned, the optimalization of treatment and consultation should be discussed with girls on beginning of their childbearing age. Since unplanned pregnancy is very often diagnosed after the most sensitive period of embryo development, when malformations are already developed, it makes no sense to change treatment. Exposure to antiepileptic drugs is not an indication for therapeutic abortion, even if they are teratogenic. Counseling is very important, because it helps to gain a realistic perspective of risk.

The frequency of seizures is essentially the same as before pregnancy, however tonic-clonic convulsions should be avoided, because they are risky for mother and fetus. Seizures can cause trauma leading to ruptured fetal membranes or abruptio placentae. Fortunately, with close monitoring and proper management, more than 90% of pregnancies in women with epilepsy will be uncomplicated.

OPTIMIZATION OF TREATMENT[12,16]

Optimization of treatment should be made before pregnancy. Diagnosis of epilepsy should be confirmed and indication for treatment with AEDs re-assessed. The possibility of AED gradual withdrawal should be considered in appropriate clinical setting prior to conception. The AED treatment should be optimized also prior to conception. Selection should be made the most appropriate for patient. Changing during pregnancy is rarely justified, risk probably overweight potential gain. To ascertain whether epilepsy remains in remission enough time before conception is required.

Drugs of choice during pregnancy are considered lamotrigine and carbamazepine.

Drugs should be given in monotherapy with the lowest effective dose. Polytherapy should be avoided because of proved increase of risk. Effective dose and optimal concentration of the drug before pregnancy should be documented. Monitoring of drug plasma concentration have to be more frequent, minimally once during trimester. Good compliance with treatment is essential. Lamotrigine, levetiracetam, and topiramate plasma levels are changing (decreasing) during pregnancy, so adjustment of therapeutic dose during pregnancy is needed. Valproic acid should be avoided, if it is possible. However, adequate seizure control is the primary goal. If it is only drug giving satisfactory control of seizures, valproic acid should be used of the lowest possible day dose (optimum under 600 mg/day) divided into three doses to minimize negative influence to fetus. Pregnancy should be considered of high-risk and must have appropriate follow-up (Ornoy, 2009).

The second level (expert) ultrasonography may justified normal development or detect most neural tube defects and about twothird of other major malformations.

FOLIC ACID SUPPLEMENTATION[20-23]

Low serum folic acid level in epileptic mothers is associated with an increased risk of congenital malformations in their offspring (Ogava et al. 1991). Population studies demonstrate benefit from fortification of cereal products by folic acid (De Walls et al. 2007) or supplementation before planed pregnancy. Daily consumption of supplements containing 400 μg of folic acid in the periconception period may reduce the risk of neural tube defects in general population by as much as 70% (Morin et al. 2002). If risk of malformation is higher in women with low plasma level of folic acid, periconceptional supplementation with minimally 0.4 mg folic acid per day in AEDs exposed population is considered prophylactic. The measurement that determines intraerythrocythal level of folic acid may help with definition of optimal dose. *Results suggest, that 5 mg/day folic acid as preconception supplementation in women with epilepsy is effective to balance the impact of AEDs on folate metabolism* (Bauer et al. 2010). Folate prophylaxis is recommended to all women taking antiepileptic drugs. Treatment with dose up to 5 mg/day should start before planned pregnancy and continued minimally to the end of first trimester.

VITAMIN K SUPPLEMENTATION

Management strategies include also the prenatal use vitamin K. Vitamin K 10 mg per day orally should be administered in the last 4 weeks of pregnancy for women taking hepatic enzyme-inducing AEDs (phenytoin, phenobarbital, primidone, carbamazepine, topiramate, and oxcarbazepine). The newborn should receive vitamin K 1 mg intravenously or intramuscularly regardless of maternal AED exposure.

REFERENCES

1. Meadow SR. Anticonvulsant drugs and congenital abnormalities. Lancet. 1968;14(2) (7581):1296, ISSN: 0140-6736.
2. Žižka J. Embryopathiahydantoinica. In: Diagnostikasyndromů a malformací; 1994. pp. 98-9. Galén, ISBN: 80-85824-04-3, Prague, Czech Republic.
3. Ornoy A. Valproic acid in pregnancy: How much are we endangering the embryo and fetus? Reprod Toxicol. 2009;28(1):1-10, ISSN: 0890-6238.
4. Bromfield EB, Dworetzky BA, Wyszynski DF, Smith CR, Baldwin EJ, Holmes LB. Valproate teratogenicity and epilepsy syndrome. Epilepsia. 2008;49(12):2122-4. ISSN: 0013-9580.
5. Holmes LB, Harvey EA, Coull BA, Huntington KB, Khoshbin S, Hayes AM, Ryan LM. The teratogenicity of anticonvulsant drugs. N Engl J Med. 2001;344(15):1132-8, ISSN: 0028-4793.
6. Steinlein OK. Gene polymorphism and their role in epilepsy treatment and prognosis. Naunyn-Schmied Arch Pharmacol. 2010;382(2):109-18, ISSN: 0028-1298.
7. Malm H, Artama M, Gissler M, et al. Selective serotonin reuptake inhibitors and risk for major congenital anomalies. Obstet Gynecol. 2011;118:111-20.
8. Verrotti A, Tana M, Pelliccia P, Chiarelli F, Latini G. Recent advances on neural tube defects with special reference to valproic acid. Endocrine, metabolic and immune disorders - Drug target. 2006;6(1):25-31, ISSN: 1871-5303 31.5.2011. Available on *www.benthamdirect.org/pages/b_viewarticle.php*
9. Buehler BA, Rao V, Finnell RH. Biochemical and molecular teratology of fetal hydantoin syndrome. Neurol Clin. 1994;12(4):741-8, ISSN: 0733-8619.
10. Azarbayjani F, Danielsson BR. Pharmacologically induced embryonic dysrythmia and episodes of hypoxia followed by reoxygenation: A common teratogenic mechanism for antiepileptic drugs? Teratology. 1998;57(3):117-26, ISSN: 0040-3709.
11. Danielsson B, Sköld AC, Azarbayjani F, Ohman I, Webster W. Pharmacokinetic data support pharmacologically induced embryonic dysrhythmia as explanation to Fetal Hydantoin Syndrome in rats. Toxicol Appl Pharmacol. 2000;163(2):164-75, ISSN: 0041-008X
12. Gelineau-van Waes J, Bennett GD, Finnell RH. Phenytoin-induced alterations in craniofacial gene expression. Teratology. 1999;59(1):23-34, ISSN 0040-3709.
13. Kluger BM, Meador KJ. Teratogenicity of antiepileptic medications. Semin Neurol. 2008;28(3):328-35, ISSN: 0271-8235.
14. Shepard TH, Lemire RJ. Clonazepan. Catalog of teratogenic agents. The John Hopkins University Press Baltimore, Maryland, USA; 2004. pp. 96 (11th ed.), ISBN: 0- 8018-7953-1
15. Meador KJ, Penovich P, Baker GA, Pennell PB, Bromfield E, Pack A, et al. Antiepileptic drug use in women of childbearing age. Epilepsy Behav. 2009;15(3):339-43, ISSN:1525-5050.
16. Almgren M, Källén B, Levebratt C. Population-based study of antiepileptic drug exposure *in utero*-Influence on head circumference in newborns. Seizures. 2009;18(10):672-5, ISSN: 1059-1311.
17. Akšamija A, Habek D, Stanojevic M, Ujevic B. Fetal malformation associated with the use of methylphenobarbital and carbamazepine during pregnancy. Fetal Diag Ther. 2009;25(1):79-82, ISSN: 1015-3837.
18. Jones KL. Fetal hydantoin syndrome, fetal valproate syndrome Smith's Recognizable Patters of Human Malformation (5th edn). WB Saunders co. Philadelphia, Pennsylvania, USA. 1997. pp. 559-67. ISBN 0-72166115-7.
19. Kuhnz W, Koch S, Jakob S, Hartmann A, Helge H, Nau H. Ethosuximide in epileptic women during pregnancy and lactation period. British Journal of Clinical Pharmacology. 1984;18(5):671-7. ISSN: 0306-5251.
20. Ogawa Y, Kaneko S, Otani K, Fukushima Y. Serum folic acid levels in epileptic mothers and their relationship to congenital malformations. Epilepsy Res. 1991;8(1):75-8, ISSN: 0920-1211.
21. De Wals P, Tairou F, Van Allen MI, Uh SH, Lowry RB, Sibbald B, et al. Reduction in neural-tube defects after folic acid fortification in Canada. N Engl J Med. 2007;357(2):135-42. ISSN: 0028-4793.
22. Morin P, De Wals P, StCyr-Tribble D, Niyonsenga T, Payette H. Pregnancy planning: a determinant of folic acid supplements use for the primary prevention of neural tube defects. Can J Public Health. 2002;93(4):259-63. ISSN: 0008-4263.
23. Bauer J, Bös M, Rück J, Stoffel-Wagner B. Folsäure substitution bei Frauen mit epilepsie. Evaluation des. Substitutions effektes durch intraery throzytäre Folsäure be stimmung. Nervenartzt (July 2010). DOI:10.1007/s00115-010-3077-6, ISSN: 0028-2804, 15.3.2011.

SECTION

7

Prenatal Operative Scope

CHAPTER

33

Principles of Fetal Surgery

Rajeev Redkar, Shirin Joshi

Fetal surgery involves operating on the fetus or the placenta during the midgestation period with the aim of altering the natural history of the disease that is diagnosed *in utero*. Most of the fetal abnormalities can be addressed after the birth of the child, especially preferred, after the lungs of the baby have achieved maturity. However, sometimes it may be useful to intervene in the antenatal period to prevent permanent organ damage or to allow complete development of the affected organ. This would be dependent on the natural history or the pathology of the malformation.

The fetal surgical specialty has recently emerged and has been practiced to prevent neonatal death due to irreversible organ damage secondary to anomalies diagnosed in fetal life. With the recent imaging technology, mainly ultrasonography and magnetic resonance imaging (MRI), it is possible to diagnose these conditions before the organ damage is done and to choose the fetus which will benefit from antenatal surgical intervention. These modalities also help us define the pathophysiology of some of the complex pediatric surgical conditions.The rationale of fetal surgery is to restore normal development of the affected fetus and thus prevent neonatal morbidity and mortality. However, while the fetal issues are being addressed, the fetal surgical clinician has to address the issue of almost eliminating a potential maternal risk. Hence, mostly, the conditions which are life-threatening to the fetus are usually managed prenatally. Fetal surgery, on the other hand, has also been successfully applied to some nonlethal conditions like meningomyelocele (MMC) and spina bifida to prevent their neurological sequelae.

The 'Maternal-fetal' surgery includes a broad-spectrum of procedures which include ultrasound guided ventriculo-peritoneal and vesicoamniotic shunt placement, Fetoscopy procedures, open fetal surgeries and EXIT (*ex utero* intrapartum treatment) treatment procedure (Fig. 33.1). Minimally invasive procedures, which are also treatment called as Fetendo surgeries, are recently introduced which involve percutaneous procedures, sometimes under local anesthesia, which help in reducing maternal morbidity than open fetal surgery.

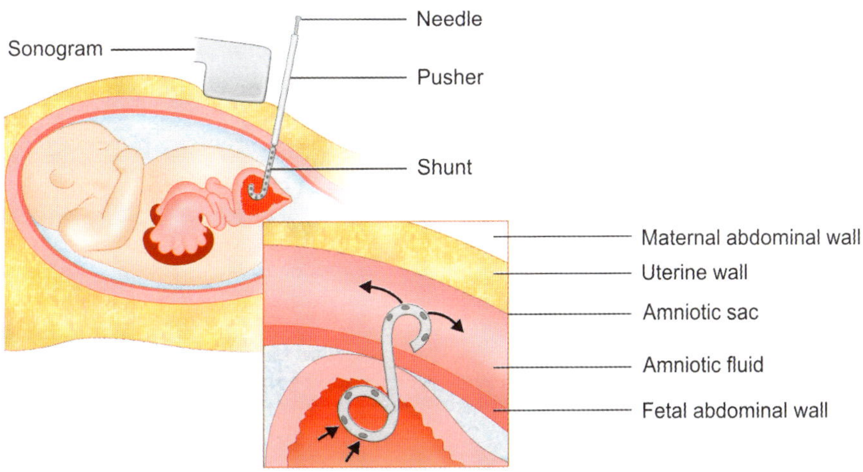

Fig. 33.1 Vesicoamniotic shunt introduction

A detailed assessment of both maternal and fetal condition is made prior to any intervention. The views and wishes of both the parents are taken into account. It is possible to ascertain maternal risk factors and fetal prognosis by a detailed history, clinical examination and relevant investigations. Exclusion of chromosomal anomalies is important and should be discussed with parents. It may be possible that the type of structural abnormality that the fetus has, carries a specific risk of a chromosomal anomaly, that can adversely affect the prognosis. For example in a fetus with a congenital diaphragmatic hernia, one needs to assess the 'ultrasound markers' or maternal age, which in turn, increases the chance of a co-existent anomaly which could be very derogatory to the final outcome.[1,2] Similarly, fetal blood sampling is a relatively rapid and simple method of assessing the fetal karyotype, which will evaluate the risk of the 'wellbeing' of the fetus.[3]

The benefits and risks of fetal therapies need to be discussed with the parents at length. The information should be provided in understandable language considering patients' education and ethnic background. There is some evidence that a taped copy of the discussions surrounding the case, given to the parents to keep and replay at a later date, may enhance understanding and help in avoiding subsequent medicolegal issues.[4]

There have been randomized controlled multicenter clinical trials conducted recently which support fetal intervention. One is the 'Management of meningomyelocele study' (MOMS) to improve neurological morbidity of MMC and another is a European trial which demonstrated efficacy of fetoscopic laser separation versus amnioreduction in twin-to-twin transfusion syndrome (TTTS).

CENTERS PRACTICING FETAL SURGERY

The first operation on a human fetus was carried out in 1981 at the University of California.[5] The fetal surgery is still at experimental stage and practiced in very few centers over the world. Below is the list of centers that have been doing fetal interventional surgeries.

- *Fetal Treatment Center at the University of California, San Francisco:* The main work in this field has been carried out by Professor Michael Harrison, a pediatric surgeon mostly in cases of congenital diaphragmatic hernia (CDH). Other therapeutic prenatal surgeries carried out there have included formation of an iatrogenic gastroschisis[6] and fetal surgery on cystic adenomatoid malformation of the lung.[6,7]
- *The Childrens' Hospital of Philadelphia:* The center for fetal diagnosis and treatment at the children's hospital of Philadelphia has operated on 18, 190 fetal surgical cases since their induction in 1995. The surgical cases include congenital diaphragmatic hernia (1234 cases), gastrointestinal anomalies (1415 cases), congenital heart disease (1854 cases), genitourinary defects (1820 cases), myelomeningocele (Spina Bifida) (1925 cases), lung lesions (1882 cases), abnormalities related to neurosurgical issues (2262 cases), complicated neck masses (346 cases), hematologic/immune problems (55 cases), sacrococcygeal teratoma (296 cases).
- *King's College Hospital, London:* The Harris Birth right Unit at King's College Hospital is one of the largest fetal medicine units the world, seeing 15,000 women and their unborn babies each year. Led by Professor Kypros Nicolaides, the unit provides specialist testing and treatment for babies with abnormalities in the womb, including Down's syndrome, heart defects and twin-to-twin transfusion syndrome (TTTS).
- The St Louis Fetal Care Institute SSM Cardinal Glennon Children's Medical Center in St Louis, Missouri.
- Fetal Care Center of Children's Hospital in Boston.
- The Center for Advanced Maternal Fetal Care at Vanderbilt.
- The Fetal Care Center at Cincinnati.
- The Fetal Treatment Center at Northeast Ohio.
- The Texas Center for Fetal Surgery.

Indications for Fetal Surgery

The list of fetal conditions for which antenatal surgery is considered currently include:

- Lower urinary tract obstruction (obstructive uropathy) like posterior urethral valves
- Twin-twin transfusion syndrome
- Myelomeningocele (Spina bifida)
- Congenital diaphragmatic hernia
- Neck masses occluding the trachea
- Congenital cystic adenomatoid malformation of the lungs
- Sacrococcygeal teratoma when associated with developing fetal hydrops
- Twin reversed arterial perfusion sequence (TRAP)
- Aqueductal stenosis of the ventricular system of the brain
- Valvular obstruction of the heart
- Congenital high airway obstruction syndrome (CHAOS)
- Cervical teratoma
- Gastroschisis
- Cleft lip and palate
- Metabolic and cellular defects
- Stem cell or enzyme defects.

Anesthesia for Fetal Surgery

Fetal surgery requires teamwork. The disciplines that interact may include pediatric general surgery, obstetrics, pediatric anesthesia, obstetric anesthesia, cardiology, radiology, geneticist, otolaryngology, neonatology, neonatal nursing, and operating room nursing.

Providing anesthesia for fetal surgery is challenging for many reasons. It requires integration of both obstetric and pediatric anesthesia practice. Two patients must be anesthetized for the benefit of one, and there is little margin for error.

PREOPERATIVE PREPARATION

Maternal Factors

Mother is evaluated for respiratory or circulatory compromise by the gravid uterus, as evidenced by symptoms of shortness of breath or light-headedness.

More severe symptoms of aortocaval compression would call for meticulous left uterine displacement and would raise the level of suspicion in a mother with persistent hypotension after induction of anesthesia.

Severity of gastroesophageal reflux may change the anesthetic plan in minimally invasive operations where maternal sedation is considered. Aspiration prophylaxis in the obstetric population includes oral sodium citrate, histamine receptor blockers or proton pump inhibitors and prokinetic agents such as metoclopramide.

Open operations should not proceed without immediately availability of cross-matched blood for the mother and warm type O-negative blood for the fetus.

Fetal Factors

The location of the placenta affects patient positioning. The placenta should not be punctured or damaged at all during the fetal intervention.

The estimated fetal weight is used to determine dosage of fetal drugs.

The actual disease process and pathophysiology, and the extent of anatomic or physiologic derangement will give the team an idea of the physiologic reserve of the fetus.

Preoperative fetal studies include ultrasound, echocardiography, and fetal magnetic resonance imaging.

Lung lesions in a fetus may grow or shrink, airway obstruction may worsen or resolve, cardiac outputs may change, hydrops fetalis may ensueand polyhydramnios may develop. These have to be meticulously and serially monitored.

There is a considerable ethical and scientific debate over the issue of fetal pain.[8]

Minimally Invasive Interventions

These are the most frequently performed fetal surgical procedures. The uterine cavity is accessed percutaneously with needles and small trocar sheaths. Visualization of structures is provided by ultrasound or by a fetoscope inserted through a trocar. The access may be as minimal as one small gauge radiofrequency probe or may be as involved as multiple trocars for a complex fetoscopic procedure.[9] Endoscopes range from 1.0 to 3.8 mm external diameter.[10] The timing of minimally invasive procedures is typically in early or midgestation.

An anesthetic plan can range from local anesthetic infiltration and sedation to neuraxial or general. Medications can be given directly to the mother by the anesthesia team and, thus, indirectly to the fetus by placental transfer. Medications can also be given directly to the fetus by the surgical team. Route of direct administration can be variable, and intramuscular, intravenous, and intracardiac routes have been described.[11, 12]

Fetal monitoring is typically limited to measurement of the fetal heart rate by the obstetricians with an ultrasound. Echocardiography may be used in cardiac interventions.

The Fetendo procedures are now done under sedation. The current practice includes maternal fasting, one intravenous (IV) catheter, aspiration prophylaxis, and tocolysis with preoperative indomethacin. Initially, tocolysis involved preoperative indomethacin, postoperative magnesium infusions and postdischarge oral nifedipine or subcutaneous terbutaline. Postdischarge tocolysis is now rare. Severe intravenous fluid restriction is no longer required and is avoided. Light sedation is administered to the mother to provide maternal comfort and decreased fetal movement.

The location of the placenta influences the surgical approach, which must avoid trespass of the placenta. Intraoperative ultrasound scans are used by the operators to guide them in introduction and manipulation of the surgical instruments. If the placenta is implanted on the anterior surface of the uterus, trocars and curved instruments are inserted in the lateral aspect of the uterus if possible, or a laparotomy is made, the uterus exteriorized, and the instruments passed through the posterior uterus. If instruments are to be introduced laterally, positioning the mother may involve "bumps" for left or right uterine displacement, or even placing the mother in full lateral decubitus position (Figs 33.2A and B).

Open Midgestation Surgery

Open midgestation surgery requires significant uterine relaxation (Figs 33.3 and 33.4). Complete uterine relaxation is mandatory for fetal manipulation and decreases the likelihood of the initiation of labor from uterine surgical manipulation. General endotracheal anesthesia with high dose volatile anesthetic gases (2MAC) is most often used to achieve uterine relaxation for open surgery. Nitroglycerin can

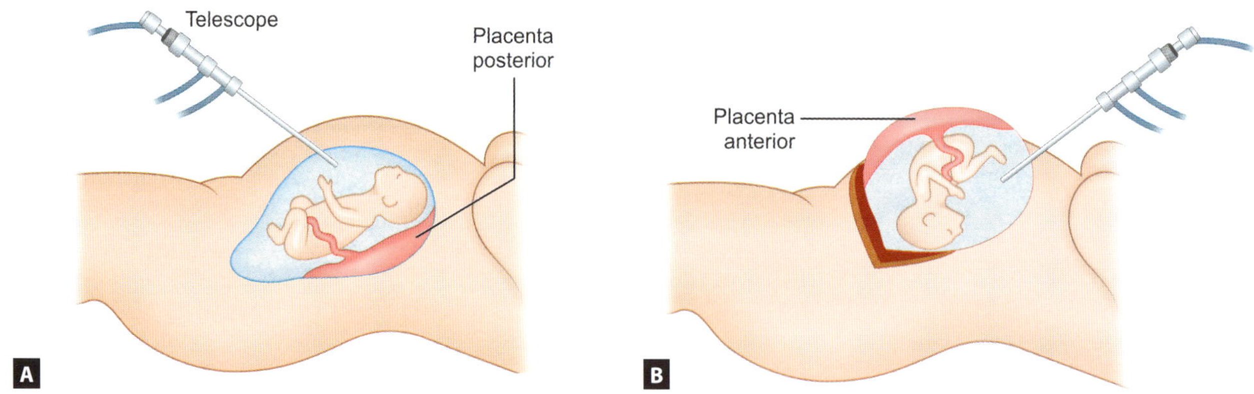

Figs 33.2A and B Introduction of instruments in relation to the position of the placenta

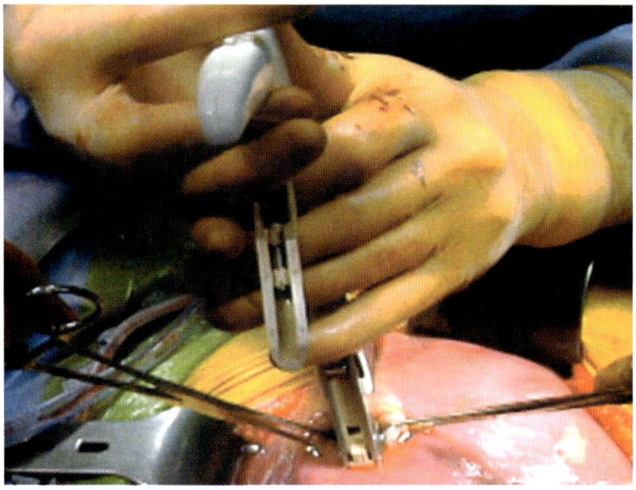

Fig. 33.3 Opening of the uterus for open fetal surgery

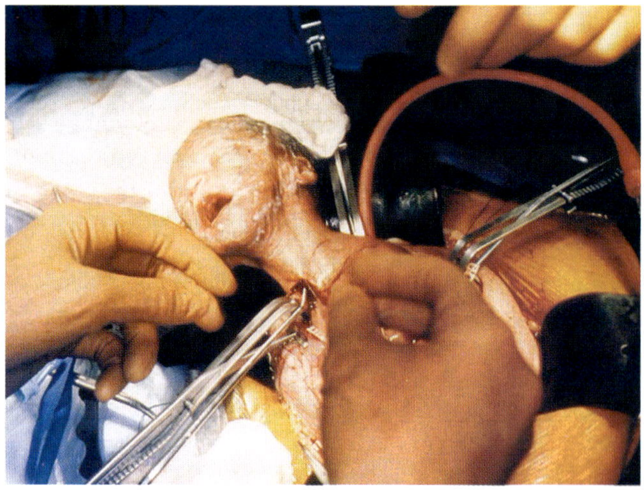

Fig. 33.4 Open fetal surgery in progress

also be used to relax the uterus. Relaxation will allow increased uterine blood flow as long as maternal blood pressure is maintained, and nitroglycerin results in less fetal exposure to volatile anesthetic agents. After adequate fasting and a placement of a peripheral intravenous access, oral tocolysis, and aspiration prophylaxis, a high lumbar epidural is placed for postoperative analgesia.

With standard monitors, a left uterine displacement and preoxygenation, rapid sequence induction and intubation takes place. An orogastric tube and a self-retaining urinary catheter are placed. Because of the risk for rapid bleeding, a second large bore peripheral intravenous line is placed. An arterial catheter is inserted to monitor small changes in maternal blood pressure which may have dramatic effects on fetal perfusion, heart rate and function. Intravenous crystalloid administration is kept to a minimum because of the risk of maternal pulmonary edema after fetal surgery.[13]

The maternal blood pressure improves with exteriorization of the uterus and with surgical manipulation. Phenylephrine and ephedrine should be prepared. Vasopressin infusions allow for smoother blood pressure control.

After exposure of the fetus, an intramuscular injection of fentanyl (20 μg/kg), atropine (20 μg/kg), and vecuronium (0.2 mg/kg) is given by the surgical team. Amniotic fluid is lost through the hysterotomy, but it is replaced with a continuous pressurized infusion of warmed crystalloid.

If fetal intravenous access is necessary it is obtained, and intravenous tubing is handed over the drapes to the anesthesia team. Monitoring of the fetus in these operations includes direct observation, fetal echocardiography, and pulse oximetry.[14,15] If a pulse oximeter is placed by the surgical team, the hand is covered with sterile foil to prevent artefact from the operating room lights, and a sterile cable is passed to the anesthesia team. The usual fetal oxygen saturation ranges from 40% to 70%.[16,17]

Fetal echocardiography is performed continuously to monitor cardiac filling, contractility and rate, along with patency of the ductus arteriosus. Umbilical blood gas measurement may be used in selected cases. The anesthesia team must watch closely for fetal bradycardia, maternal or fetal bleeding, and maternal blood pressure changes. A decrease in fetal oxygen saturation is an indicator of fetal distress.[14,18] A common sign of fetal distress is bradycardia. Blood products should be readily available. Prior to resection of large chest lesions, a transfusion of packed red blood cells may improve fetal hemodynamic stability.

A maternal laparotomy is performed. The location of this laparotomy incision is usually transverse, and more cephalad than performed for a lower uterine segment cesarean section. Once the uterus is exposed, the placental edges are mapped carefully with sterile ultrasound to plan the hysterotomy. Implantation of the placenta on the anterior or posterior aspect of the uterus will impact surgical approach, and an anterior placenta necessitates exteriorization of the uterus for a posterior or fundal hysterotomy. The fetus is exposed, but only the necessary anatomy is delivered via the hysterotomy. For example, in a meningomyelocele (MMC) closure, the lesion is exposed, while the rest of the fetus remains bathed in amniotic fluid in the uterus. If a fetal thoracotomy is planned, an arm is delivered, and the shoulder and chest are exposed while the rest of the fetus remains in the uterus. After surgery and skin closure, the fetus is replaced in the uterus antibiotics are instilled into the amniotic fluid. The uterus is closed and a flap of omentum is sewn over the uterine closure to further seal the hysterotomy closure.

With the closure of the uterus, tocolysis is begun with a bolus of intravenous magnesium sulfate, the epidural block is initiated, and the volatile anesthetic is reduced. The maternal abdomen is closed, and the mother is extubated awake. Postoperative tocolysis continues with a magnesium infusion which is transitioned to oral nifedipine.

EX-UTERO INTRAPARTUM TREATMENT PROCEDURE

This is an operation carried out as near term as it is practically possible. The fetal lungs have to be mature which is complete by around 32 weeks of gestation. The principle in this operation is that the fetus is delivered through a cesarean section and is operated upon when it is still anatomically and physiologically connected to the mother with the placenta and the umbilical cord. Once the surgical procedure on the baby is completed, then the umbilical cord is clamped and the baby separated from the mother (Fig. 33.5).

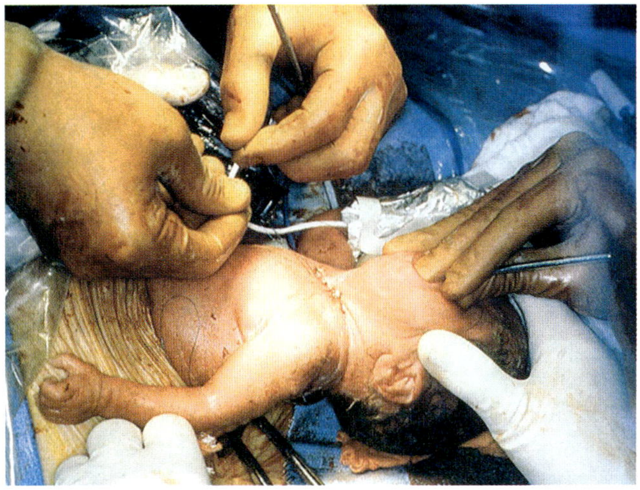

Fig. 33.5 EXIT procedure in progress

Multiple specialized personnel and teams are involved in this intricate and multispecialty venture which are enlisted below.

Preoperative Evaluation Team

- High risk obstetricians
- Pediatric surgeons
- Social workers
- Anesthesiologists
- Radiologists
- Fetal cardiologists
- Neonatologists.

Intraoperative Team

- Maternal anesthesiologist
- Fetal anesthesiologist
- Scrub nurses—2
- Circulating nurses—2
- Airway cart nurse
- Maternal-fetal medicine specialists
- Fetal cardiologist for intraoperative echocardiography
- Pediatric surgeons
- Obstetrician
- Extracorporeal membrane oxygenation (ECMO) team.

Neonatal Team

- Neonatologist
- Surgical advanced practice nurses
- Neonatal nurses
- Second operating room team on standby in adjacent operation theater.

Indications

Large tumors such as cervical teratomas or lymphangiomas, oropharyngeal masses, severe micrognathia, congenital high airway obstruction syndrome (CHAOS), large lung lesions, large mediastinal masses, special circumstances with thoraco-omphalopagus conjoined twins, and ex-utero intrapartum technique (EXIT)-to-ECMO (Extra Corporeal Membrane Oxygenerator) for severe congenital diaphragmatic hernia. Additional indications include unilateral pulmonary agenesis with airway stenosis.[18,19]

Anesthesia

Since the fetus will be delivered at the end of the operation, these procedures are performed at or near term to optimize lung maturity. Before the umbilical cord is clamped, surgical intervention is performed that will facilitate successful transition to extrauterine life.[20] This intervention may involve laryngoscopy, rigid bronchoscopy and intubation, tracheostomy. Fetal well-being is monitored with pulse oximetry, heart rate and echocardiography.

Uterine relaxation is only needed intraoperatively, not postoperatively. In case, magnesium sulphate is not given, pulmonary edema is less likely. It is important in the EXIT that no ventilation of the lungs occurs until the umbilical cord is clamped. Ventilation of the lungs will initiate the cascade of events leading to a transitional/neonatal circulation, and the benefits of operating on "placental support" are lost.

The surgical team passes sterile items like tubing for intravenous fluids, pulse oximeter cables and oxygen tubing for a sterile Mapleson circuit off the field for the anesthesia team after the patient has been adequately anesthetized.

Distinguishing fetal fluids and medication from maternal fluids and drugs is important, to avoid confusion, especially, in emergency or urgent parts of the procedure.[21]

Procedure

Following maternal laparotomy, placental mapping and hysterotomy, the fetal head, arms, and upper torso are delivered while the lower torso and legs remain in the uterus to maintain intrauterine volume. An intramuscular injection is often given depending on the surgical plan (intubation versus lesion resection). Once the airway is secured or lesion resected, surfactant may be given to the fetus and the lungs are ventilated.

Once the umbilical cord is divided, and the placenta is delivered, uterine relaxation must be promptly reversed. Administration of oxytocin and rapidly decreasing the inspired concentration of volatile anesthetic is adequate in most cases, but methyl ergonovine and prostaglandin F2 a should be readily available. After uterine tone is established, the hysterotomy is closed. After maternal hemodynamic stability is ensured, the epidural catheter is dosed to provide postoperative analgesia. The mother is extubated awake.

After completion of the procedure, the newborn is passed to an adjacent room for further resuscitation and then subsequent management in an intensive care unit.

Intraoperative Fetal Resuscitation

Intraoperatively, fetal distress may occur resulting from cord compression or kinking, placental separation, high uterine tone, maternal hypotension, hypothermia, hypoxia, hypovolemia or anemia. Placental abruption may cause fetal distress and new onset maternal hypotension which may manifest as intrauterine bleeding.

Cardiac dysfunction may result from prolonged exposure to high doses of volatile anesthetic agents.

Aortocaval compression should be avoided and the integrity of the uteroplacental unit must also be confirmed . The umbilical cord must be patent.

The surgical team will be able to confirm adequate uterine relaxation, and fetal echocardiography will inform the team about cardiac filling, function and patency of the ductus arteriosus.

Resuscitative measures will depend on how much access the surgical and anesthesia teams have to the fetus, and may include ensuring left uterine displacement, and adequate uterine blood flow, administration of maternal vasopressors, or administration of medications or blood directly to the fetus. In open cases, emergency medications such as atropine and epinephrine are handed over in a sterile fashion to the surgical team for intravenous or even intracardiac administration. Fetal cardiac compressions under fetal echocardiographic guidance may be needed.[22]

Practical Points

- First do no harm to the mother or the fetus and remember maternal safety as a priority.
- The anesthetic plan should be based on understanding of maternal and fetal physiology and the needs of the mother and fetus.
- Interdisciplinary communication is vital. Minimally invasive operations present the widest range of anesthetic possibilities.
- Open midgestation operations require complete intra-operative uterine relaxation and postoperative tocolysis.

ETHICAL ISSUES IN PERFORMING FETAL SURGERY

The fetus as a patient is getting accepted with the widespread use of many techniques. Clinical ethical judgment and decision making about invasive and transplacental fetal therapy are complex matters.[23]

With the application of concepts and language of medical ethics, these matters are conceptually and clinically manageable.

The clarified obligations owed to the pregnant woman and to the fetal patient are mandatory. They provide the basis for the identification of when it is appropriate to recommend such therapy and to which patient.

As experience grows in the management of complex problems *in utero*, the concepts and language of medical ethics will be an essential dimension of the developing field of invasive/transplacental fetal therapy.

Some centers have convened a Fetal Ethics Committee (comprising of an obstetrician, a pediatric surgeon, a perinatologist, a neonatologist and a lay person).

LIMITATIONS OF FETAL SURGERY

Problems that have yet to be completely overcome include:

- Inability to identify ideal fetal candidates for antenatal intervention,
- To determine the optimal timing of intervention
- To prevent preterm birth after fetal surgery.[5]

REFERENCES

1. Howe DT, Kilby MD, Sirry H, et al. Structural chromosome anomalies in congenital diaphragmatic hernia. Prenat Diagn. 1996;16:1003-9.
2. Whittle MJ. Ultrasonographic 'soft markers' of fetal chromosomal defects. BBr Med J. 1997;314:918.
3. Maxwell DJ, Johnson P, Hurley P, et al. Fetal blood sampling and pregnancy loss in relation to indication. Br J Obstet Gynaecol. 1991;98:892-7.
4. Cope CD, Lyons AC, Donovan V, et al. Providing letters and audio-tapes to supplement a prenatal diagnostic consultation: effects on later distress and recall. Prenat Diagn. 2003;23: 1060-7.
5. Wenstrom KD, Carr SR. Fetal surgery: principles, indications, and evidence. Obstet Gynecol. 2014;124(4):817-35.
6. Montgomery LD, Belfort MA, Saade GR, et al. Iatrogenic gastroschisis decreases pulmonary hypoplasia in an ovine congenital diaphragmatic hernia *in utero*, V. Initial clinical experience. J Pediatr Surg. 1990;25:57-5.
7. Adzick NS, Harrison MR, Flake AW, et al. Fetal Surgery for cystic adenomatoid malformation of the lung. J Pediatr Surg. 1993;28:806-12.
8. Glover V, Fisk N. Do foetuses feel pain? We don't know; better to err on the safe side from mid gestation. Br Med J. 1996;313: 796.
9. Kohl T, Tchatcheva K, MerzWetal. Percutaneous fetoscopic patch closure of human spina bifida aperta : advances in fetal surgical technique may obviate the need for early postnatal neurosurgical intervention. Surg Endosc. 2009;23:890-5.
10. Klaritsch P, Albert K, Van Miehgem T, et al. Instrumental requirements for minimal invasive fetal surgery. BJOG. 2009;116:188-97.
11. Tworetzky W, Bulich LA, Mizrahi Arnaud A, et al. Pathophysiology, management and outcomes of fetal hemodynamic instability during prenatal cardiac intervention. Pediatr Res. 2007;62:325-30.
12. Deprest J, Jani J, Gratacos E, et al. Fetal intervention for congenital diaphragmatic hernia: the European experience. Semin Perinatol. 2005;29:94-103.
13. Di Federico EM , Burlingame JM, Kilpatrick SJ, Harrison M, Matthay MA. Pulmonary edema in obstetric patients is rapidly reloved except in the presence of infection or of nitroglycerine in tocolysis after open fetal surgery. Am J Obstet Gynecol. 1998; 179:925-33.
14. Luks FI, Johnson BD, Papadakis K, Traore M, Piasecki GJ. Predictive value of monitoring parameters in fetal surgery. J Pediatr Surg. 1998;33:1297-301.
15. Keswani SG, Cromble Holme TM, Rychik J, et al. Impact of continous intraoperative monitoring on outcomes in open fetal surgery. Fetal Diagn Ther. 2005;20:316-20.
16. Helwig JT, Parer JT, Kilpatrick SJ, Laros Jr RK. Umbilical cord blood acid-base state: what is normal? Am J Obstet Gynecol. 1996;174:1807-12 (discussion 1812-1814).
17. Johnson N, Johnson VA, Fisher J, Jobbings B, Bannister J, Lilford RJ. Fetal monitoring with pulse oximetry. Br J Obstet Gynaecol. 1991;98:36-41.
18. Muller F, Dommergues M, Mandelbrot L, et al. Fetal urinary biochemistry predicys post natal renal function in children with bilateral obstructive uropathies. Obstet Gynecol. 1993;82:(8203);28:1433-9.
19. Julie S, Moldenhauer. Ex utero intrapartum therapy. Seminars in pediatric surgery. 2013;22:44-9.
20. Mychaliska GB, Bealer JF, Graf JL, Rosen MA, Adzick NS, Harrison MR. Operating on placental support: the ex utero intra partum treatment procedure. J Pediatr Surg. 1997;32: 227-30.
21. Elaina E, Lin M, et al. Anesthesia for fetal surgery. Seminars in pediatric surgery. 2013;22;50-5.
22. Yao AC, Moinian M, Lind J. Distribution of blood between infant and placenta after birth. Lancet. 1969;2:871-87.
23. Smith-Levitin M, Kowalik A, Birnholz J, et al. Selective reduction of multifetal pregnancies to twins improves outcome over non reduced triplet gestations. Am J Obstet Gynecol. 1996;175:878-82.

CHAPTER

34

Fetal Surgery: Why, When and Where?

Rajeev Redkar, Anant Bangar, Swathi Krishna

INTRODUCTION

Advances in prenatal and perinatal imaging have opened the doors for prenatal interventions on the fetuses, resulting in decrease in mortality and morbidity of many congenital malformations. But, every coin has two sides and these advances have led to the significant parental anxiety and apprehensions. It is usually a team effort comprised of sonologist, obstetrician, pediatrician, pediatric surgeon, and geneticist. As a physician, knowing the facts is important assets in helping the parents to understand the anomaly. A study by Gupta et al. (Table 34.1) summarizes the distribution of antenatally diagnosed congenital anomalies referred to a pediatric surgeon.[1] Urologic anomalies (47%) form the most common anomalies detected antenatally and referred to pediatric surgical opinion. It is beyond the scope of this chapter to discuss all the anomalies, albeit we will be discussing some common antenatally diagnosed congenital surgical anomalies.

ANTENATALLY DETECTED HYDRONEPHROSIS

Ultrasonographic examination is the most common and first-line tool for evaluation of fetus. Improvements in fetal USG have led to detection of renal pelvic dilatation—a very common occurrence. Even though this is the most common anomaly detected in the fetus, management and treatment remain controversial in terms of patient outcome.

Fetal hydronephrosis is defined as a dilatation of the renal pelvis with or without dilation of the renal calyces. It can be detected as early as the 12–14 weeks of gestation. The incidence of antenatal renal pelvic dilatation is around 0.5–1% of all pregnancies and varies depending on the criteria used for the diagnosis.

The common causes of fetal hydronephrosis are enumerated in Table 34.2.[2]

Table 34.1 Congenital anomalies diagnosed antenatally

95 anomalies in 91 cases (% of cases)	Antenatal diagnosis	N = 95
Urological—43 (47%)	Pyelocaliectasis (PUJO)	27
	Posterior urethral valve	9
	Multicystic kidney disease	4
	Polycystic kidney disease	2
	Renal agenesis	1
Gastrointestinal—12 (13%)	Esophageal atresia	1
	Meconium peritonitis	2
	Duplication cyst	1
	Omphalocele	4
	Gastroschisis	2
	Choledochal cyst	2
Cranial—17 (19%)	Hydrocephalus	12
	Dandy-Walker syndrome	2
	Porencephalic cyst	2
	Mega cisterna magna	1
Spinal—10 (11%)	Meningomyelocele	8
	Diastematomyelia	2
Thoracic—7 (8%)	CCAM	3
	CDH	3
	Lung cyst	1
Tumor—3 (3%)	Neuroblastoma	1
	Sacrococcygeal teratoma	1
	Rhabdomyosarcoma	1
Cleft lip		1
Multiple (>2) anomalies		1

Abbreviations: PUJO, pelvi-ureteric junction obstruction; CCAM, congenital cystic adenomatoid malformation; CDH, congenital diaphragmatic hernia

Thus, antenatally detected hydronephrosis resolves in 41–88% (transient hydronephrosis) of the patients. This implies that we really need to distinguish the patient with significant abnormality that will require intervention from those with transient hydronephrosis. This distinction is achieved by monitoring the fetal ultrasound parameters augmented by additional investigations, if required.

Table 34.2 Common causes of fetal hydronephrosis

Etiology	All cases (%)
Transient hydronephrosis	41–88
Pelvi-ureteric junction obstruction	10–30
Vesicoureteric reflux	10–20
Vesicoureteric junction obstruction, megaureter	5–10
Multicystic dysplastic kidney	4–6
Duplex kidneys (±ureterocele)	2–7
Posterior urethral valves	1–2
Others: urethral atresia, urogenital sinus, prune belly syndrome, tumors	Uncommon

Table 34.3 Classification of renal pelvic anteroposterior diameter (APD)

Grade	Second trimester	Third trimester
Mild	4–6 mm	7–9 mm
Moderate	7–10 mm	10–15 mm
Severe	>10 mm	>15 mm

If abnormality is detected on a screening ultrasound, then a more detailed ultrasonic evaluation of the renal system is done. This involves evaluation of renal collecting system, renal size and architecture, parenchymal echogenicity, bladder cycling and amniotic fluid volume. Important finding in the sonographic evaluation of fetal hydronephrosis is the measurement of renal pelvis anteroposterior diameter (APD), which is measured in the transverse axial image of the renal pelvis at the level of the renal hilum. Usually, the degree of hydronephrosis is graded as shown in Table 34.3 as per the Society for Fetal Urology grading.[3] APD is a surrogate marker/measure used to predict potential for disease, but cannot specifically identify pathology. Even severe cases of antenatally detected hydronephrosis (ANH) have the potential to resolve without any postnatal abnormality, while mild degree of ANH can progress into a significant pathology.

Other important things to be evaluated in ultrasound are renal size, parenchymal echogenicity, renal cortical cysts, and corticomedullary differentiation that can herald the presence of renal dysplasia or severe and irreversible damage to the renal unit. Presence of unilateral or bilateral hydronephrosis is an important finding in prognostication (Figs 34.1 and 34.2). Differentiation of obstructive and nonobstructive antenatal hydronephrosis is somewhat possible by evaluation of calyceal anatomy. The most important determinant of fetal well-being and survival is amniotic fluid volume. Amniotic fluid volume is maintained by fetal urine and remains constant throughout the gestation. Oligohydramnios results in pulmonary hypoplasia and compression deformities of the head, thorax, and extremities and is associated with poor prognosis. Presence or absence of other structural anomalies is an important factor in prognostication of these fetuses.

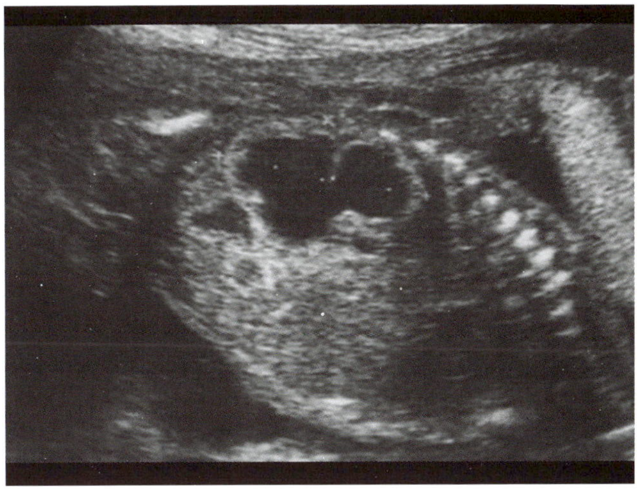

Fig. 34.1 Unilateral severe hydronephrosis

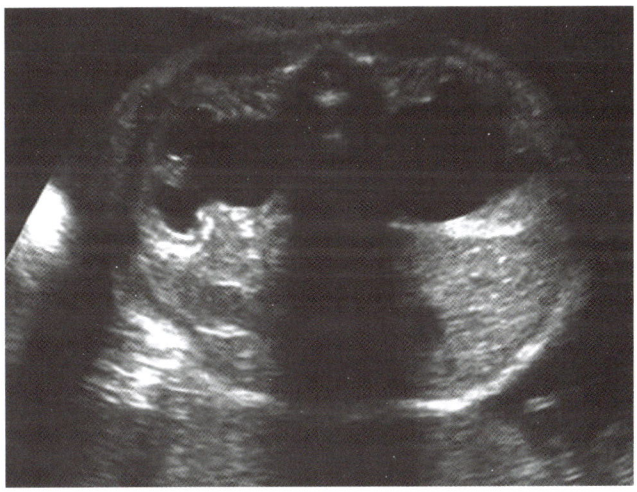

Fig. 34.2 Bilateral severe hydronephrosis

Sometimes further evaluation is required for prognostication. This usually involves evaluation for chromosomal anomalies, usually achieved by chorionic villus sampling, amniocentesis and sampling maternal blood. The other invasive method involved is fetal urine sampling. These invasive methods are rarely used in clinical practice as risk involved needs to be weighed against the benefits.

Natural History of Antenatal Hydronephrosis

If hydronephrosis resolves or improves during the antenatal period, then it is less likely to have significant postnatal sequelae. In contrast, fetuses in whom the hydronephrosis was stable or persistent or worsened during pregnancy, the outcome was variable. There is some correlation of severity of grades of hydronephrosis and subsequent postnatal abnormalities requiring surgical intervention. Underlying diagnosis may be variable, but usually, the trend is for earlier resolution with milder grades of hydronephrosis, with the majority of Society of Fetal Ultrasound (SFU) grade 1–2 hydronephrosis resolving by 18 months of age.[4] Usually fetuses diagnosed in the first trimester with hydronephrosis are more likely to have a poor outcome, whereas those diagnosed during the second trimesters have an overall favorable prognosis. In contrast, those diagnosed in the 3rd trimester appear to have higher rates of postnatally confirmed pathology which may require operative intervention.[5] If hydronephrosis increases, it generally does so in early age, usually in infancy. With higher degrees of hydronephrosis (SFU grade 3–4), severe pathology and surgical intervention are much more common[6]; however, multiple studies have also shown that surgical intervention was required in those with mild degrees of hydronephrosis.[7]

Follow-up and Evaluation during Antenatal Period

If there is isolated unilateral hydronephrosis, at least one follow-up ultrasound in the third trimester is required, whereas fetal ultrasound should be repeated every 4–6 weeks depending on findings of severity of hydronephrosis, when it was detected, and the amount of liquor. Findings suggestive of lower urinary tract obstruction might require even more frequent monitoring.[8] If the diagnosis is uncertain, fetal magnetic resonance imaging (MRI) may provide better anatomical information.

Postnatal Evaluation

All newborns with a history of ANH, irrespective of prenatal resolution, should undergo evaluation by ultrasonography 3–7 days postnatally or before discharge from hospital. But, those suspected to have lower urinary tract obstruction may need more urgent evaluation with first 24–48 hours of life. If the first ultrasound is normal then a repeat ultrasound needs to be done at 4–6 weeks. If two postnatal ultrasounds are normal, it excludes significant renal disease in most of the cases. If the first postnatal ultrasound is abnormal, then the further evaluation depends on the findings of the abnormal ultrasound. Sometimes these infants may need micturating cystourethrogram or nuclear renal scan depending on the findings of the ultrasound.

Postnatal Management

Postnatal management depends on the cause of the antenatal hydronephrosis. Discussion of each cause is beyond the scope of this chapter. But irrespective of cause, the parents of these infants should be counseled about the risk of urinary tract infection and need for prompt treatment. Antibiotic prophylaxis is usually required, if there is suspicion of vesicoureteric reflux, dilated ureters or high-grade hydronephrosis.

Posterior Urethral Valves

Posterior urethral valve (PUV) is the most common cause of lower urinary tract obstruction in male child. Its incidence is noted to be around 1 in 8000–25000 live births.[9] PUV is a common cause for significant morbidity, mortality and continuing renal damage in male infants and children. Treatment of this condition is challenging and starts from infancy (sometimes in utero) to adulthood. The aim of the treatment is to prevent renal damage and deterioration of upper and lower urinary tract. The etiology of PUV is not known, but it appears as a multifactorial gene mediated embryopathy. According to Youngs classification, there are three types of PUV with type 1 being the most common.[10]

Pathophysiology

In the fetus, due to obstruction of urethra, there is severe oligohydramnios or anhydramnios. This compresses fetal thorax and interferes in pulmonary growth. Fetal demise can happen due to significant oligohydramnios, azotemia and pulmonary hypoplasia. PUV causes elongated dilated posterior urethra, bladder muscle hypertrophy and hyperplasia, high intravesical pressure and changes in collagen structure of bladder wall. These changes usually result in high intravesical pressure, high voiding pressures, significant residual urine; and these changes may persist even after ablation of valves. PUV are also associated with vesicoureteric reflux and ureterovesical junction obstruction. These patients also have significant renal damage due to early fetal renal dysplasia or secondary to obstructive uropathy.

Antenatal Evaluation

On antenatal USG, the important signs are distended fetal urinary bladder with dilated proximal urethra, called as the key hole sign (Fig. 34.3). Bladder is thick walled. Amount of liquor is important to note. Fetal bladder tap for urinary electrolytes and beta 2 microglobulin can be done to evaluate fetal renal function.

Postnatal Evaluation

Urgent ultrasonography within first 24–48 hours of life, followed by micturating cystourethrogram should be done. Classic USG findings are thick walled bladder, dilated elongated posterior urethra, unilateral or bilateral hydroureteronephrosis, with or without echogenic kidneys with cysts within. Micturating cystourethrogram will show

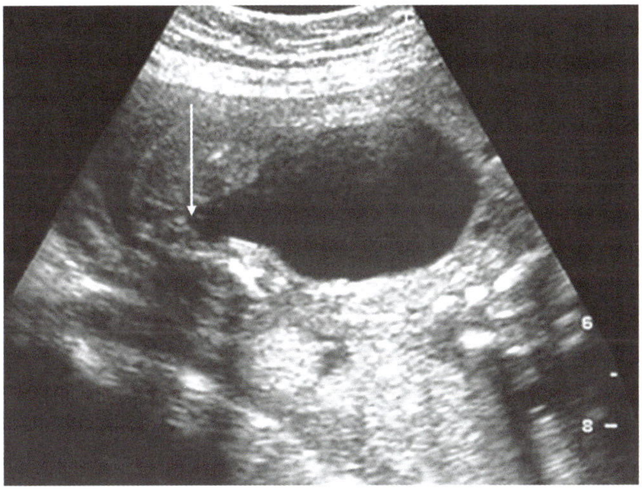

Fig. 34.3 Key hole sign

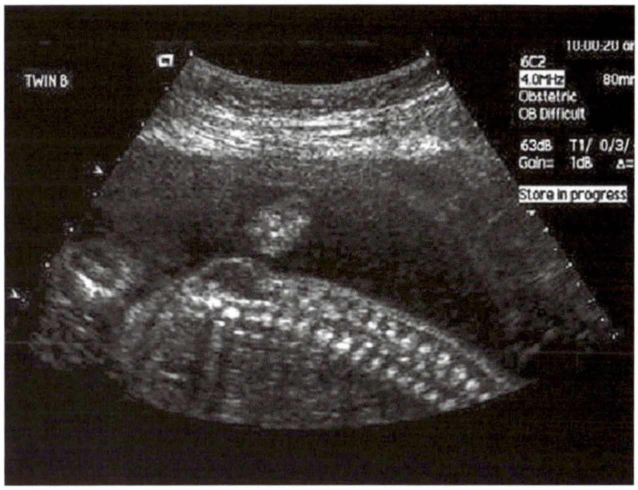

Fig. 34.4 Lumbosacral spinal defect

thickened trabeculated bladder with dilated elongated posterior urethra with bladder neck hypertrophy. Renal function tests should also be done.

Antenatal Interventions

Vesicoamniotic shunt placement, endoscopic fetal valve ablation or fetal vesicostomies are the various options available. Fetal interventions carry significant risk to the fetus and does not change long-term prognosis of renal function despite favorable antenatal features.[11]

Postnatal Interventions

Temporary bladder drainage by catheter with stabilization of neonate followed by valve ablation is a standard treatment care. Urinary diversion is rarely required.

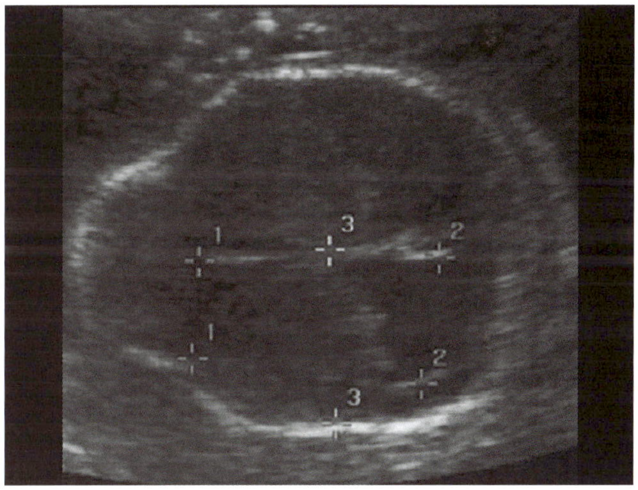

Fig. 34.5 Lemon sign

NEURAL TUBE DEFECT

Introduction

Neural tube defects (NTD) remain the most common congenital malformation in India despite recognition that periconceptional folic acid consumption can decrease the incidence significantly. NTDs result from failure of neural tube closure between 3–4 weeks in embryonic development. NTDs are spectrum of anomalies ranging from anencephaly to open or closed neural tube defect. Myelomeningocele that constitutes extrusion of neural tissue along with meninges is the most common defect.

Pathophysiology

Myelomeningocele results in neurological weakness below the level of lesion, bowel bladder incontinence, and skeletal deformities and is associated with hydrocephalus and Arnold Chiari Malformation. Neurological weakness is permanent and results in lifelong disability.

Antenatal Evaluation

Antenatal ultrasound can show the defect and bulging lesions (Fig. 34.4). Ultrasound signs such as lemon sign and banana sign are also antenatal features of NTDs (Fig. 34.5). Maternal serum alfa fetoproteins and acetylcholinesterase are also used for screening of open neural tube defect.

Postnatal Evaluation

Clinical evaluation for level of lesion and newborn well-being is important. Newborn should be evaluated for associated anomalies. They also need evaluation for presence of hydrocephalus. In later life, they need evaluation for neurogenic bladder.

Treatment

Usually the back lesion closure is performed in 24–72 hours of life. If hydrocephalus is present at birth, then ventriculoperitoneal shunt placement may be required early. They also need future management of hydrocephalus and surgeries for shunt complications. Orthopedic management and physiotherapy for mobility issues is an important part of management. Urologic evaluation for neurogenic bladder and various treatment modalities are done in later life after age of toilet training to achieve social continence. Rehabilitation is an important issue in management of these children.

Role of Fetal Surgery

In recent years, fetal surgery for back lesion closure has come a long way in few centers across the globe. This in utero surgery does not affect postnatal neurologic outcome but decreases the incidence of associated hydrocephalus and its associated complications significantly.

Role of Folic Acid

Role of periconceptional folic acid needs to be recognized. With this simple action, significant decrease in the incidence can be achieved.

Summary

The in utero treatment of myelomeningocele contributes to improved outcomes in children with reduction of hindbrain herniation, less need for VP shunt and enhanced motor outcomes. Further research and improved techniques are still needed to minimize the risks to both the fetus and mother. Future directions include the use of stem cells or biomaterials such as cellulose scaffolds to improve the neurologic outcomes and provide coverage during fetal myelomeningocele repair.[12]

CONGENITAL DIAPHRAGMATIC HERNIA

Introduction

The incidence of congenital diaphragmatic hernia (CDH) is about 1 in 2,200–5,000 livebirths.[13,14] Prenatally diagnosed CDH has mortality of around 50–75%.[15-17] CDH is being more commonly diagnosed antenatally. In the last century, advances in medical management of CDH has improved outcomes, but our ability to diagnose prenatally has not affected the grim prognosis of defects associated with fatal pulmonary hypertension. Fetal interventions for CDH is still under research and not available currently in our country. However, the pediatric surgeon will be asked to counsel families carrying pregnancies complicated by CDH. The fallout of this antenatal diagnosis is usually considering delivery at a tertiary referral center, neonatal intensive care, likelihood of extracorporeal membrane oxygenation (ECMO) and other resuscitative measures, and even termination of the pregnancy.

Diagnostic Modalities and Prognostic Indicators

Fetal Ultrasonography

Presence of diaphragmatic hernia can be confirmed by visualization of abdominal structures at the same level as the four-chamber heart view (Fig. 34.6).[13] In some cases, one can visualize the defect in the diaphragm, making the diagnosis very clear. Differential diagnoses include congenital cystic adenomatoid malformations, pulmonary sequestration, bronchogenic cysts or thoracic teratomas. Various prognostic sonographic markers are used for planning the management of pregnancy and counseling of parent. The presence of liver herniation reproducibly predicts a worse outcome for CDH.[18,19] The lung-to-head ratio (LHR) is another important prognostic indicator. The observed-to-expected ratio for LHR (O/E LHR) based on what the mean expected LHR should be for a specific gestational age in fetuses is more specific marker. Prenatal pulmonary artery (PA) measurements and Doppler waveform analysis are also used for predicting possibility of pulmonary hypertension.

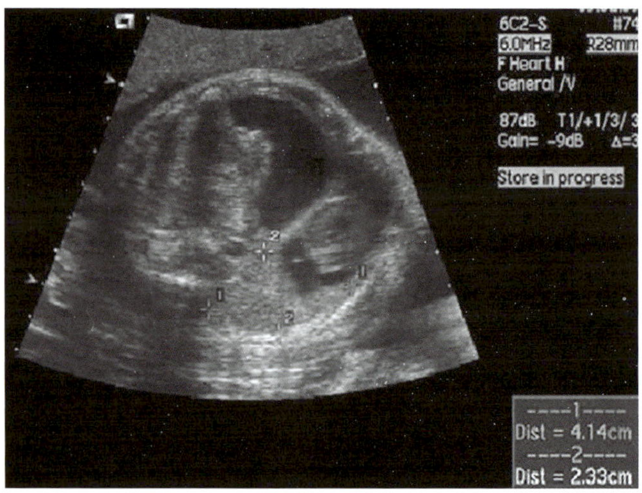

Fig. 34.6 Left diaphragmatic hernia with stomach and small bowel in thorax

Fetal Magnetic Resonance Imaging

In many institutions, fetal MRI is performed at age of diagnosis and late gestation (32–36 weeks). Prenatal MRI easily discriminates between lung, herniated liver, other herniated intra-abdominal organs, and mediastinal structures. The early imaging confirms the presence of CDH, identifying herniated tissue, lung distribution, and associated malformations.[20] Late gestation MRI is primarily obtained for lung volumes analysis. The most important measurement obtained, and studied, by MRI is the percent predicted lung volume (PPLV)—also known as the observed to expected fetal lung volume (O/E FLV).[21,22] Exactly how the PPLV should be interpreted is not agreed upon; there is a lot of variations in cut-off used by various centers.

Imaging for Associated Anomalies

It is important that an assessment be made to determine if there are any associated anomalies, as these have a significant, negative impact on survival. In fact, 95% of stillborns with CDH have an associated anomaly.[23] These anomalies can include congenital heart disease, genitourinary abnormalities, intestinal atresia, bronchopulmonary sequestrations and neurologic defects—most of which can be detected through prenatal ultrasound.[14] Further delineation of suspected anomalies may be better assessed by fetal MRI, especially if this information would impact the management of the pregnancy. Amniocentesis should be offered for karyotyping, as well as comparative genomic hybridization microarray, to identify chromosomal abnormalities. This information may be helpful for families making decisions regarding the pregnancy and postnatal care.

Fetal Interventions

Fetal surgery is offered under investigative protocols to patients who meet certain criteria at selected academic medical centers. Generally, patients deemed appropriate for fetal intervention are those who would not survive with postnatal therapy alone.[24] The three types of fetal surgeries are: (1) open fetal repair, (2) open tracheal occlusion, and (3) fetoscopic tracheal occlusion. Open fetal repair is directed toward open, in utero, repair with one-stage surgical correction of the anatomical defect. Complications after open repair include preterm labor and fetal death. Open tracheal occlusion can be done to promote fetal lung growth. If human fetuses have undergone *in utero* tracheal occlusion, the *ex utero* intrapartum treatment procedure (EXIT) is then used to deliver and intubate the fetus and safely remove the tracheal plug. At present, tracheal occlusion using a clip on the trachea (Fetendo clip), or an intratracheal balloon appears to be the best fetal surgery option.

Outcomes

The vast majority of prenatal evaluations will not be candidates for a fetal intervention; therefore, families will expect counseling on what to anticipate during the neonatal period and beyond. Clinicians should be prepared to have an in-depth discussion with families during prenatal consultation that encompasses worst- and best-case scenarios, operative timing and types of repair, ECMO and long-term outcomes. The immediate post-natal management for CDH is beyond the scope of this text. Survival has been the primary outcome analyzed repeatedly to determine the best strategies for managing CDH; however, CDH covers a broad-spectrum of severity, and it can be difficult to predict which end of the spectrum each case will fall. Overall survival is still quoted at 50%, and if the defect is prenatally diagnosed, mortality may be as high as 75%.[15-17] Survivors are still at risk for other long-term problems.

CONGENITAL LUNG LESIONS

Introduction

Congenital lung lesions (CLLs) comprise a diverse spectrum of pathologic conditions. These conditions range from small cystic lung lesions that are asymptomatic to large lesions which may lead to a lethal outcome in utero. Many of these lesions arise along a spectrum of developmental pathways with the most common being the congenital pulmonary airway malformation (CPAM). CPAM was formerly termed cystic adenomatoid malformation (CCAM). Bronchopulmonary sequestration (BPS) and bronchial atresia should also be considered in the differential for any CLL. The diagnosis and management of these lesions may be challenging in the prenatal period, and some may require urgent fetal intervention.

Associated Anomalies

Congenital pulmonary airway malformations are most sporadiac and usually isolated, but 15–20% of patiets may have associated anomalies, commonly cardiac and renal.[25] Comparatively bronchopulmonary sequestration (BPS) has more common associated anomalies than CPAM. In 40–50% of patients abnormalities of the chest wall, lung, diaphragm, spine, intestine, and heart have been reported. Both these conditions usually do not have association with chromosomal abnormalities.[26,27]

Fetal Imaging for CLLs

The diagnosis and characterization of congenital lung lesion are made primarily by the use of ultrasound. The initial categorization of CLLs is as a solid or cystic mass. Cystic

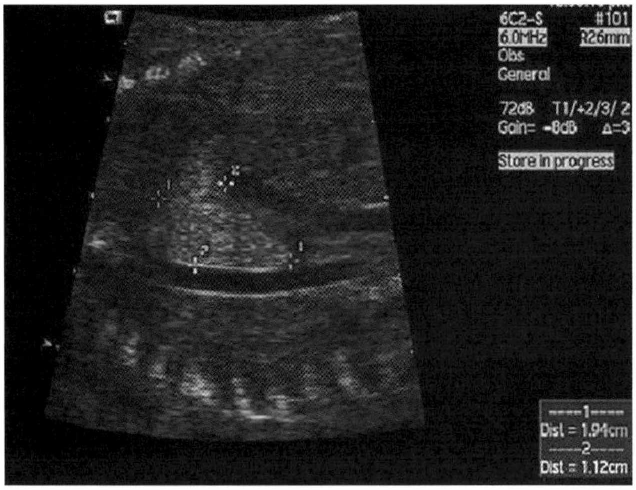

Fig. 34.7 Pulmonary sequestration

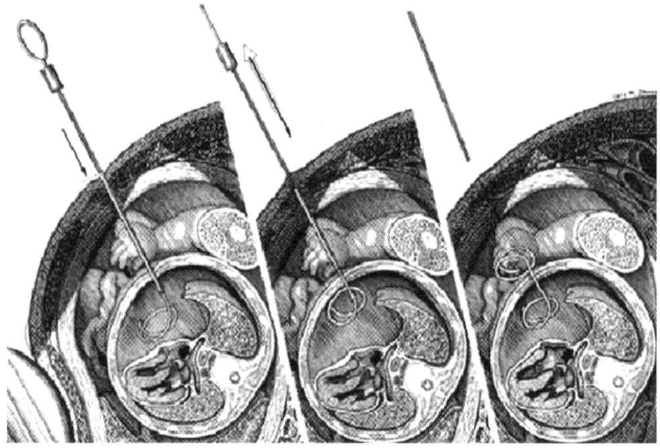

Fig. 34.8 Insertion of a pleuroamniotic shunt

lesions can be macrocystic, microcystic or hybrid lesions (Fig. 34.7). Sequestrations appear as a echogenic solid lesion. Using Doppler, the systemic feeding vessel can often be identified in these lesions. Most centers recommend that fetal patients with CLL should undergo an initial ultrasound. Findings of ultrasound determine the need for fetal MRI and fetal echocardiogram. The CVR (CCAM volume to head circumference ratio), presence of hydrops, mediastinal shift, reversal of flow within the umbilical vein and abnormal cardiac echo are all useful parameters to aid in the determination of whether fetal therapy may be beneficial. Fetal hydrops is often a harbinger of poor fetal or postnatal outcomes. Finally, the presence of placentomegaly (>5 cm in thickness) can be a harbinger of imminent in utero demise.

Fetal Therapy

There are no absolute criteria for fetal intervention; however, fetal therapy is reserved for only the most severe congenital lung lesions (i.e. expect significant respiratory distress at birth or high risk of *in utero* demise). Smaller (CVR < 2.0) lesions or asymptomatic (non-hydropic) larger lesions can be safely followed with weekly or bi-monthly ultrasound. Because certain CLLs can undergo rapid expansion up to 28 weeks, this is a crucial time period to monitor for any changes in the baby's physiologic status. Various fetal interventions/ therapy available are maternal steroids (betamethasone), cyst drainage for large, symptomatic macrocystic disease, use of a thoracoamniotic shunt and open fetal surgery and *ex utero* intrapartum treatment (EXIT). Maternal steroid therapy has been described in several case series, yielding a variable but definite response.[28] Although there are currently no definitive recommendations and no conclusive data to support the use of prenatal steroids for symptomatic CLLs, several centers have independently noted lesion regression and hydrops reversal after administration. Most centers would employ a minimally invasive approach to decompress the large lesions. This can be accomplished via ultrasound-guided cyst aspiration or deployment of a thoraco-amniotic shunt (Fig. 34.8). The use of a thoraco-amniotic shunt has been described with excellent survival rates in patients with macrocystic disease.[29,30] Open fetal surgery has been employed for resection of prenatally diagnosed high-risk lung lesions and can be offered when there is impending fetal demise. These procedures are offered prior to 30 weeks gestation. In patients greater than 30 weeks gestation, the EXIT procedure is used to provide a transition from fetal to postnatal life.

Maternal Mirror Syndrome

A fetus with a large lung mass that has developed hydrops and placentomegaly may also place the mother at significant risk for maternal mirror syndrome.[31] Mirror syndrome is a maternal complication which results in the mother's heath state mirroring that of the fetus. The mother can develop symptoms such as hypertension, vomiting, pulmonary edema and proteinuria. Untreated, these symptoms can progress in severity and can potentially threaten the life of the mother. The only treatment for the severe form of this syndrome is delivery of the baby.[32]

Summary (Indian Scenario)

With the lack of fetal intervention therapies, depending on gestational age, termination of pregnancy can be offered if diagnosed early, especially in the setting of associated anomalies, abnormal karyotype, or early-onset circulatory compromise.

SACROCOCCYGEAL TUMORS

Sacrococcygeal tumor (SCT) is a rare neoplasm that is being diagnosed with increasing frequency in utero. Fetuses with SCT are susceptible to intrauterine fetal demise (IUFD). SCTs can grow to a tremendous size in relation to the fetus and can cause high-output cardiac failure and nonimmune hydrops through vascular shunting. Rarely, tumors can hemorrhage internally or externally, resulting in fetal anemia, hypovolemia and IUFD. Other potential problems for a fetus with a large SCT are dystocia and preterm labor. Delivery can be particularly difficult when the diagnosis has not been made prenatally. A traumatic delivery may result in tumor rupture and/or hemorrhage. Most clinicians favor cesarean delivery for fetuses with large SCTs. Thus, prenatal diagnosis and careful obstetrical planning are critical in the appropriate management of such pregnancies (Figs 34.9 and 34.10).

Tumor Volume to Fetal Weight Ratio

Recent evidence has identified the tumor volume to fetal weight ratio (TFR) as an important prognostic indicator for SCT.[33]

Referral for Prenatal Therapy

The fetus with large SCT has a high risk for mortality especially when associated with nonimmune fetal hydrops. A fetus with SCT and a TFR > 0.12 should be evaluated, monitored closely in an experienced center to determine the need for fetal intervention. SCT interventions to date have included fetal surgery, radiofrequency ablation (RFA) and EXIT-to-resection. Outcomes of fetal intervention are mixed with survival ranging from 38% to 75%.[34,35] Survival in hydropic SCT patients not undergoing fetal intervention is likely <10%.[36] A predominantly cystic lesion may be amenable to percutaneous drainage or shunt placement; however, that is usually unnecessary as cystic SCTs carry a more favorable prognosis. Decompression of a large, cystic SCT may be indicated just prior to delivery to prevent dystocia or to facilitate cesarean delivery. Tumor debulking using percutaneous coagulation techniques such as radiofrequency ablation or laser coagulation to decrease the vascular shunt are minimally invasive alternatives to open resection that have been reported and may warrant further investigation; however, long-term complications noted in the survivors due to injury to adjacent structures demand a better understanding of the application of these techniques for SCTs.[36]

SUMMARY

Fetal diagnosis and counseling has gradually evolved from a niche practice to something that most pediatric surgeons should be involved in to some extent. While very few will be involved in prenatal treatment, most pediatric surgeons will care for anomalies and malformation detected prenatally. This chapter provides concise information about some of the more common fetal anomalies relevant to the pediatric surgeon. Our knowledge needs to be updated as newer diagnostic capabilities and treatment modalities are discovered. Comparisons of fetal versus postnatal surgery must consider the safety of the mother, yet limited comparative data exist. The issue is particularly complicated because while congenital defects are relatively common in aggregate, individual congenital abnormalities occur infrequently, making effective study very difficult.

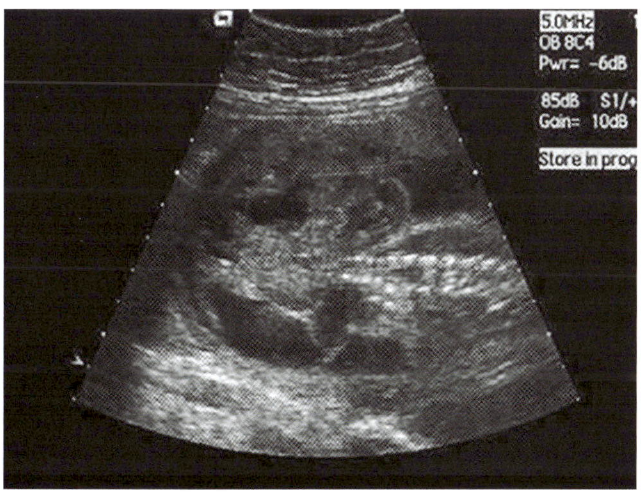

Fig. 34.9 Sacrococcygeal teratoma with solid and cystic elements

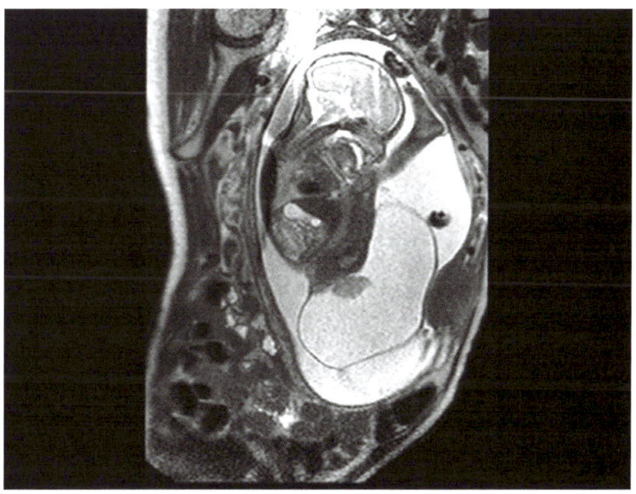

Fig. 34.10 Fetal MRI of sacrococcygeal teratoma

REFERENCES

1. Gupta DK, Sharma S, Gupta M. Outcome of antenatally referred congenital surgical anomalies—a pediatric surgeon's perspective. Journal of Pediatric Surgical Specialties. 2007; 1(1).
2. Nguyen HT, et al. The Society for Fetal Urology consensus statement on the evaluation and management of antenatal hydronephrosis. J Pediatr Urol. 2010; 6:212-31.
3. Nguyen HT, Herndon CD, Cooper C, Gatti J, Kirsch A, Kokorowski P, et al. The Society for Fetal Urology consensus statement on the evaluation and management of antenatal hydronephrosis. J Pediatr Urol. 2010;6:212-31.
4. Mallik M, Watson AR. Antenatally detected urinary tract abnormalities: more detection but less action. Pediatr Nephrol. 2008;23:897.
5. Wollenberg A, Neuhaus TJ, Willi UV, et al. Outcome of fetal renal pelvic dilatation diagnosed during the third trimester. Ultrasound Obstet Gynecol. 2005;25:483.
6. Palmer LS, Maizels M, Cartwright PC, et al. Surgery versus observation for managing obstructive grade 3 to 4 unilateral hydronephrosis: a report from the Society for Fetal Urology. J Urol. 1998;159:222.
7. Noe HN, Magill HL. Progression of mild ureteropelvic junction obstruction in infancy. Urology. 1987;30:348.
8. Sinha A, Bagga A. Revised Guidelines on Management of Antenatal Hydronephrosis. Indian Pediatrics. 2013;50:215.
9. Dinneen MD, Duffy PG (1996). Posterior urethral valves. Br J Urol. 78:275-81.
10. Young HH, Frontz WA, Baldwin JC. Congenital obstruction of the posterior urethra. J Urol. 1919;3:289-65. 2002;167:265-8.
11. Holmes N, Harrison MR, Baskin LS. Fetal surgery for posterior urethral valves: long-term postnatal outcomes. Pediatrics. 2001;108(1):E7.
12. Sanchez e Oliveira Rde C, Valente PR, Abou-Jamra RC, Araujo A, Saldiva PH, Pedreira DA. Biosynthetic cellulose induces the formation of a neoduramater following pre-natal correction of meningomyelocele in fetal sheep. Acta Cir Bras. 2007;22(3):174-81.
13. Chinn DH, Filly RA, Callen PW, et al. Congenital diaphragmatic hernia diagnosed prenatally by ultrasound. Radiology. 1983;148:119-23.
14. Bianchi DW, Crombleholme TM, D'Alton ME, Malone FD (Eds). Fetology, 2nd edn. New York, NY: McGraw-Hill; 2010. pp.278-92.
15. Skari H, Bjornland K, Haugen G, Egeland T, Emblem R. Congenital diaphragmatic hernia: a meta-analysis of mortality factors. J Pediatr Surg. 2000;35:1187-97.
16. Nakayam DK, Harrison MR, Chinn DH, et al. Prenatal diagnosis and natural history of the fetus with congenital diaphragmatic hernia: initial clinical experience. J Pediatr Surg. 1985;20: 118-24.
17. Adzick NS, Vacanti JP, Lillehei CW, et al. Fetal diaphragmatic hernia: ultrasound diagnosis and clinical outcome in 38 cases from a single medical center. J Pediatr Surg. 1981;24:654-60.
18. Harrison MR, Langer JC, Adzick NS, et al. Correction of congenital diaphragmatic hernia *in utero*. V Initial Clinical Experience. J Pediatr Surg. 1990;25:47-55.
19. Deprest JA, Hyett JA, Flake AW, et al. Current controversies in prenatal diagnosis 4: should fetal surgery be done in all cases of severe diaphragmatic hernia. J Pediatr Surg. 2009;29:15-9.
20. Leung JWT, Coakley FV, Hricak H, et al. Prenatal MR imaging of congenital diaphragmatic hernia. AJR Am J Roentgenol. 2000;174:1607-12.
21. Mahieu-Caputo D, Sonigo P, Dommergues M, et al. Fetal lung volume measurement by magnetic resonance imaging in congenital diaphragmatic hernia. J Obstet Gynecol. 2001;108: 863-8.
22. Victoria T, Bebbington MW, Danzer E, et al. Use of magnetic resonance imaging in prenatal prognosis of the fetus with isolated left congenital diaphragmatic hernia. Prenatal Diagnosis. 2012;32:715-23.
23. Puri P, Gorman F. Lethal nonpulmonary anomalies associated with congenital diaphragmatic hernia: implications for early intrauterine surgery. J Pediatr Surg. 1984;19:29-35.
24. Cass DL. Fetal surgery for congenital diaphragmatic hernia: the North American experience. Semin Perinatol. 2005;29(2):104-11.
25. Laje P, Liechty KW. Postnatal management and outcome of prenatally diagnosed lung lesions. Prenat Diagn. 2008;28:612-8.
26. Azizkhan RG, Crombleholme TM. Congenital cystic lung disease: contemporary antenatal and postnatal management. Pediatr Surg Int. 2008;24:643-57.
27. Wilson RD, Hedrick HL, Liechty KW, et al. Cystic adenomatoid malformation of the lung: review of genetics, prenatal diagnosis, and *in utero* treatment. Am J Med Genet A. 2006;140:151-5.
28. Curran PF, Jelin EB, Rand L, Hirose S, Feldstein VA, Goldstein RB, et al. Prenatal steroids for microcystic congenital cystic adenomatoid malformations. J Pediatr Surg. 2010;45(1):145-50.
29. Wilson RD, Baxter JK, Johnson MP, King M, Kasperski S, Crombleholme TM, Flake AW, Hedrick HL, Howell LJ, et al. Thoracoamniotic shunts: fetal treatment of pleural effusions and congenital cystic adenomatoid malformations. Fetal Diagn Ther. 2004;19(5):413-20.
30. Schrey S, Kelly EN, Langer JC, Davies GA, Windrim R, Seaward PG, et al. Fetal thoracoamniotic shunting for large macrocystic congenital cystic adenomatoid malformations of the lung. Ultrasound Obstet Gynecol. 2012;39(5):515-20.
31. Adzick NS, Harrison MR, Crombleholme TM, et al. Fetal lung lesions: management and outcome. Am J Obstet Gynecol. 1998;179(4):884-9.
32. Braun T, Brauer M, Fuchs I, Czernik C, Dudenhausen JW, Henrich W, et al. Mirror syndrome: a systematic review of fetal associated conditions, maternal presentation and perinatal outcome. Fetal Diagn Ther. 2010;27(4):191-203.
33. Rodriguez MA, Cass DL, Lazar DA, et al. Tumor volume to fetal weight ratio as an early prognostic classification in fetal sacrococcygeal teratoma. J Pediatr Surg. 2011;46:1182-5.
34. Hedrick HL, Flake AW, Crombleholme TM, et al. Sacrococcygeal teratoma: Prenatal assessment, fetal intervention, and outcome. J Pediatr Surg. 2004;39:430-8.
35. Adzick NS. Open fetal surgery for life-threatening fetal anomalies. Semin Fetal Neonatal Med. 2010;15:1-8.
36. Ruano R, Duarte S, Zugaib M. Percutaneous laser ablation of sacrococcygeal teratoma in a hydropic fetus with severe heart failure - too late for a surgical procedure? Fetal Diagn Ther. 2009;25:26-30.

CHAPTER

35 Prenatal Diagnosis and Postnatal Therapy of Surgical Anomalies

Vivek Rege

The availability of excellent sonography machines and extremely well trained Sonologists to interpret individual findings, the detection of surgical anomalies in a fetus has become routine. The frequency of major birth defects is about 3% in live newborns. Of these defects, more than 50% affect the central nervous system (CNS), about 20% are genitourinary; 15% are of the gastrointestinal tract; and 8% are cardiovascular. Today, we are able to pick-up surgical defects earlier and more accurately than before.[1] This has led to a number of ways to counsel the parents:

- The choice to continue the pregnancy or terminate it in case of a poor prognostic anomaly like anencephaly
- The timing of the delivery by the obstetrician, i.e. to go in for an early induced labor, or allow the pregnancy to proceed to term and then deliver the fetus
- The mode of delivery, i.e. a normal vaginal delivery or an elective cesarean
- The place of delivery, i.e. either a major institute or hospital with all facilities to treat a critical neonate immediately after birth, or a smaller nursing home.

The nature of the defect or anomaly also determines the perinatal management.[1]

Defects managed by elective termination of pregnancy (< 20 weeks)

- Anencephaly, hydrancephaly
- Severe and poor prognostic chromosomal defects like Trisomy 13
- Bilateral renal agenesis, infantile polycystic kidney disease (IPKD)
- Severe untreatable inherited metabolic disorders (Tay-Sachs Disease)
- Lethal bone dysplasia (Thanatophoric dysplasia)

Defects requiring induced preterm delivery

- Progressive hydronephrosis
- Progressive hydrocephalus
- Gastroschisis or ruptured omphalocele
- Intestinal ischemia and necrosis (Volvulus)
- Immune hydrops fetalis.

Defects requiring cesarean section delivery

- Conjoined twins
- Giant omphalocele, gastroschisis
- Large sacrococcygeal teratoma or cervical cystic hygroma.

Defects requiring correction after term delivery

- Esophageal, intestinal, anorectal atresias
- Enteric duplications and cysts
- Meconium ileus
- Small intact omphalocele
- Small intact meningomyelocele, spina bifida
- Unilateral multicystic dysplastic kidney, hydronephrosis
- Simple cystic hygroma, sacrococcygeal teratoma
- Benign cysts—choledochal, ovarian, mesenteric

Defects that may require EXIT procedure

- Congenital high airway obstruction syndrome
- Large cervical tumor, e.g. teratoma
- Mass obstructing trachea or mouth, e.g. cystic hygroma
- Conditions that may require immediate extracorporeal membrane oxygenation (ECMO) cannulation
- Chest mass preventing lung expansion.

The importance of detection of these surgical anomalies early is:

- Prognosis of the child can be given based on the gestation and severity
- Follow-up with progress or regress of the defect on the system with gestation
- Rate of progress of defect like hydronephrosis—slow, moderate or rapid
- Indications for fetal intervention and what form it should be
- Guidelines for other investigations like alpha-fetoprotein (AFP), karyotype, etc.

- Counseling for the present pregnancy, follow-up; future pregnancy recurrence.

There are also the disadvantages of prenatal sonography:[1]

- Misuse for sex determination and female feticide
- *Error in diagnosis*: Diaphragmatic hernia—lung cyst; duodenal dilated/hydronephrosis
- Missing of other system anomalies while concentrating on the one detected
- *Error in judgment*: Not all meningomyelocele may be paraplegic/incontinent

Considering all the above factors, the ideal thing to do is to send the pregnant lady to a well-trained Sonologist at 14th–16th week of gestation specifically for fetal anomaly screening to look for any of the anatomical defects that can be picked up, since:

- Almost all anomalies can be detected as they have been formed embryologically
- There is adequate amniotic fluid by now for the Sonologist to pick-up defect(s)
- A second opinion may be taken in case of doubt to confirm the defect(s)
- Prognosis and progress can be followed up by a second scan after 3 weeks
- Time is available to the family to take a decision regarding continuing the pregnancy with regular follow-up as advised, or termination after proper counseling (legal limit 20 weeks)
- This has definitely improved the approach and the results of many surgical anomalies in terms of mortality and morbidity.

FETAL INTERVENTION

This is being done for very selected indications in fetuses in few centers abroad. However, in India only 1 or 2 centers have been doing limited fetal intervention with mixed results. These procedures are dangerous for both the fetus as well as the mothers, and hence only highly trained; dedicated teams are doing these interventions and have a number of cases to show their results. Since, we do not do these procedures writing about them would be theoretical. I shall write about postnatal interventions in antenatally diagnosed surgical defects.

In this Chapter, one shall be mainly writing about postnatal interventions in antenatally diagnosed surgical defects. I propose to write by anomaly. It would be difficult to cover all possible surgical defects, so I propose to cover only some important, common anomalies and their postnatal approach in short here.

The various surgical anomalies detectable antenatally are:

Gastrointestinal
Intestinal atresias:
Esophageal, pyloric, jejunal, ileal,
Abdominal wall defects:
Omphalocele, Gastroschisis
Duplications/Cysts:
Intestinal, mesenteric, choledochal
Meconium ileus, peritonitis

Genitourinary
Renal: Agenesis, dysplasia, hydronephrosis, tumor
Ureteral: Dilatation, duplication, ureterocele
Bladder: Obstructed, diverticulum, urachal anomalies
Urethra: Valves, megaurethra

Central nervous system
Anencephaly
Hydrancephaly,
Holoprosencephaly
Choroid plexus cyst
Hydrocephalus, Dandy-Walker cyst
Encephalocele
Meningomyelocele, Diastematomyelia

Chest:
Congenital cystic, adenomatoid malformation
Diaphragmatic hernia
Cardiac anomalies: Vessels, valves
Cystic hygroma

Miscellaneous:
Sacrococcygeal teratoma
Cystic hygroma neck, axilla
thyromegaly

PRENATAL DIAGNOSIS AND APPROACH TO DIAPHRAGMATIC HERNIA

Diaphragmatic Hernia

Definition: This is a group of diaphragmatic defects in which some portion of the abdominal contents protrude into the chest cavity-frequently through a posterolateral or retrosternal defect.

This defect can be easily picked up a well-trained sonologist.[1]

Sonography (Fig. 35.1)

Fetus: A *left sided* diaphragmatic hernia may show the following:

- Deviation of the heart to the right side
- Stomach is in the chest alongside the heart (best seen transverse section)
- Liver may also be partially in the chest

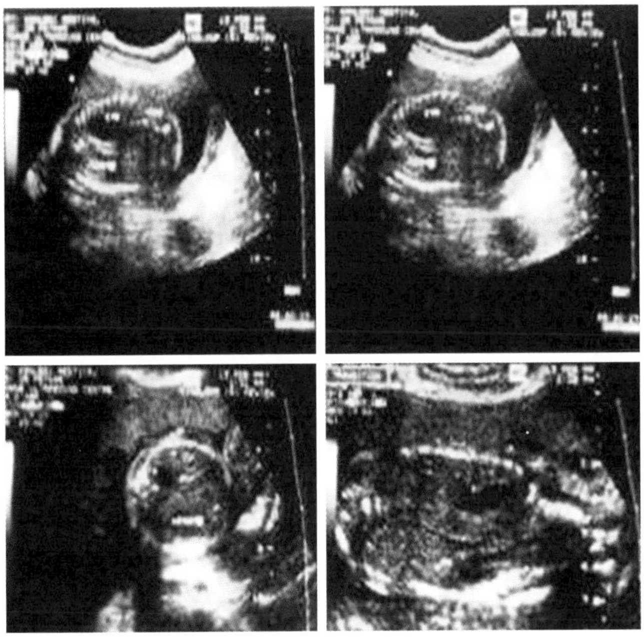

Fig. 35.1 Ultrasound: diaphragmatic hernia

- *Small bowel in the chest has a mottled pattern*: May look like lung
- Peristalsis seen in the chest
- Left diaphragm may not be clearly demarcated and visible

A *right sided* diaphragmatic hernia may show the following:

- Heart deviated to the left
- Liver seen in the chest
- Possible to see lung—liver interface above site of normal diaphragm
- Stomach alignment is abnormal; stomach towards right and horizontal
- Portal vessels can be tracked within the liver into the chest

Amniotic fluid: Usually the amniotic fluid volume is normal, unless bowel is obstructed in which case there is polyhydramnios. This may be correlated with pulmonary hypoplasia and hence is a bad prognostic sign.

Placenta: Usually no abnormality is seen.

Pitfalls in Diagnosis

Lung changes are easily overlooked, especially if stomach is in abdomen may be diagnosed as dextrocardia as lung changes may be subtle. Heart may be difficult to examine in presence of hernia.

Cystic adenomatoid disease may be missed for diaphragmatic hernia.

Prognostic Features of Diaphragmatic Hernia Diagnosed Antenatally

This is very important for counseling the parents for the future of this fetus—to predict the prognosis of the defect and allowing them to take a decision based on them[2]

- Diaphragmatic hernia detected before 24 weeks of gestation has shown to have a very poor prognosis—with a high chance of bilateral pulmonary hypoplasia. Those detected first beyond 24 weeks and nearer to term have a far better outcome post-delivery with better lung function[2]
- Liver found to be in the thoracic cavity is again a very poor prognostic sign, the survival in many series was only 43% vs 93% in those who had their liver down
- Chromosomal disorder like trisomy and/or associated major anomalies shows a poor prognosis from both short-term and long-term survival
- Bilateral diaphragmatic hernia has worse prognosis than unilateral and in unilateral right side has a worse prognosis than the left side
- Presence of polyhydramnios was shown in series to have a poorer prognosis since in most lung hypoplasia was associated
- Stomach up in the chest was a poor prognostic sign in some series with only 11% survival, but was not so in other series which showed no difference
- *Lung to head ratio (LHR)*: If this ratio is low, i.e. < 1 this was a poor prognosis, however, a ratio >1.35 is an excellent prognosis. LHR between 0.9 and 1.4 shows 80% survival, if the mother is delivered at a tertiary care center.[3,4]
- Mediastinal shift at level of atria on transverse scan is also important prognostically—severe shift—poor prognosis
- Under development of the left side heart is shown to have a poor prognosis
- Abdominal circumference below the 5th percentile is also considered a poor prognostic sign

This knowledge of the prognostic criteria is extremely useful in counseling the patient, and also when it comes to treating these critical newborns soon after birth. The approach to the type, time and place of delivery varies with the severity of the defect. In selected centers abroad, there have been numerous mothers who have undergone fetal interventions during their pregnancy for a prenatally diagnosed diaphragmatic hernia.

The basis of antenatal diagnosis in fetuses with diaphragmatic hernia is multiple:

- Prognostic evaluation depending on the various factors[4]
- Termination of pregnancy if detected before 20 weeks of gestation

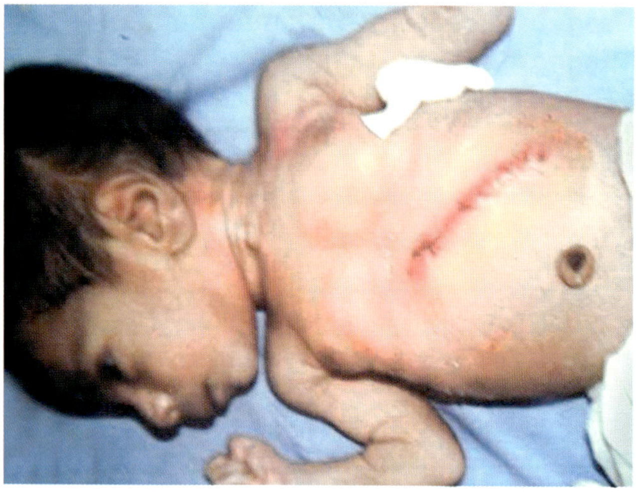

Fig. 35.2 Neonate postoperative

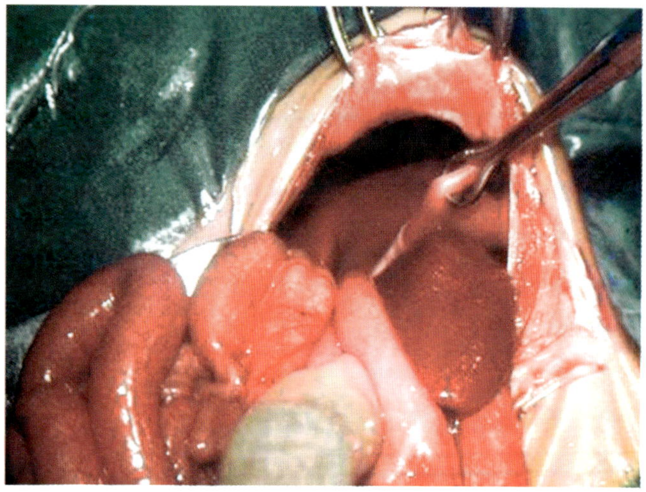

Fig. 35.3 Intraoperative defect seen

- *If too late for termination*: Look for other anomalies and chromosomal defects
- Fresh USG every 4 weeks for follow-up, with measurements of LHR
- Advice regarding delivery is the most important in India, at least this must be done, i.e. the mother is asked to be admitted in a tertiary care center where all facilities for neonatal intensive care unit (NICU), neonatal surgeon are available for the newborn immediately after birth and no risk of transportation of the critical child from a smaller hospital to a proper center.
- Immediate resuscitation after normal delivery (no need for a cesarean section)
- Stabilization of the newborn either with plain oxygen (by hood), or ventilator if necessary till parameters are within normal limits like the pO_2, pCO_2, ventilatory index. Other investigations to look for other anomalies—like plain X-ray chest, 2D echo, sonography to look for anomalies in kidneys, ureters, bladder, Doppler for looking at the diameter of the 2 pulmonary arteries, etc. Oxygen should *never* be administered by mask in a newborn with suspected diaphragmatic hernia as it may cause the child to swallow the air and distend the stomach and cause further respiratory distress. Insertion of an infant feeding tube to decompress the bowel is a must very early after birth to prevent abdominal distension, vomiting or aspiration of the bowel contents into the already poor lungs (Fig. 35.2).
- Child is taken up for surgery only after some stabilization to get the best results. At times we may have to put the child on a high frequency ventilator to keep the pressure very low. The biggest problem with ventilators in diaphragmatic hernia is pneumothorax following high pressures used in order to get proper oxygen values. Nitric oxide has also been used successfully in few cases here.
- Surgical correction of the defect has to be done based on the findings, either by primary interrupted sutures to close the defect, or, if the defect is very wide, by putting a patch—mesh and suturing it in place with sutures after reduction of the bowel and other contents (if any). Look for malrotation of the gut as it is associated with diaphragmatic hernia (Fig. 35.3).
- Postoperatively too, this child must be kept on a ventilator for about 3 days and gradually weaned off as the child is able to breathe on its own and is maintaining oxygen levels. Intravenous antibiotics and fluids need to be given for 10–15 days depending on how fast or slow is the recovery of the child after the surgical procedure.

INTESTINAL OBSTRUCTION

This is commonly picked up on antenatal ultrasonography as dilated bowel loops and this should be a clue to look for intestinal obstruction (Fig. 35.4).

Advantages of early prenatal diagnosis[1]

- Prepared for early surgery soon after confirming diagram.
- Management begins before occurrence of vomiting and aspiration
- Management of electrolyte imbalance is minimum
- Early surgery when child is in best condition
- Better convalescence and result

Once you know that this fetus is having some obstruction in bowels depending on the number of loops seen, we may be able to predict high bowel obstruction, or low bowel

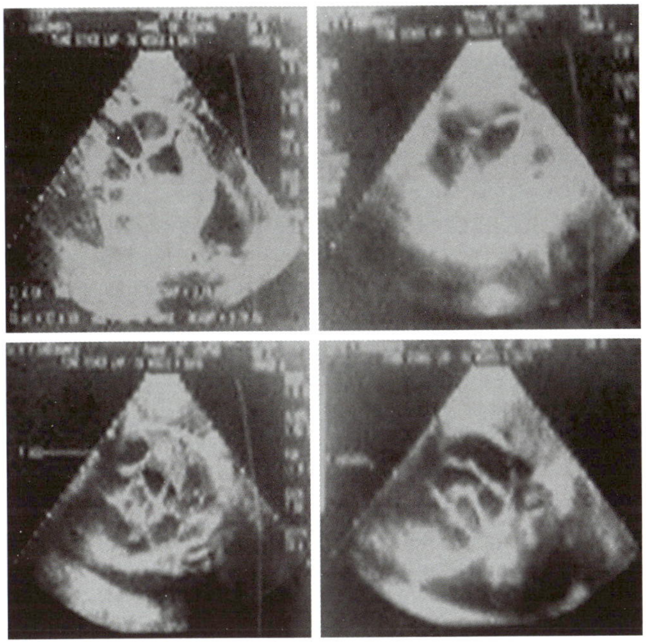

Fig. 35.4 Antenatal dilated bowel

obstruction. Prenatally, if there is polyhydramnios, and few dilated loops it is more in favor of high bowel obstruction. Multiple loops and no polyhydramnios is in favor of low or distal bowel obstruction.

Postnatally

- Clinical examination for distension, but also rule out anorectal malformation
- Insertion of nasogastric (NG) tube and aspiration to avoid aspiration
- *Investigate for surgery*: Electrolytes, blood group, complete blood count (CBC)
- Inject 20–30 mL air through NG tube for contrast X-ray abdominal and look for number of air fluid levels
- If two bubbles—think of duodenal atresia, if more than two but less than 4 jejunal atresia, if more than 6 air fluid levels, think of distal ileal or colonic; if one large fluid level more than half the abdomen, think of pouch colon with atresia.
- Exploration of neonate within 24 hours if possible to relieve the obstruction.
- Surgical correction—depending on the exact type and location of atresia resection and anastamosis (Fig. 35.5)
- *Postoperative:* Nil orally, intravenous fluids, antibiotics hyperalimentation, oral feeds in 6 days
- Child can be discharged soon after tolerating oral milk feeds (Fig. 35.6).

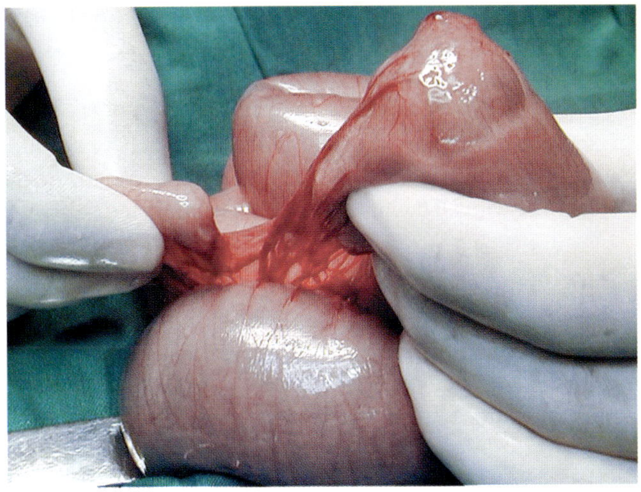

Fig. 35.5 Bowel atresia

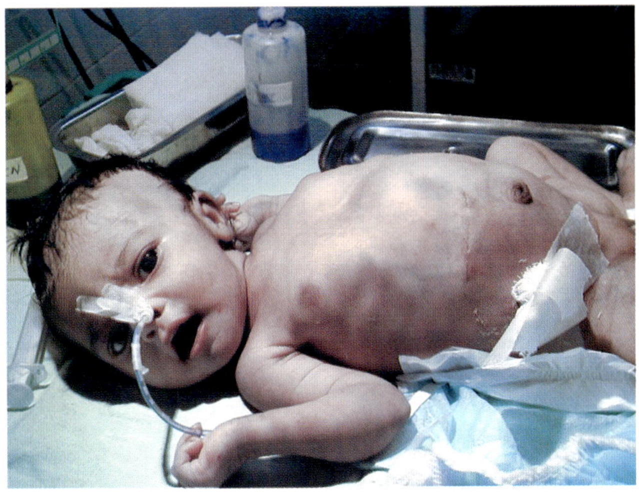

Fig. 35.6 Postoperative

Abdominal Wall Defects (Exomphalos/ Gastroschisis)

These are conditions in which there is a defect in the anterior abdominal wall of the fetus, both of which must be picked up prenatally and prognosis can be estimated on a number of factors including the actual defect, associated anomalies, other genetic syndromes, etc.[5]

Exomphalos diagnosed:

- *USG*: Abdominal wall defect (Fig. 35.7)
  - *Contents*: Bowel/fluid/liver
  - Presence of associated diaphragmatic hernia
- *Amniocentesis*: Chromosomal anomalies Trisomy 13,18,21

- *Associated anomalies*: Coronary heart disease (CHD), renal, beckwith, skeletal dysplasia, pentalogy
- *Polyhydramnios*: Poor prognosis
- *USG*: 4 weekly for growth
- Shift mother to proper center/institute for delivery would be ideal as it is easier to shift a pregnant woman to an institute with all facilities than a critical neonate.

Regarding delivery the approach should be

- Elective cesarean section delivery—though not recommended in western countries, but in view of our conditions and facilities, may be preferable
- Shift to NICU—detailed clinical assessment (Fig. 35.8)
- Avoid trauma and contamination of sac
- Infant feeding tube—decompress upper gastrointestinal (GI)

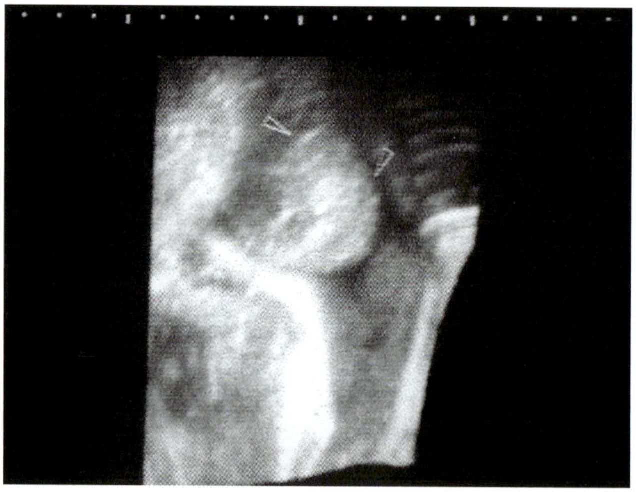

Fig. 35.7 Antenatal USG—exomphalos

- Reliable intravenous access—antibiotics, fluids, blood biochemistry
- *Investigations*: 2D echo, ultrasound-kidneys, ureters, bladder (KUB)

Postnatal approach recommended is[6]

- Warm saline and betadine soaks on exposed parts
- Hold the sac and contents vertical—prevent drag mes
- Wrap with Gladwrap—prevent desiccation and infection
- Plain X-ray chest-abdomen: rule out diaphragmatic hernia
- Investigate for surgery: Electrolytes, CBC, Blood sugar
- Insertion of NG tube and upper GI decompression
- Warm saline bowel irrigation for lower GI decompression.

SPECIFIC THERAPY

- *Conservative*: Local application betadine solution gauze
- *Conservative*: Excision of membrane and Silo
- Excision of membrane and skin closure over bowels, later repair of umbilical hernia after a year or so.
- Excision of membrane, reduction of contents, primary closure (Fig. 35.9)
- *Postoperative*: Nil orally, antibiotics, ventilator, hyperalimentation. Oral feeds gradually.

Gastroschisis

- *USG*: Abdominal wall defect
- Contents-Usually only bowels
- *Polyhydramnios; look for intestinal atresia-associated anomaly*: dilated loops
- Look for intrauterine growth restriction (IUGR) as pregnancy progresses
- Dilated bowels not good prognosis[6]

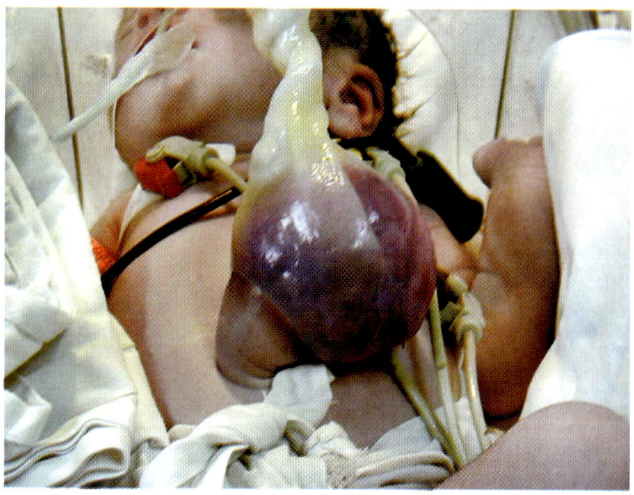

Fig. 35.8 Neonate exomphalos

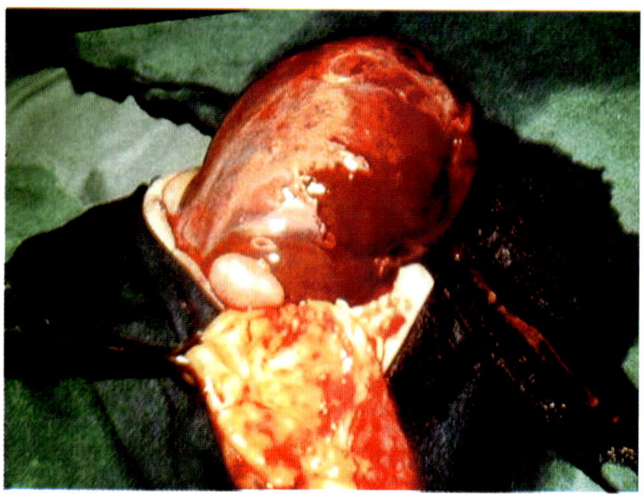

Fig. 35.9 Intraoperative exomphalos

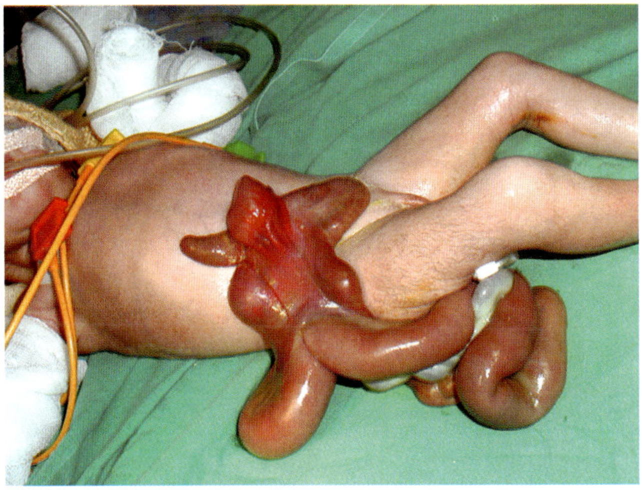

Fig. 35.10 Gastroschisis

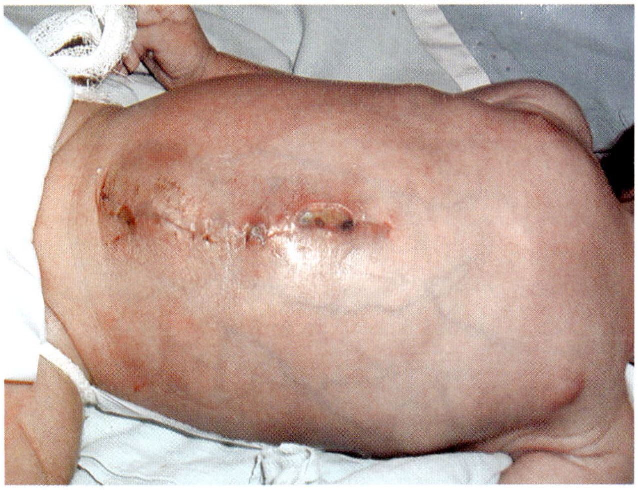

Fig. 35.11 Postoperative gastroschisis

- Chromosomal/associated anomalies rare unlike exomphalos
- Shift mother to proper center/institute for delivery
- High incidence of atresia of intestine.

Delivery and postnatal management:

- Elective cesarean section delivery—early/term better suited for our conditions
- Shift to NICU—detailed clinical assessment (Fig. 35.10)
- Avoid trauma and contamination—plastic wrap
- Infant feeding tube-decompress upper GI tract easy reduction
- Rectal warm saline irrigation—decompress lower GI
- *Reliable intravenous access*: Antibiotics, fluids, plasma, biochemistry.

The definitive therapy would be:

- Single stage closure primary
- Delayed primary closure
- Postoperative ventilator, intravenous fluids, antibiotics, parenteral hyperalimentation
- Prolonged ileus-hyperalimentation
- Oral feeds gradually begun and slowly progressed
- Wound care till healing complete to see for dehiscence or herniation (Fig. 35.11)

Sacrococcygeal Teratoma

This is another obvious anomaly that can be detected of which 47% are located externally, 34% are external with some components in the pelvic presacral space, 19% are located only within the pelvic cavity in front of the sacrum.[7] Of these tumors, 80% are benign, but 20% are undifferentiated and malignant. More commonly seen in girls ratio of males to females is 1:3 (Fig. 35.12).

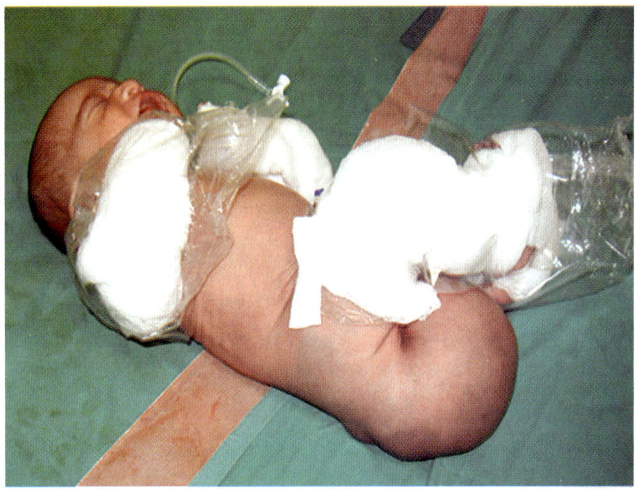

Fig. 35.12 Sacrococcygeal teratoma

Ultrasound findings: Lesion seen at the distal end of the vertebral column, that may appear to be a cystic, partly solid or purely solid lesion. Calcifications may be detected. Tumors as described above may be external, partially internal or rarely even presacral.

Prognosis is based on all these factors, cystic are usually benign, calcification also likely to be benign. Blood flow patterns are also vital for anticipating complications

Problems inherent

- Mortality > 50% neonatal-5% especially large vascular tumors
- AV shunting—hyperdynamic circulation congestive cardiac failure (CCF), maternal mirror syndrome
- Polyhydramnios-preterm labor and delivery
- Alfa fetoproteins levels also show differentiated or not.

- Nonimmune hydrops common—poor prognosis if develops before 28 weeks
- Serial monitoring of fetus vital for increase in hydrops poor prognosis
- *Watch for disseminated intravascular coagulation (DIC) after birth*: Bleeding, trauma during delivery, tumor rupture.

Postnatal approach:
- Delivery at an Institute with facilities and back up for surgery and critical care
- May require early delivery if severe as shunting in lesion[8]
- USG to get dimensions of tumor, extent, vascularity, arteriovenous shunting, etc.
- Rule out DIC, other anomalies, control CCF
- Early devascularization internal iliac artery and the middle sacral artery
- Staged resection of the tumor, or complete excision in one stage if compact
- Sacrococcygeal teratomas overall 7% malignant at birth if detected or treated late, by 2 years 50% are malignant thus, it is a dynamic situation and early surgery is required.

Urological Anomalies

These are one of the most common anomalies picked up antenatally and need to be followed up properly and systematically to come to a proper diagnosis and then planned therapy[9]
- 50% of all antenatally diagnosed lesions are urological
- 50% of all antenatally diagnosed urinary tract dilatations are pelvi-ureteric junction (PUJ) obstructions
- Obstructive urological anomalies are common in males ratio of M:F is 4:1; left side is more common (Figs 35.13 and 35.14).
- Bilateral PUJ obstruction may be present 21–36%
- Multicystic dysplastic kidney (MCDK) has contralateral PUJ obstruction.

Whenever a renal anomaly is detected it should be looked at in to
- Is it unilateral or bilateral
- Is there oligohydramnios and if so when was it detected early gestation or late
- *Severity of renal parenchyma damage*: Bright/multiple cysts, etc.[10]
- Presence of associated ascites—urinary ascites
- Serial scans at 3–4 weeks interval to detect progress (if any) and whether rapid or slow
- Details of the parenchymal thickness and progress, bladder size large or small.

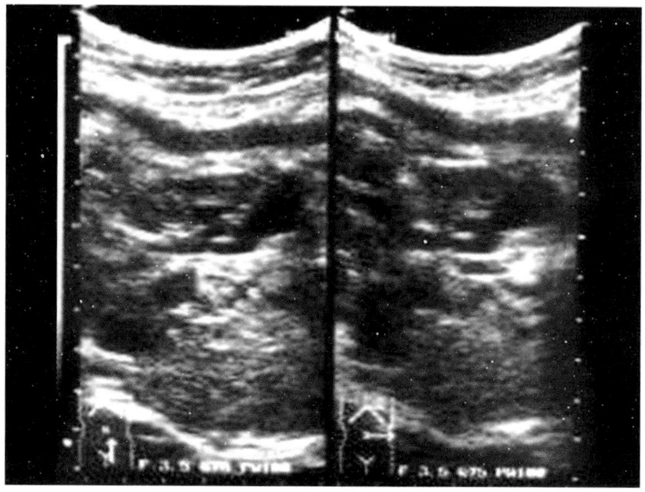

Fig. 35.13 Hydroureteronephrosis

The goals of treatment of renal anomalies are:
- Differential diagnosis of anomaly
- Look for associated anomalies of other systems
- Assess risk/prognosis for the fetus/neonate
- Begin therapy early and preserve renal function, prevent infection.

A broad clarity of possible diagnosis in bilateral hydronephrosis is correlated with size of the bladder as follows:

Normal bladder
- PUJ obstruction
- Multicystic kidney
- Retrocaval ureter
- Primary obstructive megaureter
- Nonrefluxing, nonobstructive megaureter
- Mid ureteral stricture
- Bilateral vesicoureteral reflux (VUR)

Distended bladder
- VUR
- Ectopic ureterocele
- Posterior urethral valves (PUV)
- Prune Belly Syndrome
- Urethral Atresia
- Hydrocolpos
- Pelvic Tumor Cloacal Anomaly

Follow-up of a detected renal anomaly will be done as follows:
- Follow-up progress
- Size of the renal pelvis–anteroposterior (AP) diameter; parenchymal thickness
- *Ratio of renal pelvis*: Kidney
- Amniotic fluid index (AFI)
- Renal function tests: Urinary electrolytes
Urine output
Beta-2 microglobulin levels

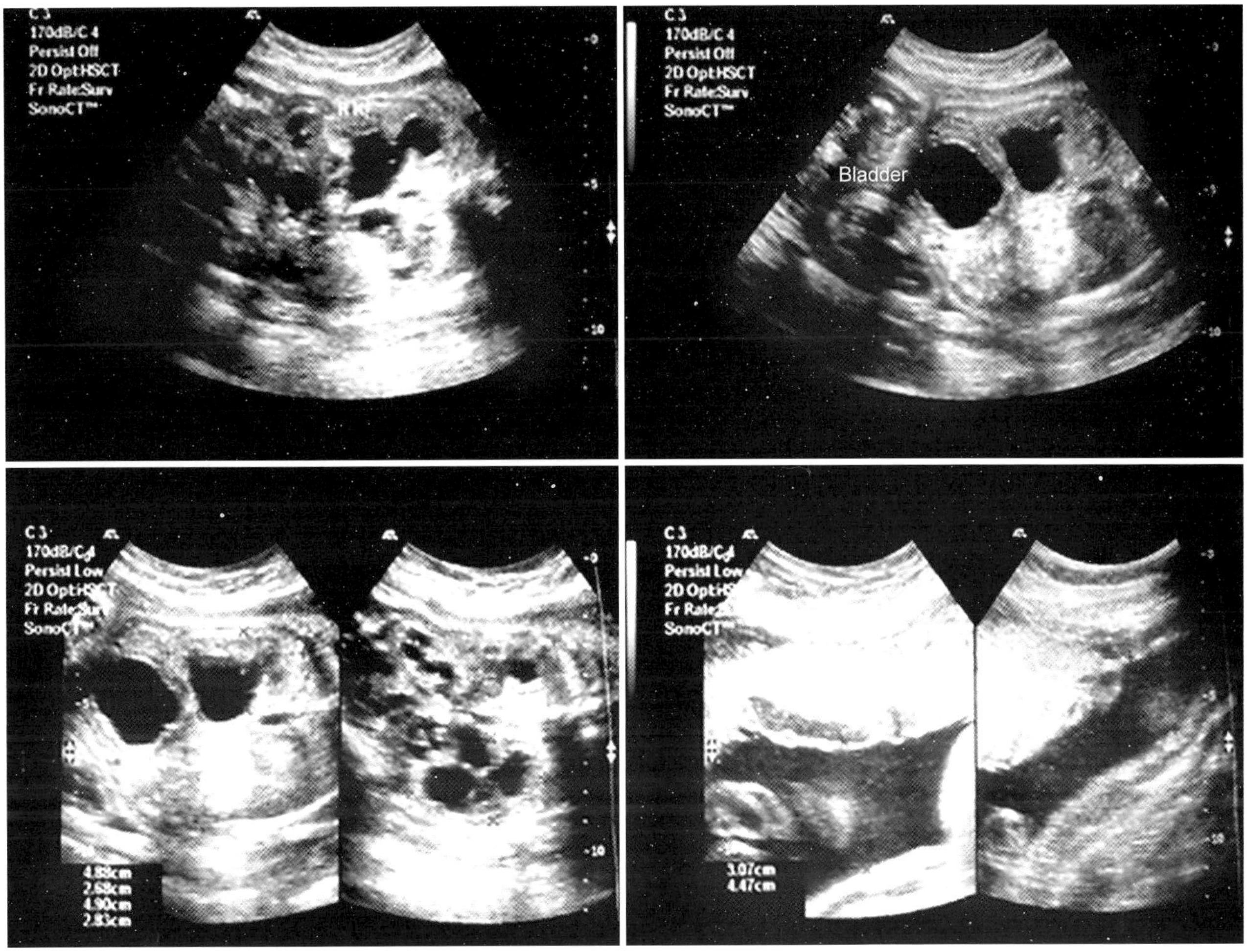

Fig. 35.14 Hydronephrosis

Overall prognosis of a particular case of renal anomaly can be assessed as:

- Prolonged oligohydramnios—bad prognosis
- Bilateral—worse than unilateral
- Bright kidneys both sides poor prognosis[11]
- Parenchyma thickness (thin)/cortical cysts poor prognosis
- Loss of corticomedullary differentiation
- Age at diagnosis <24 weeks
- Ascites and other anomalies present—poor prognosis
- Reduced thoracic—abdominal circumference
- *Elevated urinary*: Na; Cl; osmolality if high—poor prognosis
- Elevated serum/urinary beta-2 microglobulin

However, we must be careful to avoid some errors that may occur in diagnosis of hydronephrosis:

- Multicystic dysplastic kidney
- Duodenal obstruction (large duodenum mistaken for dilated pelvis)
- Gastric outlet obstruction
- Prune belly syndrome.

Postnatal approach would be:

Clinical

- *Renal mass*: MCK; PUJ obstruction suspected
- *Palpable bladder*: PUV; ureterocele obstruction.

Radiological

- USG detailed report with dimensions
- Micturating cystourethrogram (MCU) in unilateral or bilateral hydroureteronephrosis
- Renal nuclear scan at 4–6 weeks after birth for obstruction/cortical function.

Biochemical

- *Renal function tests*: Blood urea nitrogen (BUN), creatinine, electrolytes.

Hydronephrosis Pelviureteric Junction Obstruction

The most common renal anomaly detected as described above is pelviureteric junction obstruction (PUJO) and needs to be followed up carefully, both prenatally as well as postnatally and once severity of obstruction is without doubt, surgical intervention is called for to give the best long-term result.[12] Antenatal ultrasound must show the signs given below:

- Unilateral hydronephrosis, no hydroureter
- *Pelvic AP diameter*: Below 33 weeks >4 mm, above 33 weeks: >7 mm significant
- Parenchymal thickness in upper, mid and lower pole; compare with normal side
- No oligohydramnios, ascites or distended bladder seen
  These children may be delivered at term with neither induction of early delivery, nor lower segment cesarean section (LSCS).
  After delivery:
- First ultrasound to be done after 72 hours
- All details of renal pelvic AP diameter; parenchymal thickness measured
- Compare with normal unaffected side AP diameter, parenchymal thickness as reference for severity
- Get urine study done to look for infection
- Get renal function tests done at 7 days of life
- Renal radionuclear scan DTPA/EC/MAG3 to be done at 4–6 weeks of life
- If affected side function <40%, T1/2 life >20 minutes; obstructive pattern: surgery
- If above are not in favor of obstruction, then repeat USG and scan at 3 months and compare to see if diameter increasing, thickness decreasing, function falling >5%, or goes below 40%, or obstructive pattern comes, in which case surgery to be done, if not, repeat as before at 6 months and follow-up.

These children need to be followed up for at least 5 years even if not operated upon to increase the chances of detecting dynamic obstruction occurring later.

Posterior Urethral Valves

This is another well-known entity with a very guarded prognosis and, like diaphragmatic hernia has the worst prognosis if diagnosed early. Long-term results are also not good despite antenatal diagnosis.[13] The anomaly is picked up on ultrasound findings:

- Bilateral hydronephrosis and hydroureters
- Large distended bladder with thickened wall[10]
- Dilated posterior urethra seen as key hole phenomenan (Fig. 35.15)
- If detected before 24 weeks—usually poor prognosis
- Oligohydramnios—poor prognosis severe obstruction

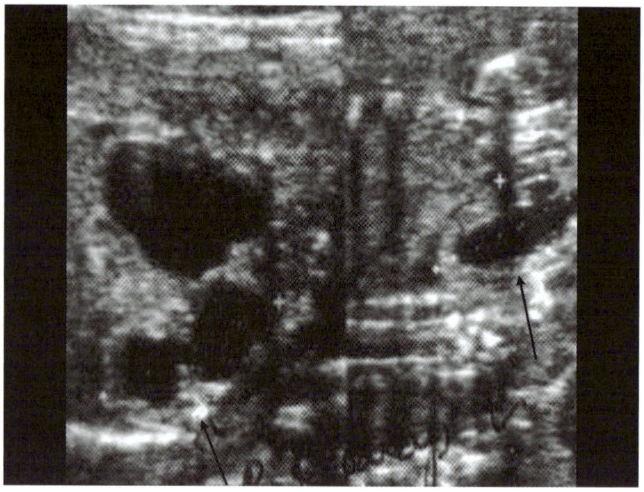

Fig. 35.15 Keyhole bladder posterior urethral valves

- Bright kidneys—poor prognosis
- Kidneys with absence of corticomedullary junction—not good prognosis
- Urinary ascites-guarded prognosis—severe obstruction
- Look for associated anomalies in other systems too.

Prognosis and progress can be estimated by:

- Progressive oligohydramnios, or development of oligohydramnios
- Bladder puncture and sending urine for electrolytes.

Na: <100 mEq;Cl: <90 mEq; Osmolality < 210 mOsm: good prognosis.

MANAGEMENT BASED ON PROGNOSIS

Poor Renal Function/Pulmonary Hypoplasia

- Nonaggressive obstetric management
- No fetal intervention.

Good/Equivocal Renal Function/ Fetal Lung Mature

- Transfer mother to tertiary care unit for delivery
- Early delivery and ex-utero correction
- *In utero intervention*: V-A shunt/fetal surgery/fetal cystoscopy and fulguration
  Risks: Diagnostic error—30–40%
  Danger to mother/fetus (Comp–45%)
  Dysplastic kidney/pulmonary hypoplasia.

Postnatal Approach

Clinical Examination

- *Palpable bladder*: Thickened, hypertrophied detrusor
- *Urinary stream*: Poor

- Residual urine post-void—large
- Palpable lump in abdomen—enlarged kidneys.

Investigations

- *Sonography*: Dimensions—pelves, ureters, bladder wall thickness, ascites
- *Urine*: Routine and culture; electrolytes.
- Renal function tests; serum electrolytes
- *Voiding cystourethrogram*: Valves, diverticuli, reflux (Fig. 35.16)
- *Renal scan*: DTPA for differential function and obstruction.

Interventions

- Catheterization of the bladder—decompress UT
- Antibiotics, repeat renal function tests
- *Cystoscopy and fulguration*: Neonatal resectoscope and loop-catheter 3 days.
- *Urethra too small/Scope too big*: Vesicostomy
- Later cystoscopy and fulguration of valves
- Renal function not improving on catheter
- Higher diversion—Ureterostomy. Later cystoscopic ablation of valves.

Follow-up

- This requires long-term follow-up as boy can develop renal failure anytime up to age of 10 years or later too[13]
- Regular ultrasound for increasing or persisting hydronephrosis

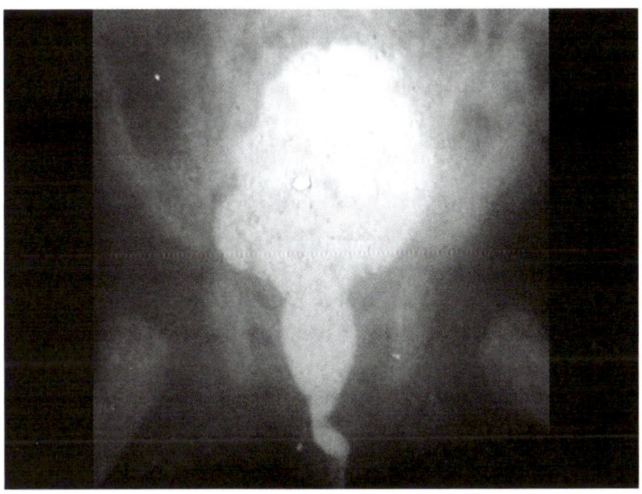

Fig. 35.16 Micturating cystourethrography: Posterior urethral valves

- Radio nuclear scan to look for decreasing function on any one side
- Renal function tests to look for early signs of failure
- Late signs of incontinence due to various causes
- Residual hydroureteronephrosis/increasing hydronephrosis
- In this condition it is the bladder which is the problem, the valves can be ablated but the problem of bladder needs to be tackled properly or else these boys can grow up with impending renal failure.

REFERENCES

1. Adzick NS, Krumel TM, et al. Prenatal diagnosis and fetal therapy. In: Hanmin Lee, Shinjiro Hirose, Michael Harrison (Eds). Pediatric Surgery, 7th Edition. Elsevier; 2012.pp.77-88.
2. Merz E, Miric TD, Bahlmann F, et al. Prenatal sonographic chest and lung measurements for predicting severe pulmonary hypoplasia. Prenat Diagn. 1999;19:614-9.
3. Danzer E, Hedrick HL. Controversies in management of severe diaphragmatic hernia. Semin Fetal Neonatal Med. 2014;19:376-84.
4. Geogescu R, Chiutu L, Nemes R, et al. Possibilities and limits in the treatment o congenital diaphragmatic hernia. J Med Life. 2014;15:433-7.
5. Gamba P, Midrio P. Abdominal wall defects: prenatal diagnosis, newborn management and long-term outcomes. Semin Pediatr Surg. 2014;23:283-90.
6. Prefumof F, Izzi C. Fetal abdominal wall defects. Best Pract Res Clin Obstet Gynecol. 2014;28:391-402.
7. Saygili-Yilmaz ES, Incki KK, Turgut M, Kelekci S. Prenatal diagnosis of type I sacro coccygeal teratoma and its management. Clin Exp Obstet Gynecol: 2008;35:153-5.
8. Holcroft CJ, BlakemoreKJ, Gurewitsch ED, et al. Large fetal sacrococcygeal teratomas: could early delivery improve outcome? Fetal Diagn Ther. 2008;24:55-60.
9. DeGraw AM, Den Dekker HT, De Mol AC, et al. The diagnostic value of routine antenatal ultrasound screening for congenital uropathies. J Matern Feal Neonatal Med. 2014;26:1-5.
10. Kumar M, Thakur S, Puri A, et al. Fetal renal anomaly: factors that predict survival. J Pediatr Urol. 2014;10:1001-07.
11. Liu DB, Armstrong WR, Maizels M. Hydronephrosis prenatal and postnatal evaluation and management. Clin Perinatol. 2014;41:661-78.
12. Dias T, Sairam S, Kumarariri S. Ultrasound diagnosis of fetal renal abnormalities. Best Pract Res Clin Obstet Gynecol. 2014; 21:18-26.
13. Sarhan OM, Helmy TE, Alotay AA, et al. Did antenatal diagnosis protect against chronic kidney disease in patients with posterior urethral valves? Multicenter study. Urology. 2013;82:1405-9.

CHAPTER

36 Fetal Autopsy for Better Prenatal Diagnosis: Illustrative Cases

Ratna D Puri

With improving antenatal care in developing countries the ultrasound detection of fetal malformations is increasing. Families are unprepared for the news of an anomalous ultrasound. The threshold of continuing a pregnancy in the presence of a fetal abnormality is low in India and therefore appropriate counseling and comprehensive care are an essential integral part of management in the event of fetal malformations identified on autopsy.

Examination of the fetus with congenital anomalies is essential to identify the nature of the defect and determine if they constitute a part of a recognized abnormality of development and morphogenesis. A structured approach, including a comprehensive history and details of the anomalies present, assists in making a definitive diagnosis. Syndrome diagnosis in the fetus may be a challenge as the complete phenotype may not be manifest, coupled with the possibility of subtle dysmorphism that is difficult to recognize.

Correlation of the antenatal scan findings with those at autopsy, combined with the experienced eye of a clinical geneticist, is helpful in making a syndrome diagnosis. Specialized databases, reference textbooks and previously published malformation syndromes are important aids for the geneticist.

The field has expanded exponentially, especially over the last decade, with application of advanced molecular techniques, which in addition to defining new malformation syndromes, has also made it possible to understand the underlying cause of birth defects and syndromes.

An accurate diagnosis is important to counsel families of the prognosis, available treatment options and recurrence risks in future conceptions. New technologies for genetic testing are available to confirm a diagnosis and consequently it is vital that appropriate fetal samples are stored in all cases. A team approach with expert input from a fetal medicine specialist, perinatal pathologist, geneticist, radiologist and the genetics laboratory are important components of fetal dysmorphic syndrome identification.

Despite recent advances in the field of minimally invasive fetal autopsy with postnatal CT scan and MRI, fetal autopsy remains the gold standard for evaluation. This is especially relevant in resource poor countries where expertise of antenatal ultrasound diagnosis varies greatly between centers and adequate counseling to prevent recurrence would depend on detailed, systematic fetal autopsy. Postnatal CT scan and MRI modalities for evaluating fetuses are expensive and special expertise required for this is still unavailable in developing countries.

Where these resources are not available, a goal should be to document phenotypic data as thoroughly as possible and collect and store tissue samples appropriately so that interpretation and ancillary testing can be done later, if needed.

Appropriate autopsy practices for different indications and its utility with prototype examples will be discussed.

One would consider four clinical situations for which autopsy is asked for:

1. Single or multiple malformations in the fetus
2. Nonimmune hydrops fetalis
3. Intrauterine death or stillbirth
4. Abnormalities of limbs.

MALFORMATIONS

A *malformation* is an abnormality of form or structure that occurs during development. A malformation can be major or minor. A *major malformation* is severe and interferes with function, e.g. neural tube defects, holoprosencephaly, cardiac defects, cleft lip and palate.

Common causes of congenital malformations include a genetic etiology due to chromosomal or single gene defects, environmental etiology comprising intrauterine infections, drugs and medications, maternal metabolic disorders, ionizing radiation and the multifactorial group. For some birth defects and malformation syndromes etiologies are not

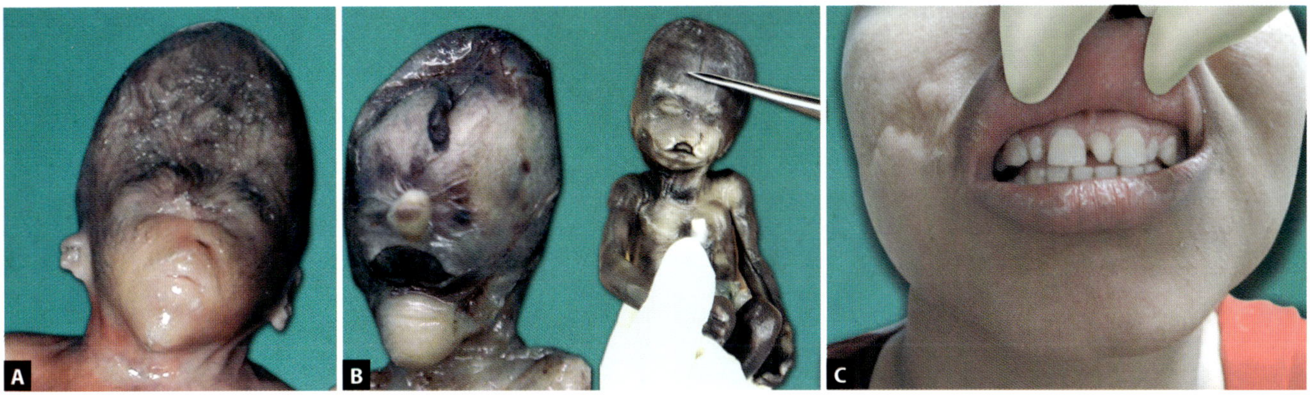

Figs 36.1A to C Spectrum of facial manifestations of holoprosencephaly. (A) Cyclopia—single or fused eye with absent nasal structures; (B) Median cleft lip and palate; (C) Single central incisor

still defined. Evaluation of malformations involves identification of the abnormality and its etiopathogenesis.

When a major malformation is identified at autopsy evaluating for a possible etiology is important for counseling the families. An example is illustrated with holoprosencephaly.

This malformation results from absent or incomplete division of the embryonic forebrain—the prosencephalon. It is of three major forms—alobar, semi-lobar and lobar. Either forms can be associated with a spectrum of facial manifestations that include cyclopia, ethmocephaly, cebocephaly, midline cleft lip, hypertelorism and single central incisor (Figs 36.1A to C). The milder forme fruste can be present in an asymptomatic, carrier parent and should be looked for.

The etiology of holoprosencephaly is varied and detailed history taking, fetal examination and appropriate tests for identification of the etiology are depicted in Table 36.1.

In another situation where detailed fetal autopsy may not be possible due to logistic reasons is depicted in Case 1. A third gravida was detected to have a possible craniosynostosis syndrome in the third trimester scan. Her first baby had died in the neonatal period and was described by the parents to have an abnormal shape of the head and ambiguous genitalia. As appropriate consultation had been sought prior to delivery, which was conducted in a facility where fetal autopsy was not possible, she was advised to stored appropriate samples after delivery for chromosomal analysis and DNA storage. It was also recommended that photographs and radiographs of the neonate after delivery be taken and all malformations recorded by the attending doctor be noted in detail (Figs 36.2A and B).

This helped us to make a diagnosis of Carpenter syndrome in the fetus, identify the mutation by sequencing the *RAB23* gene in the stored fetal DNA (Fig. 36.2C) as well as provide prenatal testing in the next pregnancy as there was a 25% recurrence risk for Carpenter syndrome.

Table 36.1 Etiology of holoprosencephaly and the relevant investigations

Etiology of holoprosencephaly	Relevant evaluation	Genetic tests
Teratogenic Maternal diabetes Retinoic, salicylates	Echocardiography HbA_{1C}	None
Chromosomal (30–50%)	T-13 (75%), T-18	Karyotype microarray
Malformation syndromes (18–25%) >25 different syndromes		Pallister-Hall, CHARGE, Meckel, SLOS Rubinstein-Taybi, Pseudotrisomy 13
Familial	ID, CL/CP, microcephaly, single central incisor Hypotelorism	*SHH*, *ZIC2*, *SIX3*, *TGIF1*, *GLI1*, *PTCH*

INTRAUTERINE DEATH AND STILLBIRTH

Postmortem examination is a standard investigation to attempt to identify the cause of unexplained IUD and a systematic evaluation results in ascertainment in majority of cases. In addition to detailed fetal examination to identify malformations and fetal dysmorphism, placental histopathology examination and karyotype in all cases is recommended. Infections, umbilical cord abnormalities and maternal fetal hemorrhage are some of the other less common etiologies of intrauterine death. An example is a case identified to have Trisomy 21 on clinical examination and karyotype testing in a fetus with unexplained intrauterine death at 34 weeks gestation (Figs 36.3A and B). In the current case the first trimester screen and NT scan as well as the second trimester genetic sonogram were normal.

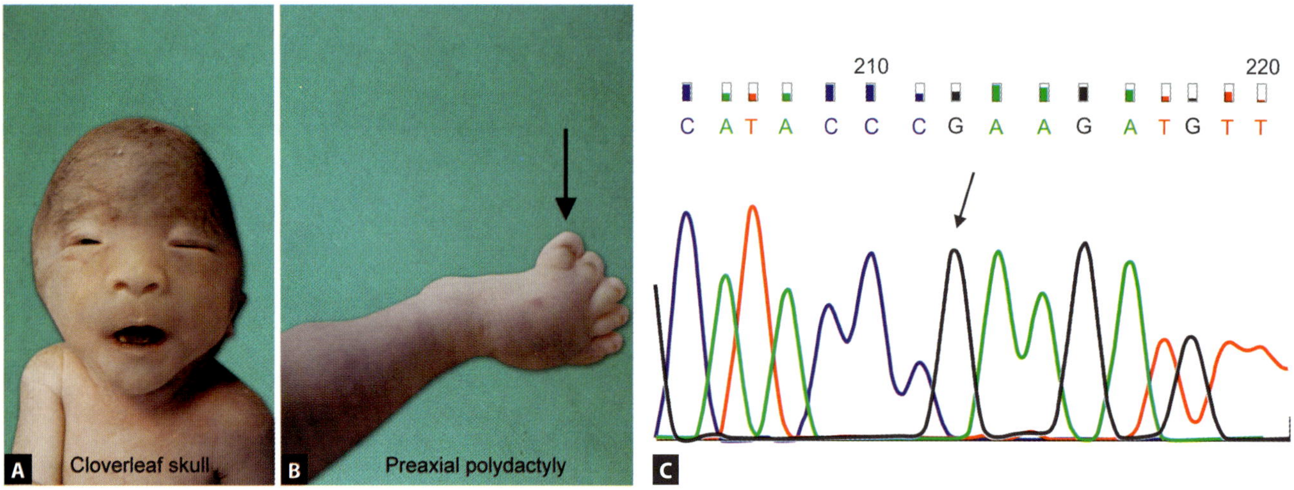

Figs 36.2A to C (A and B) Craniosynostosis and polydactyly—Carpenter syndrome; (C) *RAB23* gene mutation in Carpenter syndrome—sequence chromatogram

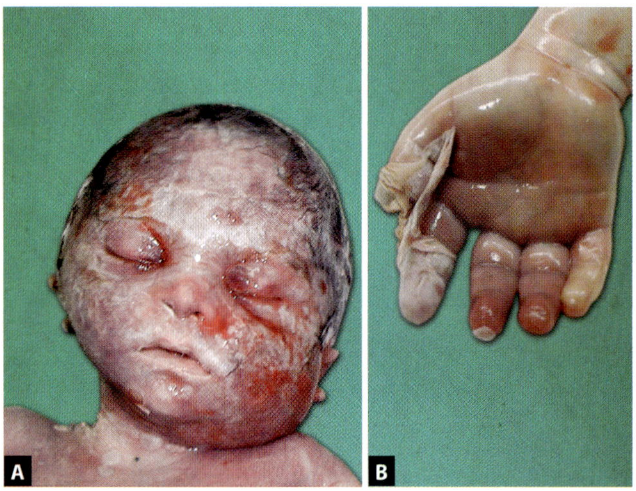

Figs 36.3A and B Fetus with intrauterine death. Trisomy 21 identified on autopsy. (A) Upslant palpebral fissure hypertelorism depressed nasal bridge low set ears; (B) Single palmar crease

This diagnosis not only allows the family to apprehend the cause of the unexplained mishap, come to terms with the loss, as well as seeks definitive counseling for recurrence risks and prevention in the next pregnancy.

Another case depicts the identification of enlarged, cystic, horseshoe shaped kidneys with numerous cysts in kidney in all regions. As for all cases with renal cystic disease, an ultrasound of the couple, identified adult onset polycystic kidney disease in the husband. The antenatal scan in this case identified a 17 weeks fetus with severe oligoamnios, fetal growth restriction and intrauterine death. The fetal autopsy not only established a diagnosis, but also enabled counseling of at risks individuals and preventive management before onset of renal disease and failure. In this case, the risk of recurrence in each pregnancy was 50% and prenatal testing can be offered after the familial mutation in the *ADPKD* gene identified.

NONIMMUNE HYDROPS FETALIS

The causes and evaluation of nonimmune hydrops fetalis are many and it is difficult to evaluate for all. A detailed history and clinical setting in which NIHF has occurred, aids to streamline the investigations. After exclusion of immune causes, the other common etiologies to evaluate for include fetal cardiac rhythm disorders, malformations, especially cardiac, skeletal dysplasia and metabolic disorders. If fetal anemia is suspected on ultrasound examination, alpha thalassemia and fetal infections should be suspected, investigated and treated as the outcomes may not be dismal in all cases. Antenatal cord blood sampling after 18 - 20 weeks of pregnancy is preferred, or an amniotic fluid sample with appropriate tests for the clinical situation are able to delineate the diagnosis in about 50% cases of nonimmune hydrops fetalis (NIHF).

ABNORMALITIES OF LIMBS

These include malformations of the limbs and skeletal dysplasias. Limb malformations can be isolated, single malformations like congenital talipes equinovarus (CTEV), ectrodactyly or multiple malformations can be part of a multiple malformations syndrome. An illustrative example is of a family with a second ongoing pregnancy where an

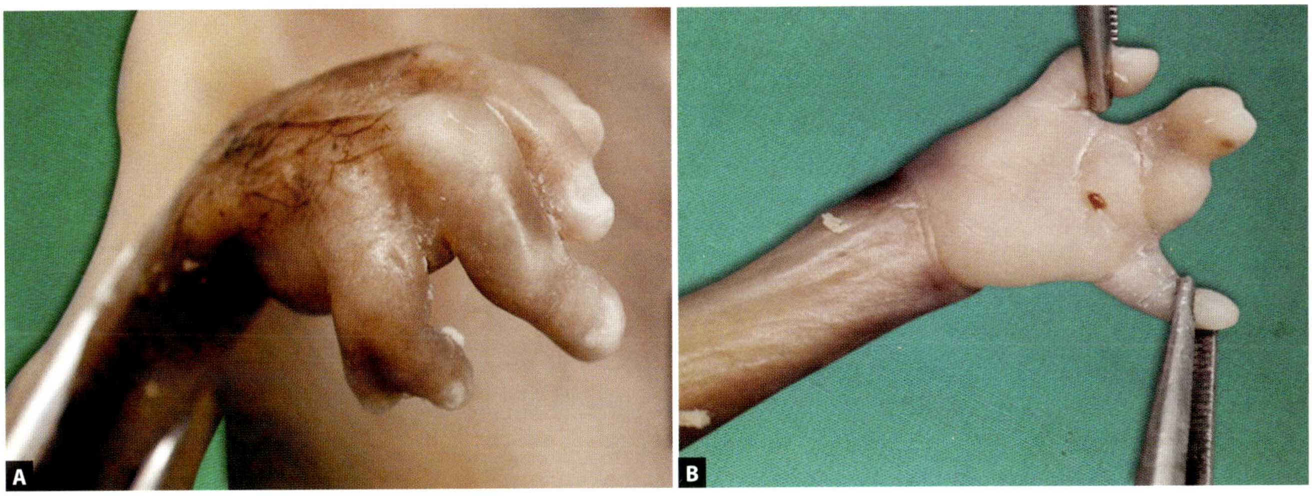

Figs 36.4A and B Autosomal recessive oligosyndactyly: Cenani-Lenz syndrome. (A) Syndactyly and camptodactyly; (B) Oligosyndactyly

amniocentesis was performed because of an increased nuchal translucency of 3 mm at 12 weeks gestations. The fetal chromosomes were normal. A follow-up level II scan identified camptodactyly of the left hand and ectrodactyly of the right hand. A previous pregnancy of this couple had been discontinued for similar malformations of the limb and unilateral renal agenesis. Fetal examination was not performed after termination of the first pregnancy. In view of a recurrence of similar malformations in two pregnancies an autosomal recessive disorder was suspected. Fetal examination after discontinuation of the second pregnancy identified syndactyly of the right hand, oligosyndactyly of left hand and 2nd and 3rd toes syndactyly bilaterally (Figs 36.4A and B).

An autosomal recessive disorder with oligosyndactyly and renal agenesis was searched and a possibility of a rare malformation syndrome, Cenani-Lenz syndrome was considered. This occurs because of biallelic mutations in the *LRPV4* gene. This gene was sequenced in the stored fetal DNA and the clinical diagnosis was confirmed with identification of two mutations in the *LRPV4* gene in the fetus and heterozygous mutations in the carrier parents. With this information, the family was offered reproductive counseling, risk estimates of recurrence in subsequent pregnancies, as well as cascade carrier screening for persons at risk. In the absence of a detailed fetal postmortem examination and fetal DNA none of this would have been possible.

Other common conditions requiring detailed fetal examination include radial ray malformations for the spectrum of differential diagnosis and arthrogryposis.

Lethal skeletal dysplasias are a heterogeneous group of rare but important causes of perinatal morbidity and mortality characterized by abnormal growth and development of bone and cartilage. Antenatal ultrasound identifies if the disorder is lethal or not. Detailed fetal examination is essential to determine the kind of dysplasia and confirm by molecular diagnosis. For this fetal external examination, radiographs in anteroposterior and lateral position and stored fetal DNA are essential. In this context an example is of a common lethal skeletal dysplasia-osteogenesis imperfecta (OI). Type II OI is lethal with high morbidity and mortality and most families opt to discontinue the pregnancy after identification of this dysplasia (Figs 36.5A and B). All decreased bone density on the antenatal scan is not OI and other disorders like lethal hypophosphatasia should to be considered (Figs 36.6A and B).

Osteogenesis impertecta (OI) commonly occurs due to mutations in one of many genes, either heterozygous or biallelic mutations. There are three situations, an affected parent with a 50% risk of recurrence, a de novo mutation where there is no family history of similar disease and micromelia, under mineralized skeleton and fractures are identified on an antenatal scan. The third scenario is of recurrence of OI in subsequent pregnancies suggesting mutation in a gene known to cause autosomal recessive OI or heterozygous mutations with gonadal mosaicism. In the latter two scenarios recurrence risks are 25% and 6% respectively. Therefore, fetal examination and elucidation of the mutations is important for counseling families and understanding the etiopathogenesis of the disease.

CONCLUSION

The above illustrative situations describe the importance of fetal examination to confirm the antenatal ultrasound findings, provide reproductive counseling to the families and improve prenatal diagnosis in subsequent pregnancies. The consent

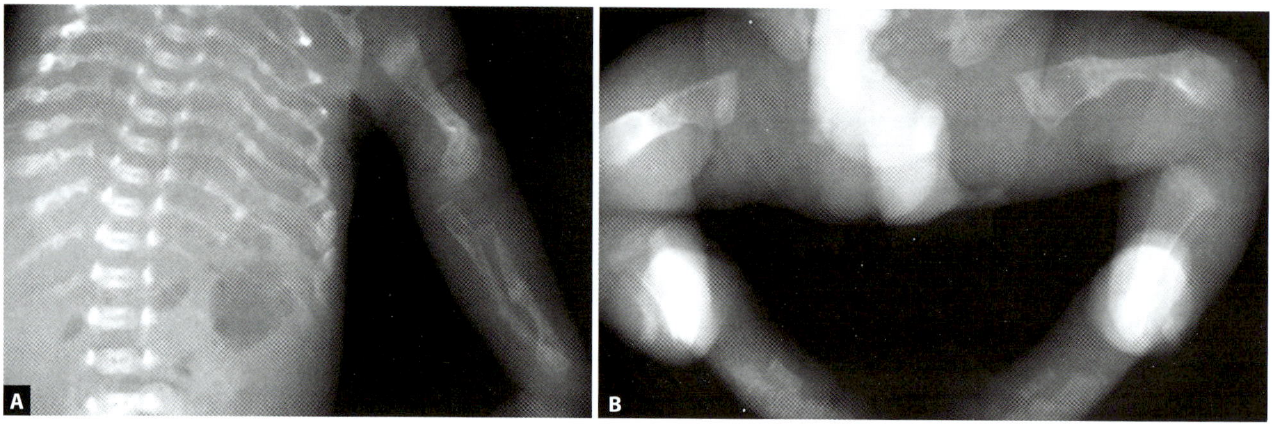

Figs 36.5A and B Osteogenesis imperfecta

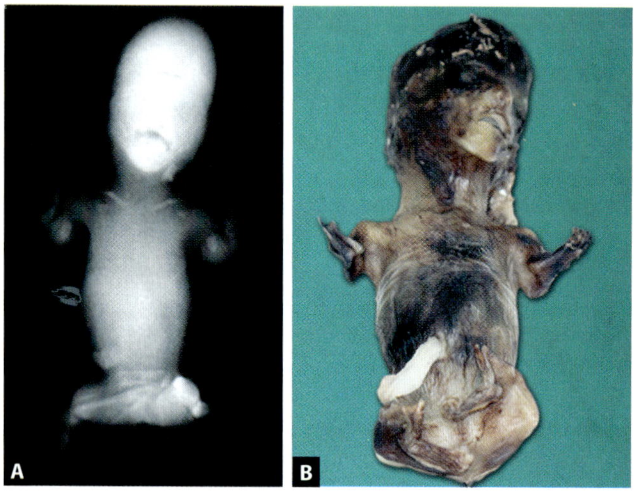

Figs 36.6A and B Lethal hypophosphatasia

for fetal autopsy improves if the obstetrician understands the utility and discusses the same with the grieving family. Prior consultation with the geneticist or pathologist who performs the autopsy and appropriate samples improves outcomes. In our experience antenatal fetal samples are preferred and avoid maternal tissue contamination. Advanced genetic technology now enables cost-effective molecular testing, but appropriate samples and detailed clinical examination is important for interpretation of testing results. Information of the utility of fetal examination to improve patient outcomes and prenatal diagnosis is well-established and appropriate counseling by obstetricians would improve uptake for fetal postmortem examination.

MAJOR RECOMMENDATIONS

1. Standard autopsy should ideally be an essential part of fully investigating fetal loss, stillbirths, and neonatal deaths associated with non-chromosomal fetal malformations.
2. Clinicians and healthcare providers approaching parents for autopsy consent should discuss the options for a full, limited, or step-wise postmortem examination; the issue of retained fetal tissues; and the value of autopsy and the possibility that the information gained may not benefit them but may be of benefit to others. This information should be provided while respecting the personal and cultural values of the families.
3. If parents are unwilling to give consent for a full autopsy, alternatives to full autopsy that provide additional clinical information must be presented in a manner that includes disclosure of limitations.
4. External physical examination, medical photographs, and standard radiographic or computed tomography should be offered in all cases of fetal anomaly(ies) of non-chromosomal etiology.
5. Well-designed, large prospective studies are needed to evaluate the accuracy of postmortem magnetic resonance imaging. It cannot function as a substitute for standard full autopsy.
6. The fetal and perinatal autopsies should be performed by trained perinatal or pediatric pathologists.
7. The need for additional sampling is guided by the results of previous prenatal and/or genetic investigations, as well as the type of anomalies identified in the fetus. Fibroblast cultures may allow future laboratory studies, particularly in the absence of previous karyotyping or if a biochemical

disorder is suspected, and deoxyribonucleic acid (DNA) analysis.

8. In cases requiring special evaluation, the most responsible health care provider should have direct communication with the fetopathologist to ensure that all necessary sampling is performed in a timely manner.
9. The most responsible healthcare providers must see the families in follow-up to share autopsy findings, plan for the management of future pregnancies, obtain consent for additional testing, and offer genetic counseling to other family members when appropriate.

SECTION

8

Ethical and Medicolegel Aspects

CHAPTER

37 Ethical and Medicolegal Issues of Prenatal Genetic Diagnosis

Ajit N Patil

ETHICS OF PRENATAL GENETIC DIAGNOSIS

Last few years have seen revolutionary changes in the way, prenatal screening is being offered. Ultrasound resolution has reached new heights. At the same time, plethora of tests are now available in genetic and molecular diagnosis. This paradigm shift is occurring at a very rapid speed with which clinicians are not able to cope with. It is raising lot of issues surrounding "quest for fitness".

Though Darwin[1] pointed out that in the struggle for existence, it is the fittest of the species which will survive; this was an environmental pressure, which brought about a change in the genes. But the technology has made now possible to understand this even before the baby is born, making it possible to "choose before birth". To what extent, is the race towards a perfect individual is right, we do not know.[2,3]

Let us take a case of echogenic bowel[4] discovered on ultrasound and whose karyotype and infection screen comes negative? What the doctor should talk and what the parents should decide? Should the pregnancy be terminated for a small increased risk of complications, which may be seen in late trimester? What about the anxiety and agony if the pregnancy is being continued? What if they demand for termination? What the doctor should do? Do our legal system permits such a termination?

So what are the ethics surrounding screenings? What benefits does it "offer"?

Reassurance

This is the whole reason of screening, currently. With so much being told and described even in lay press, pregnancy has become a state of anxiety rather than joy. But with a good ultrasound examination coupled with few biochemical tests, a negative result (which is most cases will be), parents will be relieved of this anxiety. To understand that the baby is structurally normal and to also understand its genetic risks being low, parents are more relieved.

Reduce the Fear of Selected Birth Defects

This holds true, neural tube defects being one of the common anomalies seen. A methodical structural scan carried out at hands of an experienced and trained sonographer rules out life-threatening abnormalities and has a potential to reduce the economic burden of giving birth to such abnormalities especially in our population where the costs of medical care are born entirely by the family with no governmental or insurance support.

Reproductive Autonomy

This is an era of "Choice". Women desire and demand information and knowledge about their reproductive choices, either for: (a) preventing disability, or (b) enhances experience of pregnancy—sign of responsible parenting. And those who do not opt for tests might sense a less sympathy and support. This in fact limits the so-called autonomy of decision making.

But this language of "choice and control is too simplistic and attractive. Prenatal diagnosis is therefore considered as search and destroy mission". It is not so.

Are babies akin to a "production line" separating out those products which we wish to develop from those we wish to discontinue?

For a few selected issues like Down's syndrome, this strategy may be right.

But for a vast majority, it does not take into account why reassurance is being sought, how do we select the "at risk" groups and to decide who is eligible for all this.

Choice

Choice, therefore, is a very tricky issue. Who decides this choice, are women empowered enough to make a decision on their choice? Take the example of echogenic bowel. What choice should the doctor make, what choice should the woman and her family make, what if these choices are in conflict, should the doctor refuse or accept their choice if it is conflicting with his choice, especially if family requests termination and doctor does not feel so? And if family decides to continue but fetus develops a problem, on whose shoulders does the onus lie?

Counseling

The example cited underlines the importance of counseling. It is easy to say that counseling should be "non-directional" but is difficult. Counseling skills include medical and social consequences. This presumes a certain level of expertise. There is lack of proper-trained counselors in our country. The responsibility of counseling is in hands of the average obstetricians who are not been trained in this field. It is then an obligation to improve their skills.

Inability of Offer Treatment

The risk for many illnesses can be screened today. This is not akin to diagnosis. The positive screening test simply raises the possibility of acquiring a disease. But we still lack in effective intervention. Pre-eclampsia risk can be calculated today but there is no effective pharmacological intervention (though trials about low-dose aspirin are initiated).

The human genome sequencing is a reality. With a salivary swab, host of risks can be calculated in an adult. Days are not long when the same tests will be applied to fetus. By doing the genome sequencing, it may be possible to know what is the risk of fetus developing diabetes or a coronary disease or a malignancy. This is going to a Pandora's Box.

Insurance Cover

Congenital abnormalities are not covered by insurance. If a woman decides to continue pregnancy with a prior knowledge of an abnormality, she has to bear the burden. Extending this logic will insurance companies, in future demand such information from the healthcare providers? It is but natural for the third party people to get involved in the most private decisions about pregnancy.

Social Injustice

Economic constraints limit the use of prenatal diagnosis to all strata of society. This is ironical as most diseases are seen in the low SE group who cannot afford prenatal diagnosis. These inequalities reflect society's problems with access to prenatal care in general. The affluent have disproportionate access to invasive procedures. This will lead to increase in the 'non-invasive' screening technologies, which have a poor detection rates. This is not a correct use of healthcare resources. The technology of prenatal diagnosis may not appear essential to public health as a technology that provides cure.

As Botkin points out, "This technology will force us to examine the fundamental relationship between parent and child. How much control can we legitimately exert over the biologic structure of our children, how they view us and how they view themselves?"

As perinatal medicine advances more interventions will be possible. Will it mean better care to the fetus, we still do not know. Thus, the responsibilities of obstetric professional are enormous. A rational choice will have to be made to identify the goals of a particular test in consideration. Doctors will have to play a more important role is assisting the couples in understanding their own preferences and help them to come a well-considered decision.

MEDICOLEGAL ISSUES OF PRENATAL GENETIC DIAGNOSIS

India has seen the dark side of prenatal screening. Ultrasound was being used to screen out female fetuses and sex selective abortions were rampant. There was an alarming decline in sex ratios. This prompted Indian Parliament to pass a law to curb sex selection. This is called now as the Pre-Conception and Pre-Natal Diagnostic Techniques (PCPNDT) law. It governs all aspects of prenatal diagnosis. The objectives of the law are very clear and it lays down, in detail the conditions for setting up clinics as well as the conduct of the clinics. The information needs to be collected in Form F and monthly submission to the Appropriate Authority (AA) is a must. Most of states in India now have made it compulsory to submit an online data, where authorized software is used to fill-up the data and generate the consent form. Once this declaration is filled by the pregnant woman, she proceeds for the USG/ procedure. After the procedure is over, the results are again filled in the form F and it is submitted online. The law also points out the various deficiencies.

As a disciplined partner of the society and the nation, it is important that all obstetricians follow the Act in its true spirit and avoid legal hassles. Towards this, many checklists of what to do are available. It is our duty to see that these are properly implemented.

There have been demands, these days of graded punishments and this is under review. Till the changes come into force, the existent rules remain so.

An example of checklist is given in Table 37.1.

There have been incidences where the doctors feel aggravated by the actions taken by the AA. There has been over zealous attempt by AAs in implementing the Act. It is not followed in the true spirit of the PCPNDT Act. Mere technical error does not equate to a sex determination but the punishments are the same. It is high time to have review of the provisions and make changes so that doctors will not feel harassed.

For the information, the Table 37.2 mentions the various deficiencies and the clauses and the punishments these contraventions attract.

Table 37.1 Checklist of prenatal genetic diagnosis
• Display registration certificate in the waiting room and in the ultrasound room/procedure room • Board in English/Hindi/regional languages saying that sex determination is not done here • Copy of Act available in the reception area • Obtaining proper written consents • To fill up Form F properly and put signatures • Submit the forms regularly • Have an internal audit of the process periodically and overcome the deficiencies

Table 37.2 Violations under the PNDT Act and the penalties[5-7]

Violations	Section/Rule of the PNDT Act	Penalties
1. Minor Offences • Non-availability of copy of the PNDT Act in the registered center • Non-display of registration certificate of center • Non-display of Board in the premises in English and Local Language that 'Disclosure of the sex of the fetus is prohibited under law'	 Rule no. 17(2) Rule no. 6(2) Rule no. 17(1)	**For minor offences:** Case may be launched in the court of JMIC under section of the Act Punishment may extend to 3 months or with fine, which may extend to Rs 1,000/- for first offence. Additional fine up to Rs 500/- per day for the period of contravention for subsequent offence Or Show cause notice under Section 20(1), (2) for temporary suspension of registration Or Under Section 20(3)
2. Advertisement Relating to Preconception and Prenatal Determination of Sex	Section 22(1),(2)	Under Section 22(3) of the PNDT Amendment Act, imprisonment which may extend to 3 years and with fine which may extend to Rs 10,000/- Case is to be launched in the court under Section 28 of the Act
3. Unregistered Centers. It includes all such centers where any portable equipment capable of detecting sex before or after conception is used. The owner of such equipment may be having a registered facility somewhere else	Section 3	Any such equipment has to be sealed and seized by the Appropriate Authority concerned He/She may launch the case in the court u/s 28 of the Act Register such center after receiving 5 times the registration fee as penalty and after taking a undertaking as per the PNDT Rules—Rule11(2)
4. Irregularities in Registered Center • Owner/employee conducting the ultrasonography not qualified • More ultrasound machines/equipments whereas less number register • Minor deficiency in record keeping	 Section 3(2) and Rule 3(b) Under Rule 4,6 and as per Form 'A'. Sr. No. 8 Under Rule 9	The Appropriate Authority or person authorized thereupon may: Issue show cause notice under Section 20(1)(2) of the Act and with the endorsement of the Advisory Committee, may suspend (for a reasonable period) or cancel the registration, as per the magnitude of the violation May take Suo Moto action under Section 20(3) and suspend the registration without issuing show cause notice *Note:* 1. During the period of suspension registration, the equipment needs to be sealed and signed and kept with the owner. After cancellation of registration, the equipment has to be sealed and seized Any body aggrieved by the above decision may appeal to the higher-level Appropriate Authority within 30 days of the action. The appeal shall be disposed of by the higher authority within 60 days of its receipt
5. Record Keeping Irregularities in record keeping as per revised form 'F' are a major offence	Section 4, 29 and Rule-9	Contravention (a major offence) of provision of section 5 and 6 of the Act and punishable under Section 23(1) of the PNDT Act
6. Sex Selection	Section 3A. 4(5). 6 read with section 2(0)	Violation of section 5 and 6 of the Act and punishable under Section 23 of the Act

Note:

All offences under the Act are cognizable, non-bailable and non-compoundable (Section 27).

Even a case has been registered by the police, no court shall take cognizance except the complaint has been filled by the AA or by the person/group who had served a legal notice of 15 days to the AA already (Section 28).

Action under Section 20 and filling of criminal complaint 28 can go simultaneously (Section 20).

Meanwhile, what the best a doctor can do to give justice to his patients as well as respect law, we need to understand.

When You are Liable?

The liability is a tricky issue especially in branch of obstetrics where physician attends to need of two, one the mother and the other, the fetus to whom he has only indirect access. This is a limitation to the standards of care but taken as a "breach of duty".

The standard of care means, the level of care expected of a reasonable and prudent practitioner with the same level of training, and in similar circumstances. Usually, an expert will be invited to opine on this issue. Any deviation from those can be labeled as medical malpractice.

However, poor or unexpected result may not constitute malpractice, but it is often the reason patients and families consult with an attorney.

Claims Related to Prenatal Diagnosis

Wrongful birth: When parents say that the child should never have been born.

Wrongful life: When the child himself/herself says he/she should never have been born into a life of misery.[8]

Possible ways of getting sued for prenatal USG are depicted in Table 37.3.

The complications from invasive technique under ultrasound control is given in Table 37.4.

Table 37.3 Possible ways of getting sued for prenatal USG

- Missing the sonographic finding
- Misinterpretation of the sonographic finding
- Failure to compare findings with previous ultrasound
- Failure to communicate the sonographic report properly to the referring physician or the patient
- Failure to examine the patient personally or to take a proper history
- Incorrect sonographic approach for a specific condition
- Incomplete examination
- Inadequate quality of records
- Slip and fall injuries

Table 37.4 Complications from invasive techniques under ultrasound control

- Failure to obtain informed consent
- Complications of ultrasound such as induced vaginal bleeding or abortion
- Failure to recommend additional sonographic or radiologic studies or tests
- Loss of records/inadequate archiving
- Abuse (sexual, physical, or mental) of patient by sonologist or sonographer
- Miscellaneous anxiety produced by misdiagnosis, invasion of privacy, or other issues

Prenatal Ultrasound and Record Keeping

This is important. By law also it is mandatory to keep plates of the USG examination. "Absence of visual image documentation eliminates the possibility of future review or clinical reintegration and weakens the defense against an allegation that an incomplete or inadequate study was performed" ACOG, 2004

Precautions to be Taken While Performing Scans/Procedures

- Should have evidence of training in obstetric ultrasound.
- Should have requisite training and certification when performing specific scans such as nuchal translucency (NT) scans, (FTS), anomaly scans, etc.
- *Keep in mind, common missed abnormalities:* Central nervous system (CNS)—Agenesis of the corpus callosum (ACC), posterior cranial fossa abnormalities, spine defects, cardiovascular system (CVS)—Duct dependent lesions, e.g. transposition of great asteries (TGA), critical pulmonary stenosis (PS), facial clefts, limb defects.

Prenatal genetic diagnosis is specialized situation and breach of duty may arise, if:

- Failure to offer aneuploidy screening
- Failure to offer appropriate carrier testing
- Failure to convey results appropriately
- Failure to counsel adequately for invasive procedures
- Failure to obtain informed consent.

The best steps to avoid being sued therefore appear to be:

- Understanding duties
- Having an open attitude of conveying what prenatal diagnosis means and what are its limitations?
- Use of information brochures for the parents to read
- Keep proper records as required by the law
- Obtain training and be well read
- Obtain a second opinion in case of difficulties.

CONCLUSION

Prenatal medicine is a rapidly expanding field with numerous indications coming up for evaluation. Duties of clinician are therefore enormous. On one side are the laws and on the other side are the ethics. In order to balance things, being knowledgeable is the only solution.

REFERENCES

1. Darwin Charles. On Origin of Species, 1854.
2. ACOG committee opinion: Ethical issues in genetic testing, June 2008.
3. ACOG committee opinion: Cell free DNA screening for fetal aneuploidy: no. 640, Sept 2015.
4. SOGC Clinical Practice guidelines: Fetal soft markers on obstetric ultrasound, no. 162, June 2013.
5. Pre-Conception and Pre-Natal. Diagnostic Techniques Act, 1994 and Rules with Amendments Ministry of Health and Family Welfare, Government of India.
6. Pre-Conception and Pre-Natal Diagnostic Techniques (Prohibition Of Sex Selection) Act. Ministry of Health and Family Welfare, Government of India. June 2012.
7. Goel A. Preconception and Prenatal Diagnostic Techniques Act. Radiopaedia. May 2015.
8. Rhinehart KE, The Debate Over Wrongful Birth and Wrongful Life, 26 Law & Psychol. Rev. 141 (2002).

CHAPTER

38 Amended Pre-Conception and Pre-Natal Diagnostic Techniques Act

RN Goel

WHY THIS ACT?

An Act to provide for the prohibition of sex selection, before or after conception, and for regulation of prenatal diagnostic techniques for the purposes of detecting genetic abnormalities or metabolic disorders or chromosomal abnormalities or certain congenital malformations or sex-linked disorders and for the prevention of their misuse for sex determination leading to female feticide and for matters connected therewith or incidental thereto.

PRENATAL DIAGNOSTIC TECHNIQUES

Prenatal diagnostic techniques include:
- *Prenatal diagnostic procedures* means
- *Prenatal diagnostic tests* means
- *Sex selection*

As per Notification in Gazette on 7.2.12 by GDR 80(E) the following were inserted in definition:
- *"Mobile medical unit" means a mobile vehicle which provides specialized facilities for the patients.*
- *"Mobile genetic clinic" means a mobile medical unit where ultrasound machine or imaging machine is used.*

Under this Act there is provision of Registration in 3 categories as under:

1. *Genetic counseling center (GCC):* The qualifications of the employees, for a genetic counseling center shall be as under rule 3 (1):
   - a gynecologist or a pediatrician having six months experience or four weeks training in genetic counseling or a medical geneticists
2. *Genetic laboratory (GL):* The qualifications of the employees, the requirement of equipment, etc. for a *genetic laboratory* shall be as under rule 3 (2):
   a. Any person having adequate space and being or employing
      - a medical geneticist and
      - a laboratory technician, having a BSc degree in biological sciences or a degree or diploma in medical laboratory course with at least one year experience in conducting appropriate prenatal diagnostic techniques, tests or procedures

   b. Such laboratory should have or acquire.
3. *Genetic clinic/ultrasound clinic/imaging center:* The qualifications of the employees, the requirement of equipment, etc. for a *genetic clinic/ultrasound clinic/imaging center* after GSR 13(E) 2014. Rule 3 (3):
   - Any person having adequate space and being or employing
      - Gynecologist having experience of performing at least 20 procedures, *Or*
      - a sonologist or imaging specialist or *registered medical practitioner having postgraduate degree or diploma* or six months training duly imparted in the manner prescribed in the preconception and prenatal diagnostic techniques (Prohibition of sex selection) (Six months training) Rules, 2014; *Or*

        A medical geneticist may set up a genetic clinic/ultrasound clinic/imaging center.

For in vitro fertilization (IVF) center, there is no separate category. In IVF center we are giving genetic counseling, prenatal diagnostic procedure and test. So registration in all three category is sufficient for IVF center.

Amendment 2012 by notification in gazette on 7.2.2012

3B (1). *Regulation of portable machines:* The use of portable ultrasound machine or any other portable machine or device which has the potential for selection of sex before conception or detection of sex during pregnancy shall be permitted only in the following conditions, namely:
- The portable machine being used, within the premises it is registered, for providing services to the indoor patients.
- As part of a mobile medical unit, offering a bouquet of other health and medical services; explanation—for the

purpose of this sub-rule, the expression "other health and medical services" means the host of services provided by the mobile medical unit.

Registration of genetic counseling center, genetic laboratory, ultrasound clinic and genetic clinic:

- An application for registration shall be made to the *appropriate authority, i.e. DM/CMO* in duplicate, in Form A.
- The appropriate authority, or any person in his office authorized in this behalf, shall acknowledge receipt of the application for registration, in the *acknowledgment slip provided at the bottom of Form A,* immediately if delivered at the office of the Appropriate Authority, or not later than the next working day if received by post.
  As per Notification date 4-6-2012
  Fee for registration in one category......................₹ 25000/
  Fee for registration in two or three category.........₹ 35000/
  For five year

RENEWAL FEE IS HALF OF REGISTRATION

Ultrasound machine, sonologist and place of doing ultrasound are registered together. In case of mobile ultrasound machine, place of doing obstetric ultrasound should also be registered separately.

REGISTRATION OR REJECTION

Grant of certificate of registration or rejection of application for registration shall be communicated to the applicant as specified in Form B or Form C, as the case may be, within a period of seventy days from the date of receipt of application for registration.

Renewal of Registration

An application for renewal of certificate of registration shall be made in duplicate in Form A, to the Appropriate Authority thirty days before the date of expiry of the certificate of registration. Acknowledgement of receipt of such application shall be issued by the Appropriate Authority in the manner as for registration. In the event of failure of the Appropriate Authority to renew the certificate of registration or to communicate rejection of application for renewal of registration within a period of seventy days from the date of receipt of application for renewal of registration, the certificate of registration shall be deemed to have been renewed (GSR 119 E).

Appropriate Authority and Advisory Committee–As per Rule 17

- The Central Government shall appoint, by notification in the Official Gazette, one or more Appropriate Authorities for each of the Union territories for the purposes of this Act.
- The State Government shall appoint, by notification in the Official Gazette, one or more Appropriate Authorities for the whole or part of the State for the purposes of this Act having regard to the intensity of the problem of prenatal sex determination leading to female foeticide.

District Advisory Committee

- Three medical experts from amongst gynecologists, obstetricians, pediatricians and medical geneticists;
- One legal expert;
- One officer to represent the department dealing with information and publicity of the State Government or the Union territory, as the case may be;
- Three eminent social workers of whom not less than one shall be from amongst representatives of women's organizations.

Appropriate Authority

The Appropriate Authority shall have the following functions, namely:

- To grant, suspend or cancel registration of a genetic counseling center, genetic laboratory or genetic clinic;
- To enforce standards prescribed for the genetic counseling center, genetic laboratory and genetic clinic;
- To investigate complaints of breach of the provisions of this Act or the rules made there under and take immediate action; and
- To seek and consider the advice of the Advisory Committee, constituted under sub-section (5), on application for registration and on complaints for suspension or cancellation of registration.

Offences and Penalties

Prohibition of advertisement relating to preconception and prenatal determination of sex.

Owner of the place or any employee (permanent or honorary)

- For first contravention—imprisonment up to 3 years and with fine which may extend to 10,000 rupees.
- For subsequent contravention—imprisonment up to 5 years and with fine which may extend up to ₹ 50,000

- The name of the Registered Medical Practitioner shall be reported by the A.A. to the State Medical Council concerned for taking necessary actions.
- Suspension of registration—if the charges are framed by the Court and till the case is disposed off.
- Removal of the name from the register of the council
  - For Five Years — for the first conviction
  - Premanently — for subsequent offence

Contravention of any provisions or any rules for which no penalty has been elsewhere provided in this act punishment is imprisonment up to 3 months or fine up to ₹ 1000/- Or both.

Continuing contravention additional ₹ 500 for every day during which such contravention continues after conviction for the first such contravention.

Any person who seeks the aid of any ultrasound clinic or imaging clinic for sex selection or for conducting prenatal diagnostic techniques on any pregnant women for the purposes other than those specified in subsection (2) of Section 4, *he shall, be punishable with imprisonment for a term which may extend to three years and with fine which may extend to fifty thousand rupees for the first offence* and for any subsequent offence with imprisonment which may extend to five years and with fine which may extend to one lakh rupees.

DUTIES OF REGISTERED CENTER

Person conducting ultrasonography on a pregnant women shall keep complete record thereof in the clinic/center in Form-F and any deficiency or inaccuracy found therein shall amount to contravention of provisions of section 5 or section 6 of the Act, unless contrary is proved by the person conducting such ultrasonography.

Facilities for Inspection–Rule No. 11

- Every genetic center, genetic lab, genetic clinic, ultrasound clinic, imaging center, nursing home, hospital, institute or any other place where any of the machines or equipment capable of performing any procedure, technique or prenatal determination of sex or selection of sex before or after conception is used, shall afford all reasonable facilities for inspection of the place, equipment and records to the Appropriate Authority or to any other person authorized by the Appropriate Authority in this behalf for registration of such institutions, by whatever name called, under the Act, or for detection of misuse of such facilities or advertisement therefore or for selection of sex before or after conception or for detection/disclosure of sex of fetus or for detection of cases of violation of the provisions of the Act in any other manner.
- The Appropriate Authority or the officer authorized by it may seal and seize any ultrasound machine, scanner or any other equipment, capable of detecting sex of fetus, used by any organization if the organization has not got itself registered under the Act. These machines of the organizations shall be confiscated and further action shall be taken as per the provision of the Section 23 of the Act. As per Amendment Rule 2011 by Notification dated 31-5-2011.

Intimation of Changes in Employees, Place or Equipment–Rule 13

Every genetic clinic shall intimate every change (Addition/Removal) of employee, place, address and equipment installed, to the Appropriate Authority within a period of seven days of such change. As per Delhi High Court order dated 27-6-2012 in CM NO, 8402 of writ petition no. 4009/2012.

New Registration not required .... **Rule 13)**

Public Information.........................Rule 17

- Every genetic counseling center, genetic laboratory and genetic clinic shall prominently display on its premises a notice in English and in the local language or languages for the information of the public, to effect that disclosure of the sex of the fetus is prohibited under law.
- At least one copy each of the bare Act and these rules shall be available on the premises of every genetic counseling center, genetic laboratory and genetic clinic, and shall be made available to the clientele on demand for perusal.

Code of Conduct..........................Rule 18

*Wear name tag yourself and every employee working at the US Clinic. Write full name and designation under signatures.....**(Rule 18-viii and ix)**

*Should not indulge in sex determination and female feticide and do not commit any other act of professional misconduct.....**(Rule 18-x and xi)**

Appear .... Rule 19

Appeal against charge sheet can be filed to DAC/SAC within 30 days and decision has to be taken within 90 days .... **(Rule 19-1-3)**.

Maintenance and Preservation of Records ....Rule 9

- Genetic Clinic shall maintain a register showing, in serial order, the names and addresses of the women given genetic counseling, subjected to prenatal diagnostic procedures or prenatal diagnostic tests, the names of their husbands or fathers and the date on which they first reported for such counseling, procedure or test (Rule 9.1).

- *For genetic counseling center:* Patient records shall be kept as specified in Form-D (Rule 9.2)
- *For genetic laboratory:* Patient records shall be kept as specified in Form-E (Rule 9.3)
- For genetic/US clinic patient records shall be kept as specified in Form-F (Rule 9.4)
- For interventional process consent form should be filled Form-G (Rule 9.5)
- Picture of sonographic image sgould pe preserved in soft/hard copy (Rule 9.6)
- Every genetic clinic/ultrasound clinic shall send a complete report in respect of all pre-conception or pregnancy related procedures/techniques/tests conducted by them in respect of each month by 5th day of the following month to the concerned appropriate authority even zero report (Rule 9.8).

SEARCH

Whenever an appropriate authority or any other authorized officer has reason to believe that an offence under the Act has been or is being committed, he may search a *genetic counseling center*, a *genetic laboratory or genetic clinic or any other place which is suspected of conducting prenatal diagnostic techniques.*

The scope of the powers of the appropriate authority to search and seize is very wide and it includes the power to:

- Enter freely into the place of search.
- Search at all reasonable times.
- Examine and inspect all documents like:
  - Registers
  - Records including consent forms, referral slips, charts, laboratory results, microscopic pictures
  - Forms
  - Books
  - Pamphlets
  - Advertisements
  - Material objects like sonographic plates or slides
  - Equipment like ultrasonography machines, needles, fetoscope, etc.
- Seize and seal any document, record, material object or equipment, etc. If there is reason to believe that it may furnish evidence of commission of an offence punishable under the Act.
- Further the appropriate authority may seal and seize any offending equiment if the facility has not registered itself.

SEARCH AND WITNESSES

- During the search *at least two independent witnesses of the locality* should be present.
- If no such persons are available or willing to be witness to the search, then two such persons of another locality should be present.
- The search should be made in the presence of the two or more independent witnesses.
- The witnesses are to be selected by the appropriate authority or the officer duly authorized to conduct search.
- The witnesses so selected should be unprejudiced and uninterested as the object of the section is to ensure fair dealing and a feeling of confidence and security amongst public.
- The witnesses may be summoned by Court to appear as witnesses.
- Any person suspected of having any object on his person may also be searched.

However, if such person, is a woman than, the search can be done only by a female officer.

SEIZURE AND PREPARATION OF LIST

- A list of documents, records, material objects, etc. seized during the search should be prepared in duplicate and both copies of such list shall be signed on every page by the appropriate authority or the officer authorized and the witnesses to the seizure.
- Assistance of your office staff can always be taken during the process of search and seizure.
- The list should be prepared at the place affecting the seizure and if it is not practicable to do so at the place affecting the seizure then for reasons to be recorded in writing it can be done in any other place, but it has to be in the presence of the witnesses.
- A copy of the list prepared must be handed over to the person from whose custody the document, record or material object, etc. is being seized or his representative under acknowledgment or sent by registered post to him if he is not available at the place of effecting the seizure.
- The person from whose custody the document, record or material object, etc. is being seized or his representative should be permitted to attend during the search and seizure.

- The appropriate authority or the officer duly authorized in this behalf may seize any document, material object, record or equipment and take the same into safe custody.
- It is preferable that along with the preparation of list of objects seized, a slip is made and pasted on each object seized along with the date, time and the signature of the witnesses.
- After a list of seizure is prepared the same must be sent to the Magistrate having jurisdiction or incharge of the case within 24 hours of the seizure by the appropriate authority or officer duly authorized. Permission to retain the seized objects should be obtained from the Court. The owner of the seized object may make an application to the court for the release of the same. The court may do so after imposing conditions for custody and taking a bond to the effect that, the objects must not be misused for conducting sex-determination tests and that the objects must be produced in Court as and when required, etc.
- Police aid can be taken if the appropriate authority apprehends a law and order problem during the process of search and seizure.

SEALING

- If any material object seized is perishable in nature then arrangements shall be made promptly by the appropriate authority or officer duly authorized for sealing, identification and preservation of the same and send the same to a facility for test if so required.
- And till such arrangements for safe removal are made the refrigerator or other equipment used by the genetic counseling center, genetic laboratory or genetic clinic for preservation of such material object seized shall be sealed; In case of such sealing it is important to mention the same in the list of seizure prepared.
- If the search and seizure is not completed in a day then the appropriate authority or officer duly authorized may either seal the premises or mount a guard for safe keeping to prevent any tampering of the documents, records, material objects, etc.
- After seizure the seized objects can be removed to your own premises or may be left in the custody of a respectable person of the locality. If it is not possible to remove the seized objects, they may be retained where they are found after taking a bond from the owner that the same would be produced before the court as and when required.
- The appropriate authority is duty bound to maintain systematic records of the search and seizure and the same would also safeguard the appropriate authority against any allegations of abuse.

COLLECTION OF EVIDENCE

The evidence that needs to be collected in order to make out a case under the PNDT Act varies depending upon the nature of the violation and in some cases the pieces of evidence can overlap.

- **Illegal advertisement**
  The documentary evidence will include:
  - The paper cutting of the advertisement, the name of the newspaper or magazine or any other document which carries the advertisement, the date of the issuance of the advertisement;
  - The name of the advertiser, his place of business;
  - The name of the owner of the clinic, center or laboratory issuing such advertisement, the address of the said center, laboratory or clinic;
  - The name of the distributor, his place of business;
  - The photograph of the advertisement, the photograph of the hoarding, board, wall on which the advertisement is present, etc.
  - The letters heads, memorandum of association, annual reports, statements showing organizational structure and ownership of the newspaper, or 17 Rule 11(2) under the amended PNDT Rules, distributorship, or the center. This information has to be collected in order to link the person to the violation.
- *In case of conducting a test for determination of sex or communication of the sex of the fetus: The documentary evidence will include*
  - Referral slips
  - Consent forms
  - Laboratory results
  - Microscopic pictures
  - Sonographic plates or slides
  - Registers containing names and addresses of patients and their families
  - Case history of the patient
  - Records of clients maintained on the computer or other electronic equipment can be taken on a floppy or a printed copy of the same
  - Floppy or printed copy of the ultrasound image of the fetus
  - Receipt of fee paid for the test, details of cheque payment, etc.

- *In case of non-registration, cancellation or suspension of registration:*

  The documentary and oral evidence will include:
  - Copy of the registration certificate
  - Copy of the affidavit given by the owner that he will not conduct prenatal determination of sex.
  - Copy of the particulars given about the qualifications of the employees while registration
  - Documents collected from the MCI, the degree certificate of the medical practitioners (employees of the center), etc.
  - Statements of decoy witnesses
  - The tape and video recording
  - Other materials collected as evidence in case of conducting tests.

The complete evidence to be submitted before the Magistrate would include:

- A copy of the complaint
- A statement showing the list of witnesses both witnesses of the search and seizure and decoy witnesses
- The report of the search and seizure or commonly called Panchnamah
- A copy of the all the documents collected.
- Statements of witnesses if any.
- Most essential would be the complete address of the *genetic counseling center, genetic clinic* or *genetic laboratory*.

FORM A

[See rules 4(1) and 8(1)]
(To be submitted in Duplicate)

With supporting documents as enclosures, also in duplicate form of application for registration or renewal of registration of a genetic counseling center/genetic laboratory/genetic clinic.

1. **Name of the applicant** (specify Shri./Smt./Km./Dr.)
2. **Address of the applicant**
3. **Type of facility to be registered** (specify Genetic Counseling Center/Genetic Laboratory/Genetic Clinic/any combination of these)
4. **Full name and address/addresses** of Genetic Counseling Center/Genetic Laboratory/Genetic Clinic with Telephone/ Telegraphic
   Telex/Fax e-mail numbers.
5. **Type of ownership and organization**
   (Specify individual ownership/partnership/company/cooperative/any other). In case of type of organization other than individual ownership, furnish copy of articles of association and names and addresses of other persons responsible for management, as enclosure.
6. **Type of institution**
   (Government Hospital/Municipal Hospital/Public Hospital/Private Hospital/Private Nursing Home/Private Clinic/Private Laboratory/any other to be started.)
7. **Specific prenatal diagnostic procedures/tests for which approval is sought**
   (For example amniocentesis, chorionic villi aspiration/chromosomal/biochemical/molecular studies, etc.)
   Leave blank if registration sought for genetic counseling center only.
8. **Equipment available with the make and model of each equipment**
   List to be attached on a separate sheet.
9. (a) **Facilities available in the counseling center**:
   i. Ultrasound
   ii. Amniocentesis
   iii. Chorionic villi aspiration
   iv. Fetoscopy
   v. Fetal biopsy
   vi. Cordocentesis

   (b) **Whether facilities are available in the Laboratory/Clinic for the following tests**:
   i. Chromosomal studies
   ii. Biochemical studies
   iii. Molecular studies
10. **Names, qualifications, experience and registration number of employees may be furnished as an enclosure (Refer Schedules I, II or III).**
11. State whether the Genetic Counseling Center/Genetic Laboratory/Genetic Clinic qualifies for registration in terms of minimum requirements laid down in Schedule I, II and III and if not, reasons therefore.
12. **For renewal applications only**:
    Registration No.
    Date of issue and date of expiry of existing certificate of registration.
13. **List of Enclosures:**
    Please attach a list of enclosures giving the supporting documents enclosed to this application.

Date:
Place

(............................)
Name and signature of applicant

DECLARATION

I, Sh/Smt/Kum/.............................. son/daughter/wife of .... aged .... years resident of.. hereby declare that I have read and understood the Prenatal Diagnostic Techniques (Regulation and Prevention of Misuse) Act, 1994 (57 of 1994) and the Prenatal Diagnostic Techniques (Regulation and Prevention of Misuse) Rules, 1995.

I also undertake to explain the said Act and Rules to all employees of the Genetic Counseling Center/Genetic Laboratory/ Genetic Clinic in respect of which registration is sought and to ensure that Act and Rules are fully complied with.

Date:
Place

(.......................)
Name and signature of applicant

ACKNOWLEDGMENT

[See Rules 4(2) and 8(1)]

The application in Form A in duplicate for grant*/renewal* of registration of Genetic Counseling Center*/Genetic Laboratory*/Genetic Clinic* by ....(Name and address of applicant) has been received by the Appropriate Authority .... On (date).

*The list of enclosures attached to the application in Form A has been verified with the enclosures submitted and found to be correct.

OR

On verification it is found that the following documents mentioned in the list of enclosures are not actually enclosed.

This acknowledgment does not confer any rights on the applicant for grant or renewal of registration.

Date:

(...............................)
Signature and Designation of Appropriate Authority,
or authorized person in the
Office of the Appropriate Authority

Seal
Original
Duplicate for Display

FORM B

[See Rules 6(2), 6(5) and 8(2)]

CERTIFICATE OF REGISTRATION

(To be issued in duplicate)

1. In exercise of the powers conferred under Section 19 (1) of the Prenatal Diagnostic Techniques (Regulation and Prevention of Misuse) Act, 1994 (57 of 1994), the Appropriate Authority .... hereby grants registration to the Genetic Counseling Center/Genetic Laboratory/Genetic Clinic named below for purposes of carrying out Genetic Counseling/Prenatal Diagnostic Procedures/Prenatal Diagnostic Tests as defined in the aforesaid Act for a period of five years ending on ....
2. This registration is granted subject to the aforesaid Act and Rules there under and any contravention thereof shall result in suspension or cancellation of this Certificate of Registration before the expiry of the said period of five years.
   A. Name and address of the Genetic Counseling Centre/Genetic Laboratory/Genetic Clinic.
   B. Name of Applicant for registration.
   C. Prenatal diagnostic procedures approved for (Genetic Clinic).
      i. Ultrasound
      ii. Amniocentesis
      iii. Chorionic villi biopsy
      iv. Fetoscopy
      v. Fetal skin or organ biopsy
      vi. Cordocentesis
      Any other (specify)
   D. Prenatal diagnostic tests* approved (for Genetic laboratory)
      i. Chromosomal studies
      ii. Biochemical studies
      iii. Molecular studies
      iv. Registration no. allotted
      v. For renewed Certificate of Registration only
      vi. Period of validity of earlier Certificate From ...... to ......, Or Registration.

Signature, Name and Designation of the Appropriate Authority

Date:

Seal

DISPLAY ONE COPY OF THIS CERTIFICATE AT A CONSPICUOUS PLACE AT THE PLACE OF BUSINESS

FORM C

[See Rules 6(3), 6(5) and 8(3)]

REJECTION OF APPLICATION FOR REGISTRATION OR RENEWAL OF REGISTRATION

In exercise of the powers conferred under Section 19(2) of the Prenatal Diagnostic Techniques (Regulation and Prevention of Misuse) Act, 1994, the Appropriate Authority .... Hereby rejects the application for grant/renewal of registration of the Genetic Counseling Center/Genetic Laboratory/Genetic Clinic named below for the reasons stated.

Name and address of the Genetic Counseling Center/Genetic Laboratory/Genetic Clinic

Name of Applicant who has applied for registration

Reasons for rejection of application for registration

Date: **Signature, Name and Designation of the Appropriate Authority**

Seal

FORM D

[See rule 9(2)]

NAME, ADDRESS AND REGISTRATION NO. OF GENETIC COUNSELING CENTER RECORD TO BE MAINTAINED BY THE GENETIC COUNSELING CENTER

1. Patient's name
2. Age
3. Husband's/Father's name
4. Full address with Tel. No., if any
5. Referred by (Full name and address of Doctor(s) with registration No.(s) (Referred note to be preserved carefully with case papers)
6. Last menstrual period/weeks of pregnancy
7. History of genetic/medical disease in the family (specify) Basis of diagnosis:
   a. Clinical b. Bio-chemical c. Cytogenetic d. Other (e.g. radiological)
8. Indication for prenatal diagnosis
   A. Previous child/children with:
      i. Chromosomal disorders
      ii. Metabolic disorders
      iii. Congenital anomaly
      iv. Mental retardation
      v. Hemoglobinopathy
      vi. Sex linked disorders
      vii. Any other (specify)
   B. Advanced maternal age (35 years)
   C. Mother/father/sibling has genetic disease (specify)
   D. Others (specify)
9. Procedure advised
   i. Ultrasound
   ii. Amniocentesis
   iii. Chorionic villi biopsy
   iv. Fetoscopy
   v. Fetal skin or organ biopsy
   vi. Cordocentesis
   vii. Any other (specify)
10. Laboratory tests to be carried out
   i. Chromosomal studies
   ii. Biochemical studies
   iii. Molecular studies
11. Result of prenatal diagnosis. If abnormal give details. Normal/Abnormal
12. Was MTP advised?
13. Name and address of Genetic Clinic to which patient referred.
14. Dates of commencement and completion of genetic counseling.

Date:

Name, Signature and Registration no. of the Medical Geneticist/Gynecologist/Pediatrician

FORM E

[See Rule 9(3)]

NAME, ADDRESS AND REGISTRATION NO. OF GENETIC LABORATORY RECORD TO BE MAINTAINED BY THE GENETIC LABORATORY

1. Patient's name
2. Age
3. Husband's/Father's name
4. Full address with Tel. No., if any
5. Referred by/sample sent by (full name and address of Genetic Clinic) (Referral note to be preserved carefully with case papers)
6. Type of sample: Maternal blood/chorionic villus sample/amniotic fluid/fetal blood or other fetal tissue (specify)
7. Specify indication for prenatal diagnosis
   A. Previous child/children with
      i. Chromosomal disorders
      ii. Metabolic disorders
      iii. Malformation(s)
      iv. Mental retardation
      v. Hereditary hemolytic anemia
      vi. Sex linked disorder
      vii. Any other (specify)
   B. Advanced maternal age (-35 years)
   C. Mother/father/sibling has genetic disease (specify)
   D. Other (specify)
8. Laboratory tests carried out (give details)
   i. Chromosomal studies
   ii. Biochemical studies
   iii. Molecular studies
9. Result of prenatal diagnosis
   If abnormal give details. Normal/Abnormal
10. Date(s) on which tests carried out.
    The results of the prenatal diagnostic tests were conveyed to ....on................

Date: **Name, Signature and Registration no. of the Medical Geneticist**

NEW FORM F

[See Provision to section 4(3), Rule 9(4) and Rule 10(1A) as per GSR 77 (E) dated 31.1.2014]

FORM FOR MAINTENANCE OF RECORDS IN CASE OF A PREGNANT WOMAN BY GENETIC CLINIC/ULTRASOUND CLINIC/IMAGING CENTER

Section A: *To be filled in for all Diagnostic Procedures/Tests*

1. Name and complete address of Genetic Clinic/Ultrasound Clinic/Imaging center: ______
2. Registration No. (*Under PC and PNDT Act*).______
3. Patient's name ______Age______
4. Total number of living children:______
   a. Number of living sons with age of each living son (in years or months): ______
   b. Number of living daughters with age of each living daughter (in years or months): ___
5. Husband's/Father's/Mother's Name :______
6. Full postal address of the patient with contact number, if any______ ______
7. a. Referred by (Full name and address of Doctor(s)/Genetic Counseling Center):______

   (Referral slips to be preserved carefully with Form F)

   b. Self Referral by Gynecologist/Radiologist/Registered Medical Practitioner conducting the diagnostic procedures: ______

   (Referral note with indications and case papers of the patient to be preserved with Form F)
   (Self-referral does not mean a client coming to a clinic and requesting for the test or the relative/s requesting for the test of a pregnant woman)
8. Last menstrual period,
   OR weeks of pregnancy:______

Section B: *To be filled in for performing non-invasive Diagnostic Procedures/Tests only*

9. Name of the doctor performing the procedure/s: ______
10. Indication/s for diagnosis procedure ______ (*specify with reference to the request made in the referral slip or in a self-referral note)*
    (Ultrasonography prenatal diagnosis during pregnancy should only be performed when indicated. The following is the representative list of indications for ultrasound during pregnancy.
    (Put a "Tick" against the appropriate indication/s for ultrasound)
    1. *To diagnose intrauterine and/or ectopic pregnancy and confirm viability.*
    2. *Estimation of gestational age (dating).*
    3. Detection of number of fetuses and their chorionicity.
    4. Suspected pregnancy with IUCD *in situ* or suspected pregnancy following contraceptive failure/MTP failure.
    5. Vaginal bleeding/leaking.
    6. Follow-up of cases of abortion.
    7. Assessment of cervical canal and diameter of internal os.
    8. Discrepancy between uterine size and period of amenorrhea.
    9. Any suspected adenexal or uterine pathology/abnormality.
    10. Detection of chromosomal abnormalities, fetal structural defects and other abnormalities and their follow-up.
    11. To evaluate fetal presentation and position.
    12. Assessment of liquor amnii.
    13. Preterm labor/preterm premature rupture of membranes.

14. *Evaluation of placental position, thickness, grading and abnormalities (placenta praevia, retro placental hemorrhage, abnormal adherence, etc.).*
15. *Evaluation of umbilical cord – presentation, insertion, nuchal encirclement, number of vessels and presence of true knot.*
16. *Evaluation of previous Cesarean Section scars.*
17. *Evaluation of fetal growth parameters, fetal weight and fetal well-being.*
18. *Color flow mapping and duplex Doppler studies.*
19. *Ultrasound guided procedures such as medical termination of pregnancy, external cephalic version, etc. and their follow-up.*
20. *Adjunct to diagnostic and therapeutic invasive interventions such as chorionic villus sampling (CVS), amniocenteses, fetal blood sampling, fetal skin biopsy, amnio-infusion, intrauterine infusion, placement of shunts, etc.*
21. *Observation of intra-partum events.*
22. *Medical/surgical conditions complicating pregnancy.*
23. *Research/scientific studies in recognized institutions.*

11. Procedures carried out (Non-invasive) (Put a "Tick" on the appropriate procedure)
    i. Ultrasound
    (***Important note:*** *Ultrasounds not indicated/advised/performed to determine the sex of fetus except for diagnosis of sex-linked diseases such as Duchenne muscular dystrophy, hemophilia A and B, etc.)*
    ii. Any other (specify) __________
12. Date on which declaration of pregnant was woman obtained:____________________
13. Date on which procedures carried out:___________________________________
14. Result of non-invasive procedure carried out *(report in brief of the test including ultrasound carried out)* ______________
    ____
15. The result of prenatal diagnostic procedures was conveyed to ____________on_____
16. Any indication for MTP as per the abnormality detected in the diagnostic procedures/tests ________________________
    ____

Section C: *To be filled for performing invasive Procedures/Tests only*

17. Name of the doctor/s performing the procedure/s:______________________________
18. History of genetic/medical disease in the family (specify):__________________________
    Basis of diagnosis ("Tick" on appropriate basis of diagnosis):
    a. Clinical b. Bio-chemical
    c. Cytogenetic d. Other (e.g. radiological, ultrasonography, etc. specify)
19. Indication/s for the diagnosis procedure ("Tick" on appropriate indication/s):
    A. Previous child/children with:
       i. Chromosomal disorders ii. Metabolic disorders
       iii. Congenital anomaly iv. Mental disability
       v. Hemoglobinopathy vi. Sex linked disorders
       vii. Single gene disorder viii. Any other (specify)
    B. Advanced maternal age (35 years)
    C. Mother/father/sibling has genetic disease (specify)
    D. Other (specify) ____
20. Date on which consent of pregnant woman was obtained in Form G prescribed in PC&PNDT Act, 1994 :______________
    ____
21. Invasive procedures carried out ("Tick" on appropriate indication/s)
    i. Amniocentesis
    ii. Chorionic villi aspiration
    iii. Fetal biopsy
    iv. Cordocentesis
    v. Any other (specify)

22. Any complication/s of invasive procedure (specify)______________________________
23. Additional tests recommended (Please mention if applicable)
    i. Chromosomal studies   ii. Biochemical studies
    iii. Molecular studies   iv. Pre-implantation gender diagnosis
    v. Any other (specify)
24. Result of the procedures/tests carried out (report in brief of the invasive tests/procedures carried out)________________
    ____
25. Date on which procedures carried out:__________________________________
26. The result of prenatal diagnostic procedures was conveyed to ____________on_________
27. Any indication for MTP as per the abnormality detected in the diagnostic procedures/tests
    ____

Date:

Place:

Name, Signature and Registration Number with Seal of the Gynecologist/Radiologist/Registered Medical Practitioner Performing Diagnostic Procedure

Section D: *Declaration*

DECLARATION OF PREGNANT WOMAN UNDERGOING ULTRASONOGRAPHY/IMAGE SCANNING

I, Mrs ____________________(name of the pregnant woman) declare that by undergoing ultrasonography/image scanning, etc. I do not want to know the sex of my fetus.

Date:

Signature/Thumb impression of pregnant woman

In case of thumb impression:
Identified by (Name)__________________________ __________Age:______Sex:_______
Relation (if any):___________Address and Contact No.:_______________________________
____

Date: _____________

Signature of a person attesting thumb impression: ________________

DECLARATION OF DOCTOR/PERSON CONDUCTING DIAGNOSTIC PROCEDURE/TEST

I, _____________________________ (name of the person conducting ultrasonography/image scanning) declare that while conducting ultrasonography/image scanning on Ms.__________________ (name of the pregnant woman), I have neither detected nor disclosed the sex of her fetus to anybody in any manner.

Date:

Signature: __________________________

Name in Capitals, Registration Number with Seal of the Gynecologist/Radiologist/Registered Medical Practitioner Conducting Diagnostic Procedure

FORM G

[See Rule 10]

FORM OF CONSENT

I, ... wife/daughter of .... Age .... years residing at .... hereby state that I have been explained fully the probable side effects and after effects of the prenatal diagnostic procedures. I wish to undergo the prenatal diagnostic procedures in my interest to find out the possibility of any abnormality (i.e. deformity or disorder) in the child I am carrying.

I undertake not to terminate the pregnancy if the prenatal procedure and any prenatal tests conducted show the absence of deformity or disorders. I understand that the sex of the fetus will not be disclosed to me.

I understand that breach of this undertaking will make me liable to penalty as prescribed in the prenatal diagnostic techniques (Regulation and Prevention of Misuse) Act, 1994 (57 of 1994).

Date: **Signature**

Place:

I have explained the contents of the above consent to the patient and her companion (Name .... Address .... Relationship .... in a language she/they understand.

Date: **Name, Signature and/Registration number of Gynecologist**

Name, Address and Registration number of Genetic Clinic

FORM H

[See Rule 9(5)]

PERMANENT RECORD OF APPLICATION FOR REGISTRATION, GRANT OF REGISTRATION REJECTION OF APPLICATION FOR REGISTRATION AND RENEWALS OF REGISTRATION

1. Serial number
2. File number of Appropriate Authority.
3. Date of receipt of application for grant of registration.
4. Name, Address, Phone/Fax, etc. of Applicant:
5. Name and address(es) of Genetic Counseling Center/Genetic Laboratory/Genetic Clinic.
6. Date on which case considered by Advisory Committee and recommendation of Advisory Committee, in summary.
7. Outcome of application (state granted/rejected and date of issue of orders).
8. Registration number allotted and date of expiry of registration.
9. Renewals (date of renewal and renewed up to).
10. File number in which renewals dealt.
11. Additional information, if any.

Designation and Signature of Appropriate Authority

Guidance for Appropriate Authority

a. Form H is a permanent record to be maintained as a register, in the custody of the Appropriate Authority.
b. Means strike out whichever is not applicable.
c. Against item 7, record date of issue of order in Form B or Form C.
d. On renewal, the Registration Number of the Genetic Counseling Center/Genetic Laboratory/Genetic Clinic will not change. A fresh registration Number will be allotted in the event of change of ownership or management.
e. No registration number shall be allotted twice.
f. Each Genetic Counseling Center/Genetic Laboratory/Genetic Clinic may be allotted a folio consisting of two facing pages of the Register for recording Form H.
g. The space provided for 'additional information' may be used for recording suspension, cancellations, rejection of application for renewal, change of ownership/management, outcome of any legal proceedings, etc.
h. Every folio (i.e. 2 pages) of the Register shall be authenticated by signature of the Appropriate Authority with date, and every subsequent entry shall also be similarly authenticated.

SECTION

9

The Future of Prenatal Diagnosis

CHAPTER 39

Current Status of Fetal Genomic Diagnosis in Fetal Medicine, Progress and Challenges

Amit Chakravarty, Sudipa Chakravarty

ABSTRACT

Prenatal genetic diagnostic technology is advancing at an astonishingly rapid pace. Of the 117 references cited in this paper, 53 (45%) of them have been published in the past 2 years. Professional education and guidelines for incorporating new genetic tests into current practice are urgently needed. High-level economic analyses are also required to assess the benefits and limitations of current compared to future approaches. Multidisciplinary research teams consisting of basic and translational scientists, clinicians, ethicists and parents should be formed to consider many of the issues raised here. Time is of the essence because the commercial sector has already made some of these tests, such as fetal sex and determination of paternity, directly available to pregnant women.

For the past 30 years, the goal of prenatal diagnosis has been to provide an informed choice to prospective parents. That paradigm is now shifting. We are now at a point where that goal can and should be expanded to incorporate genetic and genomic data to pave the way for a personalized approach to fetal treatment.

INTRODUCTION

Prenatal diagnosis or prenatal screening (note that *prenatal diagnosis* and *prenatal screening* refer to two different types of tests) is testing for diseases or conditions in a fetus or embryo before it is born.[1] The aim is to detect birth defects such as neural tube defects, Down syndrome, chromosome abnormalities, genetic disorders and other conditions, such as spina bifida, cleft palate, Tay-Sachs disease, sickle cell anemia, thalassemia, cystic fibrosis, muscular dystrophy, and fragile X syndrome. Screening can also be used for prenatal sex discernment. Common testing procedures include amniocentesis, ultrasonography including nuchal translucency ultrasound, serum marker testing, or genetic screening.[2-5] In some cases, the tests are administered to determine if the fetus will be aborted, though physicians and patients also find it useful to diagnose high-risk pregnancies early so that delivery can be scheduled in a tertiary care hospital where the baby can receive appropriate.

We first discuss these technological advances and provide examples of how they have provided a greater understanding of the genetic basis of specific fetal disorders (Table 39.1). In the prenatal setting, pure fetal material may be obtained invasively through amniocentesis or chorionic villus sampling or noninvasively through maternal blood. The invasive diagnostic techniques are generally safe and accurate, although they need to be performed by obstetricians with specific expertise, and they carry with them a small but measurable chance of miscarriage.[4] There is expanding interest in noninvasive techniques of fetal assessment using cell-free DNA and RNA molecules that circulate in the maternal blood. Maternal venipuncture has no associated risk of fetal loss; however, maternal blood contains a mixture of both fetal and maternal nucleic acids, which increases the downstream analytic complexity care.

Fetal genomic analyses are also beginning to be applied to prenatal diagnosis; these analyses can provide a dynamic view of fetal and placental development. We would like to discuss advances in this area and how such approaches might be used to find new biomarkers for fetal diseases or provide insights into the functional pathways involved in a particular disorder. We also discuss the practical and ethical challenges facing the field of fetal diagnostics, including how these new technologies should be incorporated into clinical practice, as well as how to move forward to translate these insights to provide new therapeutic strategies for fetal disease and achieve the goal of fetal medicine.

Current Status of Invasive Diagnosis by Fetal Chromosome Analysis

Cytogenetic diagnosis is in a transition from the microscopic analysis of chromosomes in metaphase to the analysis

Table 39.1 Overview of advances in molecular testing that affect fetal diagnostics and treatment

Genetic material analyzed	Type of testing	Consequences
Chromosomal DNA	Chromosome microarray analysis	Detection of submicroscopic fetal chromosome abnormalities. Detection of copy number variation in the genome.
Cell-free DNA in maternal blood	Real-time PCR amplification; massively parallel sequencing	Noninvasive prenatal diagnosis of fetal sex, RhD genotype, aneuploidy, other submicroscopic chromosome abnormalities and single-gene disorders.
Cell-free RNA in amniotic fluid	Gene expression microarray analysis; comparative transcriptomic analyses between normal and affected individuals	Improved knowledge of fetal functional development in health and in disease states. Development of new biomarkers. Identification of new therapeutic targets.
RNA in maternal blood	Gene expression microarray analysis; comparative transcriptomic analyses between normal and affected individuals; quantitative miRNA analysis	Improved knowledge of fetal functional development in health and in disease states. Development of new biomarkers. Identification of new therapeutic targets.
RNA in placenta	Gene expression microarray analysis; comparative transcriptomic analyses between normal and affected individuals	Improved knowledge of fetal functional development in health and in disease states. Development of new biomarkers. Identification of new therapeutic targets.
RNA in cord blood	Gene expression microarray analysis; comparative transcriptomic analyses between normal and affected individuals	Improved knowledge of fetal functional development in health and in disease states. Development of new biomarkers. Identification of new therapeutic targets.

of DNA within chromosomes using microarrays. In the postnatal setting, a chromosomal microarray analysis is now considered to be the first-tier cytogenetic diagnostic test for individuals with congenital anomalies, intellectual disability or both.[6] Even before the International Standard Cytogenomic Array (ISCA) Consortium (*https://www.iscaconsortium.org/*) published their evidence-based summary of 33 studies involving over 21,000 children and adults in 2010,[6] there was a demand for applying this technology prenatally. Therefore, in 2007 the *Eunice Kennedy Shriver* National Institute of Child Health and Human Development (NICHD) funded a clinical trial comparing the accuracy of microarrays to that of standard cytogenetic analyses (NCT01279733).

Current Status of Noninvasive Prenatal Testing for Fetal Aneuploidy

(*Recommended by The American College of Obstetricians and Gynecologists Committee on Genetics; The Society for Maternal-Fetal Medicine Publications Committee*)

Noninvasive prenatal testing that uses cell free fetal DNA from the plasma of pregnant women offers tremendous potential as a screening tool for fetal aneuploidy. Cell free fetal DNA testing should be an informed patient choice after pretest counseling and should not be part of routine prenatal laboratory assessment. Cell free fetal DNA testing should not be offered to low-risk women or women with multiple gestations because it has not been sufficiently evaluated in these groups. A negative cell free fetal DNA test result does not ensure an unaffected pregnancy. A patient with a positive test result should be referred for genetic counseling and should be offered invasive prenatal diagnosis for confirmation of test results.

Indications for Considering the Use of Cell Free Fetal DNA

- Maternal age 35 years or older at delivery
- Fetal ultrasonographic findings indicating an increased risk of aneuploidy
- History of a prior pregnancy with a trisomy
- Positive test result for aneuploidy, including first trimester, sequential, or integrated screen, or a quadruple screen
- Parental balanced Robertsonian translocation with increased risk of fetal trisomy 13 or trisomy 21.

Conclusion

- Patients at increased risk of aneuploidy can be offered testing with cell free fetal DNA. This technology can be expected to identify approximately 98% of cases of Down syndrome with a false-positive rate of less than 0.5%.
- Cell free fetal DNA testing should not be part of routine prenatal laboratory assessment, but should be an informed patient choice after pretest counseling.
- Cell free fetal DNA testing should not be offered to low-risk women or women with multiple gestations because it has not been sufficiently evaluated in these groups.
- Pretest counseling should include a review that although the cell free fetal DNA test is not a diagnostic test, it has high sensitivity and specificity. The test will only screen for the common trisomies and, at the present time, gives no other genetic information about the pregnancy.

- A family history should be obtained before the use of this test to determine if the patient should be offered other forms of screening or prenatal diagnosis for familial genetic disease.
- If a fetal structural anomaly is identified on ultrasound examination, invasive prenatal diagnosis should be offered.
- A negative cell free fetal DNA test result does not ensure an unaffected pregnancy.
- A patient with a positive test result should be referred for genetic counseling and offered invasive prenatal diagnosis for confirmation of test results.
- Cell free fetal DNA does not replace the accuracy and diagnostic precision of prenatal diagnosis with CVS or amniocentesis, which remain an option for women.

FETAL GENOME ANALYSIS

Background

The advantages of microarray testing over the current standard, metaphase karyotyping, include a higher sensitivity to detect chromosome deletions, duplications and unbalanced rearrangements and a shorter turn around time. This shorter time is because the DNA isolation procedures can be automated, and there is no need to culture the fetal cells. Whereas metaphase analyses using banding techniques can identify chromosome deletions and duplications in the range of 5–10 Mb, the higher resolution provided by microarrays can detect changes as small as 50–100 kb.[7] The disadvantages of microarrays include their inability to detect a balanced chromosome rearrangement or a triploid karyotype. The design of the array is crucial. Oligonucleotide and bacterial artificial chromosome arrays provide less coverage of the genome but are specifically designed to identify known chromosomal aberrations that are associated with clinically significant disease. Whole-genome arrays provide sequence information without complete knowledge of the long-term prognostic implications of all of the variants detected. Such sequence information, however, may be permanently archived and used as a reference source to advance our knowledge of the health of individuals and populations, human development and disease.

Advanced genetic and genomic techniques in the prenatal setting is that genomic variation can be identified and precise genetic counseling could be offered for further fetal management. Outline of the three major current technology for analyzing fetal genome are as follows:

1. Molecular cytogenetics.
2. Array CGH.
3. Whole genome microarray.

MOLECULAR CYTOGENETICS

Fetal cells are cultured and analyzed during cell division in metaphase. Chromosomes are analyzed under the microscope for the presence of dark and light staining bands. The staining patterns are compared with normal reference standards. Only relatively large deviations from normal (~5–10 Mb) can be detected. The DNA within the fetal chromosomes, rather than the fetal chromosome itself, is compared to reference genomes.

Fluorescence *in situ* Hybridization (Fig. 39.1)

The *in situ* hybridization technique involves making the nucleic acid in the target chromosomes or nuclei single stranded and incubating it with a short (e.g. 3 kbp) single stranded complimentary probe. With fluorescence *in situ* hybridization (FISH), the probe labels may be fluorochromes or other molecules that are subsequently detected with fluorescent affinity reagents. After hybridization, the numbers, intensity and spatial distribution of the fluorecent signals are analyzed. This gives an understanding of how the target nucleic acid sequences are distributed within the cells and chromosomes.

Metaphase and Interphase FISH

Metaphase FISH is used to map the location of a DNA sequence on a chromosome, using fluorescence microscopy. Metaphase FISH identifies the position of DNA sequences ranging in length from IMAGE clones to yeast artificial chromosomes (YACs). Chimerism and sequence homology can also be established. The location of integrated sequences can be determined via metaphase FISH using probes made from the transfected products in combination with chromosome banding or painting. Two, three and four color FISH is used to determine clone order. Similarly, the DNA probe sequence can also be visualised within the cell nucleus using interphase FISH (Fig. 39.2).

Fiber FISH

FISH to DNA fibers with bacterial artificial chromosome (BAC) and PAC allows rapid visualization of the extent of overlaps and gaps in contigs. Small clones can be hybridized against larger YAC clones to confirm clone order over longer distances. Fiber FISH with transfected clones allows the quantitation of integrated sequences and can be used to demonstrate the final integrity of the construct (Fig. 39.3).

Choice and Resolution of FISH Techniques

- Metaphase FISH resolves probes over approximately 2 Mbp apart and is suitable for chromosome and band assignment

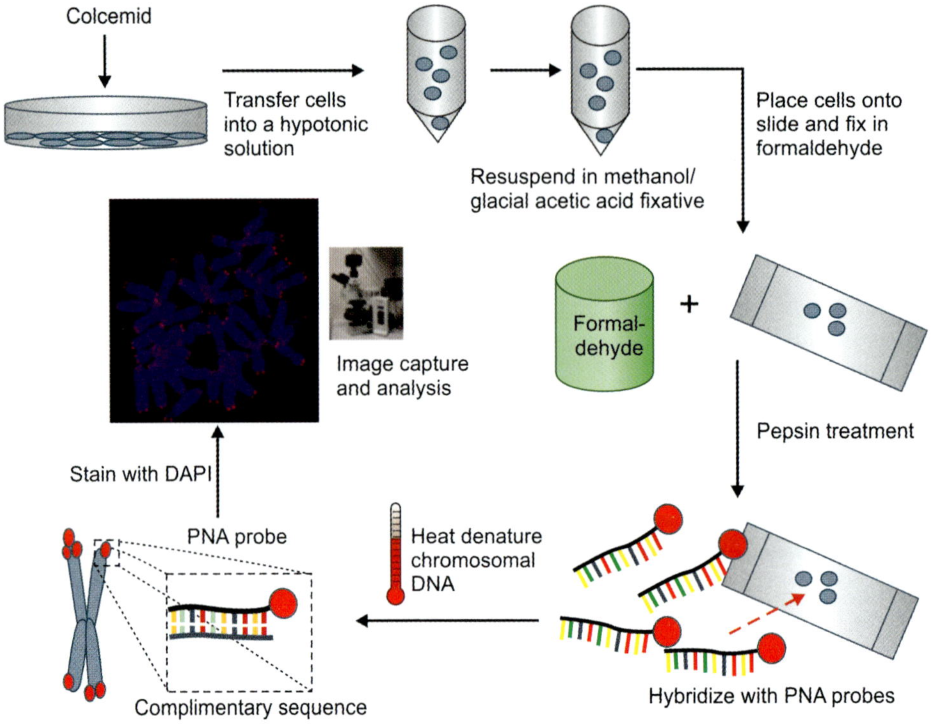

Fig. 39.1 FISH is an important molecular cytogenetic tool used for the identification of genetic disorders and the detection of chromosomal (DNA) genetic abnormalities[14]
Abbreviations: DAPI, 4; 6-diamidino-2-pherylindole; PNA, peptide nucleic acid

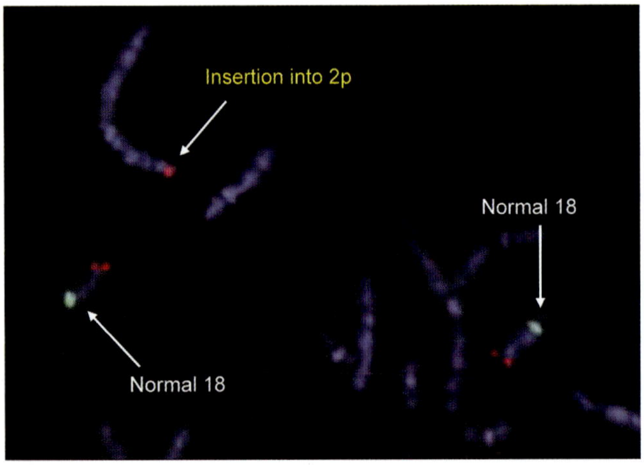

Fig. 39.2 Duplicated region of chromosome 18, which is present on chromosome 2p due to an insertional translocation Green = 18 centromere, Red = 18q23;
Source: Molecular Cytogenetics; *http://www.well.ox.ac.uk/molecular-cytogenetics-2*

- Interphase FISH resolves probes 100 Kbp–2 Mbp apart and is suitable for clone ordering and orientation
- Fiber FISH resolves probes 10 Kbp–500 Kbp apart and is suitable for clone ordering and to assess overlaps and gaps in contig maps.

M-FISH and CGH

Multiplex fluorescence *in situ* hybridization (M-FISH) and comparative genomic hybridization (CGH) are complementary fluorescent molecular cytogenetic techniques. M-FISH acquires images of each human or mouse chromosome in a different color, allowing semi-automatic karyotyping and the identification of chromosomal aberrations (Figs 39.4 and 39.5).

ARRAY COMPARATIVE GENOMIC HYBRIDIZATION

Array comparative genomic hybridization (Array-CGH) allows for the detection of a large number of genetic and epigenetic

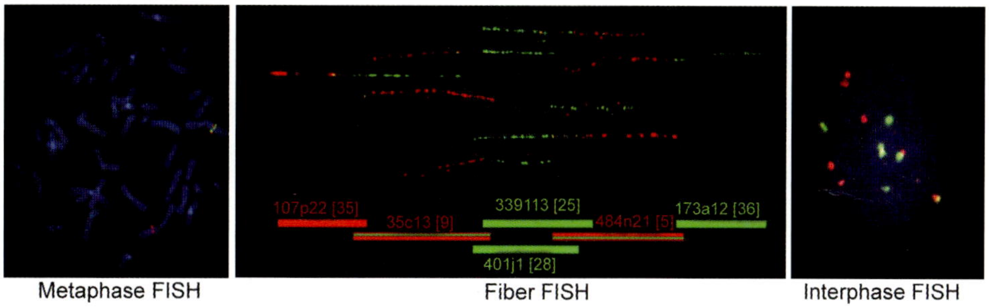

Fig. 39.3 FISH metaphases
Source: Molecular cytogenetics; *http://www.well.ox.ac.uk/molecular-cytogenetics-2*

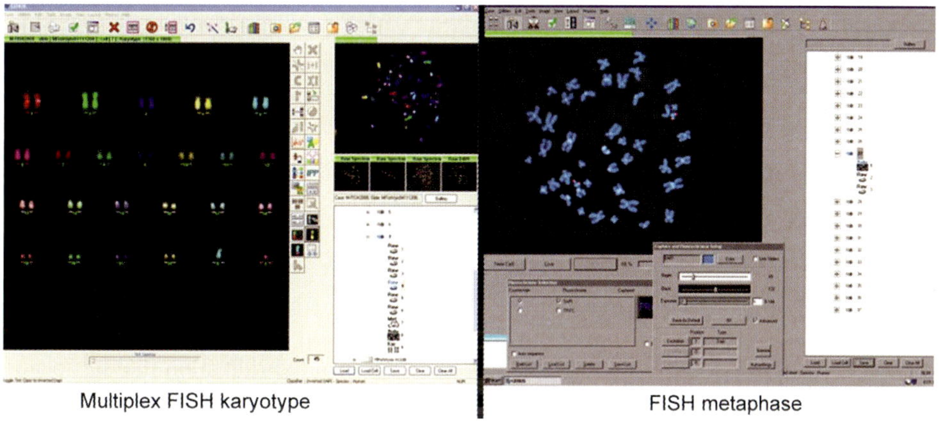

Fig. 39.4 The complimentary technique of CGH visualizes the hybridization of differentially labeled reference DNA sequences to generate a high resolution map of DNA copy number changes in the genome. The Wellcome Trust Center for Human Genetics (WTCHG) can further investigate copy number variation using the *Affymetrix GeneChip* Cytogenetics Array system

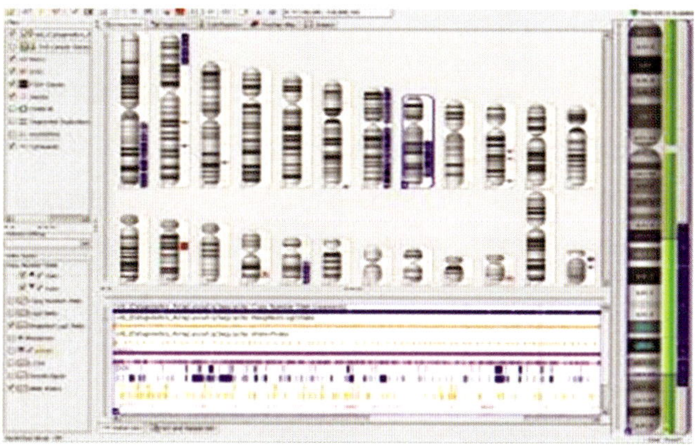

Fig. 39.5 In addition there are routine classical cytogenetics techniques like Giemsa DNA staining for chromosome banding image acquisition and semi-automatic human chromosome karyotyping[11]
(*Source:* The Wellcome Trust Centre for Human Genetics; Roosevelt Drive; Oxford; OX3 7BN; United Kingdom

alterations to be assessed in a single experiment. Array-CGH (or microarray) can be utilized to evaluate DNA copy number changes (gain/loss) observed in tumor genomes.

In an array-CGH assay, the evaluation of DNA copy number changes is performed by comparing a DNA test isolated from the tissue of interest (patient sample including cancer cells) against a normal reference DNA without cancer cells. The genomic DNA from the test tissue is fluorescently labeled with a red dye whereas the reference DNA is fluorescently labeled with a green dye. Both sets of genomic DNA are hybridized to thousands of probes printed on a glass slide or microarray. After removal of the excess labeled DNAs, the intensity of hybridized DNAs is measured and compared. The ratio between the test and reference DNAs define the presence of copy number changes for a particular locus. The signal on the microarray can vary from red (gain) to green (loss) with yellow being the balance between red/green (no change, ratio=1) (Fig. 39.6).[1]

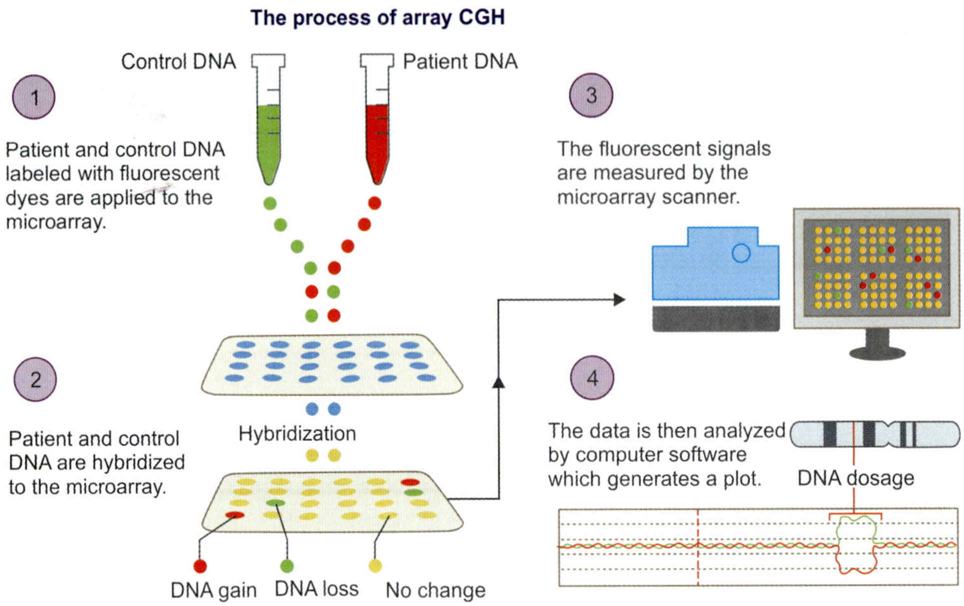

Fig. 39.6 Array CGH[16]

Advantages of Array-CGH Methodology

- Higher resolution than FISH (1–2 Kb vs 100 Kb)
- Detects multiple distinct genomic aberrations in one hybridization (gain and loss)
- Identifies alterations not currently assessable by other techniques
- Identifies more abnormalities than FISH. For instance, MatBA®-CLL/SLL detects more abnormalities than FISH in 30% of CLL cases.[2]

WHOLE GENOME MICROARRAY

Principle of cDNA Microarray Assay of Gene Expression

A microarray is a set of short expressed sequence tags (ESTs) made from a cDNA library of a set of known (or partially known) gene loci. The ESTs are spotted onto a cover-slip-sized glass plate, shown here as an 8 × 12 array. In practice, microarrays of many thousand ESTs are possible.

A complete set of mRNA transcripts (the transcriptome) is prepared from the tissue of an experimental treatment or condition, e.g. fish fed a high-protein diet, or an individual with breast cancer. Complementary DNA (cDNA) reverse transcripts are prepared and labelled with a (red) fluorescent dye. A control library is constructed from an untreated source, e.g. a standard fish diet, or noncancerous breast tissue; this library is labelled with a different fluorescent [green] dye. The experimental and control libraries are hybridized to the microarray. A dual-channel laser excites the corresponding dye, and the fluorescence intensity indicates the degree of hybridization that has occurred. Relative gene expression is measured as the ratio of the two fluorescence wavelengths. Increased expression or "up-regulation" of genes in the experimental transcriptome relative to the control will be visualized as a "hotter" red "pseudo-color," and decreased expression or "down-regulation" shows as a "cooler" green. Intensity of color is proportional to the expression differential. Unchanged, constitutive expression (1:1 ratio of experimental to control) shows as a neutral black (Fig. 39.7).

Microarrays Offer Advantages over Conventional Karyotyping

The advantages of microarray testing over the current standard, metaphase karyotyping, include a higher sensitivity to detect chromosome deletions, duplications and unbalanced rearrangements and a shorter turn around time. This shorter time is because the DNA isolation procedures can be automated, and there is no need to culture the fetal cells. Whereas metaphase analyses using banding techniques can identify chromosome deletions and duplications in the range of 5–10 Mb, the higher resolution provided by microarrays can detect changes as small as 50–100 kb.[7] The disadvantages of microarrays include their inability to detect a balanced chromosome rearrangement or a triploid karyotype. The design of the array is crucial. Oligonucleotide and

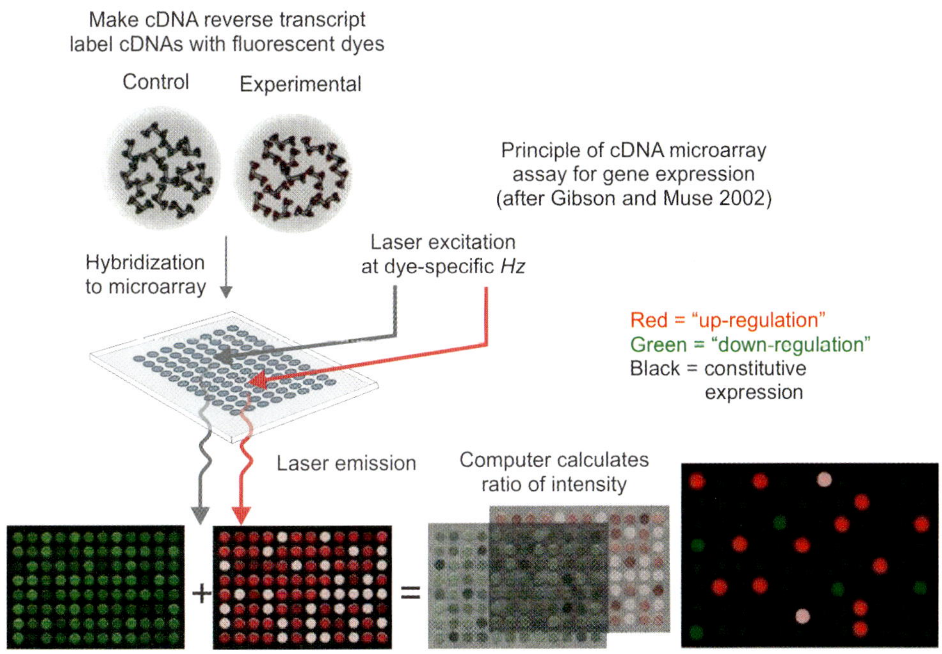

Fig. 39.7 DNA microarray
Source: Gibson & Muse ©2002; text material ©201by Steven M. Carr[19]

bacterial artificial chromosome arrays provide less coverage of the genome but are specifically designed to identify known chromosomal aberrations that are associated with clinically significant disease. Whole-genome arrays provide sequence information without complete knowledge of the long-term prognostic implications of all of the variants detected. Such sequence information, however, may be permanently archived and used as a reference source to advance our knowledge of the health of individuals and populations, human development and disease.

A major concern regarding the widespread application of chromosome microarray technology to low-risk pregnancies is the possibility of detecting copy number variants (CNVs) that have unknown clinical consequences. This is a problem because the phenotype of the fetus cannot be completely assessed while in the womb, so it can be difficult to determine the functional consequences of these genetic changes. When an indeterminate CNV is detected, several factors increase the probability of its pathogenicity. These include being absent in the parents (*de novo*), having a size of larger than 1 Mb, being a deletion rather than a duplication or involving a gene-rich area of the genome. A final consideration is whether there is a similar phenotype that involves genes within the same pathway.[7] When a *de novo* CNV is found in the fetus, publicly available references can be consulted to interpret its clinical implications, such as the database of Genotypes and Phenotypes (dbGAP) (*http://www.ncbi.nlm.nih.gov/gap*)[8] or the Database of Chromosomal Imbalance and Phenotype in Humans using Ensembl Resources (DECIPHER) (*http://decipher.sanger.ac.uk/*).[9] However, most clinicians do not have adequate training to perform such interpretations of CNVs.

Comment on Karyotype and Microarray Analyses to Maximize Information

In the prenatal setting, there is uncertainty as to whether it is better to use an array that only detects findings of known clinical meaning or one that has the greatest possible resolution.[10] Despite this uncertainty, a consensus exists with regard to the essential need for counseling before and after testing as well as the clinical scenarios in which microarrays are a useful adjunct to metaphase karyotyping. For example, in the settings of miscarriage[11] and stillbirth,[12,13] in which tissue culture frequently fails, the quality of the chromosome preparation is suboptimal or both, microarrays have been shown to improve the detection of genomic alterations in the fetus. Similarly, the addition of a microarray analysis when there is a fetal structural anomaly and a normal metaphase karyotype results in the detection of 1–16% additional clinically relevant chromosome abnormalities.[14-21] The lower end of the range reflects the use of lower density arrays,[14-18] and the higher percentages are derived from the studies that used whole-genome platforms.[19-21] The use of microarrays has shown that up to 25% of apparently balanced translocations analyzed by metaphase karyotyping are in fact unbalanced

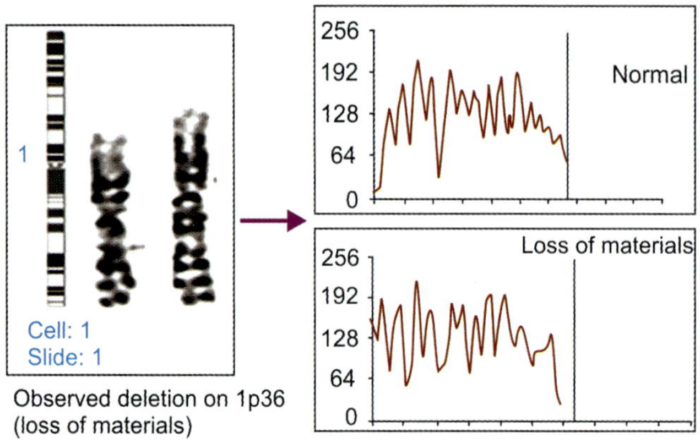

Fig. 39.8 Abnormal karyotype; 1p36; Structural defects observed (New novel techniques to detect submicroscopic deletion (1–5 Mb deletion; CytoVision 3.4
Source: DeP et al Int J Ped. Genetics. 3(2014)

and contain substantial aberrations in regions of the genome known to encode for essential genes.

A recent retrospective study performed in Israel compared antenatal karyotyping to microarrays; both options were routinely offered to couples undergoing invasive procedures.[22] This study illustrated the potential added value of a microarray analysis in a prenatal context. Of the 269 fetuses examined, 254 had a normal metaphase karyotype and 15 had abnormal metaphase findings of unknown clinical meaning (Fig. 39.8). In the former group, 36 out of 254 fetuses had an abnormal microarray result, and 33 of these 36 fetuses were found to have benign CNVs. The remaining three fetuses had *de novo* duplications (two of them also had sonographic abnormalities). All three of the women carrying these fetuses opted for termination. The overall risk of having an unbalanced genomic finding after a normal karyotype was 1 in 84, or 1.1%. The microarray results were normal in 11 of the 15 fetuses (73.3%) with an abnormal metaphase finding; all of these pregnancies were continued. In four fetuses, unbalanced abnormalities in the karyotype were confirmed by a microarray analysis; the women chose to terminate their pregnancies in these instances. In the entire study, clinically relevant genetic or genomic changes that had not been previously detected were found in 18 out of 269 (6.5%, or 1 in 15) fetuses (Table 39.2). Thus, the addition of genomic data allowed the physicians to better define the expected prognosis for the child, which substantially influenced subsequent pregnancy management and parental decisions.

Table 39.2 Limitation of the current technologies in fetal genome analysis are to be considered during the genetic counseling season

Method	Technical limitation
Routine karyotype (GTB)	• Possible to detect <5 Mb deletion • Detect mosaicism and balanced translocation • Result (8–10 days)
Molecular cytogenetics (FISH)	• Metaphase FISH resolves probes 100 Kb–2 Mbp • Fiber FISH resolves probes 10 Kbp–500 Kbp • Detect mosaicism and balanced translocation
Array CGH	• Higher resolution than FISH (1–2 Kb) • Detect multiple genomic aberration in one hybridization (gain or loss) except mosaicism and balance tranlocation • Need DNA from unculture cell and shorter turn around time
Genome microarray	• Higher resolution than FISH (50–100 Kb) • Detect multiple genomic aberration in one hybridization gain or loss) except mosaicism and balance translocation • Need DNA from unculture cell and shorter turn around time

Current Status of Noninvasive Prenatal Diagnosis

The clinical experience with microarrays illustrates the immediate impact that rapid advances in technology can have on clinical care, even before the completion of a prospective blinded trial. The same phenomenon occurred with the noninvasive diagnosis of fetal sex and the Rhesus D blood group (RhD) using circulating nucleic acids. In 1997, Lo and his colleagues first found that cell-free fetal DNA circulates in maternal plasma and serum by showing that gene sequences that are unique to the fetus could be amplified from maternal plasma.[23] Maternal blood contains a mixture of maternal and fetal (predominantly placental)[24-30] cell-free nucleic acids. Therefore, fetal DNA can be isolated from maternal blood and analyzed noninvasively (Fig. 39.9).

Cell-free DNA analysis to diagnose fetal disorders. Cell-free DNA from maternal plasma is a mixture of maternal and fetal DNA. When testing is being performed for the diagnosis of the presence or absence of a uniquely fetal gene, the relatively low-cost method of real-time quantitative PCR can be used (left). Primers and probes that map uniquely to the fetal genome can be used to amplify the gene of interest to allow, for example, the detection of the *RHD* gene.[31-34] For diagnosing aneuploidies such as Down's syndrome, the total cell-free DNA in maternal plasma is sequenced (right). The DNA is fragmented and analyzed in 36-bp lengths known as reads. These 36-bp reads are aligned against the human genome sequence and counted. The amount of DNA in chromosomes of interest, for example, those involved in common fetal aneuploidies such as those of chromosomes 13, 18 and 21, is normalized against the DNA from other chromosomes to determine the relative number of reads present in a given sample. The lower right image shows an

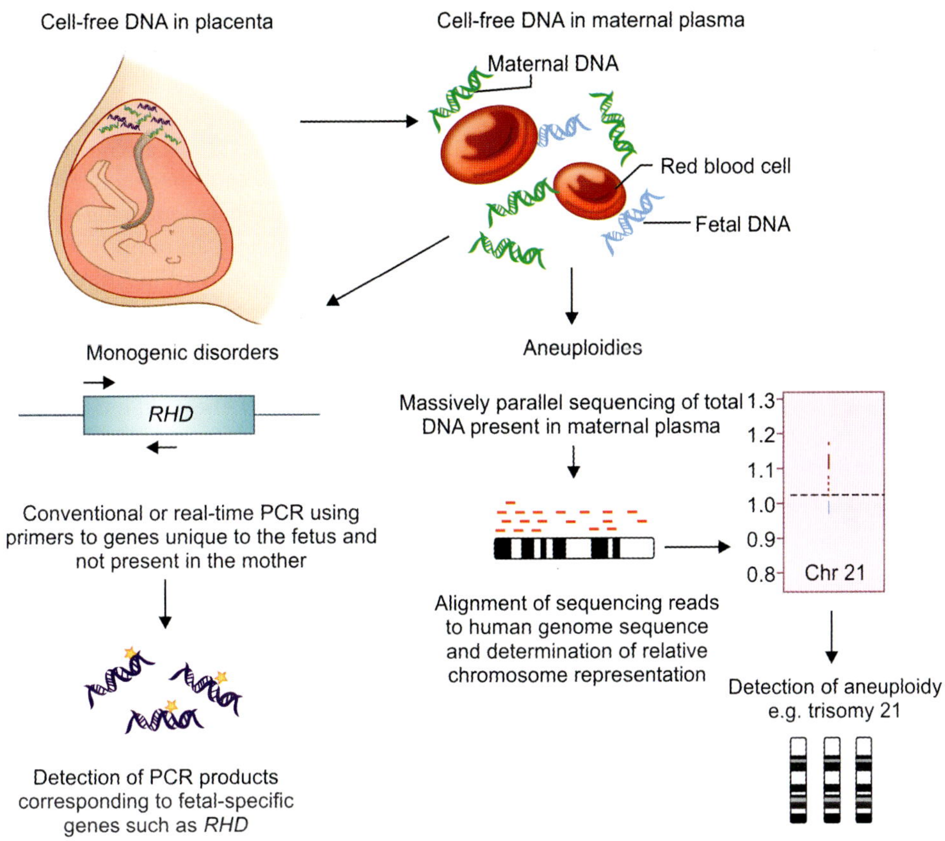

Fig. 39.9 Fetal DNA isolated from maternal blood and analyzed noninvasively[14]

increased number of sequences derived from chromosome (chr) 21 (in red) plotted against what should normally be present, indicated by the dashed line slightly above 1.0. This result is consistent with a fetus that has trisomy 21.[35-37]

Noninvasive Diagnosis of Sex-linked Disorders

Similarly, PCR amplification of cell-free DNA in maternal blood has been used as a noninvasive alternative to cytogenetic diagnosis after an invasive procedure to determine fetal sex. Such diagnostic tests are recommended when knowledge of fetal sex is needed for the management of X-linked conditions or of ambiguous genitalia detected by sonogram. Furthermore, knowledge of fetal sex helps determine which women need to take steroids to prevent the masculinization of a female fetus that is at risk for congenital adrenal hyperplasia. The widespread availability of this technology over the internet and in pharmacies in the United States, however, raises substantial ethical concerns.[4] To determine the analytic and clinical validity of diagnosing fetal sex, a recent meta-analysis of 80 discrete datasets from 57 studies and 6,541 singleton fetuses showed that the overall diagnostic performance of noninvasive testing was high (with a 95.4% sensitivity and a 98.1% specificity) when maternal blood samples were obtained after 7 weeks of gestation.[38] The variables that had the biggest effect on test performance were gestational age and DNA amplification methodology. Currently in the United States, noninvasive fetal DNA testing is not available at point of care, and this testing is not approved by the Clinical Laboratory Improvement Amendments (CLIA) or reimbursed by insurers, despite the results of this meta-analysis.[38] In contrast, in the UK, this approach has already been incorporated into prenatal care and has led to a reduction in invasive prenatal diagnostic procedures for sex-linked disorders.[39]

Prenatal Testing for Fetal Aneuploidies by Noninvasive Prenatal Testing

Antenatal recognition of fetuses with trisomy 21 is a major goal of all screening programs in the developed world.[40] Whereas noninvasive prenatal testing (NIPT) of fetal sex and *RHD* genotype can be performed using the relatively straightforward technique of real-time PCR, identification of fetal trisomy 21 using maternal plasma is much more complicated because there are no unique fetal gene sequences to be detected. Multiple attempts over the past two decades have used intact fetal cells in maternal blood,[41,42] cell-free DNA[43] or cell-free RNA[44,45] to noninvasively diagnose Down's syndrome. The subsequent development of digital PCR techniques led to the ability to quantify the amount of nucleic acids in a maternal sample by counting amplifications from single molecules. Digital PCR has been applied to the molecular detection of aneuploidy using cell-free RNA[46] or DNA.[47]

Although some of the early studies achieved success on a small scale, the arrival of massively parallel sequencing techniques and instrumentation substantially changed the landscape for this type of research. In 2008, two independent reports published 2 months apart each showed that fetal aneuploidy could be accurately diagnosed using DNA isolated from maternal plasma samples by mapping and aligning short sequence tags to a reference human genome, followed by counting and bioinformatics analyses.[48,49]

Subsequently, progress has been rapid. Since January 2011, at least ten independent large-scale clinical trials involving NIPT of trisomies 21, 18 and 13 have been published.[50-55] Three of these studies were prospective.[54-55] So far, all of them were performed with study subjects that were at a high-risk for fetal aneuploidy and incorporated a case-control study design in which an independent third party matched known euploid fetuses with fetuses that had a variety of chromosomal abnormalities. The teams that performed the sample processing, sequencing and bioinformatics analyses were blinded. All of the studies achieved similar, near-perfect rates of detection of trisomy 21, including in two sets of twins (in which at least one was affected),[52] three cases of mosaic trisomy 21 and several cases caused by an unbalanced translocation. All of the studies had very low false-positive rates (<1%). The various studies, however, differed in their bioinformatics analytical approaches. In some of them, the number of sequence tags on the chromosome of interest was normalized to the number of tags on all chromosomes in the particular sequencing run (the *z*-score).[49-51,53-55] In other studies,[52] a normalized chromosome value (NCV) was used to calculate the ratio of the number of counts on the chromosome of interest (for example, 21) in a specific sample to the number of counts on a reference chromosome or a chromosome set derived from an unaffected group of samples. The NCV is a fixed ratio that removes variation within and between sequencing runs. A third approach incorporates information on the fraction of fetal DNA present in the sample to calculate an individual risk of trisomy.

By late 2011, NIPT of trisomy 21 by sequencing of maternal plasma DNA began to be offered on a clinical and commercial basis in the United States and China at approximate costs ranging from $475 to $1,900, depending on the patient's insurance. This development prompted a rapid response statement to be issued by the International Society for Prenatal Diagnosis, which cautioned that before routine population screening for fetal Down's syndrome is introduced, additional trials are needed, particularly in low-risk populations. Despite these concerns, noninvasive testing using massively parallel sequencing of maternal plasma DNA is now a clinical reality. As of April 2012, over 25,000 clinical tests have been performed in China and several thousand have been performed in the United States (*http://www.genomeweb.com/mdx/non-invasive-t21-testing-space-abuzz-firms-jockey-share-1b-market-battle-over-ip*).

Compared with the antenatal diagnosis of Down's syndrome, the diagnosis of other commonly occurring fetal aneuploidies, such as trisomies 13 and 18, is more challenging because the accuracy of aneuploidy detection is affected by the GC base content of an individual chromosome. Whereas chromosome 21 has a midrange percentage of GC content, chromosomes 18 and 13 have a lower percentage, which increases the coefficient of variation in the sequencing reactions of these chromosomes. Specific quantitative correction of the GC content bias in the sequencing data using modified *z*-score equations has resulted in improved sensitivity and specificity in the detection of trisomies 13 and 18. The NCV analytic method was sensitive enough to detect a case of mosaic trisomy 9, an 11q21-23 deletion, partial trisomy of 6q12-16.3 and several sex chromosome abnormalities, suggesting this method may have expanded clinical utility as compared to the *z*-score.

CONCLUSION

Prenatal genetic diagnostic technology is advancing at an astonishingly rapid pace. Of the 117 references cited in this paper, 53 (45%) of them have been published in the past 2 years. Professional education and guidelines for incorporating new genetic tests into current practice are urgently needed. High-level economic analyses are also required to assess the benefits and limitations of current compared to future approaches. Government organizations, such as the United States Food and Drug Administration and also Indian Organization (ICMR), need to be more proactively involved to ensure the quality and safety of the tests. Multidisciplinary research teams consisting of basic and translational scientists, clinicians, ethicists and parents should be formed to consider many of the issues raised here. Time is of the essence because the commercial sector has already made some of these tests, such as fetal sex and determination of paternity, directly available to pregnant women.

For the past 30 years, the goal of prenatal diagnosis has been to provide an informed choice to prospective parents.

That paradigm is now shifting. We are now at a point where that goal can and should be expanded to incorporate genetic and genomic data to pave the way for a personalized approach to fetal treatment.

TAKE HOME MESSAGES

- Current prenatal diagnostic technologies (Noninvasive and invasive) need proper understanding and training to all practicing clinicians for patient counseling.
- Fetal genome analysis would be a multidisciplinary approach so good coordination and understanding is essential to avoid misunderstandings and medicolegal problems in India.
- International guidelines and respectives professional organization databases could be a great help to all clinicians and scientist for patient counseling and management in featal medicine.

REFERENCES

1. Khoury MJ, et al. The scientific foundation for personal genomics: recommendations from an NIH-CDC multidisciplinary workshop. Genet Med. 2009;11:559-67.
2. Ferguson-Smith MA, Bianchi DW. Prenatal diagnosis: past, present, and future. Prenat Diagn. 2010;30:601-4.
3. Wolfberg AJ. Genes on the web-direct-to-consumer marketing of genetic testing. N Engl J Med. 2006;355:543-5.
4. Bianchi DW. At-home fetal DNA gender testing: caveat emptor. Obstet Gynecol. 2006;107:216-8.
5. Hawkins AK, Ho A. Genetic counseling and the ethical issues around direct to consumer genetic testing. J Genet Counsel. 2012;21:367-73.
6. Miller DT, et al. Consensus statement: chromosomal microarray is a first-tier clinical diagnostic test for individuals with developmental disabilities or congenital anomalies. Am J Hum Genet. 2010;86:749-64.
7. Friedman JM. High-resolution array genomic hybridization in prenatal diagnosis. Prenat Diagn. 2009;29:20-8.
8. Mailman MD, et al. The NCBI dbGAP database of genotypes and phenotypes. Nat Genet. 2007;39:1181-6.
9. Firth HV, et al. DECIPHER: Database of Chromosomal Imbalance and Phenotype in Humans Using Ensembl Resources. Am J Hum Genet. 2009;84:524-33.
10. ACOG Committee Opinion No. 446: array comparative genomic hybridization in prenatal diagnosis. Obstet Gynecol. 2009;114:1161-3. Anonymous.
11. Schaeffer AJ, et al. Comparative genomic hybridization-array analysis enhances the detection of aneuploidies and submicroscopic imbalances in spontaneous miscarriages. Am J Hum Genet. 2004;74:1168-74.
12. Raca G, et al. Array-based comparative genomic hybridization (aCGH) in the genetic evaluation of stillbirth. Am J Med Genet A. 2009;149A:2437-43.
13. Harris RA, et al. Genome-wide array-based copy number profiling in human placentas from unexplained stillbirths. Prenat Diagn. 2011;31:932-44.
14. Shaffer LG, et al. Comparison of microarray-based detection rates for cytogenetic abnormalities in prenatal and neonatal specimens. Prenat Diagn. 2008;28:789-95.
15. Coppinger J, et al. Whole-genome microarray analysis in prenatal specimens identifies clinically significant chromosome alterations without increase in results of unclear significance compared to targeted microarray. Prenat Diagn. 2009;29:1156-66.
16. Van den Veyver IB, et al. Clinical use of array comparative genomic hybridization (aCGH) for prenatal diagnosis in 300 cases. Prenat Diagn. 2009;29:29-39.
17. Park JH, et al. Application of a target array comparative genomic hybridization to prenatal diagnosis. BMC Med. Genet. 2010;11:102.
18. Kleeman L, et al. Use of array comparative genomic hybridization for prenatal diagnosis of fetuses with sonographic anomalies and normal metaphase karyotype. Prenat Diagn. 2009;29:1213-7.
19. Tyreman M, et al. High resolution array analysis: diagnosing pregnancies with abnormal ultrasound findings. J Med Genet. 2009;46:531-41.
20. Faas BH, et al. Identification of clinically significant, submicroscopic chromosome alterations and UPD in fetuses with ultrasound anomalies using genome-wide 250k SNP array analysis. J Med Genet. 2010;47:586-94.
21. D'Amours G, et al. Whole-genome array CGH identifies pathogenic copy number variations in fetuses with major malformations and a normal karyotype. Clin Genet. 2012;81: 128-41.
22. Maya I, et al. Diagnostic utility of array-based comparative genomic hybridization (aCGH) in a prenatal setting. Prenat Diagn. 2010;30:1131-7.
23. Lo YM, et al. Presence of fetal DNA in maternal plasma and serum. Lancet. 1997;350:485-7.
24. Tjoa ML, Cindrova-Davies T, Spasic-Boskovic O, Bianchi DW, Burton GJ. Trophoblastic oxidative stress and the release of cell-free feto-placental DNA. Am J Pathol. 2006;169:400-04.
25. Alberry M, et al. Free fetal DNA in maternal plasma in anembryonic pregnancies: confirmation that the origin is the trophoblast. Prenat Diagn. 2007;27:415-8.
26. Bischoff FZ, Lewis DE, Simpson JL. Cell-free fetal DNA in maternal blood: kinetics, source and structure. Hum Reprod Update. 2005;11:59-67.
27. Masuzaki H, et al. Detection of cell free placental DNA in maternal plasma: direct evidence from three cases of confined placental mosaicism. J Med Genet. 2004;41:289-92.
28. Sekizawa A, et al. Evaluation of bidirectional transfer of plasma DNA through placenta. Hum Genet. 2003;113:307-10.
29. Chim SS, et al. Detection of the placental epigenetic signature of the maspingene in maternal plasma. Proc Natl Acad Sci. USA. 2005;102:14753-8.
30. Chan KC, et al. Hypermethylated RASSF1A in maternal plasma: a universal fetal DNA marker that improves the reliability of noninvasive prenatal diagnosis. Clin Chem. 2006;52:2211-8.

31. Bennett PR, et al. Prenatal determination of fetal RhD type by DNA amplification. N Engl J Med.1993;329:607-10.
32. Lo YM, et al. Prenatal diagnosis of fetal RhD status by molecular analysis of maternal plasma. N Engl J Med. 1998;339: 1734-8.
33. Finning KM, Martin PG, Soothill PW, Avent ND. Prediction of fetal D status from maternal plasma: introduction of a new noninvasive fetal RHD genotyping service. Transfusion. 2002;42:1079-85.
34. Bianchi DW, Avent ND, Costa JM, van der Schoot EM. Noninvasive prenatal diagnosis of fetal Rhesus D: ready for prime(r) time. Obstet Gynecol. 2005;106:841-4.
35. Scheffer PG, van der Schoot CE, Page-Christiaens GC, de Haas M. Noninvasive fetal blood group genotyping of rhesus D, C, E and of K in alloimmunised pregnant women: evaluation of a 7-year clinical experience. BJOG. 2011;118:1340-8.
36. Daniels G, Finning K, Martin P. Noninvasive fetal blood grouping: present and future. Clin Lab Med. 2010;30:431-42.
37. Clausen FB, et al. Report of the first nationally implemented clinical routine screening for fetal RHD in D-pregnant women to ascertain the requirements for antenatal D prophylaxis. Transfusion. 2012;52:752-8.
38. Devaney SA, Palomaki GE, Scott JA, Bianchi DW. Noninvasive fetal sex determination using cell-free fetal DNA. J Am Med Assoc. 2011;306:627-36.
39. Hill M, et al. Non-invasive prenatal determination of fetal sex: translating research into clinical practice. Clin Genet. 2011;80:68-75.
40. ACOG Committee on Practice Bulletins ACOG practice bulletin no. 77: screening for fetal chromosomal abnormalities. Obstet Gynecol. 2007;109:217-27.
41. Bianchi DW, et al. Fetal gender and aneuploidy detection using fetal cells in maternal blood: analysis of NIFTY I data. National Institute of Child Health and Development Fetal Cell Isolation Study. Prenat Diagn. 2002;22:609-15.
42. Bianchi DW, Hanson J. Sharpening the tools: a summary of a National Institutes of Health workshop on new technologies for detection of fetal cells in maternal blood for early prenatal diagnosis. J Matern Fetal Neonatal Med. 2006;19: 199-207.
43. Lo YM. Noninvasive prenatal detection of fetal chromosomal aneuploidies by maternal plasma nucleic acid analysis: a review of the current state of the art. BJOG. 2009;116:152-7.
44. Lo YM, et al. Plasma placental RNA allelic ratio permits noninvasive prenatal chromosomal aneuploidy detection. Nat Med. 2007;13:218-23.
45. Tsui NB, et al. Synergy of total PLAC4 RNA concentration and measurement of the RNA single-nucleotide polymorphism allelic ratio for the noninvasive prenatal detection of trisomy 21. Clin Chem. 2010;56:73-81.
46. Lo YM, et al. Digital PCR for the molecular detection of fetal chromosomal aneuploidy. Proc Natl Acad Sci. USA. 2007;104:13116-21.
47. Fan HC, Quake SR. Detection of aneuploidy with digital polymerase chain reaction. Anal Chem. 2007;79:7576-9.
48. Fan HC, Blumenfeld YJ, Chitkara U, Hudgins L, Quake SR. Noninvasive diagnosis of fetal aneuploidy by shotgun sequencing DNA from maternal blood. Proc Natl Acad Sci. USA. 2008;105:16266-71.
49. Chiu RW, et al. Noninvasive prenatal diagnosis of fetal chromosomal aneuploidy by massively parallel genomic sequencing of DNA in maternal plasma. Proc Natl Acad Sci. USA. 2008;105:20458-63.
50. Chiu RW, et al. Non-invasive prenatal assessment of trisomy 21 by multiplexed maternal plasma DNA sequencing: large scale validity study. Br Med J. 2011;342:c7401.
51. Ehrich M, et al. Noninvasive detection of fetal trisomy 21 by sequencing of DNA in maternal blood: a study in a clinical setting. Am J Obstet Gynecol. 2011;204:205.e1-11.
52. Sehnert AJ, et al. Optimal detection of fetal chromosomal abnormalities by massively parallel sequencing of cell-free fetal DNA from maternal blood. Clin Chem. 2011;57: 1042-9.
53. Chen EZ, et al. Noninvasive prenatal diagnosis of fetal trisomy 18 and trisomy 13 by maternal plasma DNA sequencing. PLoS ONE. 2011;6:e21791.
54. Palomaki GE, et al. DNA sequencing of maternal plasma to detect Down syndrome: an international clinical validation study. Genet Med. 2011;13:913-20.
55. Palomaki GE, et al. DNA sequencing of maternal plasma reliably identifies trisomy 18 and trisomy 13 as well as Down syndrome: an international collaborative study. Genet Med. 2012;14:296-305.

CHAPTER

40

Array-based Comparative Genomic Hybridization: Future in Prenatal Diagnosis

Usha P Dave, Dhanlaxmi L Shetty

INTRODUCTION

Karyotype or chromosomal testing is the most common genetic test used for number of structural and numerical chromosomal aberrations in varied genetic, cancer, neurologic, developmental and reproductive disorders; often conducted to give diagnosis. No doubt, it is still referred as the "gold standard" test in genetic practice. Though karyotyping is partially automated in most cytogenetic laboratories, the highly experienced technical person is necessary to offer reliable chromosomal diagnosis. Additionally, conventional G-banding karyotyping has limitation of detecting the aberrations of about 5–10 Mb. The molecular and cytogenetic techniques such as fluorescence *in situ* hybridization (FISH) and Multiplex Ligation-dependent Probe Amplification (MLPA) were developed with relatively better resolution for specific microdeletions, or chromosomal alterations to increase the sensitivity and specificity of targeted genetic abnormalities. The telomeric and subtelomeric chromosomal abnormalities, often missed by conventional karyotype due to its limitation can be detected using these techniques. However, there still existed a dire need of identifying the precise locus on chromosomes involved in aberrant gene function or in other words to increase the resolution at molecular level covering the whole genome or targeted genes by increasing the detection power.

The advances in genomic technology coupled with powerful bioinformatics tools has led to the discovery of new molecular approaches to study the chromosomal aberrations in a variety of disorders spanning the entire protein coding region of the human genome. The comparative genomic hybridization (CGH) was first used to detect DNA amplification in tumors.[1] In array CGH, small fragments of DNA called probes are chemically attached to a glass slide and used as targets while hybridization with patient's DNA occurs and comparison takes place. This allowed the multifold resolution and became popular in tumor cytogenetics in the last decade.[2,3] It was later that array-based comparative genomic hybridization (array CGH) technology revolutionized the cytogenetic field by detecting the chromosomal imbalances such as gain or loss of genetic material at molecular level and ascertaining the possible genes involved to result into a particular phenotype. Soon it is considered to be the first line genetic test for genome wide copy number variation replacing conventional karyotyping.[4]

ARRAY-BASED COMPARATIVE GENOMIC HYBRIDIZATION

Chromosomal microarray analysis (CMA) or array CGH is a technique that simultaneously detects submicroscopic DNA copy number changes at several loci across the genome. It is a high resolution whole-genome screening method of measuring gains and losses of DNA throughout the human genome. The small genomic deletions and duplications are called copy-number variants (CNVs) which are not routinely seen on the standard cytogenetic analysis. Copy-number variants result in a variation from the expected number of copies of a segment of DNA (i.e. the number in a normal genome). These changes at molecular level (e.g. CNVs found), can either be benign or pathogenic, depending on their location and genetic content. The DNA variants are identified with the use of chromosomal microarray analysis in which a test sample of DNA from the patient is compared directly or indirectly with a reference (normal) genome. The certain copy number variants (CNVs) have been observed in many individuals with no phenotypic associations and are believed to be clinically insignificant. Another type of DNA alteration is a single-nucleotide polymorphism (SNP). A SNP is a DNA variation in which a single nucleotide (A, T, C or G) in the genome sequence is altered. This can occur between two different individuals or between paired chromosomes of the same individual and may or may not cause disease.

In the aCGH method, the patient's DNA is sex matched with control DNA which are differentially labeled with fluorescence dyes and are simultaneously hybridized *in situ* to cytogenetically 'normal' reference human DNA on glass slide. At a particular wavelength of laser (649 for Cy5 and 553 for Cy3), the fluorescent dyes are excited and the emission by fluorescent signal—green or red is measured using appropriate filters. The intensity ratio of the fluorescence is analyzed using special softwares which can delineate DNA variation in terms of duplication, deletion, amplifications, monosomies or trisomies. As shown in Figure 40.1, the gains are universally represented by green color and loss by red color. These variations are of magnitude of 3–5 Mb which in other words are very high resolution banding of patient's chromosomes (Fig. 40.1). Chromosome Analysis Suite (ChAS) software is designed by cytogeneticists for cytogeneticists. The most popular ChAS software is tailored to cytogenetic research analysis and reporting.

WHAT ARE ARRAYS?

The known genomic spot or chromosome target smeared on glass slide is described as *array* which can be of different types based on our requirements. The artificially synthesized small fragments of known DNA sequences are recently developed and referred as BAC (Bacterial Artificial Chromosome) or PAC (P1-derived Artificial Chromosome) arrays. The arrays can range from 150 kb to 200 kb and can detect as small as 2 Mb deletions. There are usually 3 types of microarrays:

1. *Whole genome oligonucleotide array-CGH* with millions of probes with high resolution of 20–30 kb and increased density of probes in coding region of genome;
2. *Single nucleotide polymorphism (SNP) microarrays* which will enable to detect homozygosity or heterozygosity (identical or different length of DNA e.g. LOH) without quantitative DNA imbalances as required in oncogenic sample analysis; and
3. *Targeted array*—means only specific region of interest of genome is focused (e.g. subtelomere region or microdeletion/duplication) and probes are accordingly designed to detect CNVs known to cause the pathologic condition and the whole genome is not covered.

The various arrays are, thus commercially available for the diagnostic purposes to identify major chromosomal aneuploidy as well as the location and type of specific genetic changes that are too small to be detected by conventional karyotyping. For example, one CytoScan 750K array contains probes for more than 750,000 markers for copy number analysis which consist of 550,000 unique nonpolymorphic probes and approximately 200,000 SNPs that fully genotype with greater than 99% accuracy. It provides the power to detect copy-neutral LOH, uniparental isodisomy (UPD), and regions identical-by-descent. It is the first FDA-cleared whole-genome diagnostic test to aid physicians in identifying the underlying genetic cause of developmental delay, intellectual

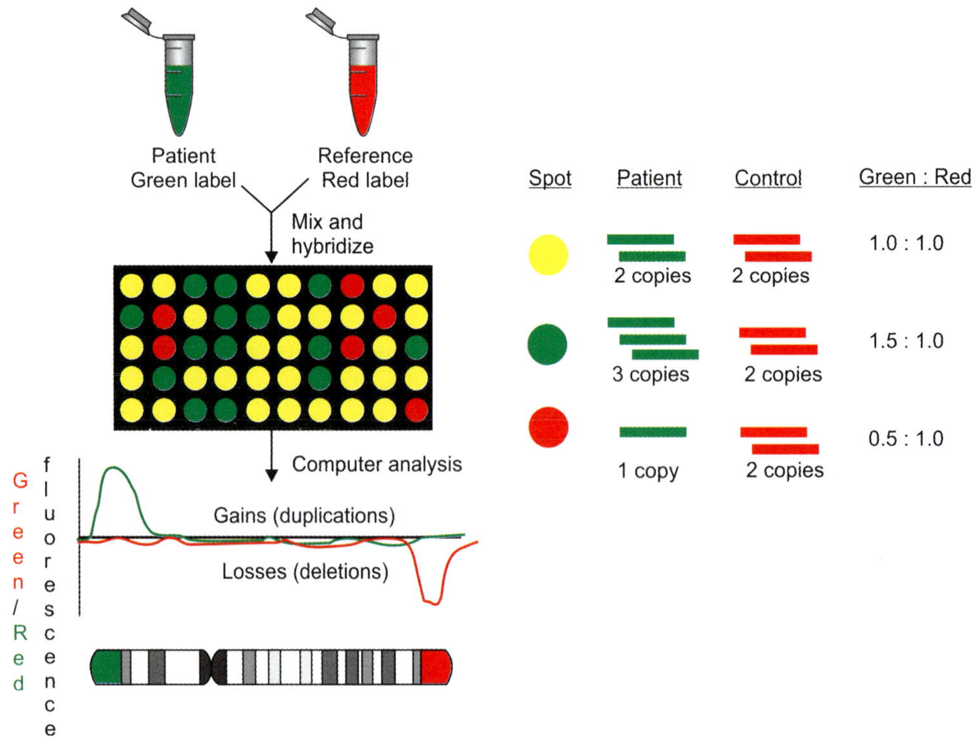

Fig. 40.1 Diagrammatic representation to explain principles of CMA. In prenatal diagnosis, the DNA is from fetal tissue instead of patient's DNA

disability, congenital anomalies, or dysmorphic features in children. The detection of breakpoints, allelic confirmation of copy number changes, and >5 Mb of LOH are other advantages. Since large number of data is generated with any of the microarrays, the bioinformatics tools are integral part of this technology and are useful to determine whether the specific CNVs have been previously reported as pathologic, benign or the new CNV of uncertain clinical significance.

CLINICAL UTILITY OF CHROMOSOMAL MICROARRAY

Because of its genome-wide capability, greater sensitivity, higher resolution, and greater diagnostic yield chromosomal microarray analysis (CMA) has been increasingly used in many congenital and acquired genetic diseases.[5] The recommendations and guidelines for utilization of array-based technology in medical genetic practice for detection of chromosomal abnormalities are provided for professional practice.[6] The study on trends has revealed the prevalence of children with developmental disability to be 13.87% in US children.[7] These occur across all racial, ethnic, and socioeconomic groups. It has been reported that 1 in 33 babies is born with congenital anomalies in the USA.[8] The subtelomeric fluorescence *in situ* hybridization (FISH) has been replaced by chromosomal microarray analysis since it covers the whole genome.[6]

The submicroscopic chromosomal rearrangements are responsible for majority of genetic disorders and estimated to be as high as 15%.[9] Microarray-based whole genome analysis detects submicroscopic alterations in intellectually disabled (ID) patients at higher resolution than routine chromosomal analysis. It is considered to be first-tier test in the genetic evaluation of infants and children, where conventional chromosomal analysis is normal, especially in children with unexplained intellectual disability, congenital anomalies, or autism spectrum disorder. The diagnostic genomic profiling by aCGH has been well depicted by de Vries and group in intellectually disabled children showing the increased diagnostic yield.[10] Similarly, the use of array CGH has been emphasized in evaluation of dysmorphology, malformations, developmental delay and idiopathic mental retardation with normal karyotype.[11] The causative genomic imbalances or genetic mutations in as many as 15% of children with a normal conventional karyotype were shown. Frequently, developmental delay and/or intellectual disability (DD/ID) present with one or more congenital anomalies or dysmorphic features. These affected individuals have lifelong challenges, including motor disabilities, learning and behavior problems and/social interaction deficits. Intellectual disability might be present as the only manifestation of a disease or may be associated with other manifestations mentioned earlier causing a clinical syndrome.[12] Some syndromes are genetically heterogeneous and may be caused by aberrations in several genes with distinct roles in common biological pathways. In such a situation, the specific gene testing proves most of the time uninformative in diagnosis.

Besides environmental factors and nutritional deficiencies as are known causative factors of ID, the largest specific etiology of ID is genetic.[13] According to the American Academy of Neurology, the Child Neurology Society, and the American College of Medical Genetics, a chromosomal microarray analysis (CMA) is considered the first-line genetic test to aid in the diagnostic evaluation of ID when patient history and physical examination do not provide an obvious syndrome diagnosis.[4,6,14] These guidelines for CMA to replace traditional karyotype as first-line genetic testing for unexplained ID are due to its greater sensitivity, higher resolution, and greater diagnostic yield.[15]

Advantages

The limit of light microscopy karyotyping is up to 5–10 Mb and the higher resolution by chromosomal microarray analysis is the important advantage over the conventional karyotype as it yields more genetic information. Furthermore, DNA can be easily obtained from uncultured cells and therefore results are usually available more quickly than with karyotyping, which requires cultured cells.[14] Because chromosomal microarray analysis does not require dividing cells, it may be useful in the evaluation of fetal demise or stillbirth, in which the culturing of macerated tissue is frequently unsuccessful[16] and in third-trimester amniocentesis. The karyotyping involves microscopic examination of stained chromosomes and may be more subjective and prone to human error, while chromosomal microarray analysis is a standardized procedure that involves the use of computerized analysis.

Limitations

Unlike conventional karyotyping, chromosomal microarray analysis cannot detect balanced inversions, balanced translocations, point mutations or all cases of tissue mosaicism. In addition, not all microarrays can detect triploidy, although most triploid fetuses can be identified by ultrasonography. A limitation of chromosomal microarray analysis is the potential to identify copy number variants of unknown clinical significance.[17] Such cases are referred as likely "benign" or likely "pathogenic". The clinical evaluation is of utmost importance while analysing the exponential data. In some cases, evaluation of parental samples can help clarify whether or not this is inherited finding or a new finding in the offspring; however, the clinical outcome may still remain unclear.

CHROMOSOMAL MICROARRAYS IN PRENATAL DIAGNOSIS

The utility of microarray in the diagnosis of genetic abnormalities in infants and children stimulated interest in its application in the prenatal setting. The fetal DNA to be studied is typically derived from amniocytes or chorionic villi samples. With CGH, the fetal DNA is labeled with one color of fluorescent dye, while the control DNA (of known genetic sequences) is labeled with another color as explained in Figure 40.1. The relative intensity of the different colors (the relative amount of fetal DNA versus control DNA) is compared. Duplications or deletions are detected as regions with a higher or lower hybridization signal than the control sample. Single-nucleotide polymorphism (SNP) arrays detect homozygosity or heterozygosity (identical or different stretches of DNA) and, therefore, can demonstrate the extent of consanguinity (shown as regions of homozygosity), as well as triploidy and uniparental disomy. It is important that the arrays used for prenatal testing should contain SNP probes that can reliably identify triploidy. Arrays can be "targeted" and can focus on copy number variants of known pathogenicity instead of testing the entire genome. In contrast, whole genome arrays are designed to provide greater coverage across the genome. As there is large number of potential findings, databases are used to determine if specific copy number variants have been previously reported and whether they are considered pathogenic, benign, or of unknown significance.

Many studies have demonstrated the potential benefit of chromosomal microarray analysis for fetal abnormalities beyond conventional fetal karyotyping. Genomic imbalances in fetuses with multiple malformations have been demonstrated prenatally.[18] The clinical usefulness of array comparative genomic hybridization (aCGH) for prenatal diagnosis has been shown in 300 cases.[19] Similarly, the diagnostic utility of aCGH in prenatal setting has been proved with evidences.[20] A systematic review and meta-analysis study has shown that comparative genomic hybridization technology offers additional information over conventional karyotyping in prenatal diagnosis.[21] From previous studies array CGH identified additional clinically significant abnormalities in approximately 6% fetuses with ultrasonographic abnormalities and a normal karyotype[22] and in 1.7% of fetuses with a normal ultrasonographic abnormalities and a normal karyotype.[17] Using SNP-based platform, twice the number of stillbirths were found to have genetic abnormalities compared with conventional cytogenetics.[16] The American College of Obstetricians and Gynecologists and the Society for Maternal- Fetal Medicine have given recommendations regarding the application of chromosomal microarray technology in the prenatal setting.[23] The laboratory reporting practices for regions of homozygosity indicating parental relatedness by SNP microarray testing has also been discussed.[24]

GENETIC COUNSELING

The preconceptional and prenatal genetic counseling plays an important role while using chromosomal microarray technology. The clinically uncertain and complicated findings during pregnancy can result in great anxiety in patient when genetic changes identified may or may not cause disease. There also lies a possibility of detecting genetic abnormalities associated with adult-onset disorders (e.g. BRCA mutations) which may be inherited from an asymptomatic parent. This may raise ethical issue and it is beyond the scope of the present topic. Some types of arrays can identify evidence of consanguinity and nonpaternity. Hence, there is a critical need for comprehensive pre-test and post-test genetic counseling by the qualified geneticist or genetic counselor explaining the benefits, disadvantages and interpretation of results so that patients can make informed decisions. The type and amount of information reported varies depending on the type of array used as well as the policy of the laboratory that performs the microarray analysis.[24] Therefore, genetic counseling and informed consent is essential before patients undergo prenatal microarray testing.

ARRAY COMPARATIVE GENOMIC HYBRIDIZATION RECOMMENDATIONS

Microarrays are gaining importance in prenatal diagnosis of rare genetic disorders when conventional karyotype is normal and ultrasonography shows abnormal finding. The College and Society for Maternal–Fetal Medicine provided the following recommendations for the use of chromosomal microarray analysis in prenatal diagnosis:[23]

- In patients with a fetus with one or more major structural abnormalities identified on ultrasonographic examination and who are undergoing invasive prenatal diagnosis, chromosomal microarray analysis is recommended. This test replaces the need for fetal karyotype.
- In patients with a structurally normal fetus undergoing invasive prenatal diagnostic testing, either fetal karyotyping or a chromosomal microarray analysis can be performed.
- Most genetic mutations identified by chromosomal microarray analysis are not associated with increasing maternal age; therefore, the use of this test for prenatal diagnosis should not be restricted to women aged 35 years and older.

- In cases of intrauterine fetal demise or stillbirth when further cytogenetic analysis is desired, chromosomal microarray analysis on fetal tissue (i.e. amniotic fluid, placenta, or products of conception) is recommended because of its increased likelihood of obtaining results and improved detection of causative abnormalities.
- Limited data are available on the clinical utility of chromosomal microarray analysis to evaluate first-trimester and second trimester pregnancy losses; therefore, this is not recommended at this time.
- Pre- and post-test counseling from qualified personnel is essential. It should not be ordered without informed consent, which should be documented in the medical record and include discussion of the potential to identify findings of uncertain significance, nonpaternity, consanguinity, and adult-onset disease.

The 2 cases are illustrated below to indicate a significant role of cytogenetic microarray analysis in preconceptional and prenatal genetic counseling.

Case 1

The couple approached for preconceptional genetic counseling with a daughter having developmental delay. The index case diagnosis was inevitable; clinical and laboratory investigations were as below:

Their daughter was 3 years old with mild autistic features, craniofacial dysmorphism and multiple congenital anomalies, born of FTND from a nonconsanguineous marriage. Her birth weight was 3.0 kg and perinatal birth history was normal. Her linguistic skills were at eight to ten months level. Repetitive behaviors and tactile seeking behaviors were noted, indicative of moderate autistic features. She had squint since birth and vision assessment showed amblyopia and anisometropia and morning glory disc anomaly for which she was prescribed spectacles for constant use. She had constant horizontal sensory nystagmus. Electroretinogram showed no evidence of retinal disease in both eyes. Physical examination revealed hypotonia, soft palate fissure, microphthalmia, microcornea, frontal bossing, anteverted nares, small ears and syndactyly of left thumb (Fig. 40.2A). The karyotype showed normal female (46,XX) karyotype. On brain MRI, no significant findings were identified and metabolic profiles were within normal limits.

The couple was informed about microarray testing, its benefits and disadvantages. The informed consent was taken. SNP microarray analysis was performed and imbalances related to common microdeletion/microduplication syndromes, subtelomeric deletions or duplications, as small as 30 kb with an average marker spacing of 6.2 kb were studied and karyoview was captured (Fig. 40.2B). The results showed 226 kb duplication at cytoband 17p12p11.2 with clinical significance (Fig. 40.2C). A copy neutral LOH (Loss of heterozygosity) on chromosomes 15 (Fig. 40.2D) and 11 (Fig. 40.2E) representing about 0.25% of the genome was noticed. The literature search and clinical correlation helped to identify this patient as having Potocki-Lupski syndrome (PTLS) [MIM 610883].[25,26] The precise diagnosis, and further genetic counseling was feasible to prevent the recurrence risk in the family only due to SNP microarray analysis. The post-test counseling was also done. So far 50 cases have been described worldwide in the medical literature but to the best of our knowledge, none from India.

Case 2

A young couple had 7 years old male child going to 1st Std. in school with a strong clinical diagnosis of muscular dystrophy (MD). The progressive deterioration in muscular activities and no therapy for their child had depressed the couple and they approached for genetic counseling and to explore the reproductive options. There was no family history of DMD and no other sibs. The extensive clinical and laboratory investigation was already conducted. The clinical evaluation revealed delayed motor milestones with Gower's sign +, hypertrophy of calves/brachioradialis, recently more muscle weakness with increasing difficulty in walking, toe walking, knee jerks absent and restless. He falls easily, cannot run or climb now. The serum CPK was high (10604 IU/L) suggestive of muscular disorder. The DMD phenotype was confirmed. The mental function was normal. The neurologist had recommended *DMD* gene deletion study and muscle biopsy for immunohistochemistry (IHC) study, the latter was not done by parents due to cost factor. The MLPA test for 79 exons for dystrophin gene was found negative. The diagnosis was inconclusive and the prenatal diagnosis would have been difficult in the absence of the marker in the index case.

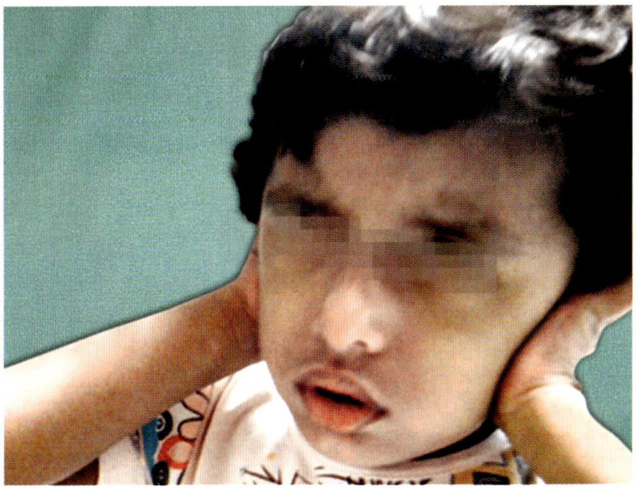

Fig. 40.2A Index case diagnosed with Potocki-Lupski syndrome using chromosomal microarray analysis

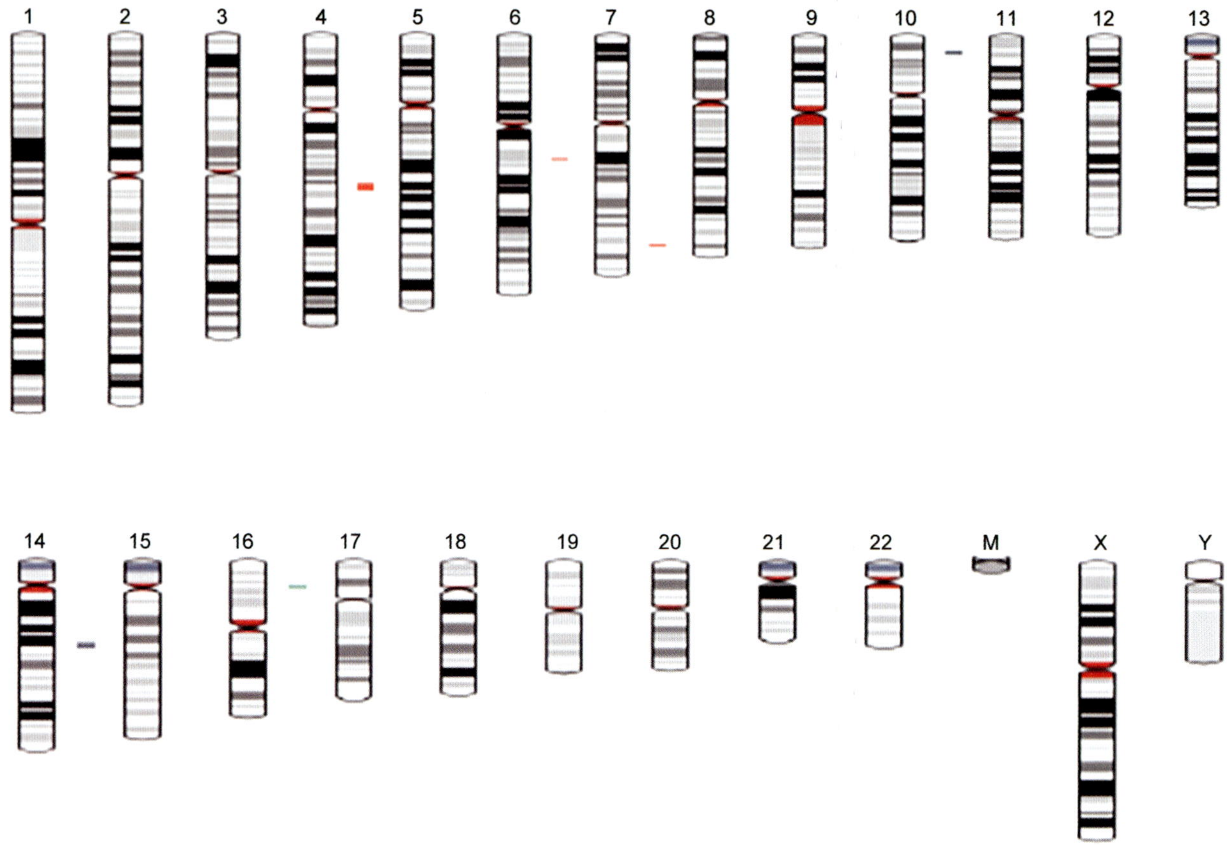

Fig. 40.2B Karyoview of case-1 (PTLS syndrome)

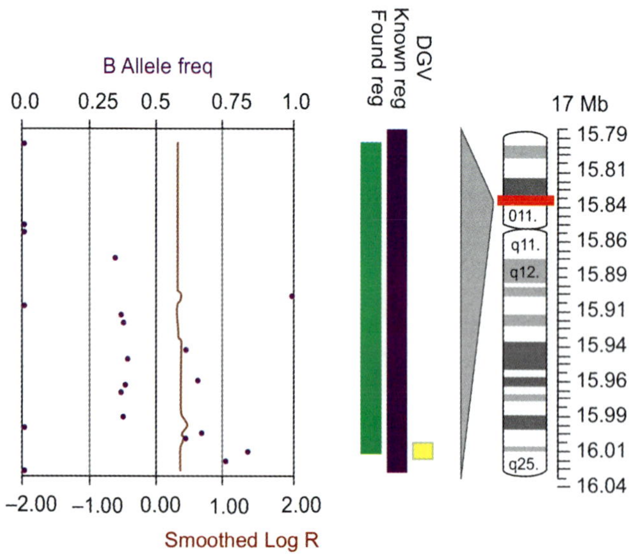

Fig. 40.2C Duplication of 226 kb at cytoband 17p12p11.2

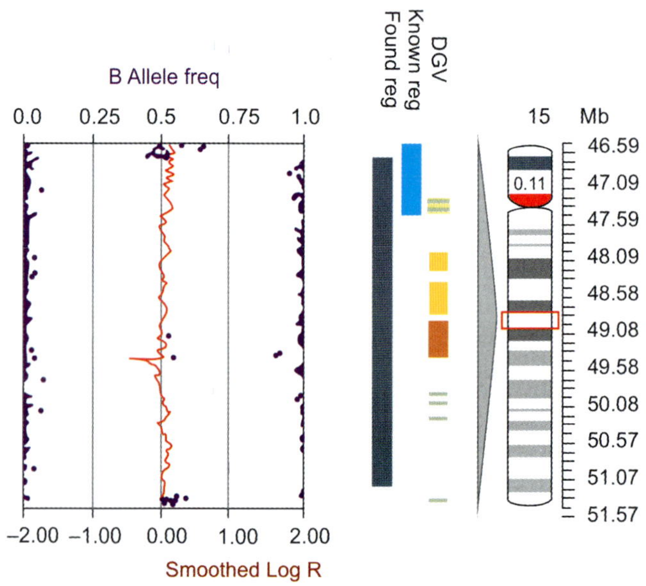

Fig. 40.2D Copy neutral loss of heterozygosity on chromosome 15

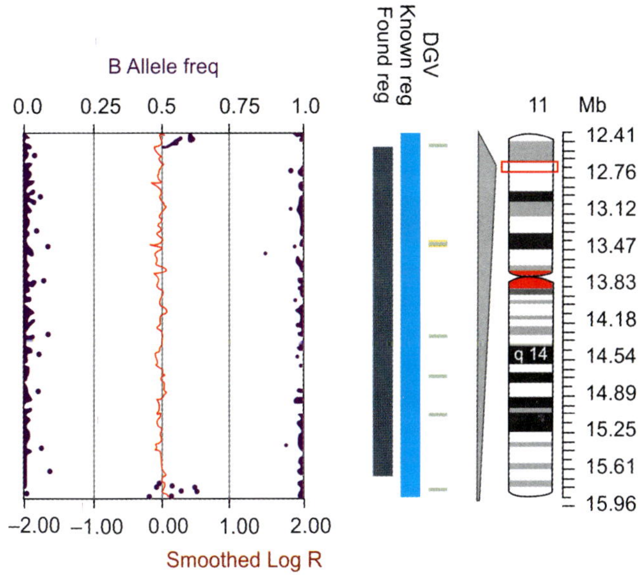

Fig. 40.2E Copy neutral loss of heterozygosity on chromosome 11

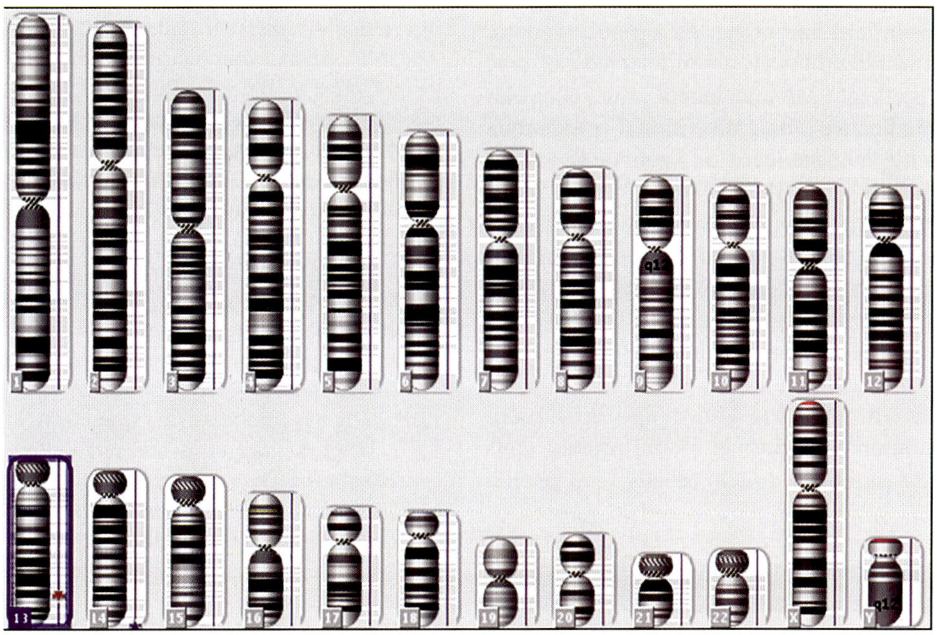

Fig. 40.3 Karyoview of case-2 showing 1.81 Mb deletion on chromosome 13 (13q31.3) shown in red color dot which includes *GPC5* (OMIM 602446) and *GPC6* (OMIM 604404) genes

The couple was counseled about CMA test, its benefits and limitations. They agreed to undergo the microarray testing in their son. The informed consent was taken.

The genomic DNA of child revealed a male karyotype with intact *DMD/BMD* gene at the exon intron level, ruling out suspected DMD in this patient. However, the 1.81 Mb deletion was seen on chromosome 13 (13q31.3) (Fig. 40.3) which includes *GPC5* (OMIM 602446) and *GPC6* (OMIM 604404) genes having a role in cell-cell adhesion. *GPC6* gene is mainly associated with craniofacial abnormalities and limb deformities (congenital, or Omodysplasia Type 1) and *GPC5* is associated with musculoskeletal diseases. Considering the present clinical findings in this patient, it could be inferred that gene *GPC5* and *GPC6* could play a role in causing musculoskeletal abnormalities manifested by the present progressive muscular deterioration (similar to that seen in

DMD) resulting into difficulty in motor activities like sitting, walking, etc. The CMA completely changed the diagnostic scenario and even the possibility of DMD/BMD X-linked disorder—was ruled out. The post-test counseling was done and the couple now opted for prenatal CMA diagnosis.

TAKE HOME MESSAGE

The 21st century has witnessed a significant impact of genomic technologies on the diagnosis of human genetic diseases; one of those is array-based CGH. Not only can hundreds of well-characterized genetic syndromes be detected in a single assay, but new genomic disorders and disease-causing genes can also be discovered. Prenatal chromosomal microarray analysis (Prenatal CMA) is a diagnostic test that can detect genetic abnormalities in a fetus and is most beneficial when ultrasonography identifies fetal structural anomalies. The CMA of the index case in a family remains the prerequisite. Using amniocytes or CVS cells, it is possible to quickly and thoroughly analyze all fetal chromosomes in a single test with greater sensitivity, specificity and a level of resolution far superior to a standard karyotype. As a result, genetic abnormalities that would otherwise go undetected can now be ascertained by prenatal CMA and genetic counseling can also become more effective. The conventional cytogenetic will always remain the 'gold standard' as a genetic screening test. The disadvantages of aCGH should be kept in mind while arriving at the diagnosis, viz. inability of aCGH to detect single gene disorders, balanced translocations and inversions, trisomy from translocations, and alterations in regions other than the protein-coding region. Presently, how the information should be introduced into patient care is a challenge to both medical geneticists and fetal medicine experts. However, with growing knowledge on human genome and phenomenal progress in bioinformatics tools will definitely play a significant role in precise fetal genetic diagnosis.

ACKNOWLEDGMENTS

We are thankful to PhD student Umakant Nadkar for his help in the literature search in Case-1. We thank all our patients undergoing microarray analysis and the referring doctors for their kind support and encouragement.

REFERENCES

1. Kallioniemi A, Kallioniemi OP, Sudar D, et al. Comparative genomic hybridization: a rapid new method for detecting & mapping DNA amplification in tumours. Semi Cancer Biology. 1993;4:41-6.
2. Pinkel D, Segraves R, Sudar D, et al. High resolution analysis of DNA copy number variation using comparative genomic hybridisation to microarrays. Nature Genetics. 1998;20: 207-11.
3. Lichter P, Joos S, Bentz M, Lampel S. Comparative genomic hybridisation: uses and limitations. Semi Hematology. 2000;37:348-57.
4. Miller DT, Adam MP, Aradhya S, et al. Consensus statement: chromosomal microarray is a first-tier clinical diagnostic test for individuals with developmental disabilities or congenital anomalies. Am J Hum Genet. 2010;86(5):749-64.
5. Sheth F, Andrieux J. Array-comparative genomic hybridization (a-CGH) in constitutional and acquired anomalies. In: Sheth J, Sheth F (Eds). Genetics in Clinical Practice. Jaypee Brothers Medical Publishers (P) Ltd; 2014.pp.93-114.
6. Manning M and Hudgins L. Professional Practice and Guidelines Committee. Array-based technology and recommendations for utilization in medical genetics practice for detection of chromosomal abnormalities. Genet Med. 2010;12(11):742-5.
7. Boyle CA, Boulet S, Schieve LA, et al. Trends in the prevalence of developmental disabilities in US children. Pediatrics. 2011;127(6):1034-42.
8. Heron MP, Hoyer DL, Murphy SL, et al. Deaths: Final data for 2006. National Vital Statistics Reports. 2009;57(14):1-136.
9. Srebniak M, Boter M, Oudesluijs G, Joosten M, Govaerts L, Van Opstal D, et al. Application of SNP array for rapid prenatal diagnosis: implementation, genetic counselling and diagnostic flow. Eur J Hum Genet. 2011;19:1230-37.
10. de Vries BB, Pfundt R, Leisink M, Koolen DA, Vissers LE, Janssen IM, et al. Diagnostic genome profiling in mental retardation. Am J Hum Genet. 2005;77:606-16.
11. Stankiewicz P, Beaudet AL. Use of array CGH in the evaluation of dysmorphology, malformations, developmental delay, and idiopathic mental retardation. Curr Opinion Genet Dev. 2007;17:182-92.
12. Chelly H, Khelfaoui M, Francis F, et al. Genetics and pathophysiology of mental retardation. Eur J Hum Genet. 2006;14:701-13.
13. Leonard H, Wen X. The epidemiology of mental retardation: challenges and opportunities in the new millennium. Mental Retardation and Developmental Disabilities. Research Review. 2002;8(3):117-34.
14. Michelson DJ, Shevell MI, Sherr EH, et al. Evidence report: genetic and metabolic testing on children with global developmental delay: report of the Quality Standards Subcommittee of the American Academy of Neurology and the Practice Committee of the Child Neurology Society. Neurology. 2011;77(17):1629-35.
15. Vissers LE, Veltman JA, van Kessel AG, Brunner HG. Identification of disease genes by whole genome CGH arrays. Hum Mol Genet. 2005;14(Spec No.2): R215-23.
16. Reddy UM, Page GP, Saade GR, et al. Karyotype versus microarray testing for genetic abnormalities after stillbirth.

NICHD Stillbirth Collaborative Research Network. N Eng J Med. 2012;367:2185-93.

17. Wapner RJ, Martin CL, Levy B, Ballif BC, Eng CM, Zachary JM, et al. Chromosomal microarray versus karyotyping for prenatal diagnosis. N Eng J Med. 2012;367:2175-8.
18. Le Caignec C, Boceno M, Saugier-Veber P, Jacquemont S, Joubert M, David A, et al. Detection of genomic imbalances by array based comparative genomic hybridisation (aCGH) in fetuses with multiple malformations. J Med Genet. 2005;42:121-8.
19. Van den Veyyer IB, Patel A, Shaw CA, Pursley AN, Kang SH, Simovich MJ, et al. Clinical use of array comparative genomic hydridization (aCGH) for prenatal diagnosis in 300 cases. Prenat Diagn. 2009;29:29-39.
20. Maya I, Davidov B, Gershovitz I, Zalzstein Y, Taub E, Coppinger J, et al. Diagnostic utility of array- based comparative genomic hybridization (aCGH) in a prenatal setting. Prenatal Diagnosis. 2010;30:1131-7.
21. Hillman SC, Pretlove S, Coomarasamy A, McMullan DJ, Davison EV, Maher ER, et al. Additional information from array comparative genomic hybridization technology over conventional karyotyping in prenatal diagnosis: a systematic review and meta-analysis. Ultrasound Ostet Gynecol. 2011;37:6-14.
22. Shaffer LG, Rosenfeld JA, CDabell MP, Coppinger J, Bandholz AM, Ellison JW, et al. Detection rates of clinically significant genomic alterations by microarray analysis for specific anomalies detected by ultrasound. Prenatal Diagnosis. 2012;15:139-45.
23. The American College of Obstetricians and Gynecologists committee on Genetics Society for Maternal-Fetal Medicine. The Use of Chromosomal Microarray Analysis in Prenatal Diagnosis. Committee Opinion No. 581; 2013:1-4.
24. Grote L, Myers M, Lovell A, Saal H, Lipscomb Sund K. Variability in laboratory reporting practices for regions of homozygosity indicating parental relatedness as identified by SNP microarray testing. Genet Med. 2012;14:971-6.
25. Potocki L, Chen KS, Park SS, Osterholm DE, Wither MA, Kimonis V, et al. Molecular mechanism for duplication 17p11.2- the homologous recombination reciprocal of the Smith-Magenis microdeletion. Nature Genetics. 2000;24: 84-7.
26. Potocki L, Bi W, Treadwell-Deering D, Carvalho CMB, Eifert A, Friedman EM, et al. characterization of Potocki-Lupski syndrome [dup(17) (p11.2p11.2)] and delineation of a dosage-sensitive critical interval that can convey an autism phenotype. Am J Hum Genet. 2007;80(4):633-49.

CHAPTER

41 Future of Prenatal Diagnosis and Screening

Raju R Sahetya

INTRODUCTION

The past half-century has been witness to the application of a series of clinical and laboratory technologies that have provided remarkable insights into the human genome. It is now possible to define the human genotype at distinct biological levels, chromosome, gene, nucleotide, as well as their intrinsic and extrinsic interactions culminating in phenotype. Nowhere have these technologies, and the genetic information generated from them, been more widely applied than in the case of prenatal testing, both screening and diagnosis.

Each year hundreds of thousands of women and their partners now undergo genetic testing in the form of carrier screening for single gene mutations, prenatal screening for chromosome abnormalities, and/or diagnostic analysis following an invasive procedure (first trimester chorionic villus sample or midtrimester amniocentesis). The dynamism of the field of prenatal genetic diagnosis and screening is illustrated with the ongoing introduction of new technologies, such as noninvasive prenatal testing (NIPT), array comparative genome hybridization (aCGH), exome sequencing, whole genome amplification, and RNA sequencing. The time has come where testing of a preimplantation embryo, post-implantation embryo or a fetus has the potential of revealing not simply individual, deleterious mutations but rather a series of genes and gene interactions that impact on different stages of life in both positive and negative manners. If, as anticipated, the technologies associated with single cell analysis of the transcriptome[1-6] and the expansion of the proteotome[7] become a clinical reality, the obvious question and past designation as to who and what are "normal" may no longer have any value or utility, losing meaning both on an individual basis as well as from a population perspective and just as dynamic has been the increasing sophistication in the prenatal analyses of the genome and its products, there has been virtually no change in parental choices following identification of any genetic mutation, which at present is either termination of pregnancy or continuation with birth of affected offspring. Incorporating all of this into a meaningful discussion on the future of prenatal diagnosis and screening leads to five situations:

Situation 1: Whereas the field of reproductive genetics has achieved remarkable success in the diagnosis and screening of chromosome and single gene disorders, the goal of positive therapeutic interventions has yet to be achieved.

Situation 2: The etiology and pathogenesis of many genetic/developmental disorders are known and/or are being continuously refined and detailed.

Situation 3: There is a categorical imperative for the need to shift focus from late identification of genetic and developmental disorders of the fetus (i.e. 9 weeks gestation and beyond) to the embryonic period (i.e. preimplantation to day 58 post-conception).

Situation 4: Identification of genetic and developmental disorders in the embryonic period is insufficient; there is a need to develop therapeutic interventions that either correct, alleviate and/or minimize the phenotypic effects of any genetic and developmental disorder at the time of their potential genesis, namely, during embryogenesis.

Situation 5: Recognizing that there will be insufficient numbers of medical geneticists and genetic counselors to address the expansive genetic information generated by the multitude of technologies applicable to prenatal diagnosis and screening, the format of genetic counseling will be required to change in philosophy and in practice.

The following is a discussion elaborating on each situation:

Situation 1: Whereas the field of reproductive genetics has achieved remarkable success in the diagnosis and screening of chromosome and single gene disorders, the goal of positive therapeutic interventions has yet to be achieved.

The first situation is that, based on current approaches and practices, essentially there will be no change in the future of prenatal diagnosis and screening. Whereas over the past 50 years prenatal identification of genetic mutations and developmental malformations has become increasingly sophisticated and expansive, the choices following such identification, namely, pregnancy termination or the birth of an affected offspring, have in fact not changed. In opposition to pregnancy termination, it has been proposed that prenatal diagnosis and screening represent a failure of medicine in the classical sense. This failure of current practices of prenatal diagnosis and screening, it is claimed, was first articulated specifically in the Hippocratic Oath:

"I will prescribe regimens for the good of my patients according to my ability and my judgment and never do harm to anyone."

"I will give no deadly medicine to anyone if asked, nor suggest any such counsel; and similarly I will not give a woman a pessary to cause an abortion."

As part of the argument, it is evident that the distinction between a viable and nonviable fetus as a rationale and justification for termination of pregnancy is artificial on medical grounds alone, with no need for moral or religious considerations. Consequently, as presently conducted, it is argued, prenatal diagnosis and screening represents a violation of the basic tenet of medicine from the perspective of the fetus and ultimately is likely in many instances to be considered a failure on the part of the parents as well, especially those choosing pregnancy termination. The argument further suggests that the diagnosis of a genetic mutation and/or developmental anomaly made in the first trimester, i.e. 9–11 weeks' gestation, is also an acknowledgement of a medical failure, since from a developmental perspective, the damage, physical and/or functional, has already taken place many weeks earlier and as a result the best that can be expected from fetal therapy is partial but incomplete amelioration of the phenotypic effects of most genetic mutations and/or developmental anomalies.

Situation 2: The etiology and pathogenesis of many genetic/developmental disorders are known and/or are being continuously refined and detailed.

The human genome consists of coding and noncoding DNA sequences. Coded DNA comprises sequences that are transcribed into mRNA and eventually translated into proteins in the course of embryonic development. Whereas these coding sequences comprise less than 2% of the genome, they ultimately lead to the production of all human proteins, recognizing that other biological processes lead to the formation of many more unique proteins than the number of protein-coding genes.[7] In the case of prenatal genetic testing and evaluation, the current focus is identification of pathological conditions associated with clinically defined diseases and caused by sequence variation in genomic DNA. There are many different, clinically-significant forms of DNA sequence variation, ranging from polyploidy and aneuploidy to a change in a single nucleotide. The exact number of valid human protein-coding genes is unknown but estimates range from 2000 to 25,000; the average number of genes listed in human gene catalogs appears to be around 22,500 with uncertainty of the role of another 2000 genes, which appear to be retroposons, pseudo genes, or "orphan" DNA sequences, i.e. non-human in origin[8] In the case of pregnancy, either planned or in progress, current practices with regard to routine genetic testing can include the following, individually or combined: (1) carrier screening of prospective parent(s) of a defined set of disease-causing mutations based on population frequency, e.g. cystic fibrosis, spinal muscle atrophy, fragile X, as well as other, specific gene mutations based on family history; (2) visualization of fetal development by ultrasound, the earliest time usually no earlier than 9 weeks' gestation; (3) first trimester screening for risk assessment of chromosome abnormalities, cardiac malformations and other developmental disorders; (4) noninvasive prenatal testing (NIPT) for aneuploidy involving chromosomes 21, 18, 21, X and Y and for microduplications/microdeletions associated with specific genetic syndromes, e.g. 22q deletions; (5) second trimester screening, particularly for open neural tube defects, as well as more detailed ultrasound evaluation at 18–20 weeks' gestation; (6) diagnostic testing based on genetic analysis of chorionic villi or amniocytes, following invasive testing by first trimester chorionic villus sampling (CVS) or mid-trimester amniocentesis, respectively; and, (7) in an increasing number of cases, microarray, exonic and whole genome analyses.

A number of Mendelian genes can serve as models wherein the complete spectrum of genetic and developmental effects of individual mutations has been defined. Examples would include, but not be limited to, sickle cell disease, Tay Sachs, spinal muscle atrophy, and cystic fibrosis. In the case of sickle cell disease (SCD), for example, every component of the pathogenesis has been defined including specific changes at the nucleotide level, the altered composition of the protein coded by the mutation(s), its effect on red cell morphology, the biochemical and physiological impact on somatic development, and the overall clinical expression as a direct consequence of the mutation(s). Patients with SCD experience multisystem complications comprising recurrent and painful vaso-occlusive crises, acute chest syndrome, splenic sequestration and pulmonary hypertension; organ damage begins at a young age and reduces life expectancy to half of the general population; SCD remains a highly morbid disease caused by chronic and progressive physical damage.[9] Despite knowledge of all facets of the disease process, the only available cure for SCD is hematopoietic stem cell transplant (HSCT), which has been demonstrated to improve overall survival by reversing organ damage and stabilizing CNS vasculopathy.[10-13] There is a series of medical as well as social barriers markedly prohibiting widespread usage of this approach, including lack of suitable HLA-matched donors, the risk of transplant-related toxicities, complications and even death, and the lack of information and limited understanding of HSCT by SCD family members.[9] Alternative methods and technologies such as population-wide preimplantation genetic diagnosis and screening does not appear to be realistic or practical,[14,15] whereas current forms of prenatal genetic diagnosis and screening with termination of affected pregnancies not only has moral, religious and legal constraints but also challenges the very core of medical philosophy and practice.

Situation 3: There is a categorical imperative for the need to shift focus from late identification of genetic and developmental disorders of the fetus (9 weeks gestation and beyond) to the embryonic period (preimplantation to day 58 postconception).

It is generally understood that genetic disorders are developmental in nature and as such are formulated during embryogenesis; are already physically and/or functionally defined primarily before the beginning of the fetal stage; and, that developmental disturbances identified postnatally are in reality extensions of biological events occurring between 3 and 8 weeks' gestation. Consequently, the current practice of genetic testing following first trimester CVS or second trimester amniocentesis is applying prenatal diagnosis weeks far-too-late in pregnancy. Furthermore, as previously stated, when a genetic and/or developmental abnormality is identified using current technologies, the primary choices are usually limited to pregnancy termination or the birth of an affected offspring followed by ameliorative medical/surgical treatment.

If this scenario is to be altered with a potentially positive outcome, alternative medical approaches and interventions that are not only realistic and practical but also acceptable to major sectors of any society, must be considered. Preimplantation genetic diagnosis and screening is an obvious choice but it is proposed that in the future the focus of reproductive geneticists will be interventions during embryogenesis.

The initial impression is that preimplantation evaluation, either of gametes (i.e. polar bodies) or of embryos prior to transfer, easily meets the need of early identification of genetic and developmental disorders. There now, is a relatively extensive worldwide body of knowledge and experience defining the field of preimplantation genetic diagnosis and screening.[14] Over the past two decades, thousands of couples have undergone preimplantation diagnosis and screening for dozens of different genetic disorders following analysis either of polar body, day 3–4 embryo, or trophectoderm.[14] However, there are distinct disadvantages to this approach: preimplantation genetic diagnosis and screening is costly, labor-intensive; limited to relatively few couples, not without controversy in regard to preimplantation genetic screening[15] and, at present (2014) has a worldwide success rate of less than 25% in the "take-home-baby-rate" for each cycle of egg retrieval.[14]

Situation 4: Identification of genetic and developmental disorders in the embryonic period is insufficient; there is a need to develop therapeutic interventions that will correct, alleviate or minimize the phenotypic effects of any genetic and developmental disorder at the time of their potential genesis, namely, during embryogenesis.

A HISTORICAL PERSPECTIVE

Prior to the introduction of prenatal diagnosis in the late 1960s, prospective parents at significant reproductive risk had limited preventive choices, either having no children by aborting each pregnancy, voluntary sterilization, sexual abstinence or by adoption. At the time of introduction of prenatal diagnosis by amniocentesis, the ultimate goal articulated by health professionals was fetal gene therapy, based in part in response to the controversy and rhetoric surrounding the morality and social implications of pregnancy termination based on genetic mutations. These debates have continued unabated to the present time, with one side viewing abortion following diagnostic testing for genetic disorders as a "logical or moral precedent for infanticide"[16] and their counterparts arguing that selective abortion prevents suffering of families and reduces the economic burdens to society.[17]

Over the past two decades, there have been a series of publications focused on moral and ethical issues with respect to human fetal gene therapy.[18-23] Whereas the ethical and religious concerns about the current consequences of prenatal diagnosis and screening will likely remain unresolved, the future challenge to reproductive geneticists will be their creative ability in devising the technological means to: (1) physically and functionally define comprehensive embryonic development; and (2) be able to act on that information so as to modify specific forms of embryonic maldevelopment (e.g. open spinal defects) toward a positive outcome. There is likely to be a more general understanding and acceptance that with effective oversight, gene therapy during embryonic development is likely to be an acceptable medical goal, if it: (1) demonstrably improves the health and wellbeing of individuals who would otherwise experience irreversible physical and functional damage before birth, thereby potentially avoiding the need for alternative techniques such as gamete donation, embryo selection, abortion, adoption or non-parenthood; and (2) demonstrates that the risk of germ-line gene mutation through *in utero* gene transfer is minimal or nonexistent.[17]

There is general consensus by health professionals that whereas elective abortion following any form of prenatal testing may be expeditious, in reality, it still connotes an unsatisfactory medical response and outcome, as does the birth of a developmentally compromised newborn. The focus of the past 30 years has been on refining genetic analyses of the fetus, including the application of fluorescent *in situ* hybridization (FISH), chromosome banding, aCGH, next generation sequencing and NIPT, but all applied in distinguishing "normal" from "affected". There have been projects aimed at integrating multiple approaches to identify the functional element encoded in the human genome, e.g., ENCODE,[24] however, the focus being children and adults, its applicability to embryonic development is questionable, since it has been well established that the clinical effects of a genetic change detected *in utero* does not always match the postnatal phenotype. More recently, a data base correlating prenatal copy number variations (CNV) with postnatal outcome has been established, with a focus on the autistic spectrum disorder.[25]

When genetic testing by amniocentesis was clinically introduced in the 1960s, it was generally recognized and agreed upon that this approach was not the ultimate goal of prenatal diagnosis. While the idea of fetal gene therapy was envisioned as a distant but attainable goal, it was understood that ultimately prenatal diagnostic testing had to be complemented by some form(s) of therapy, be it genetic, medical or surgical. Fetal gene therapy is inherently flawed as the potential detrimental phenotypic effects of any genetic mutation, be it at the chromosomal or molecular level, have already occurred in the embryonic period. Albeit with some minor success, *in utero* treatment has been applied to fetuses at risk for a number of genetic and congenital anomalies, including congenital diaphragmatic hernia, cystadenomatoid malformation of the lung and sacrococcygeal teratoma, shunts for uropathies and thoracic fluids, pharmacological therapies for congenital adrenal hyperplasia and neural tube defect as well as stem cell treatment of severe combined immunodeficiency disorder.[26-30] The insights gained over the past decade with regard to stem cell biology as well as the ability to manipulate genetic sequences are two of an increasing number of technologies whereby there now are opportunities to alter the course of abnormal development during the critical time of embryogenesis, as summarized next.

FUTURE PERSPECTIVES

In the 30th Anniversary Issue of Prenatal Diagnosis published in 2010, three paradigm shifts in preimplantation and prenatal genetics were projected to occur by 2020, each in turn enhancing one ultimate goal of medical science, namely, "personalized medicine":

1. Epigenomics would become a reality in which regulatory regions of all known genes in all major cell types and their disease variants would have been analyzed and their influences would be understood during prenatal and early postnatal development when epigenetic mechanisms undergo establishment and maturation;
2. Prevention of chromosome abnormalities by defining the biological processes associated with gamete maturation including chromosome pairing, synapses and segregation of homolog's, thereby ensuring that the euploid state would be obtained at conception and maintained during early embryonic development;
3. Treatment of mendelian, mitochondrial and multifactorial diseases in the preimplantation and embryonic periods of development, which would involve cost-effective sequencing of the human genome at the single gene level, the development of databases cataloging submicroscopic copy number variants and their role in disease, a complete understanding of the pathogenesis of both single gene mutations and complex diseases, and knowledge derived from the epigenome, all of which have become a reality over the past decade.[31]

Such related technologies would make possible implementation of targeted molecular interventions and the realization of the full potential of a personalized genome analysis in the prenatal period of human development, a consequence of the synergy of epigenetics, pharmacogenetics, and the ability to physically and chemically manipulate cells, tissues or organ systems.[31] The additional challenge of germline gene therapy, rationalized in part by anticipated success in somatic gene therapy, must also be considered.[32] Such a challenge will result in debates over the moral and ethical consequence of such actions, namely, the potential and realization of altering the genome of future generations, but more importantly, addressing the categorical imperative of medicine of doing no harm, i.e. a call to re-examine germline gene therapy as a responsible way to address the consequences of somatic gene therapy.[32]

Gene therapy is likely to be first applied in preimplantation embryos, namely, in the case of mitochondrial disorders, which in turn immediately raises a recurring concern of simultaneously altering the germ line. Both in the United Kingdom and the United States, governmental approval has been requested for placing a fertilized oocyte at risk for a mitochondrial disorder into the cytoplasm with normal mitochondria, thus resulting in a conception with three genotypes, i.e. maternal, paternal and mitochondrial. The potential of manipulating the genetic inheritance of future offspring by modification of spermatozoa, oocytes and embryos prior to implantation can be criticized as being "high-tech eugenics" and experimentation on humans. This criticism is a recurring theme consistently sounded following the introduction of new prenatal technology, e.g. when amniocentesis, chorionic villus sampling, *in vitro* fertilization (IVF) and preimplantation genetic diagnosis (PGD) were each introduced. In the case of mitochondrial disorders, the combined application of several different technologies provides an opportunity for a carrier parent to ensure an offspring free of the clinical devastation as a consequence of dysfunctional mitochondria.

While the preimplantation substitution of defective mitochondria represents a heritable change by virtue of the interaction of these organelles with the recipient nuclear genome, this approach does not address nuclear genetic mutations, e.g. the over six thousand single gene mutations, the hundreds of different kinds of chromosome abnormalities, and/or any of the multifactorial traits. It is likely that any attempt at prenatal genetic therapy during embryogenesis will require different types of molecular technologies for different developmental disorder. Targeted gene therapy in metabolic disorders restricted to an organ system, e.g. the liver in phenylketonuria or in maple syrup urine disease, would appear to be an acceptable approach, implemented as early as possibly in gestation in order to minimize any potential negative impact, particularly the development and function of the central nervous system.[33]

With the ability to edit DNA at the nucleotide level by virtue of such technologies as CRISPR (Clustered Regularly Interspaced Short Palindromic Repeats), the "future is now" in the case of prenatal genetic therapy may no longer be a paradoxical statement.[34] The technology uses a nuclease, CRISPR-associated (Cas9) that complexes with small RNAs as guides (gRNA) to cleave DNA in a sequence-specific manner upstream of the protospacer adjacent motif (PAM) in any genomic location. CRISPR editing technology has been successfully applied to model organisms, including nematodes, zebra fish, fruit flies and most recently in mammals, demonstrating its broad utility and specificity for editing genes regardless of their source and type.[34] It may be possible for the CRISPR technology to be applied to genes associated with genetically-determined forms of autism, addressing the question, "Could autism be treated prenatally?"[35,36] For many genetic diseases expressed at birth and childhood, it is well recognized that their biological effects actually manifest during embryogenesis. Therefore, to be most effective, the future in prenatal diagnosis and screening should involve the development and application of technologies capable of identifying genetic disorders as early as possible in gestation, either in the preimplantation or embryonic time periods, and then to apply corrective gene therapies that minimize, if not completely eliminate, their negative phenotypic impact on somatic development and/or intellectual functions. This will be an especially arduous scientific journey, requiring novel technologies involving embryonic visualization,[37] gene manipulations[33] and/or transplantation of genetically-altered mesenchymal stem cells,[27] all with the goal to ameliorate potential physical and functional damage. It is anticipated that the first effective therapies would be applied to a collective group of monogenic disorders for the purpose of achieving phenotypic cure early in the disease process and before the development of permanent organ damage.[29]

One consequence of the development and application of individualized gene therapies will likely be challenges to the relative autonomy of parental decision-making. In fact, in societies practicing a public health model, challenges to parental autonomy concerning various aspects of genetic testing have already been accepted. In the case of private healthcare models, e.g. the United States, individual choice concerning various forms of genetic testing is often considerably modulated by the professional societies, which, in turn, influence another important factor in parental decision-making, namely, insurance coverage. Therefore, although the basic right of reproductive choice, of when, with whom, and how to reproduce, continues to be articulated by Western societies, parental autonomy has been, and will continue to be, moderated by healthcare providers, particularly as new technologies are applied in prenatal diagnosis. What has been increasingly contentious in Western societies, primarily on ethical and moral grounds, is the granting of broad autonomy to prospective parents when the choice includes abortion. Over the coming decades, it will be the medical consequences and available choices following prenatal diagnosis that will be expanded to include preimplantation and embryonic gene therapies. And, if practiced in the preimplantation embryo, it must be understood and accepted that any form of gene therapy will likely involve altering the germ line as well as the soma.

CONCLUSION

How in the near future is genomic medicine to influence pregnancy management and pregnancy outcome? New genetic technologies as well as new therapeutic strategies must be developed if embryonic care is to include expanded choices of action beyond current means.[2-7] In other words, there must be a synergy of the ability to define *in vivo* embryonic development at all biological levels, i.e. cell, tissue and organ,[38] along with the technical means to repair, alter or at least minimize the phenotypic effects of potentially negative mutations,[39-42] Thus, there should be a rapid and energetic shift in the research focus of prenatal diagnosis and screening, and a call for an expansion of all future prenatal studies to include therapeutic strategies other than current choices. This requires that the embryo must be completely defined not only at the genomic level, but also analyzed at all stages of embryonic development the transcriptome, its functional pathways, as well as its intrinsic and extrinsic interactions.[43,44] This challenge is heightened by the knowledge that the oocyte,[45] spermatozoa[46] and fertilized oocyte are characterized by high rates of spontaneous mutations, thereby diminishing the impact of familial inheritance.[47] Until new therapeutic strategies are developed and incorporated into the management of embryonic development, only then will a more complete and personalized form of medicine be attained.

REFERENCES

1. Trapnell C, Williams BA, Pertea G, Mortazavi A, Kwan G, van Baren MJ, et al. Transcript assembly and quantification by RNA-Seq reveals unannotated transcripts and isoform switching during cell differentiation. Nat Biotechnol. 2010;28;511-5.
2. Ramsköld D, Luo S, Wang Y, Li R, Deng Q, Faridani OR, et al. Full-length mRNA-Seq from single-cell levels of RNA and individual circulating tumor cells. Nat Biotechnol. 2012;30:777-82.
3. Fan J, Chen J, April CS, Fisher JS, Klotzle B, Bibikova M, et al. Highly parallel genome-wide expression analysis of single mammalian cells. PLoS One 2012, doi:10.1371/journal.pone.0030794.
4. Ramsköld D, Kavak E, Sandberg R. How to Analyze gene expression using RNA-sequencing data. In: Wang J, Tan AC, Tian T (Eds). Next Generation Microarray Bioinformatics: Methods and Protocols; Humana Press: New York, NY, USA, 2012. pp. 259-74.
5. Deng Q, Ramsköld D, Reinius B, Sandberg R. Single-cell RNA-seq reveals dynamic, random monoallelic gene expression in mammalian cells. Science. 2014;343:193-6.
6. Wang X, Lu Z, Gomez A, Hon GC, Yue Y, Han D, et al. N6-methyladenosine-dependent regulation of messenger RNA stability. Nature. 2014:505:117-20.
7. Wilson LOW, Spriggs A, Taylor JM, Fahrer AM. A novel splicing outcome reveals more than 2000 new mammalian protein isoforms. Bioinformatics. 2014;30:151-6.
8. Pertea M, Salzberg SL. Between a chicken and a grape: Estimating the number of human genes. Genome Biol. 2010, 11, doi:10.1186/gb-2010-11-5-206.
9. Thompson AL, Bridley A, Twohy E, Dioguardi J, Sande J, Hsu LL, et al. An educational symposium for patients with sickle cell disease and their families: results from surveys of knowledge and factors influencing decisions about hematopoietic stem cell transplant. Pediatr Blood Cancer. 2013;60:1946-51.
10. Shenoy S. Hematopoietic stem cell transplantation for sick cell disease: Current practice and emerging trends. Hematol Am Soc Hematol Educ Program 2011. 2011. pp. 273-9.
11. Locatelli F, Pagliara D. Allogeneic hematopoietic stem cell transplantation in children with sickle cell disease. Pediatr Blood Cancer. 2012;59:372-6.
12. Khoury R, Abboud MR. Stem-cell transplantation in children and adults with sickle cell disease: An update. Expert Rev Hematol. 2011;4:343-51. J Clin Med. 2014;3:1300.
13. Bernaudin F, Socie G, Kuentz M, Chevret S, Duval M, Bertrand Y, et al. Long-term results of related myeloblative stem-cell transplantation to cure sickle cell disease. Blood. 2007;111:2749-56.
14. Moutou C, Goossens V, Coonen E, de Rycke M, Kokkali G, Renwick P, et al. ESHRE PGD Consortium data collection XII: Cycles from January to December 2009 with pregnancy follow-up to October 2010. Hum Reprod. 2014;29;880-903.
15. Gleicher N, Kushnir VA, Barad DH. Preimplantation genetic screening (PGS) still in search of a clinical application: A systematic review. Reprod Biol Endocrin. 2014, 12, doi:10.1186/1477-7827-12-22.
16. Neel JV. Ethical issues resulting from prenatal diagnosis. Early Diagnosis of Human Genetic Defects; Health, Education and Welfare Publications: Washington, DC, USA, 1972.
17. Fletcher JC, Richter G. Human fetal gene therapy: Moral and ethical questions. Hum Gene Ther. 1996;7:1605-14.
18. Juengst ET. Germ-line gene therapy back to basics. J Med Plulos. 1991;16:593-612.
19. Lyon J, Comer P. Altered Fates WW. Norton: New York, NY, USA, 1995. p. 498.
20. Ledley FD. Prenatal application of somatic gene therapy. Obstet Gynecol Cln N Am. 1993;20:611-20.
21. Lee TF. Gene Future. Plenum Press: New York, NY, USA, 1993. p. 19.
22. Moseley R. Commentary maintaining the somatic/germline Distinction: Some ethical drawbacks. J Med Plulos. 1991;16:641-7.
23. Zimmerman BK. Human germ-line therapy. The case of its development and use. J Med Plulos. 1991;16:129-39.
24. Dunham I. ENCODE-ing the Future. Genet Eng Biotechnol News. 2013;33:38-39.
25. Prenatal Array Registry Home Page. Available online: *http://www.prenatalarray.org* (accessed on 18 August 2014).

26. Evans MI, Harrison MR, Flake AW, Johnson M. Fetal therapy. Best Pract Res Clin Obstetr Gynaecol. 2002;16:671-83.
27. Chan J, O'Donoghue K, de la Fuente J, Roberts IA, Kumar S, Morgan JE, Fisk NM. Human fetal mesenchymal stem cells as vehicles for gene delivery. Stem Cells. 2005;23:93-102.
28. Rahim AA, Buckley SM, Chan JK, Peebles DM, Waddington SN. Perinatal gene delivery to the CNS. Ther Deliv. 2011;4:483-91.
29. Mattar CN, Choolani M, Biswas A, Waddinton SN, Chan JKY. Fetal gene therapy: recent advances and current challenges. Expert Opin Biol Ther. 2011;11:1257-71.
30. Van Mieghem T, Baud D, Devlieger R, Lewi L, Ryan G, de Catte L, Deprest J. Minimally invasive fetal therapy. Best Pract Res Clin Obstetr Gynaecol. 2012;26:711-25.
31. Pergament E. By 2020. Prenat Diagn. 2010;30:710-1.
32. Fiddler M, Pergament E. Germline gene therapy: Its time is near. Mol Hum Reprod. 1996;2:75-76.
33. McKay TR, Rahim AA, Buckley SK, Ward NJ, Chan JKY, Howe SJ, Waddington SN. Perinatal gene transfer to the liver. Curr Pharm Des. 2011;17:2528-41. J Clin Med. 2014;3:1301.
34. Niu Y, Shen B, Cui Y, Chen Y, Wang J, Wang L, et al. Generation of gene-modified cynomolgus monkey via Cas9/RNA-mediated gene targeting in one-cell embryos. Cell. 2014;156:836-43.
35. Tyzio R, Nardou R, Ferrari D, Tsintsadze T, Shahrokhi A, Eftekhari S, et al. Oxytocin-mediated GABA inhibition during delivery attenuates autism pathogenesis in rodent offspring. Science. 2014:343:675-9.
36. Zimmerman AW, Connors SL. Could autism be treated prenatally? Science. 2014;343:620-1.
37. Donnelly JC, Malone FD. Early fetal anatomical sonography. Best Pract Res Clin Obstetr Gynaecol. 2012;26:561-73.
38. Papaioannou GKI, Syngelaki A, Maiz NR, Ross JA, Nicolaides KH. Sonographic markers of aneuploidies at 6–10 weeks gestation. Early Hum Dev. 2011;87:453-6.
39. Chan J, Kumar S, Fisk NM. First trimester embryo-fetoscopic and ultrasound-guided fetal blood sampling for ex vivo vial transduction of cultured human fetal mesenchyma stem cell. Hum Reprod. 2008;23:2427-37.
40. Mattaar CN, Biswas A, Choolani M, Chan JKY. The case for intrauterine stem cell transplantation. Best Pract Res Clin Obstetr Gynaecol. 2012;26:683-95.
41. Gotherstrom C, Westgre M, Shaw SWS, Astrom E, Biswas A, Byers PH, et al. Pre- and postnatal transplantation of fetal mesenchymal stem cells in osteogenesis imperfect: A two-center experience. Stem Cells Transl Med. 2014;3:1-10.
42. Trainer PA, Dixon J, Dion MJ. Treacher Collins syndrome: Etiology, pathogenesis and prevention. Eur J Hum Gene. 2009;17:275-83.
43. ENCODE Project Consortium. Bernstein BE, Birney E, Dunham I, Gree ED, Gunter C, Synder M. An integrated encyclopedia of DNA elements in the human genome. Nature. 2012:489:57-74.
44. Mehta G, Jalan R, Mookerjee RP. Cracking the ENCODE: From transcription to therapeutics. Hepatology. 2013;57:2532-5.
45. Hou Y, Fan W, Yan L, Li R, Lian Y, Huang J, Li J, et al. Genome analyses of single human oocytes. Cell. 2013;155:1492-506.
46. Lu S, Zong C, Fan W, Yang M, Li J, Chapman AR, et al. Probing meiotic recombination and aneuploidy of single sperm cells by whole-genome sequencing. Science. 2012;338:1627-30.
47. Campbell CD, Eichler EE. Properties and rates of germline mutations in humans. Trends Genet. 2013;29:575-84.

SECTION

10

Guidelines

- FIGO: Good Practice Advice
- Maternal-Fetal Medicine

CHAPTER

42

FIGO: Good Practice Advice

SCREENING FOR CHROMOSOMAL ABNORMALITIES AND NONINVASIVE PRENATAL DIAGNOSIS AND TESTING

Universal screening is a strategy applied to all individuals of a certain category to identify a high risk group to have an unrecognized disease in individuals without signs or symptoms of such disease (e.g. screening of all pregnant women to identify the high-risk group for fetal chromosomal abnormalities). A test used in a screening program, especially for a disease with low incidence, must have a high detection rate (DR) and low false positive rate (FPR). Prenatal diagnosis of fetal aneuploidies necessitates invasive testing, which is essentially carried out by chorionic villus sampling at 10–15 weeks' gestation or amniocentesis at or after 16 weeks. However, invasive testing is expensive and can cause miscarriage in about 1% of pregnancies; it is therefore reserved for cases identified by screening as being at high-risk for aneuploidies.

First-trimester screening for trisomies 21, 18 and 13 by a combination of maternal age, fetal nuchal translucency thickness (NT), fetal heart rate (FHR) and serum-free β-human chorionic gonadotropin (β-hCG) and pregnancy-associated plasma protein-A (PAPP-A) can detect about 90% of cases of trisomy 21 and 95% of those with trisomies 18 and 13, at FPR of about 5%. The performance of first-trimester screening can be improved by expanding the combined test to include other first trimester sonographic markers, such as the presence or absence of the fetal nasal bone, measurement of fetal ductus venosus pulsatility index for veins (DV-PIV) and regurgitation across the tricuspid valve.

Some countries developed a national program of screening for trisomy 21 based on the combined risk test and the offer of invasive testing at a risk cut-off which aims to maintain the invasive test rate at 3% or less. In others there are no national guidelines on screening and individual practitioners offer a variety of first and/or second trimester methods. Even worse, in some parts of Europe the rate of invasive testing is in excess of 20% based mainly on maternal age.

Recently, screening for fetal aneuploidies based on the analysis of cell free DNA (cfDNA) in the plasma of pregnant women has been introduced into clinical practice. This can be undertaken from as early as the 10th week of pregnancy with results available approximately 1 week after maternal blood sampling. Evidence suggests that analysis of cfDNA in maternal blood can detect about 99% of cases of trisomy 21, 97% of trisomy 18, and 92% of trisomy 13, with respective FPRs of 0.08%, 0.15% and 0.2%.

At present, cfDNA testing is expensive and therefore widespread uptake of the test into routine clinical practice is likely to be contingent on the results of first-line screening by another method, preferably the first-trimester combined test, rather than as a primary method of screening. Such a strategy would also retain the advantages of first-trimester testing by ultrasound and biochemistry, including accurate pregnancy dating, early detection of many major fetal defects and prediction, with the International Federation of Gynecology and Obstetrics Working Group on Best Practice on Maternal-Foetal Medicine potential of prevention, of a wide range of pregnancy complications, including preterm birth and pre-eclampsia.

The International Federation of Gynecology and Obstetrics (FIGO) recommends the following:

- Maternal age has a low performance as a screening for fetal chromosomal abnormalities with a detection rate (DR) of 30–50% for false-positive rate (FPR) of 5–20%. Therefore, invasive testing for diagnosis of fetal aneuploidies should not be carried out by taking into account only maternal age.
- First-line screening for trisomies 21, 18 and 13 should be achieved by the combined test, which takes into account maternal age, fetal nuchal translucency (NT) thickness, fetal heart rate (FHR) and maternal serum free β-human chorionic gonadotropin (β-hCG) and pregnancy-associated plasma protein-A (PAPP-A). The combined risk test has a DR of 90% for trisomy 21 and 95% for trisomies 18 and 13, at FPR of about 5%.
- The combined test could be improved by assessing additional ultrasonographic markers, including the fetal nasal bone and Doppler assessment of the fetal ductus venosus flow and tricuspid flow. If all those markers are included the DR is increased to more than 95% and the FPR decreased to less than 3%.

- Screening by analysis of cfDNA in maternal blood has a DR of 99% for trisomy 21, 97% for trisomy 18 and 92% of trisomy 13, at a total FPR of 0.4%.
- Clinical implementation of cfDNA testing should preferably be in a contingent strategy based on the results of first-line screening by the combined test at 11–13 weeks' gestation. In this case, we recommend the strategy below:
  - *Combined test risk over 1 in 100*: The patients can be offered the options of cfDNA testing or invasive testing.
  - *Combined test risk between 1 in 101 and 1 in 2,500*: The patients can be offered the option of cfDNA testing
  - *Combined test risk lower than 1 in 2,500*: There is no need for further testing.

Patients contemplating pregnancy termination following a positive result from cfDNA testing should be advised that the diagnosis should be confirmed by invasive testing before undertaking any further action.

PERICONCEPTIONAL FOLIC ACID FOR THE PREVENTION OF NEURAL TUBE DEFECTS

Neural tube defects (NTDs) are severe birth anomalies, due to lack of neural tube closure at either the upper or lower end in the third to fourth week after conception (day 26 to day 28 post-conception).

The NTD commonly occur in all population worldwide, especially in the low and middle income countries. Each year, more than 4,500 pregnancies in the European Union are affected by NTD. In the United Kingdom and Ireland, the prevalence of NTD declined from 4.5 per 1,000 births in 1980 to 1.5 per 1,000 in the 1990s. In contrast, in the rest of Europe the prevalence during the 1980s and thereafter reminded close to 1 per 1.000 births. In the USA, the incidence ranges from 1.4 to 1.6 per 1,000 livebirths and 0.8 per 1,000 births in Canada. In the Latin America, the prevalence was about 5 cases per 1,000 births in the Brazil northeastern and South region, and in the southeast, the prevalence was 1 per 1,000 births. In Mexico, the current prevalence is about 1 in 1,000 births.

There are several evidences supporting the hypothesis for the relationship between folate deficiency and NTD, such as: (a) RCT for the prevention of primary occurrence or recurrence has been confirmed that periconceptional acid folic supplementation reduces the rate of NTD with reduction rate of 72%, (b) folic acid antagonists (methotrexate, dihydrofolate reductase inhibitors and others) increase the risk for NTD; and, concentration of folate in red blood cells is lower in women which give birth to children with NTD.

Hence, folic acid supplementation is of great benefit, especially in developing country settings for several reasons. Firstly, the prevalence of NTD in developing countries is very high compared to the industrialised world. Secondly, folic acid supplements are readily available and affordable. Since iron supplementation is almost universally recommended in pregnancy, especially in developing country reproductive health programs, it would be convenient to combine the two interventions. Nevertheless, the keystone is pre-pregnancy administration the synthetic folic acid supplement, which may not be easy in public health programs geared principally towards pregnant women.

The International Federation of Gynecology and Obstetrics (FIGO) recommends that (see also Table 42.1):

- All women who plans to become pregnant or all women at childbearing age without contraceptive method and who do not present risk factors for NTD should utilize 400 μg (0.4 mg) of synthetic folic acid, beginning at least 30 days before the conception and continue daily supplements throughout the first trimester of pregnancy.
- All women in the reproductive age group should be advised about the benefits of folic acid supplementation during any medical appointment (e.g. birth control renewal, cervical cancer prevention clinic, yearly examination), especially if they are planning pregnancy in the near future, or they do not use any contraceptive method, or are using a contraceptive method that does not guarantee an optimal birth control, International Federation of Gynecology and Obstetrics Working Group on Best Practice on Maternal-Fetal Medicine.
- The healthcare providers should inform the woman at counseling that:
  - The benefit of folic acid supplementation is not limited to the reduction of risk of NTD, but include possibly the reduction of risk of other adverse outcomes, including congenital heart defects, orofacial and cleft palate defects, low birth weight, preterm birth, and autism.
  - The folic acid supplementation of 400 μg (0.4 mg) can be taken for years, without any known side effects, even in countries with mandatory staple food fortification.
  - The effects of higher intakes of folic acid are not well known but include complicating the diagnosis of vitamin B_{12} deficiency; therefore care should be taken to keep total folic acid consumption at less than 1 mg per day, except for women who are at high risk of having a pregnancy affected by a NTD.
- Women who have risk factors should be advised that synthetic folic acid supplementation at a dose of

Table 42.1 Summary of the International Federation of Gynecology and Obstetrics recommendations regarding the administration of folic acid to prevent the NTD

Population	Women who plan to become pregnant or are at childbearing age with no contraceptive method
Recommendation	Daily supplementation of synthetic folic acid at a dose of 400 µg
Time using folic acid	Supplementation should begin at least 30 days before conception and should be maintained for the first trimester of pregnancy
Risk assessment for NTD	High-risk factors include:
	• NTD affected previous pregnancy
	• Partner affected by spina bifida
	• First degree relative affected by NTD
	• Use of anticonvulsants
	• Pregestational diabetes
	• Obesity (BMI> 35 kg/m^2)
	• Use of folate antagonists (methotrexate, sulfonamides, etc.)
	• Malabsorption syndromes (including pregnant women with a history of surgery for obesity)
Note: The women at high-risk group should be instructed to use a daily dose of 4,000 µg (4 mg) for the same time recommended above	
Recommendations from other associations	The American College of Obstetricians and Gynecologists, the American Academy of Family Physicians, American Academy of Pediatrics, the National Institute for Health and Clinical Excellence (NICE) Guidance and many other organizations have similar recommendations

4,000 µg/day (4.0 mg) is recommended. It should start at least 30 days before the conception and tcontinue as daily supplements throughout the first trimester of pregnancy.

- The risk factors include women with:
  - NTD-affected previous pregnancy
  - Partner affected by NTD
  - First degree relative which had affected by NTD
  - Prepregnancy diabetes
  - Epilepsy treatment with valproic acid or carbamazepine
  - Use of folate antagonists (methotrexate, sulfonamides, etc)
  - Malabsorption syndrome
  - Obesity (BMI > 35 kg/m^2)
- Finally, The International Federation of Gynecology and Obstetrics (FIGO) encourages all efforts of public agencies worldwide towards the development of more comprehensive programs to fortify food with synthetic folic acid and more vigilance in monitoring these programs.

CERVICAL LENGTH AND PROGESTERONE FOR THE PREDICTION AND PREVENTION OF PRETERM BIRTH

At least 15 million babies are born preterm worldwide each year. Preterm birth-related deaths are one of the leading causes of infant mortality; over one million babies die each year from preterm birth complications. The rates of preterm birth range from 5–18%; over 80% of preterm babies are born between 32 and 37 weeks of gestation. The sequelae of preterm birth include respiratory distress syndrome, necrotizing enterocolitis, neonatal sepsis, neurodevelopmental disabilities, cerebral palsy and neonatal death. Despite decades of research, high rates of preterm birth and infant mortality persist in both developed and developing countries.

A sonographic short cervix diagnosed by transvaginal ultrasound is the most powerful predictor of preterm delivery (50% of women with a cervical length <15 mm will deliver prior to 32 weeks of gestation). Randomized clinical trials and systematic reviews have demonstrated that vaginal progesterone reduces significantly the rate of preterm birth by 50% and reduces neonatal morbidity/mortality. The use of cervical length screening and vaginal progesterone is cost saving.

The International Federation of Gynecology and Obstetrics (FIGO) recommends the following (Table 42.2):

- Sonographic cervical length measurement should be performed in all pregnant patients at 19–23 6/7 weeks of gestation using transvaginal ultrasound. This can be done at the same time as the ultrasound performed for the anatomical survey.
- Women with a sonographic short cervix (<25 mm) diagnosed in the midtrimester should be offered daily vaginal micronized progesterone treatment for the prevention of preterm birth and neonatal morbidity.

Table 42.2 International Federation of Gynecology and Obstetrics recommendations regarding the use of transvaginal sonographic cervical length and vaginal progesterone use for the prevention of preterm birth

Population	All pregnant women with a singleton gestation
Recommendation	Transvaginal sonographic cervical length measurement at 19–23 6/7 weeks for all pregnant patients. Vaginal progesterone administered to women with a cervical length < 25 mm
200 mg vaginal soft capsules or 90 mg vaginal gel of micronized progesterone can be used for treatment	
Time using progesterone	Treatment should begin at the time of the diagnosis of a short cervix until 36 6/7 weeks, labor or rupture of membranes
Risk assessment	Transvaginal sonographic cervical length on all patients regardless of obstetrical history
Other recommendation	When a transvaginal ultrasound is not available other devices may be used as a screening tool to measure objectively and reliably the cervical length

- The progesterone formulation to be used is vaginal micronized progesterone (200 mg vaginal soft capsules) nightly or vaginal micronized progesterone gel (90 mg) each morning.
- Universal cervical length screening and vaginal progesterone treatment (90 mg vaginal gel or 200 mg micronized vaginal soft capsules) is a cost-effective model for the prevention of preterm birth.
- In cases in which a transvaginal ultrasound is not available, transabdominal ultrasound (with different cutoff) or other devices may be used as a screening tool to measure objectively and reliably the cervical length.

CHAPTER

43 Maternal-Fetal Medicine

BEST PRACTICE ADVICES ON MAGNESIUM SULFATE USE IN OBSTETRICS

Premises

Eclampsia and cerebral palsy are both associated with significant morbidity and healthcare costs. Magnesium sulfate, a membrane stabilizer is used in the prevention of both of these conditions through the following mechanisms:

1. Magnesium sulfate sets like a non-competitive antagonist of the NMDA receptors
2. It is a potent vasodilator
3. It may also prevent neuronal death.

It is by these mechanisms that neurological sequelae are reduced in both the mother and fetus.

Magnesium Sulfate use in Severe Pre-eclampsia/Eclampsia

Cochrane reviews have demostrated that in women with either severe or mild/moderate pre-eclampsia, magnesium sulfate was better than no treatment/placebo in preventing eclampsia.

The authors also showed that in women with eclampsia, magnesium sulfate was more effective than diazepam, phenytoin or lytic cocktails in preventing maternal death and recurrence of convulsions. Babies of women treated with magnesium sulfate were less likely to require neonatal care (variously reported in the primary studies as NICU or SCBU) for more than 7 days, to be intubated at place of birth or have an Apgar score less than 7 at both 1 minute and 5 minutes from delivery. The recommendation is that magnesium sulfate be administered to women with severe pre-eclampsia and for whom delivery has been planned. Severe pre-eclampsia is diagnosed by worsening blood pressure which may be resistant to drug administration, consistent proteinuria more than 300 mg/24 hours, presence of signs and symptoms such as headache, flashing lights, nausea, vomiting, epigastric pain, hyperreflexia and clonus and worsening biochemical parameters especially thrombocytopenia, liver dysfunction and hemolysis. Local guidelines may vary in terms of diagnosis of severity and should be used alongside this recommendation.

The International Federation of Gynecology and Obstetrics (FIGO) recommends the following:

- Intravenous/intramuscular magnesium sulfate is indicated during labor and postpartum for all women diagnosed with severe pre-eclampsia/eclampsia.
- For elective cesarean delivery, magnesium sulfate is given at least 2 hours before the procedure, continued during surgery and for at least 12 hours after.
- The doses for intravenous $MgSO_4$ in 4–6 g diluted in 100 mL NS/D5W over 15–20 minutes followed by maintenance of 1–2 g/hour. For IM administration, up to 10 g can be given undiluted 50% solution divided into each buttock followed by 4–5 g every 4 hours.
- Once $MgSO_4$ has been given, monitoring of respiratory rate, presence of deep tendon reflexes and urine output is mandatory to identify magnesium toxicity. As magnesium is excreted renaly, particular attention to women who are oliguric is advised. Magnesium toxicity is treated with 10% 10 mL calcium gluconate.
- Magnesium pharmacokinetics are well established during pregnancy and in women with normal renal function the half time for excretion is 4 hours.
- There is no association between magnesium sulfate use and congenital birth defects.
- Long-term infusion may be related to sustained hypocalcemia in the fetus resulting in congenital rickets and adverse effects on fetal bone mineralization. Neonatologists should be alerted to look for signs such as neonatal neurologic depression, respiratory depression, muscle weakness or hyporeflexia.

Magnesium Sulfate use in Fetal Neuroprotection

Cerebral palsy has an incidence of 2/1000 livebirths and can result from delivery at less than 34 weeks gestation. It is caused by intraventricular hemorrhages and periventricular leukomalacia that occurs as a result of prematurity.

"The prevalence of cerebral palsy is between 1.5 and 2.5 per 1000 livebirths and has remained stable. A systematic review by Oskoui et al. found a worldwide prevalence of cerebral palsy of 2.11 per 1000 in 2013 and that prevalence is inversely related to gestational age and birth weight at delivery. Antenatal factors such us preterm birth, perinatal infection, and chronic uteroplacental insufficiency that leads to impaired growth might potentially lead to the development of cerebral palsy, which is usually seen in the setting of diffuse white matter injury or cystic periventricular leukomalacia (or both); or intraparenchymal hemorrhage and intraventricular hemorrhage.

Prevalence of cerebral palsy is highest in infants between 1000 g and 1499 g at birth (59.8/1000 livebirths) and lowest in those over 2500 g (1.33/1000 livebirths). Similarly, prevalence was higher in those born before 28 weeks of gestation (111.8/1000) than in those born after 36 weeks (1.35/1000).

Magnesium sulfate given to the mother during preterm labor can help to reduce white matter injury in the fetal brain by the mechanisms mentioned above. The results of five randomized controlled trials, 3 meta-analyses and a The Cochrane review showed that antenatal magnesium sulfate therapy given to women at risk of preterm birth substantially reduced the risk of cerebral palsy in their child [relative risk (RR) 0.68; 95%] [confidence interval (CI) 0.54 to 0.87]. The cochrane review demonstrated a relative risk reduction of 31% translates into an absolute risk reduction of 1.7%. Therefore, the number of women needed to be treated to benefit one baby by avoiding cerebral palsy is 63 (95% CI). Short-term side effects include flushing, sweating and nausea but have not been significant enough to cause discontinuation of therapy in the majority of women. Magnesium can be given regardless of indication for delivery, number of fetuses, mode of delivery, parity and does not affect the efficacy of antenatal steroids.

FIGO recommends the following:

- For imminent preterm birth which is either active labor diagnosed with or without rupture of membranes or elective delivery for maternal or fetal concerns, antenatal magnesium sulfate should be considered for fetal neuroprotection.
- Although there is controversy about the upper gestational age, antenatal magnesium sulfate should be considered from viability until 31 weeks + 6 days gestation.
- Magnesium sulfate should be discontinued, if delivery is no longer imminent or after a maximum of 24 hours of therapy.
- Magnesium sulfate should be administered as a 4 g loading dose over 30 minutes, ideally 4–6 hours before delivery followed by an infusion of 1 g/hour until delivery occurs. However, there still may be benefit if given less than 4 hours prior to delivery.
- There is insufficient evidence for use of a repeat course of antenatal magnesium sulfate for fetal neuroprotection.
- Delivery should not be delayed in order to administer antenatal magnesium sulfate, if there are maternal or fetal indications for emergency delivery.
- When magnesium sulfate is given for fetal neuroprotection, maternity care providers should use existing protocols to monitor women for signs of toxicity as those used in cases of pre-eclampsia/eclampsia.
- Neonatologists should be alerted to assess neonates for hypotonia and/or apnea as therapy with magnesium sulfate has the potential to cause hypocalcemia.

BEST PRACTICE ADVICES ON ULTRASOUND EXAMINATION IN PREGNANCY

Premises

Ultrasound is highly dependent upon the level of technology and hence the quality and performance of the equipment used, but also on the capability and knowledge of the operator. It is therefore understood that advice, guidelines and recommendations will mainly apply when and where appropriate resources and training programs can be dedicated to ultrasound in pregnancy, but also in the context of sound and appropriate referral patterns and clinical management schemes. Counseling on potential benefits and limitations of a routine ultrasound scan should therefore be provided prior to performing the examination. The evaluation of the performance of ultrasound examination in pregnancy is mainly based on low to fair level of evidence and recommendations, largely because excessively high expectations were directed solely to this technical assessment and largely failed to consider the necessary soundness for its interpretation and the action to be based-upon. Randomized controlled studies were inadequately designed to evaluate its impact on perinatal mortality, although ultrasound examination is best able to provide critical information to the perinatologists who are in the capacity to influence perinatal outcome, including: assessment of viability and gestational age (Fig. 43.1), degree and type of multiple pregnancies, fetal presentation, size and anatomy as well as placental location and cervical length. This has led to improve perinatal outcome through the identification and sound clinical management of fetal malformations and diseases, growth disturbances but also high-risk pregnancies for preterm delivery and for peripartum hemorrhage. Ultrasound is currently being investigated for the early prediction and basis for prevention of hypertensive disorders, assessment of uterine cesarean scars and identification of placenta accreta, as well as an adjunct in the management of labor and delivery. Telemedicine seeking expert opinion by using either real-time ultrasound examination or acquired images or 3D-volumes is being developed. There are several types of ultrasound examinations in pregnancy depending on the indication and on the gestational age at which they are

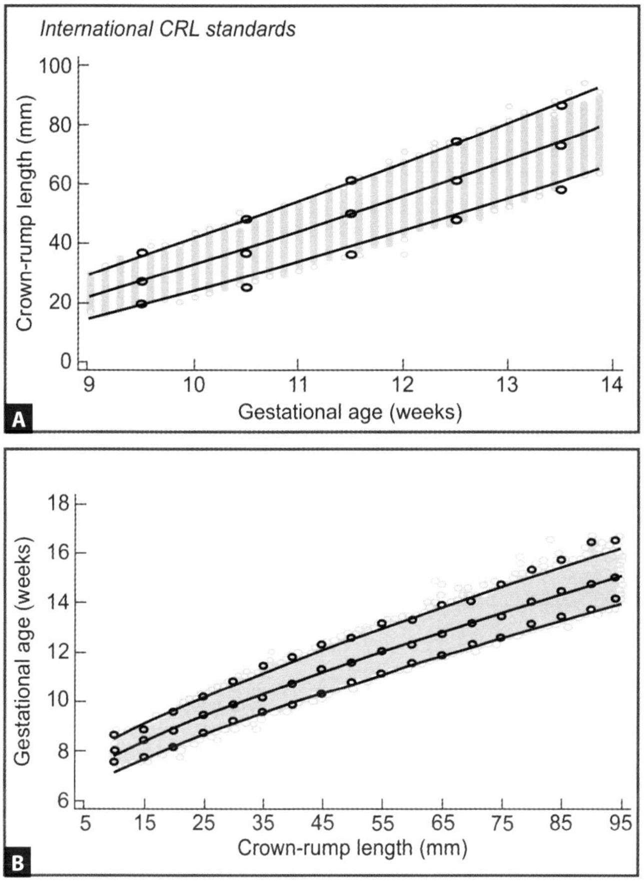

Figs 43.1A and B Determination of gestational age by crown--rump--length (CRL) measurement between 8, 6, and 13 weeks +6 days

From Ultrasound in Obstetrics & Gynecology. 2014,44;6:641-8
CRL is expressed in mm and GA in days:
GA = 40.9041 + (3.21585 × CRL0.5) + (0.348956 × CRL);
SD of GA = 2.39102 + (0.0193474 × CRL)

performed, including screening by ultrasound in the first trimester and in the mid or third trimester, which together with clinical indications can generate specialized or limited ultrasound examinations. Ultrasound is also the basis for the indication of other imaging modalities in pregnancy including 3D-4D ultrasound modalities, MRI and CT scanner.

FIGO recommends the following:

1. Ultrasound in pregnancy should be performed by specifically qualified operators and undergoing specific continuous medical education and quality assurance programs.
2. Current equipment should have the capability to perform transvaginal and Doppler ultrasound examination, and be subjected to adequate maintenance.
3. All pregnant women should be offered at least 2 ultrasound screening examination at 11–13+6 weeks and at 18–22, but optimally at least one from 20 weeks' onwards.
4. Medically indicated ultrasound examination in pregnancy is safe. It should be preceded by specific counseling and it should be documented by a comprehensive report and set of images.
5. First trimester ultrasound examination recognizes five aims and objectives:
    - Assess viability
    - Assess gestational age
    - Diagnose and characterize multiple pregnancies
    - Conduct an anatomical survey to screen for malformations amenable to first trimester US
    - Measure nuchal translucency.
6. First trimester ultrasound should also include visualization of both ovaries.
7. Mid trimester ultrasound examination recognizes five aims and objectives:
    (i) Assess gestational age if this has not been done in the first trimester
    (ii) Assess fetal biometry
    (iii) Conduct an anatomical survey to screen for malformations amenable to mid trimester US
    (iv) Assess placental location and cord insertion
    (v) Measure cervical length as part of risk assessment for preterm delivery.
8. Ultrasound and Doppler should be used liberally in the third trimester following clinical indications in order to assess:
    - Amniotic fluid volume
    - Cervical length
    - Fetal wellbeing
    - Fetal growth.
9. The result of a screening ultrasound examination in the first or second trimester can generate the indication for a specialized or focused ultrasound examination following appropriate referral patterns.
10. In multiple pregnancies, chorionicity should be optimally determined before 15 weeks.
11. The use of ultrasound in labor should be encouraged to determine fetal and placental position as well as prior to perform instrumental delivery.
12. The use of ultrasound should be encouraged in the post-partum period in cases with non-physiological bleeding or infection.

BEST PRACTICE ADVICES ON THYROID DISEASES IN PREGNANCY

Premises

Pregnancy acts like a stress for the thyroid gland and impacts its functioning profoundly. Production of T4 and T3 and daily iodine requirement can increase each by 50%. Hence, women in a hyperthyroid status during the first trimester can become, hypothyroid in later stages of gestation. Clinical symptoms and sign and thyroid hormones testing are used for diagnosing various thyroid disorders during pregnancy. Specially Figures 43.2 to 43.4 depict the different thyroid disorders during pregnancy.

FIGO recommends the following:

1. Screening for thyroid function is recommended in the first trimester particularly in countries with a deficient iodine diet and in symptomatic patients (Fig. 43.2). TSH is the superior method for screening. Free T4 and TPO Ab testing are not recommended for screening. The best reliable tests for TSH are by chemiluminescence immunoassay (CIA) or 3rd generation radioimmunoassay (RIA). Notably normal thyroid test values change in pregnancy (Fig. 43.3).
2. Treatment for hypothyroidism is recommended when TSH levels are >2.5 and >3.0 IU/L during the first and second/third trimesters respectively. The only replacement therapy is L-thyroxine. Instead treating subclinical hypothyroidism, in the presence of negative thyroid auto-antibodies, is still debatable. Importantly, women on L-thyroxine before pregnancy should increase their dosage by 30–50% when they first recognize the pregnant state.
3. Treatment of hyperthyroidism due to Grave's disease is by antithyroid drugs [(propylthiouracil (PTU) or carbimazole/methimazole (MMI)]. It is not recommended to change drugs during pregnancy symptomatic (Fig. 43.2) treatment with beta-blockers for short-term may be needed.
4. Primary, prevention of hypothyroidism is by a healthy diet and iodized fortified salt (especially in iodine deficient areas).
5. If the patient has a thyroid nodule, she should be evaluated and treated during pregnancy. The primary steps are perfomance of a thyroid ultrasonogram and a fine needle aspiration (FNA) as needed. Surgery should be preferably deferred to the postpartum period.
6. Follow-up and postpartum TSH evaluation and reduction of L-thyroxine dose to pre-pregnant levels in patients with hypothyroidism.

Symptoms	Hyperthyroid	Hypothyroid
	Nervousness	Fatigue
	Palpitations	Constipation
	Tachycardia	Weight gain
	Heat intolerance	Memory loss
	Sweating	Dry skin/cold tolerance
	Sudden paralysis	Loss of hair
	Weight loss	Irregular menstruation
	Fatigue/cramping	Hoarseness
	Changes in vision	Myalgia
	Pretibial myxedema	Reflex delay
	Freq. bowel/Diarrhea	Bradycardia

Fig. 43.2 Symptoms and signs of thyroid disease in pregnancy

FT4			
High	Primary hyperthyroid	NTI or patient on thyroxine treatment	Secondary hyperthyroid
Normal	Sub-clinical hyperthyroid	Euthyroid	Sub-clinical hypothyroid
Low	Secondary hyperthyroid	Non-thyroid illness-NTI	Primary hypothyroid
	Low	Normal	High

Fig. 43.3 Basic thyroid evaluation

Test	Non-pregnant	1st trim	2nd trim	3rd trim
Free T4 pmol/L	11–23	10–24	9–19	7–17
Free T3 pmol/L	4–9	4–8	4–7	3–5
TSH mu/L	<4	0–1.6	1–1.8	7–7.3

Fig. 43.4 Thyroid function test during pregnancy – pregnancy specific values

BEST PRACTICE ADVICES ON HYPERGLYCEMIA IN PREGNANCY

Premises

Non-communicable diseases (NCDs) and maternal health are closely linked. NCDs such as diabetes, obesity and hypertension have significant adverse impact on maternal health and pregnancy outcome; and through the mechanism of intrauterine programming, maternal health impacts the NCD burden in future generations. The cycle of vulnerability to NCDs is thus repeated with increasing risk accumulation in subsequent generations. The Millennium Development Goals (MDGs) have resulted in justifiable attention on maternal and child health (MCH) programs, especially in the developing world. These programs focused on factors that directly impact maternal, neonatal and infant mortality, resulting in improved access to maternity services and survival of 'at-risk' mothers and their offspring in many low and middle-income countries. Unfortunately, this short-term biomedical focus fails to address the root causes and the social determinants, and the very individuals saved continue to be vulnerable and are at the highest risk of NCDs in later life. Pregnancy offers a window of opportunity to provide maternal care services to not only reduce traditional maternal and perinatal morbidity and mortality indicators but to also address intergenerational prevention of NCDs, such as diabetes, hypertension, cardiovascular disease, and stroke. To improve both the short-term MCH outcomes and long-term population health, NCDs must be addressed simultaneously alongside MCH. Hyperglycemia is one of the most common health problems of pregnancy.

Hyperglycemic disorders of pregnancy are divided into:

- Diabetes mellitus (DM) in pregnancy [diabetes (type 1 or type 2) known before pregnancy, or overt diabetes (often type 2) first detected during pregnancy]
- Gestational diabetes mellitus (GDM) (hyperglycemia first detected during pregnancy not amounting to overt diabetes).

The occurrence of gestational diabetes mellitus (GDM) parallels the prevalence of impaired glucose tolerance (IGT); obesity; and type 2 diabetes in a given population. These conditions are on the rise globally. Moreover, the age of onset of diabetes and prediabetes is declining while the age of childbearing is increasing. There is also an increase in the rate of overweight and obese women of reproductive age, thus more women entering pregnancy have risk factors that make them vulnerable to hyperglycemia during pregnancy. Global hyperglycemia during pregnancy prevalence rates show variations due to ethnicity and ethnic heterogeneity of populations studied as well as the different screening and diagnosis criteria used. The International Diabetes Federation (IDF) estimates that 1 in 6 livebirths (16.8%) occur to women with some form of hyperglycemia in pregnancy and 16% of these may be due to overt diabetes in pregnancy and rest due to hypertensive disorder of pregnancy (HDP). HDP is associated with a higher incidence of maternal morbidity, including cesarean deliveries, shoulder dystocia, birth trauma, hypertensive disorders of pregnancy (or pre-eclampsia) and subsequent development of type 2 diabetes. Perinatal and neonatal morbidities are also increased; the latter include macrosomia, birth injury, hypoglycemia, polycythemia and hyperbilirubinemia. Long-term sequelae in offspring with *in utero* exposure to maternal hyperglycemia may include higher risks for obesity and diabetes later in life. In most parts of the low, low middle and upper middle-income countries, which contribute to over 85% of the annual global deliveries, the majority of women are not properly screened for diabetes during pregnancy. Many of the very same countries also account for 80% of the global diabetes burden as well as for over 90% of all cases of maternal and perinatal deaths and poor pregnancy outcomes. The interaction between hyperglycemia and poor pregnancy outcomes and the role of *in utero* imprinting in increasing risk of diabetes and cardiometabolic disorders in offspring of mothers with hyperglycemia in pregnancy, it has been demonstrated as well as, increasing maternal vulnerability to future diabetes and cardiovascular disorders. There needs to be a greater focus on preventing, screening, diagnosing and managing hyperglycemia in pregnancy globally. The relevance of HDP as a priority for maternal health and its impact on the future burden of non-communicable diseases is no longer in doubt but how best to deal with the issue remains relatively unclear as there are many gaps in knowledge on how best to prevent, diagnose and manage GDM to optimize care and outcomes. These must be addressed through future research. There should be greater attention and focus on the links between maternal health and NCDs both in the area of international research collaboration to address the knowledge gaps and on the sustainable developmental goals agenda.

FIGO recommends the following:

- All pregnant women should be tested for hyperglycemia during pregnancy. FIGO encourages its member associations to adapt and promote strategies to ensure universal testing of all pregnant women for hyperglycemia during pregnancy.
- WHO (2013) criteria for diagnosis of diabetes first diagnosed during pregnancy and the WHO (2013) and IADPSG (2010) criteria for diagnosis of gestational diabetes mellitus must be used when possible but keeping in mind the resource constraints in many parts of the developing world alternate strategies described in the attached table should also be considered equally acceptable.
- Diagnosis of HDP should be based on venous plasma samples properly collected and transported and tested in a lab. However, in primary care settings particularly

in the developing world where proper facilities to test or store and transport blood samples to a distant lab may not exist, a plasma calibrated hand held glucometer with properly stored test strips to measure plasma glucose is an acceptable alternative. Using a glucose meter in this situation may be more reliable than lab tests done on samples that have been inadequately handled and transported.

- Management of HDP should be in accordance with available national resources and infrastructure and even without high quality evidence, as it is preferable to no care.
- Nutrition and physical activity counseling are the primary tools in the prevention and management of women with HDP must include practical nutrition education and counseling that empowers them to choose the right quantity and quality of food and level of physical activity. Women with HDP must be repeatedly advised and encouraged to continue the same healthy lifestyle even after delivery in order to reduce the risk of future obesity, type 2 diabetes and cardiovascular diseases.
- When lifestyle changes are inadequate in controlling hyperglycemia, insulin may be added. Glyburide and/or metformin may be used as a safe and effective treatment option during the 2nd and 3rd trimesters in place of insulin as long as glycemic control is achieved. These medications may be initiated as a first line treatment when lifestyle modification alone fails to achieve glucose control. Insulin should be added if lifestyle and oral agents fail to control glucose levels.
- Following a pregnancy, the postpartum period (8-week visit) provides an important platform to initiate early preventive health for both the mother and the child as both are at heightened risk for future obesity, metabolic syndrome, diabetes, hypertension and cardiovascular disorders. Obstetricians must establish links with family physicians, internists and pediatricians to support post-partum follow-up of mothers linked to their children's vaccination program to ensure continued follow-up and engagement of the high-risk mother child pair.
- Public health measures to increase awareness and acceptance of preconception counseling and to increase affordability and access to preconception and antenatal services for women in the reproductive age must be put in place, as this is likely to have both immediate and lasting benefit for maternal and child health.

Options for Diagnosis of Hyperglycemia in Pregnancy

See Table 43.1.

Table 43.1 Option for diagnosis of hyperglycemia in pregnancy

Option	Strategy	Setting
1a	• Booking/first trimester; measure FPG, RBG, or HbA1c to detect diabetes in pregnancy • If negative perform 75 g 2 hour OGTT at 24–28 weeks Interpret as per IADPSG / WHO/IDF guideline	Fully resourced settings
1b	• Booking/first trimester; perform 75 g 2 hour OGTT to detect diabetes in pregnancy • Repeat at 24–28 weeks if negative. Interpret as per IADPSG / WHO/IDF guideline	Fully resourced settings dealing particularly with ethnic populations at high risk. See note below§
1c	• Perform 75 g 2 hour OGTT between 24 and 28 weeks. Interpret as per IADPSG / WHO/ IDF guideline	All settings (basic); particularly medium to low resourced settings serving ethnic populations at risk
2	• Booking/first trimester; measure FPG to detect diabetes in pregnancy. (>7.0 mmol/L or >126 mg/dL) • FPG values between 5.6 and 6.9 mmol/L, (100 and 125 mg/dL) consider as GDM • In those without Diabetes in Pregnancy perform OGTT at 24–28 weeks. Interpret as per IADPSG / WHO/IDF guideline (To reduce number of OGTTs, measure FPG at 24 to 28 weeks – value >5.1 mmol/L or >92 mg/dL diagnostic of GDM. In women with values between 4.4 mmol/L and 5.1 mmol/L perform 2 hr 75 g OGTT. Interpret as per IADPSG/ WHO/IDF guideline#	Medium to low resource settings dealing with populations at high risk in China
3	Booking/first trimester; Measure non-fasting 2 hr PG value after 75 g oral glucose; if result below 7.8 mmol/L or 140 mg/dL repeat test in second/third trimester. Reading medium to low resource settings dealing with rural/semiurban/urban ethnic populations at high-risk particularly in the International Federation of Gynecology and Obstetrics Working Group on Best Practice on Maternal-Fetal Medicine between 7.8 and 11.0 mmol/L or 140 and 199 mg/dL indicates GDM**	Indian sub-continent

Contd...

Contd...

Option	Strategy	Setting
4	Booking/first trimester; Measure fasting plasma glucose to rule out diabetes in pregnancy Value between 100 and 125 mg/dL (5.6 and 6.9 mmol/L) are considered diagnostic for GDM If negative, perform OGTT at 24–28 weeks. 2 hr 75 g glucose value > 7.8 mmol/L or >140 mg/dL is diagnostic of GDM ***	Medium-to-low resource settings in Latin America
	Booking/first trimester; Offer only women with past history of GDM or women with glycosuria of 2+ or above on 1 occasion or of 1+ or above on 2 or more occasions detected by reagent strip testing during routine antenatal care in current pregnancy: • 75 g 2-hour OGTT as soon as possible after booking (whether in the first or second trimester), if negative, perform 75 g 2-hour OGTT at 24–28 Offer women with any of the other risk factors for GDM: • BMI above 30 kg/m^2; • Previous macrosomic baby weighing 4.5 kg or above • Family history of diabetes (first-degree relative with diabetes) • Minority ethnic family origin with a high prevalence of diabetes 75 g 2-hour OGTT at 24–28 weeks FPG of 100 mg/dL or 5.6 mmol/L or above or 2-hour PG of 140 mg/dL or 7.8 mmol/L or above is diagnostic[@]	United Kingdom

**Diabetes in Pregnancy Study Group in India (DIPSI) Guideline

*** Latin America Study Group

[§] Asians are at high risk of hyperglycemia during pregnancy which may include previously undiagnosed diabetes. The proportion of previously undiagnosed diabetes is highest in the youngest age-group particularly among women. In Asian populations, fasting plasma glucose and glycosylated hemoglobin (HbA1c) concentrations have much lower sensitivity than the 2 hour post-glucose value. In a study of 11 Asian cohorts more than half of the diabetic subjects had isolated post-challenge hyperglycemia. In a study in China 46.6% of the participants with undiagnosed diabetes (44.1% of the men and 50.2% of the women) had isolated increased 2-hour plasma glucose levels after an oral glucose-tolerance test. Therefore, the need to identify postprandial hyperglycemia seems especially relevant in Asian populations.

@ National Institute for Health and Care Excellence (NICE) Diabetes in pregnancy: Management of diabetes and its complications from preconception to the postnatal period. NICE guideline—3 Feb 2015. National Collaborating Centre for Women's and Children's Health.

APPENDIX

National Institute for Health and Care Excellence (NICE) Guideline 3

NICE published an update to its 2008 guidance on Diabetes in Pregnancy on 25th Feb 2015. By the time this document became available publically the FIGO GDM initiative writing group had finalized its document and recommendations and did not have the time to fully review this document.

The key features of the NICE recommendations are the following:

- NICE guidance does not recommend universal testing for GDM.
- NICE guidance recommends early testing (as soon as possible after booking, whether in the first or second trimester) with a 75 g 2 hour OGTT only for women with history of GDM in a previous pregnancy and for women with glycosuria of 2+ or above on 1 occasion or of 1+ or above on 2 or more occasions detected by reagent strip during routine antenatal care in current pregnancy.
- NICE guidance recommends testing for GDM with a 75 g 2 hour OGTT between 24–28 weeks of gestation only for women with the risk factors given further.
  - BMI above 30 kg/m^2;
  - Previous macrosomic baby weighing 4.5 kg or above
  - Previous GDM
  - Family history of diabetes (first-degree relative with diabetes)
  - Minority ethnic family origin with a high prevalence of diabetes.
- Cut off value for diagnosing GDM are
  - FPG ≥100 mg/dL or ≥5.6 mmol/L.
- In deciding on the recommendation for risk factor based testing versus universal testing and the cut off values, the NICE Guidance apart from other available evidence, also relied on the cost-effectiveness of different testing options (universal versus risk factor based) and cut off values

primarily using data from the HAPO study centers in UK and Australia—representing the population of UK.

- NICE guidance does not distinguish between diabetes first diagnosed during pregnancy and GDM. Any level of glycemia above the cut off levels diagnosed first time during index pregnancy is considered GDM.

BIBLIOGRAPHY

Management of diabetes and its complications from preconception to the postnatal period National Institute for Health and Care Excellence (NICE) Guideline 3. Feb 2015 http://*www.nice.org.uk/guidance/ng3/evidence* accessed on 12th March 2015.

Appendix: Growth Charts

ESTIMATED FETAL WEIGHT PERCENTILE CHART

Gestational Weeks = Estimated Fetal Weight Percentile Chart +/– 1.28 Standard Deviation [A fetus is considered normal if they are between 10th and 90th percentile]			
	Average	Estimated fetal weight +/– SD 1.28	
Gestational weeks	Estimated fetal weight	10th%	90th%
16	146 g (5 oz)	121	171
17	181 g (6 oz)	150	212
18	223 g (7 oz)	185	261
19	273 g (9 oz)	227	319
20	331 g (11 oz)	275	387
21	399 g (14 oz)	331	467
22	478 g (1lb)	398	559
23	568 g (1lb 5 oz)	471	665
24	670 g (1lb 7 oz)	556	784
25	785 g (1lb 11 oz)	652	918
26	913 g (2lb)	758	1068
27	1055 g (2lb 5 oz)	876	1234
28	1210 g (2lb 10 oz)	1004	1416
29	1379 g (3lb)	1145	1613
30	1559 g (3lb 7 oz)	1294	1824
31	1751 g (3lb 13 oz)	1453	2049
32	1953 g (4lb 4 oz)	1621	2285
33	2162 g (4lb 12 oz)	1794	2530
34	2377 g (5lb 3 oz)	1973	2781
35	2595 g (5lb 11 oz)	2154	3036
36	2813 g (6lb 3 oz)	2335	3291
37	3028 g (6lb 10 oz)	2513	3543
38	3236 g (7lb 2 oz)	2686	3786
39	3435 g (7lb 9 oz)	2851	4019
40	3619 g (7lb 15 oz)	3004	4234

FETAL GROWTH PERCENTILE CHARTS

Measurement Charts

Biparietal Diameter and Head Circumference

The biparietal diameter and occipitofrontal diameter are measured on a transverse axial section of the fetal head which includes the falx cerebri anteriorly and posteriorly, the cavum septum pellucidum anteriorly in the midline and the thalami. The BPD is measured from the outer edge of the nearer parietal bone to the inner edge of the more distant parietal bone. The OFD is measured perpendicular to the BPD (Figs A-1 and A-2).

Femur and Humerus Length

The long bones are measured with the bone across the beam axis. The strong acoustic shadow behind the femoral or humeral shaft and the visualization of both cartilaginous ends indicates that the image plane is on the longest axis and is the optimal measurement plane. The calipers are placed along the diaphyseal shaft excluding the epiphysis (Figs A-3 and A-4).

Abdominal Circumference

These measurements are more appropriately used in the assessment of fetal growth, particularly in the second half of the pregnancy, than in the assessment of gestational age. It is, however, an appropriate measurement in the second trimester to demonstrate normal fetal proportions.

The abdominal circumference is measured at the level of the liver and stomach, including the left portal vein at the umbilical region (Fig. A-5).

Ultrasonic Fetal Measurement Standards

If we assume a fetus is growing normally, biometric measurements are determined by gestational age, and we can estimate the gestational age and thus the due date. When the date of the last menses preceding conception is known, it is usually a more accurate estimate (+/– 5 days) of EDC.

When using ultrasound to estimate gestational age, remember that we are assuming the fetus is growing normally. Conditions which alter fetal growth will make the estimates less reliable. Although many embryonic and fetal structures can be measured, only a few measurements are easy and repeatable enough for widespread use.

The most common are:

Gestational Sac

The first element to be measurable is the gestation sac of the early pregnancy. The gestational sac is measured in three dimensions, and the average, the mean sac diameter (MSD) used for estimating gestational age. It is useful between 5 and 8 menstrual weeks with accuracy of +/– 3 days. As a rough rule of thumb, the MSD + 30 = Menstrual age in days.

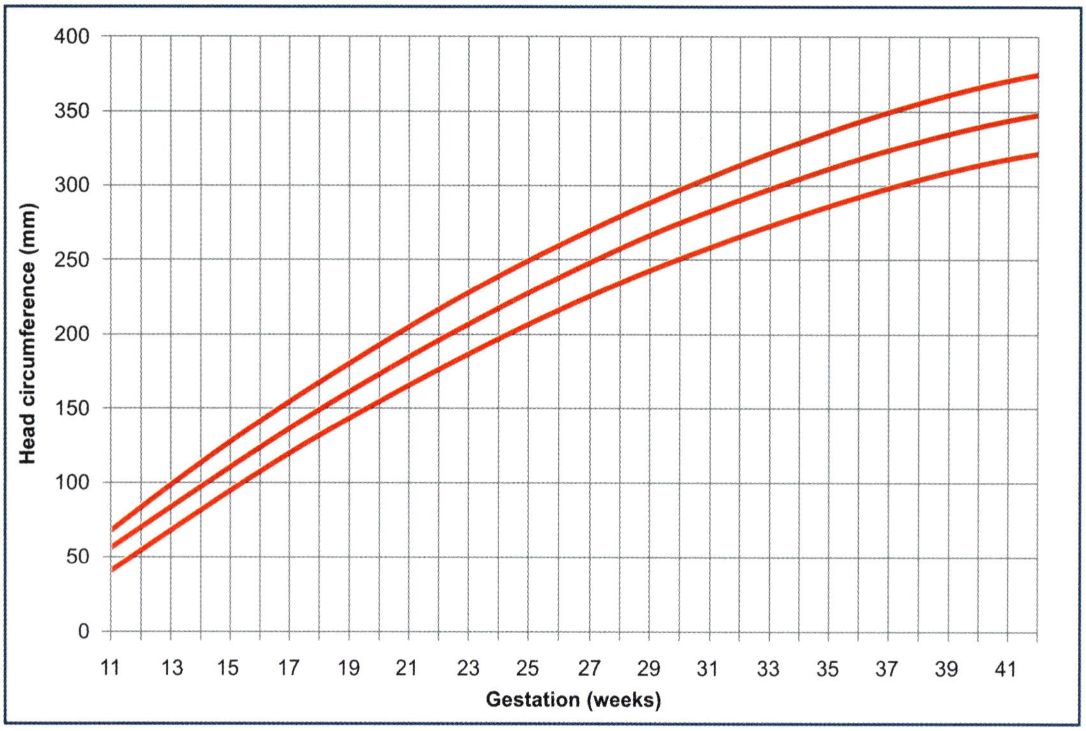

Fig. A-1 Head circumference

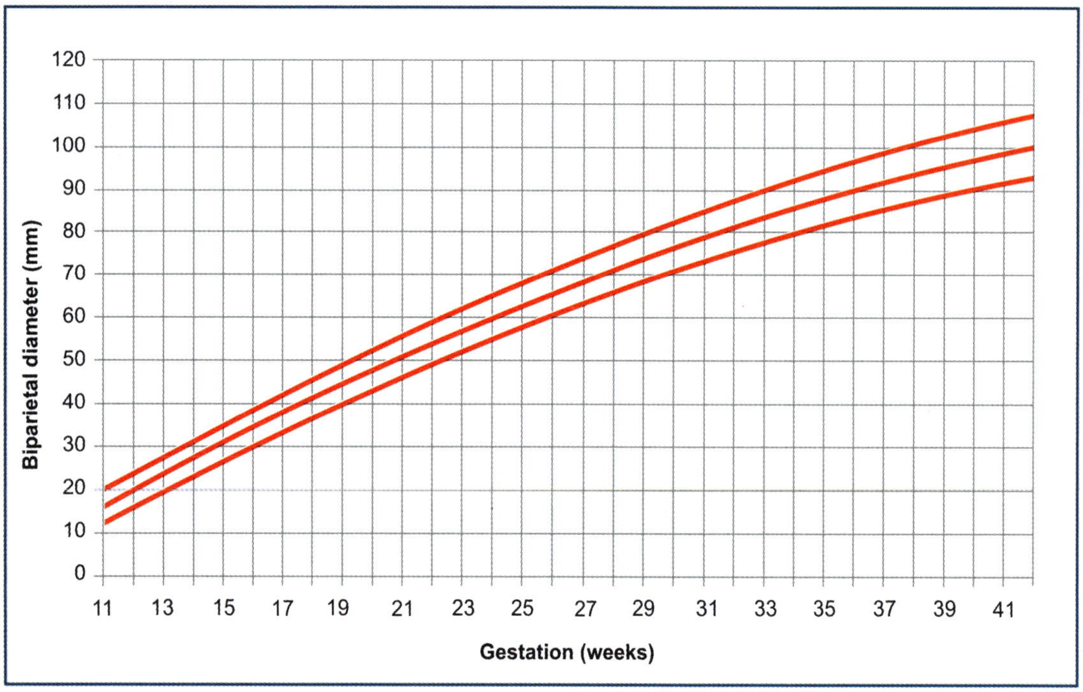

Fig. A-2 Biparietal diameter

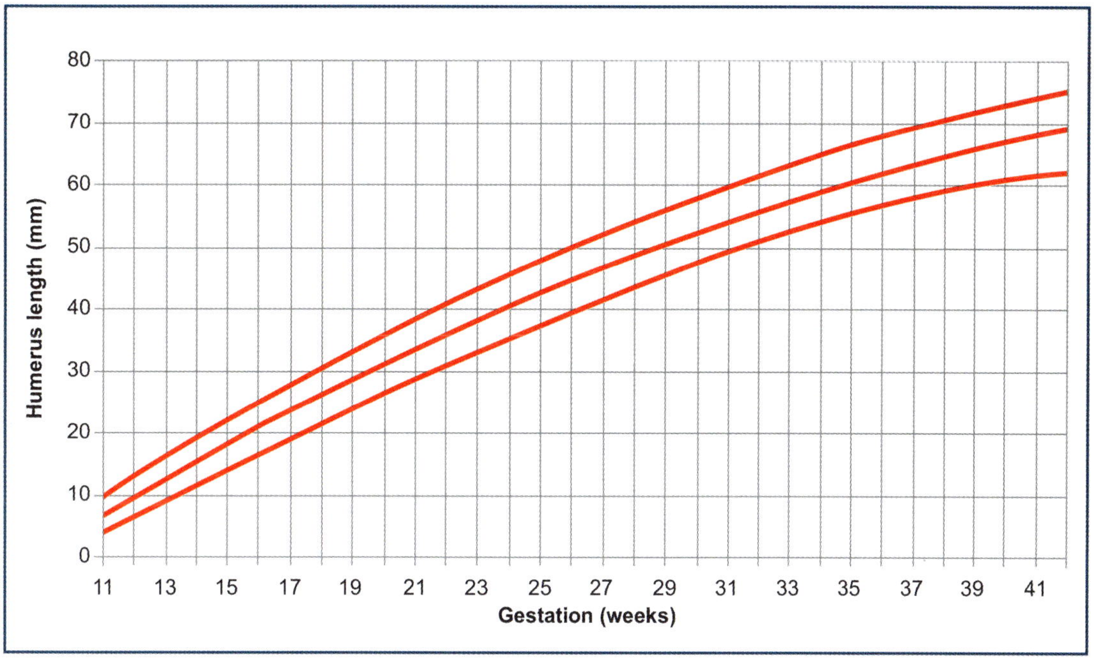

Fig. A-3 Humerus length

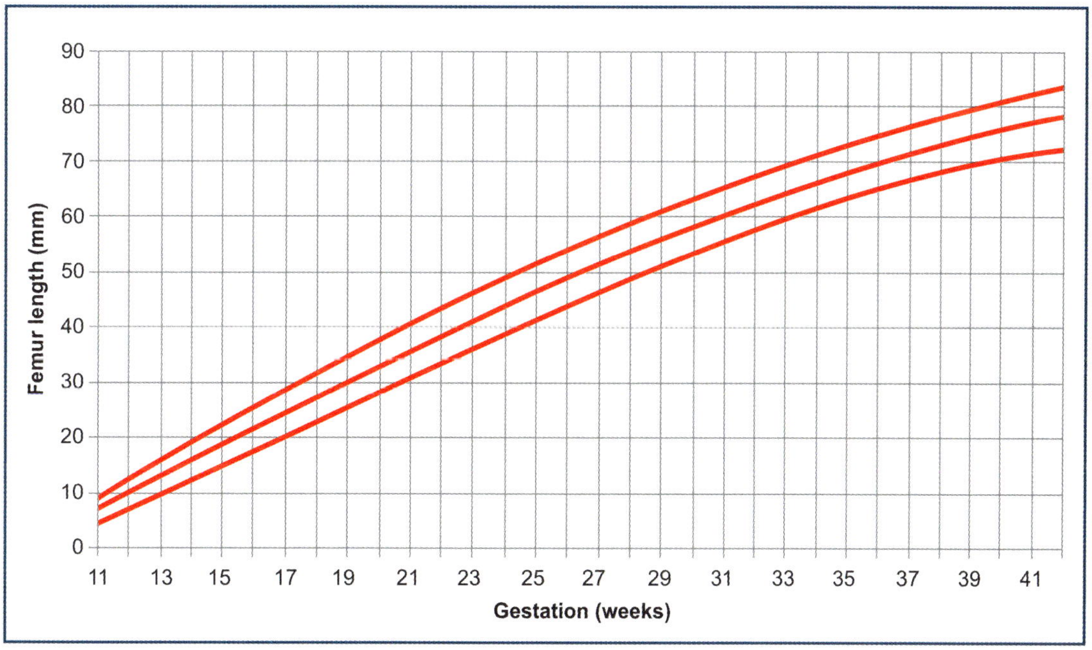

Fig. A-4 Femur length

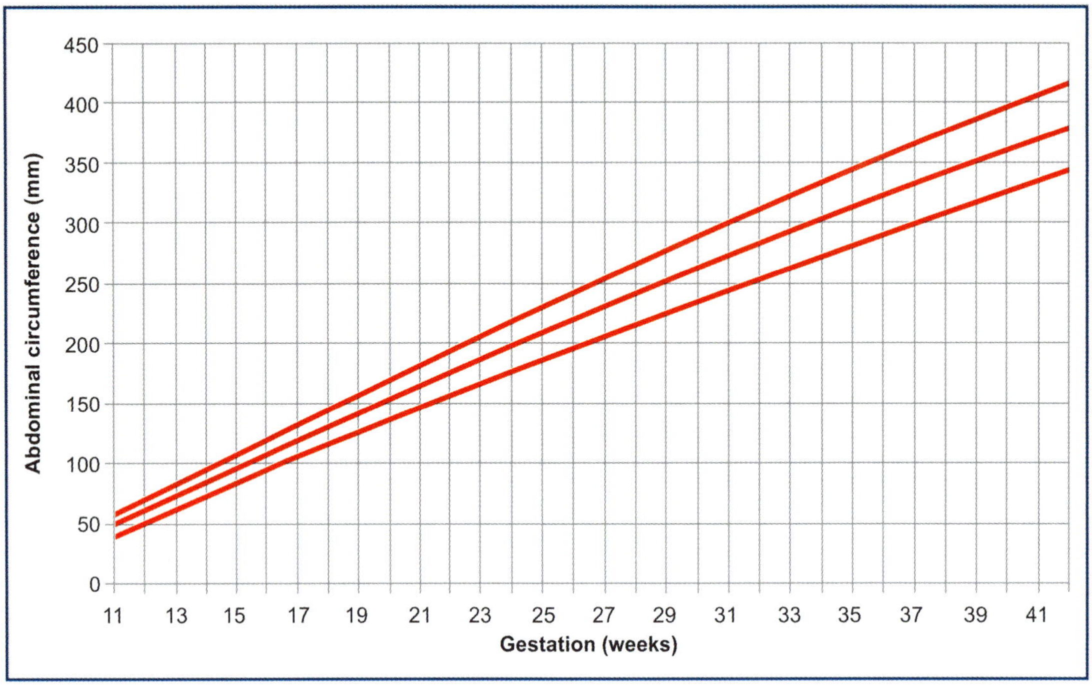

Fig. A-5 Abdominal circumference

Embryonic Crown-rump Length

The length of the embryo on the longest axis (excluding the yolk sac) constitutes the crown-rump length. This is among the best documented parameters to date the embryo, with accuracy of +/- 3-5 days. As a rough rule of thumb, the CRL + 6.5 = menstrual age in weeks.

Biparietal Diameter

The transverse width of the head at it is widest. We measure from the leading edge to leading edge of the bones, because this leading interface is most distinct. Since, the head is oval, the error induced by small errors in positioning is small, making for a repeatable, robust measure.

Head size is determined largely by brain growth which is relatively independent of nutritional (maternal/placental insufficiency) growth retarding processes, and head growth is often relatively "spared" in such growth retardation.

The BPD best used after 12 weeks.

Accuracy is +/- 1.1 week 14-20 weeks,
+/- 1.6 weeks 20-26 weeks,
+/- 2.4 week 26-30 weeks
and +/- 3-4 weeks after 30 weeks.

Femur Length

The femur length is a repeatable measurement with accuracy similar to the BPD. It is effected by skeletal dysplasias, but since these are rare, it is a reliable measurement which confirms measurements of the head. It is best measured after 14 weeks.

It is common to make at least 2 and often 4-5 measurements to estimate gestational age. In most cases, BPD, head circumference, femur length, and abdominal circumference are used.

Since all of these measurements are strongly related to gestational age, it is not usually important how they are combined. Most modern ultrasound machines include computerized biometric analysis programs used to easily calculate your estimated due date or estimated date of delivery (EDD) or estimated date of confinement (EDC).

ULTRASOUND FETAL MEASUREMENT STANDARDS CHART

Note: +/– Standard deviations shown in (brackets). Measurements are for completed weeks.

Ultrasonic Fetal Measurement Standards Chart						
Gestation (weeks)	**Biparietal diameter (BPD) (mm)**	**Occipitofrontal diameter (OFD) (mm)**	**Head circumference (mm)**	**Abdominal circumference (mm)**	**Femur (mm)**	**Humerus (mm)**
11	16 (2.0)	21 (2.0)	59 (15)	52 (10)	8 (2.0)	8 (3.0)
12	20 (4.0)	24 (2.0)	70 (15)	63 (10)	10 (2.5)	9 (2.0)
13	24 (4.0)	29 (3.0)	84 (15)	74 (10)	11 (2.5)	11 (3.0)
14	28 (4.0)	34 (3.0)	96 (15)	84 (10)	15 (3.0)	14 (4.0)
15	31 (4.0)	38 (3.0)	108 (15)	96 (10)	17 (3.5)	17 (5.5)
16	36 (5.0)	46 (3.0)	128 (15)	106 (10)	22 (4.0)	21 (4.0)
17	39 (5.0)	50 (3.0)	141 (15)	120 (15)	25 (4.0)	25 (5.0)
18	42 (4.0)	54 (3.5)	151 (20)	131 (15)	28 (5.0)	27 (5.5)
19	45 (5.0)	57 (3.5)	160 (20)	140 (15)	30 (5.0)	29 (5.0)
20	47 (4.0)	61 (3.5)	170 (20)	151 (15)	32 (6.0)	31 (5.0)
21	49 (4.0)	63 (4.0)	176 (20)	164 (20)	34 (6.0)	32 (6.0)
22	52 (5.0)	68 (3.5)	188 (20)	176 (20)	37 (5.0)	35 (6.0)
23	57 (5.0)	76 (4.0)	210 (20)	186 (20)	43 (5.0)	38 (4.0)
24	60 (6.0)	79 (4.0)	220 (20)	201 (20)	45 (4.0)	40 (6.0)
25	64 (6.0)	82 (4.5)	231 (20)	212 (20)	48 (5.0)	43 (5.0)
26	67 (4.0)	84 (4.5)	238 (20)	223 (25)	49 (5.0)	44 (4.0)
27	68 (5.0)	86 (4.5)	250 (20)	230 (25)	50 (5.0)	47 (4.0)
28	72 (4.0)	95 (5.0)	263 (20)	242 (25)	54 (4.0)	50 (5.0)
29	75 (4.0)	97 (5.5)	269 (25)	259 (25)	55 (5.5)	51 (5.0)
30	76 (4.0)	98 (5.5)	274 (25)	262 (25)	58 (6.0)	52 (5.0)
31	80 (6.0)	101 (5.0)	284 (25)	272 (30)	59 (5.5)	54 (5.0)
32	81 (4.0)	102 (5.0)	288 (25)	283 (30)	62 (6.0)	56 (5.0)
33	84 (6.0)	107 (5.5)	300 (25)	294 (30)	65 (4.0)	57 (6.0)
34	86 (6.0)	108 (5.5)	305 (25)	305 (30)	66 (4.0)	59 (5.5)
35	88 (6.5)	109 (5.5)	310 (25)	315 (30)	67 (6.0)	60 (6.0)
36	90 (6.0)	112 (5.5)	317 (25)	325 (35)	69 (6.0)	62 (5.0)
37	92 (6.5)	113 (6.0)	321 (25)	333 (35)	72 (5.0)	63 (6.0)
38	93 (6.0)	116 (5.5)	328 (25)	342 (35)	73 (5.5)	64 (6.0)
39	95 (8.0)	119 (6.0)	336 (25)	356 (35)	75 (6.0)	65 (5.5)
40	96 (8.0)	120 (6.0)	340 (25)	362 (35)	76 (4.0)	66 (6.0)
41	98 (8.0)	122 (6.0)	344 (25)	367 (35)	77 (5.0)	68 (6.0)

CROWN-RUMP LENGTH MEASUREMENTS

Gestation (weeks/days)	Crown-rump length (mm)	Gestation (weeks/days)	Crown-rump length (mm)	Gestation (weeks/days)	Crown-rump length (mm)
5.2	1	8.3	20	11.4	52
5.3	2	8.4	21	11.5	55
5.4	3	8.5	22	11.6	56
5.5	3	8.6	22	12.0	57
5.6	4	9.0	23	12.1	58
6.0	4	9.1	24	12.2	60
6.1	5	9.2	26	12.3	61
6.2	6	9.3	27	12.4	63
6.3	7	9.4	28	12.5	64
6.4	8	9.5	29	12.6	65
6.5	9	9.6	31	13.0	68
6.6	10	10.0	34	13.1	70
7.0	11	10.1	36	13.2	72
7.1	11	10.2	37	13.3	74
7.2	12	10.3	38	13.4	76
7.3	12	10.4	39	13.5	77
7.4	13	10.5	39	13.6	80
7.5	14	10.6	40	14.0	81
7.6	15	11.0	44	14.1	84
8.0	17	11.1	45	14.2	85
8.1	18	11.2	47	14.3	86
8.2	19	11.3	48	14.4	87

HOW MANY SCANS SHOULD I HAVE?

As a practical matter, ultrasound scanning has proven to be so popular with patients and also their obstetricians, that almost everyone receiving regular prenatal care ends up with at least one scan anyway. The total number of scans will vary depending on whether a previous scan has detected certain abnormalities that require follow-up assessment.

There is no hard and fast rule for the number of scans you should have during pregnancy.

In some countries, sonograms are performed just twice during pregnancy. Once at 16–18 weeks to assess fetal abnormalities, and again at 32–34 weeks to assess age and well-being.

It is now recommended that all pregnant women have a dating scan in the first trimester—ideally at 10–13 weeks of pregnancy—to confirm your dates. This is especially important if you are going to have any screening tests for Down's syndrome, as knowing the exact dates makes sure your result is accurate. Most hospitals offer a scan in the second trimester at about 20 weeks (the anomaly scan) to check that your baby is developing normally.

Index

Page numbers followed by *t* refer to table, *f* refer to figure and *fc* refer to flow chart

D

E

F

G

H

I

L

M